TODAY'S HEALTH PROFESSIONS

Working Together to Provide Quality Care

TODAY'S HEALTH PROFESSIONS

Working Together to Provide Quality Care

Patricia Lockamy Royal, EdD, MSW
Tenured Associate Professor
Department of Health Services and Information Management
Adjunct Associate Professor
Department of Public Health
Director, Health Care Administration Graduate Certificate
East Carolina University
Greenville, North Carolina

 F.A. Davis Company • Philadelphia

F. A. Davis Company
1915 Arch Street
Philadelphia, PA 19103
www.fadavis.com

Printed in the United States of America

Last digit indicates print number: 10 9 8 7 6 5 4 3 2 1
Publisher: T. Quincy McDonald
Manager of Content Development: George W. Lang
Senior Developmental Editor: Jennifer A. Pine

As new scientific information becomes available through basic and clinical research, recommended treatments and drug therapies undergo changes. The author(s) and publisher have done everything possible to make this book accurate, up to date, and in accord with accepted standards at the time of publication. The author(s), editors, and publisher are not responsible for errors or omissions or for consequences from application of the book, and make no warranty, expressed or implied, in regard to the contents of the book. Any practice described in this book should be applied by the reader in accordance with professional standards of care used in regard to the unique circumstances that may apply in each situation. The reader is advised always to check product information (package inserts) for changes and new information regarding dose and contraindications before administering any drug. Caution is especially urged when using new or infrequently ordered drugs.

Library of Congress Cataloging-in-Publication Data

Names: Royal, Patricia Lockamy, author.
Title: Today's health professions : working together to provide quality care / Patricia Lockamy Royal.
Description: Philadelphia, PA : F.A. Davis Company, [2016] | Includes bibliographical references.
Identifiers: LCCN 2015039091 | ISBN 9780803644656
Subjects: | MESH: Career Choice. | Health Occupations. | Professional Role. | Vocational Guidance.
Classification: LCC R697.A4 | NLM W 21 | DDC 610.69—dc23
LC record available at http://lccn.loc.gov/2015039091

To Tyler, Olivia, Karlie, Alexis, and Sophie—the next generation.

PREFACE

Although it is no mystery that careers in health care represent some of the most stable and lucrative positions of all professional fields, many individuals are unaware of all the diverse roles and opportunities available in health care. My purpose and goal for this textbook is to improve on this lack of awareness by educating students about the various health-care fields and the careers within them. *Today's Health Professions: Working Together to Provide Quality Care* was written to provide students with a frame of reference for those contemplating a career in health care but unsure about opportunities.

As a true believer in the interprofessional approach to health care, I also want to showcase the importance of this approach to students while providing them with the skills needed for teamwork. Quality health care depends on a collaborative approach. My personal philosophy is that health-care workers do not or should not work in isolation but rather focus on providing holistic care to patients. This same philosophy holds true in nonclinical health professionals as well. This book will help promote and encourage learning through collaboration with other disciplines. Students should understand that the ultimate goal for health-care workers is to provide quality care for patients; however, providing quality care can only occur when there is patient-centered care by all professions.

Overview of the Textbook

This textbook is divided into five sections and introduces many important concepts that allow for student knowledge and exploration in fields of health care. Throughout the text, case studies, exercises, and other learning activities are used to challenge students to begin thinking like future health-care professionals. Assimilation into an interprofessional role by completion of the activities will better prepare students for their future careers should they decide to become health-care professionals.

Section I

This section introduces the student to the environment of health care, what it is, and how it affects, and has affected, our health status. The historical component in this section

helps students recognize the technological advances that have occurred over the past 100 years.

Section II

This section provides an overview of the primary health-care professions, outlines the history of allied health professions, and introduces students to the interprofessional approach for patient care. An early appreciation of interprofessional care should enhance future interactions because familiarity often improves implementation. This section allows students to examine the impact of interprofessional care through cases and other activities and solidifies the importance of teams in achieving quality health care.

Section III

This section introduces the primary-care professions of medicine, nursing, and pharmacy. These early professions are often recognized as the forerunners to health-care careers. Each chapter provides a historical overview, allowing students opportunities to trace the beginnings of each profession to the longitudinal scope of practice that we now recognize. This section also provides information such as salaries, employment trends, and scopes of practice for each discipline.

Section IV

This section introduces many of the allied health professions that students often overlook as a possible career choice. Allied health represents a vast number of disciplines with which students may be unfamiliar. Like the previous section, this section also provides information about salaries, employment trends, and scopes of practice for each of the disciplines.

Section V

The last section ties all the chapters together by addressing factors relevant to all of the health-care professions, such as ethics, professionalism, and collaboration. Students need to understand the importance of being a professional in the work environment and the expectations associated with choosing a career in health care. This section addresses team issues, such as conflict management and decision-making strategies.

Supplemental Activities

A Day in the Life

Each of the discipline-specific chapters begins with "A Day in the Life," which provides students with a firsthand approach to what a typical day in that health-care field might entail. Students are taken on a journey that showcases the day-to-day activities, challenges, and rewards of working as a professional in that health-care field.

Cases

Each of the discipline-specific chapters, as well as other select chapters, has a case based on a real-life scenario that describes the patient or client and associated conditions that might affect the patient's care. The case always involves other professionals who need to be involved in the plan of care. Students are given thought-provoking questions that might help them to understand the complexity of the care and the need for the interprofessional team to ensure quality care.

Author Spotlight

Each of the discipline-specific authors has a feature that delivers a personal message to help connect students to the author's field. This message might describe the author's personal career journey, or it might provide the author's additional insight and feedback on the most rewarding elements of the job.

Aptitude Profile

Each discipline-specific chapter provides an aptitude profile that will help assess the student's interest in a particular field. The profile provides the characteristics and traits that help to ensure success in a given area. Students can examine their strengths and weaknesses in these concentration areas and identify potential health-care fields that are the most appropriately fitting.

Working Together

One of the main focuses in this textbook is on the need for interprofessional care and the recognition that health care is not limited to one profession but rather consists of an array of disciplines working together to achieve the best results. All discipline-specific chapters have a section that demonstrates the importance of teamwork by identifying other professionals who might contribute to the patient's plan of care.

End-of-Chapter Review

All chapters have end-of-chapter review questions to engage students and test their knowledge of the chapter.

Online Resources

Additional materials are available online at DavisPlus.com. Instructors will find helpful course tools such as an instructor guide, PowerPoint slides, and a full test bank. Students will have access to resources designed to enhance their study and understanding of the many different health professions presented in the text. Bonus chapters on three different professions are also provided for continued learning.

Personal Goal

I want students, after reading this textbook, to have a better understanding of potential health-care careers in addition to understanding the importance of interprofessional care. More important, my hope is that students become excited about careers in health care as they contemplate a future as a health-care professional who truly cares about quality patient care.

Patricia Lockamy Royal, EdD, MSW

CONTRIBUTORS

Rex A. Ameigh, MSLM, BSRT(R)

Professor, Austin Peay State University
Director, Radiologic Technology Program
Chair, Allied Health Sciences
Clarksville, Tennessee

Missy Armstrong, MS, CTRS/R

Manager, Inpatient Rehabilitation and Psychiatry,
    Rehabilitation Therapies
Harborview Medical Center
University of Washington
Seattle, Washington

Tony Burkett, MS, CES

Instructor, College of Health Professions and Social
    Work
Florida Gulf Coast University
Fort Myers, Florida

Doyle M. Cummings, PharmD, FCP, FCCP

Berbecker Distinguished Professor of Rural Medicine
Professor of Family Medicine and Public Health
Adjunct Professor of Pharmacy, UNC
East Carolina University, Brody School of Medicine
Greenville, North Carolina

Deanna Dye, PT, PhD

Eastern Idaho Regional Medical Center
Wound Care Department
Idaho Falls, Idaho

Amy Freshley-Lebkuecher, MS, RT(R)(T)

Professor, Allied Health Sciences
Austin Peay State University
Clarksville, Tennessee

Katie Walsh Flanagan, EdD

Professor
Department of Health Education and Promotion
East Carolina University
Greenville, North Carolina

Joan Glacken, EdD

Professor and Associate Dean
Florida Gulf Coast University
College of Health Professions and Social Work
Fort Myers, Florida

Annette G. Greer, PhD, MSN

Associate Professor
Department of Bioethics and Interdisciplinary Studies
East Carolina University
Greenville, North Carolina

Jennifer L. Harper, MD

Associate Professor
Department of Radiation Oncology
Medical University of South Carolina
Charleston, South Carolina

Michelle Hesse (Battista), PhD, RD

Assistant Professor
Dietetics
James Madison University
Harrisonburg, Virginia

Linda Holloway, PhD, CRC

Professor and Chair
Department of Addiction and Disability Rehabilitation
University of North Texas
Denton, Texas

Thomas G. Irons, MD, FAAP

Professor of Pediatrics
Brody School of Medicine
East Carolina University
Greenville, North Carolina

Jennifer L. Keely, MEd, RRT-ACCS

Assistant Clinical Professor
Respiratory Therapy Program
School of Health Professions
University of Missouri
Columbia, Missouri

Julie Kennel, PhD, RDN, LD

Clinical Assistant Professor
Director, Human Nutrition Dietetic Internship
Education and Human Ecology, Department of Human
  Sciences
Ohio State University
Columbus, Ohio

Mary Ann Keogh Hoss, PhD, CTRS, FACHE, FDRT

Professor, Health Services Administration
Eastern Washington University
Spokane, Washington

Kelley Lybrand, DDS

James P. Edwards College of Dental Medicine
Medical University of South Carolina
Charleston, South Carolina

Laura Melendez, BS, RMA, RT, BMO

Keiser University Regional Director
Fort Lauderdale, Florida

Amanda Moloney-Johns, MPAS, PA-C

Director of Clinical Development
University of Utah Physician Assistant Program
Department of Family and Preventive Medicine
University of Utah
Salt Lake City, Utah

Keith A. Monosky, PhD, MPM, EMT-P

Program Director, EMS Paramedicine Program
Tenured Professor, Department of Nutrition, Exercise,
  and Health Sciences
Central Washington University
Ellensburg, Washington

Tonya Orchard, PhD, RDN, LD

Director, Didactic Program in Dietetics
Assistant Professor
Ohio State University
Department of Human Sciences
Human Nutrition Program
Columbus, Ohio

Kathryn Rollins, MEd, RRT-NPS, RRT-ACCS

Adjunct Clinical Instructor, Respiratory Therapy
  Program
School of Health Professions
University of Missouri
Columbia, Missouri

Ayasakanta Rout, PhD

Assistant Professor, Department of Communication
  Science and Disorders
James Madison University
Harrisonburg, Virginia

Elaine M. Shuey, PhD, CCC-SLP

Licensed speech-language pathologist
Professor, East Stroudsburg University
East Stroudsburg, Pennsylvania

Gregory Wintz, PhD, OTR/L

Program Director and Associate Professor
Pacific University School of Occupational Therapy
Hillsboro, Oregon

Julie Zemplinski, MSH, MS, MLS(ASCP)CM

Clinical Laboratory Science Program Director
Florida Gulf Coast University
Fort Myers, Florida

REVIEWERS

Elizabeth M. Adams, PhD, CCC-A

Associate Professor
Department of Speech Pathology and Audiology
University of South Alabama
Mobile, Alabama

Connie Allen, MAED/CI-AE, CMA (AAMA)

Instructor/Clinical Coordinator
Department of Medical Assisting
Wallace State Community College
Hanceville, Alabama

Nancy H. Allen

Registered Nurse, Education Consultant
HOSA–Future Health Professionals Associate Director
Central, South Carolina

Renee Andreeff, EdD, PA-C, DFAAPA

Academic Coordinator
Physician Assisting
D'Youville College
Buffalo, New York

Debra J. Aukes, BSN, EMT, AHA

Instructor, School of Health
North Iowa School
Buffalo Center, Iowa

Richard K. Beck, MS, EMT-P

EMS Consultant, Author
Department of Emergency Medicine
AEMSTEC Center for EMS Education
St. Lucia, West Indies

Joe D. Bell, PhD

Associate Professor, Department of Kinesiology and
    Nutrition
Abilene Christian University
Abilene, Texas

Tara Leigh Bell, BS, MEd

Program Director, Health Science and Public Safety
Career and Technical Education
Colorado Community College System
Denver, Colorado

Lynn Berk, MA-CCC-SLP

Speech Language Pathology Supervisor
Department of Speech Pathology/Audiology
Kent State University
Kent, Ohio

Carole Berube, MA, MSN, BSN, RN

Professor Emerita in Nursing; Instructor in Health
    Sciences
Department of Health Sciences
Bristol Community College
Fall River, Massachusetts

Darci Brown, MSPAS, PA-C

Interim Program Director/Director of Clinical
    Education
Department of Physician Assistant Studies
Misericordia University
Dallas, Pennsylvania

John W. Burns, MS, ATC, LAT

Director, Athletic Training Program
Kinesiology Department
Washburn University
Topeka, Kansas

Hollie K. Caldwell, PhD, RN

Dean
School of Nursing
Platt College
Aurora, Colorado

W. Lynne Clarke, RN, EdD

Department Chair
Department of Health Science
AR Johnson Health Science and Engineering Magnet
    School
Augusta, Georgia

Amanda Cline, OTR/L

Program Manager/Adjunct Faculty at Saint Louis
    University
Department of Therapy
Alliance Rehab and Saint Louis University
St. Louis, Missouri

Jaclyn Conelius, PhD, FNP-BC

Assistant Professor
School of Nursing
Fairfield University
Fairfield, Connecticut

Jacqueline Cox Kazik, MA, PA-C

Physician Assistant
Emergency Department
Waukesha Memorial Hospital
Waukesha, Wisconsin

Candace A. Croft, PhD

Dean
Department of Health Sciences
Hawkeye Community College
Waterloo, Iowa

Sarah Darrell, BSN, RN, CNOR

Adjunct Faculty
Department of Health Science
Ivy Tech
Indianapolis, Indiana

Vera Dauffenbach, EdD, MSN, RN

Associate Professor
Department of Nursing
Bellin College
Green Bay, Wisconsin

Elizabeth D. Deluliis, OTD, OTR/L

Assistant Professor/Academic Fieldwork Coordinator
Department of Occupational Therapy
Duquesne University
Pittsburgh, Pennsylvania

Sarah Deshler, RN, MSN, CNE

Professor of Nursing
Department of Nursing
Central Arizona College
Coolidge, Arizona

Randy De Kler, MS, RRT

Program Director
Department of Respiratory Care
Miami Dade College
Miami, Florida

Leila Dickinson, RDH, MEd

Assistant Professor
Department of Dental Hygiene
University of Arkansas for Medical Sciences
Little Rock, Arkansas

John Chad Duncan, CRC, CPO, LPO

Chair, Prosthetics and Orthotics
Interim Program Coordinator, Rehabilitation
    Counseling and Associate Professor
Department of Prosthetics and Orthotics
Department of Rehabilitation Studies
Alabama State University
Montgomery, Alabama

Michael Durham, BSSW, LSW, LICDC-CS

Substance Abuse Counselor and Educator
Department of Counseling Services
Kenyon College
Ganbier, Ohio

Yolanda Feimster Holt, PhD, CCC-SLP

Assistant Professor
Communication Sciences and Disorders
East Carolina University
Greenville, North Carolina

Tim Feltmeyer, MS

Director—Academics
Department of Academics—Medical
Erie Business Center
Erie, Pennsylvania

Thomas F. Fisher, PhD, OTR, CCM, FAOTA

Professor and Chairman
Department of Occupational Therapy
Indiana University
Indianapolis, Indiana

Katharine Lynn Fitzharris, AuD, CCC-A, FAAA

PhD Candidate, Research and Teaching Assistant
Department of Communication Sciences and Disorders
School of Behavioral and Brain Sciences
University of Texas at Dallas
Dallas, Texas

Diana L. Gardner, MBA-HM, RHIA, FACMPE, CPC

Product Manager/Course Mentor
Department of Health Informatics
Western Governors University
Salt Lake City, Utah

Sandra Jean Graham Hobson, BSc(OT), MAEd, LLD, FCAOT

Professor Emerita
School of Occupational Therapy
University of Western Ontario
London, Ontario

Grant Goold, EdD

Program Director and Department Chair
Department of EMS Education
American River College
Sacramento, California

Lynda Harkins, PhD, RRT

Director, Clinical Education
Department of Respiratory Care Technology
McLennan Community College
Waco, Texas

Lezli K Heyland, BSRC, RRT-NPS

Program Director
Department of Respiratory Care
Francis Tuttle Technology Center
Oklahoma City, Oklahoma

Lori Diane Henrichs, RN, BSN

Secondary School Nurse/Health Academy Instructor
Clarke Community School District
Osceola, Iowa

Valerie Herzog, EdD, LAT, ATC

Graduate Athletic Training Program Director/Athletic
   Therapy Program Director
Department of Health Promotion and Human
   Performance
Weber State University
Ogden, Utah

Paulette N. Horner

Health Science Instructor/Paramedic
Department of Health Science
Maquoketa Community School District—Maquoketa
   High School
Maquoketa, Iowa

Diane Huff Pitts, PT, DPT, RN, BSN

Clinical Instructor
Physical Therapy Department
University of South Alabama
Mobile, Alabama

Randi Hunewill, MS, Ed

Education Program Supervisor
Department of Career and Technical Education
Nevada Department of Education
Carson City, Nevada

Georgia T. Jenkins, EMT-P, CC-P

Associate Professor
School of Emergency Services
Daytona State College
Daytona Beach, Florida

Stephen M. Johnson, MS, MT(ASCP)

Program Director
School of Medical Technology
Saint Vincent Hospital
Erie, Pennsylvania

Connie Keintz, PhD, CCC-SLP

Associate Professor
Department of Communication Sciences and Disorders
Florida Atlantic University
Boca Raton, Florida

Judith Kimelman Kline, RMA, AHI, CMAA, CCMA, CEKGT, NCECGT, NCPT

Medical Assistant Instructor
Department of Health Science, Medical Assisting
Miami Lakes Educational Center
Miami Gardens, Florida

Lori L. King, NRCMA

Medical Program Instructor
Department of Medical Assisting
Great Lakes Institute of Technology
Erie, Pennsylvania

Ramona B. Lazenby, EdD, FNP-BC, RN, CNE

Professor and Associate Dean
Department of Nursing
Auburn University Montgomery
Montgomery, Alabama

Jennifer Mai, PT, DPT, PhD, MHS, NCS

Associate Professor of Physical Therapy
Physical Therapy Department
Clarke University
Dubuque, Iowa

Paula Malcomson, BA, BEd

Faculty, Dental Programs
Fanshawe College
London, Ontario

George Markos, MBChB

Instructor, Career Technical Education
Baldwin Park Adult and Community Education
Baldwin Park, California

Michelle M. Maskulinski, MA, BSN, RN

Health Technologies Instructor
Fairfield Career Center
Caroll, Ohio

Gary Miller, PhD

Associate Professor
Department of Health and Exercise Science
Wake Forest University
Winston-Salem, North Carolina

Krista Moloney, RHIA

Adjunct Instructor
Department of Continuing Education, Healthcare
    Division
Trident Technical College
Charleston, South Carolina

Clarice K. W. Morris, PhD

Coordinator of the Academy of Medical Professions
Gorton High School
Yonkers, New York

**Elizabeth Motter Salinas, MEd, CTRS, TRS/TXC
(Texas Certified)**

Professor, Austin Community College
Austin, Texas

Shirley P. O'Brien, PhD, OTR/L, FAOTA

Professor, Department of Occupational Therapy
Eastern Kentucky University
Richmond, Kentucky

Kim O'Connell-Brock, MS, ATC/L

Program Director, Athletic Training Program
Department of Kinesiology and Dance
New Mexico State University
Las Cruces, New Mexico

Mari A. Ono, MSW

Student Services Director
Myron B. Thompson School of Social Work
University of Hawaii at Manoa
Honolulu, Hawaii

Barbara Peacock, BS, RT, R, CT

Radiography Clinical Coordinator
Radiography Program
Cumberland County College
Vineland, New Jersey

Kristy L. Richardson, MS, CCC-SLP

Speech-Language Pathologist
Colleyville, Texas

Leah W. Rising, BS, MS

Consultant, Department of Dentistry
Gulf Coast State College
Panama City, Florida

Georgette Rosenfeld, RRT, RN, PhD

Program Director, Department of Respiratory Care
Indian State River College
Port Saint Lucie, Florida

Karen Rourke, MSPA, PA-C

Avon, Connecticut

Denise Ruscio, M.S. CCC

Speech-Language Pathologist/Clinical Supervisor
Speech-Language-Hearing Clinic
Hofstra University
Hampstead, New York

Kathleen Cecilia Sailsbery, MA

Health Science Technology Faculty, Educational
    Administration
Department of Health Sciences
Morgan Community College
Fort Morgan, Colorado

Gary Shaver, EdD, RT (R)

Radiography Program Director
Health Sciences Division
Indian River State College
Fort Pierce, Florida

Lara Skaggs, MA

State Program Manager
Health Careers Education
Oklahoma Department of Career Tech Education
Stillwater, Oklahoma

Martha P. Smith, RN, CMA (AAMA)

Program Director
Department of Medical Assisting
Georgia Northwestern Technical College
Rock Spring, Georgia

Karen Ruble Smith, RN, BS

Health Science Consultant
Office of Career and Technical Education
Kentucky Department of Education
Frankfort, Kentucky

Ronda Sturgill, PhD, ATC, CHES

Associate Professor
Department of Health Sciences and Human
    Performance
University of Tampa
Tampa, Florida

David L. Sullivan, PhD, NRP

Professor, Health Occupations—EMS
Pasco Hernando State College
New Port Richey, Florida

Robin Thompson-McAvoy, BSc, Bed (Adult), MLT

Coordinator, Department of Medical Laboratory
    Science
St. Lawrence College
Kingston, Ontario, Canada

Kia Vang, CMA (AAMA), CPT

Department Head, Medical Assisting
Department of Medical Assisting
Randolph Community College
Archdale, North Carolina

Janice Vermiglio-Smith, RN, MS, PhD, RMA

Director of Nursing and Health Careers
Department of Nursing
Central Arizona College
Apache Junction, Arizona

Kimberly Whiter, MS, MLS(ASCP)CM

Assistant Professor
Medical Laboratory Science Program
Jefferson College of Health Sciences
Roanoke, Virginia

Laura Witte, PhD, PA-C

Associate Program Director
Physician Assisting
A.T. Still University
Mesa, Arizona

Bret A. Wood, MEd, LAT, ATC

Lecturer and Athletic Training Clinical Education
    Coordinator
Department of Kinesiology
University of North Carolina at Charlotte
Charlotte, North Carolina

Ning Zhou, PhD

Department of Communication Sciences and Disorders
College of Allied Health Sciences
Eastern Carolina University
Greenville, North Carolina

ACKNOWLEDGMENTS

As with any major undertaking, it usually takes an army to accomplish the task. That is certainly the case for this textbook. Many people played major roles in the completion of this text. Some played emotional support roles; others played social support roles; many played resource support roles. And then there were those who played all three roles. To all of those who had a hand in the creation and development of this textbook, I am truly eternally thankful.

I am grateful to Royce, and to my daughters, Cherri and Summer, for their emotional support and for their understanding of my lack of time to commit to other activities as this book took precedence many times. Whether they realize it or not, they played the largest role in my determination to succeed in writing this text.

I am grateful to my friends and colleagues, especially Tom and Bonita, who encouraged me and always had faith in me, even when I did not. They also had to endure long conversations about the stages of the book.

I want to thank my contributors, who, like me, often put their lives on hold to write their chapters, make revisions, or take those photos. Without your support, this textbook would not exist.

I want to thank my reviewers, who took their time to read, revise, and make suggestions needed to ensure a quality textbook.

Finally, I want to thank F. A. Davis Publishing, particularly Jennifer Pine, for support throughout the entire journey of the creation and development of the book. Jennifer always found a way to help me relax when I became stressed. Her soft-spoken voice often provided me with direction as well as a new commitment to the challenge. To all the others at F. A. Davis, I thank you for your support and continued belief in me.

CONTENTS

Section I
The State of the Health-Care Environment

Chapter 1   Is a Career in the Health Professions Right for You?   3
Patricia Royal, EdD

Chapter 2   The Health-Care Environment   11
Patricia Royal, EdD

Chapter 3   Types of Health-Care Facilities   25
Patricia Royal, EdD

Chapter 4   Paying for Services   33
Patricia Royal, EdD

Section II
The Divisions of Health Care

Chapter 5   Introduction to the Primary Health-Care Professions   45
Patricia Royal, EdD

Chapter 6   History of Allied Health Professions   55
Patricia Royal, EdD

Chapter 7   Interprofessional Approach to Patient Care   63
Patricia Royal, EdD

Section III
Primary-Care Professions

Chapter 8   Medicine   77
Thomas G. Irons, MD

Chapter 9   Nursing   87
Annette Greer, PhD, MSN

Chapter 10   Pharmacy   101
Doyle M. Cummings, PharmD, FCP, FCCP

Section IV
Allied Health Professions

Chapter 11   Athletic Training   115
Katie Walsh Flanagan, EdD

Chapter 12   Audiology   127
Ayasakanta Rout, PhD

Chapter 13   Clinical Laboratory Science   137
Joan Glacken, EdD, Julie Zemplinski, MSH, and Tony Burkett, MS

Chapter 14   Dental Professions   149
Kelley Lybrand, DDS

Chapter 15   Dietetics   159
Michelle Hesse (Battista), PhD, RD; Tonya Orchard, PhD, RDN, LD; and Julie Kennel, PhD, RDN, LD

Chapter 16   Emergency Medical Services   171
Keith Monosky, PhD

Chapter 17   Health Information Management   187
Patricia Royal, EdD

Chapter 18   Health Services Management   199
Patricia Royal, EdD

Chapter 19   Medical Assisting   209
Laura Melendez, BS, and Patricia Royal, EdD

Chapter 20   Occupational Therapy   219
Gregory Wintz, PhD, OTR/L

Chapter 21   Physical Therapy   233
Deanna Dye, PT, PhD

Chapter 22   Physician Assisting   247
Amanda Moloney-Johns, MPAS, PA-C

Chapter 23   Radiography   257
Amy Freshley-Lebkuecher, MS, and Rex Ameigh, MSLM

Chapter 24   Radiation Therapy   269
Jennifer L. Harper, MD

Chapter 25   Recreational Therapy   277
Mary Ann Keogh Hoss, PhD, and Missy Armstrong, MS

Chapter 26   Rehabilitation Counseling   289
Linda Holloway, PhD, CRC

Chapter 27   Respiratory Care/Cardiopulmonary   301
Jennifer Keely, MEd, RRT-AACS; and Kathryn Rollins, MEd, RRT-NPS

Chapter 28   Social Work   313
Patricia Royal, EdD, MSW

Contents

Chapter 29   Speech-Language Pathology   323
              Elaine Shuey, PhD

Section V

The Professional Work Environment

Chapter 30   Professionalism and Ethics in
              Health Care   337
              Patricia Royal, EdD

Chapter 31   Professionals Working Together   349
              Patricia Royal, EdD

Appendix   Other Health-Related Professions   365

Index   373

The State of the Health-Care Environment

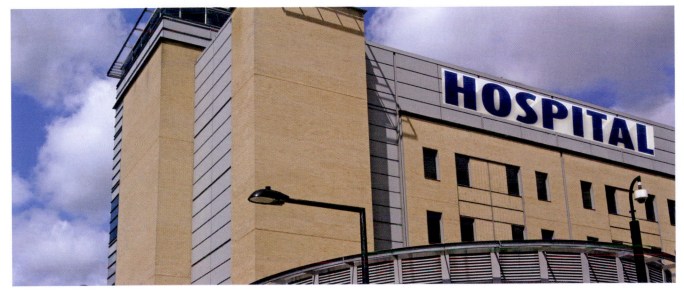

Photo credit: monkeybusinessimages/istock images/Thinkstock

Chapter 1
Is a Career in the Health Professions Right for You?

Chapter 2
The Health-Care Environment

Chapter 3
Types of Health-Care Facilities

Chapter 4
Paying for Services

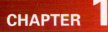
Is a Career in the Health Professions Right for You?

Patricia Royal, EdD

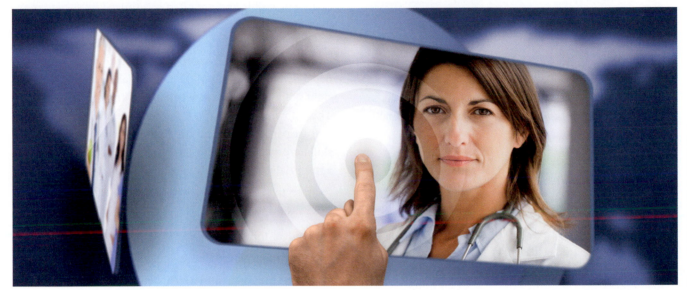

Photo credit: Wavebreak Media, LTD/Thinkstock

Learning Objectives

After reading this chapter, students should be able to:

- Identify skills and aptitude needed for a career as a health professional
- Identify self-values and interests associated with health care
- Display awareness of assessment tools that identify compatible fields
- Discuss the importance of choosing the right career

Key Terms

- Aptitude
- Work values
- Self-assessments
- Work interests

Introduction

Careers are often lifelong choices, so deciding on a career can be somewhat daunting, especially for an individual without work experience. Sometimes we follow in our parents' or grandparents' footsteps. Other times, we select a career based on potential income, prestige, importance, or other societal issues that may be trendy during a particular time period. These reasons may work for some, but for others this type of career selection process may leave us unhappy or dissatisfied in the years to come. Regardless, making a career decision should be taken seriously and be based on our own perspectives rather than on the ideology of others. Career decision-making involves many steps in determining the best fit for the individual. This first chapter will provide guidance on making a career choice in the health professions arena as well as resources that will help ensure success.

Expectations

When selecting a career, we need to be clear about our expectations for that choice. Our expectations may not be the same as those of our parents or friends. Therefore, we need to learn as much as possible about the roles and responsibilities that align with a specific job and see if our expectations match. With knowledge of the job, an understanding of ourselves, and realistic expectations, we may be able to well imagine ourselves in a specific career. Therefore, we need to start by examining our own interests, drives, values, and motivations in addition to our natural talents.

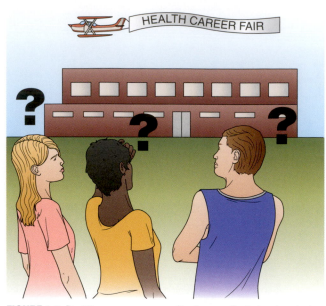

FIGURE 1-1 Deciding on a career can often be complicated and confusing.

Many of us recall, as children, imagining careers such as teachers, doctors, nurses, or some other profession that sparked our interest. When asked, "What do you want to be when you grow up?", we might have responded with an answer based on those imaginary careers. As we age, we develop certain characteristics that might match quite well in a specific career. Certain characteristics, such as a desire to help others, may guide us toward a career in health care, even if we do not yet know exactly which area of health care that will be. Although this may be the first step in choosing a career, narrowing it down to the specific discipline becomes somewhat more difficult. Fortunately, there are some general interests, values, skills, and talents that cross all boundaries

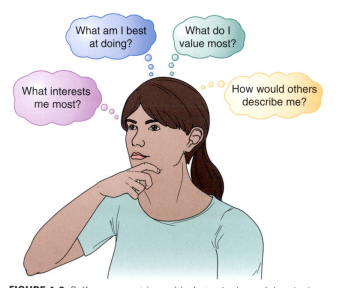

FIGURE 1-2 Self-assessment is a critical step in determining the best career match.

of health care. Before selecting a career in health care, an individual should complete a **self-assessment** to confirm that one's interests, values, and goals are closely represented in a given profession.

Skills

There are common sets of skills that cross many types of careers, such as good verbal and written communication skills, but some are more prevalent and useful for success in the field of health care than others. Health-care professionals are extremely visible and are often scrutinized by society more than those in other careers. These workers are in the public eye and must work with all types of individuals while maintaining a professional approach; therefore, success is often dependent on the skills of the individual worker. Having the right skills, in addition to specific field knowledge, is crucial. The following is a list of skills needed for many job areas but that are particularly necessary for those in health care. These skills are vital to ensure patient safety, quality care, and appropriate treatment options.

- Effective verbal and written communication skills
- Active listening skills
- Critical-thinking skills
- Time-management skills
- Sound judgment and decision-making skills
- Problem-solving skills
- Emotional maturity skills
- Team-based skills
- Leadership skills
- Project management skills

Personality

Our personality type plays an important role in helping us to obtain a well-suited career. A personality is a relatively stable set of characteristics formed early in life. These characteristics, which are influenced by hereditary and social, cultural, and environmental factors, usually remain consistent throughout various circumstances.[1] The way a person behaves in any given situation will generally be the same in a similar situation. Therefore, we are generally able to predict our behaviors based on past experiences, which help us to understand our future behaviors. For the most part, a person's personality remains unchanged; therefore, it is a strong indicator of the job for which he or she may be best suited. Knowing and understanding your personality type will be most beneficial in the selection of your career, because some personality traits can predict job satisfaction.[1]

When we think about personality traits, two of the most common characteristics are extroversion and introversion. Typically, the person who is very outgoing and energetic is known as an extrovert, whereas the quiet, shy person is usually referred to as the introvert. Although these characteristics are common, there are other personality traits that help us determine our personality, such as agreeableness, emotional stability, conscientiousness, and degree of openness.[1] Because our personalities are formed naturally, it is important to look for careers that will enhance that natural ability to help keep us motivated and energized. There is no recognized direct link between personality and skills or abilities; however, by understanding our personality, we are able to recognize and build skills that complement our natural approach.[2] A person's natural approach is anything that comes without conscious thought or effort or one's preferences for doing things a specific way, such as an individual whose natural way of learning is the visual approach or someone who has a natural ability in solving mathematical equations.

Work Values

Our personal values reflect our belief system and ideas associated with morality and the difference between right and wrong. Although similar to personal values, **work values** are associated with our desires to work in certain environments under certain conditions. Identifying our work values will help to provide clarity in our career choices. For example, if one of your work values is leisure, working as a physician may not appeal to you because of the on-call time required. In this situation, you might decide to select another direct patient approach that has few or no on-call requirements. If you view yourself as a loner and desire a job without contact with others, a job in health care still might suit you if you have an interest in laboratory science; however, you might still be expected to work in partnership with others but to a lesser degree. Health-care professionals collaborate on a regular basis and often work in team environments. Your work values will help you to determine your best fit for a career. Although not an inclusive list, other work values include the following[3]:

- Achievement—the need to see results
- Collaboration—working well with others
- Creativity—using your own ideas
- Challenge—solving difficult problems
- Job security—high employment outlook
- Recognition—being rewarded for achievements
- Compensation—receiving appropriate pay for work
- Altruistic nature—desire to help others

Understanding your values is not a guarantee of satisfaction within your career choice; however, it should promote more clarity in the selection process, which should increase your overall satisfaction in the job. To help you recognize your values, a number of job value inventories are available through career counseling centers. Volunteering, job shadowing, and internships also provide measurement tools that enhance your clarity regarding your work values.

Interests

When exploring a health career, you need to keep in mind what interests you. What are your preferences? What types of things do you enjoy doing? Like values, **work interests** help identify who you are and what your preferences are that will keep you motivated and energized in your career. For example, if you are someone who enjoys motivating and influencing others, you might do well as a counselor or a therapist. If your interest is in the area of solving practical problems and achieving results, you could opt for being a dentist or an optometrist. Some areas of career interest include creating, planning, ordering, working with numbers, investigating, and innovating.[4] Keep in mind that interests should be used in combination with work values to enhance your decision-making skills when looking for the right career.

Aptitude

Aptitude is the ability to acquire new skills required for the task at hand. People with an aptitude for math are able to understand complex formulas; however, they may not be able to relate to written communication or literature. To say someone has an aptitude for a specific task indicates that he or she has the ability to quickly absorb information related to that area. Aptitude is not the knowledge itself but rather the innate ability to comprehend and relate the knowledge or skill to the task. Aptitude is often used as a predictor for judging ability to be successful in certain disciplines. Because all occupations use some type of aptitude measurements, it is important to understand your aptitude and the relationship between it and your chosen career.[5] Not having the desired aptitude in a specific discipline does not necessarily indicate an unsuccessful career; however, it does suggest a misfit, which will likely produce dissatisfaction; this, in turn, will probably reduce performance levels. Therefore, by understanding your aptitude, you will benefit greatly when choosing your career.

Aptitude testing generally occurs in high school to provide students with ammunition for selecting possible programs for college. There are several types of aptitude tests or inventories; therefore, taking more than one is probably a good idea. Depending on age, influence, and social support, students tend to differ in their test results. Testing more than one time and using more than one type of inventory validates your answers and provides more consistency for the selection process. One type of aptitude test administered in middle or high school is the Differential Aptitude Test (DAT). This inventory is actually a composite of eight aptitude tests, which helps guide the test taker and counselor in the direction in which the student has already confirmed an interest. This particular aptitude test is closely tied to vocational careers and is used as support for the student's interest. The DAT measures the following eight areas:

- *Verbal ability*—ability to comprehend and use words
- *Numerical ability*—ability to think in numbers
- *Abstract reasoning*—ability to perceive issues and reach conclusions using generalizations rather than concrete facts (also known as *inductive reasoning*)
- *Clerical ability*—ability to find errors quickly
- *Mechanical reasoning*—ability to use mechanical concepts and reasoning
- *Spatial relations*—ability to think in three dimensions
- *Spelling*—ability to quickly recognize misspelled words
- *Grammar*—ability to write grammatically correct sentences

It is important to remember that this test does not predict aptitude in a career, but rather a relationship between a career and an area that the student previously identified as an interest. The DAT provides support for the interest but should not derail students from their career interest. Instead, students should recognize the strengths or weaknesses in the above areas and use them for guidance.[6]

Health-Care Careers

Some students have envisioned working in health care—so after taking the aptitude test they are ensured that pursuing a career in the medical environment is the right path. The thing that they might not know is the specific field in which they want to work. Some people are sure they want direct patient contact, whereas others are sure of the opposite. One

of the great things about working in health care is that there are many opportunities in either direct patient care or the nondirect patient approach. Trying to determine the appropriate fit may be problematic due to the many possibilities. There are about 100 different allied health careers, which provides many options but may also create second guessing on your choice. One approach to help alleviate some of the uncertainty is the use of health career inventories. Even if you are unsure about the exact role, you can generally narrow down the type of occupation. Health careers can be grouped into six categories or clusters. Within each category, there are various professions that have comparable characteristics[4] (see Figs. 1-3 through 1-8). The categories and examples of each are as follows:

- Treatment and diagnostics (direct practice care)
  - Physician
  - Dentist
  - Podiatrist

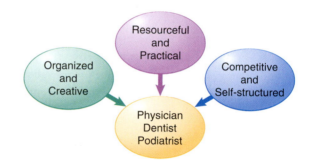

FIGURE 1-3 Direct practice career characteristics.

- Medicine-and dentistry-related careers (associated health)
  - Dietitian
  - Pharmacist
  - Registered nurse

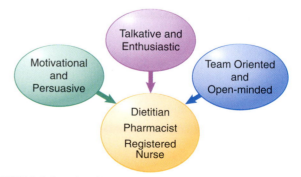

FIGURE 1-4 Associated health career characteristics.

- Technicians, assistants, and technologists (health related)
  - Clinical laboratory technician
  - Dental assistant
  - Emergency medical technician

- Administrative
  - Volunteer services director
  - Hospital public relations director
  - Admissions director

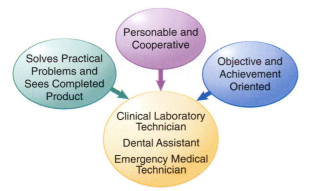

FIGURE 1-5 Technologists and technicians career characteristics.

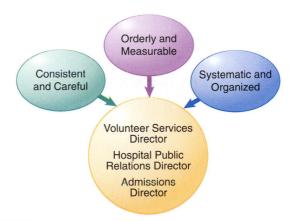

FIGURE 1-7 Administrative health–related career characteristics.

- Rehabilitation
  - Occupational therapist
  - Respiratory therapist
  - Physical therapist

- Affiliated health careers
  - Child Life Specialist
  - Health services manager
  - Mental health worker

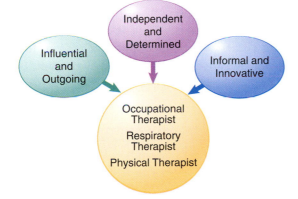

FIGURE 1-6 Rehabilitation career characteristics.

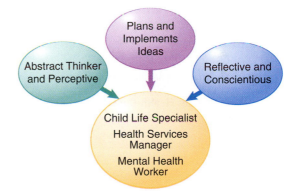

FIGURE 1-8 Affiliated health career characteristics.

Each of these careers requires certain attributes or characteristics to work in that environment. In addition to having these characteristics, you must also understand your own expectations and other related factors before starting on a career. These expectations and factors include salary, educational requirements, time commitment, occupational outlook, employment trends, and personal desire. These factors, along with the various health-care professions, will be presented in detail throughout this text.

Does Health Care Fit Me?

The world of health care is ever evolving. As the number of aging baby boomers is increasing exponentially, so are the jobs in health care. Advancements in technology have prolonged life while creating new jobs. Securing a job as a health-care professional assures you a strong, steady, and challenging career that offers many exciting opportunities for growth. The next decade promises to be full of challenges and opportunities, particularly in light of the federal government issuing more mandates and assuming more control over health care. The implementation of new federal initiatives will likely create new jobs and increase the overall employment outlook for health-care workers.

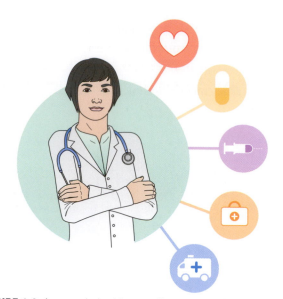

FIGURE 1-9 A career in health care offers many different avenues of practice.

Creating new jobs and having job security does not equate to everyone working in health care. It takes more than job opportunities and the promise of a weekly or monthly paycheck to create the right fit. With the amount of time, education, and money that can be spent on obtaining the credentials required for some health-care careers, you need to feel confident that your chosen career is right for you. Always use available resources to confirm or complement your choice, but a true calling is always the better fit. Take advantage of training opportunities, shadowing experience, or volunteering in health-care facilities where you have an interest. After spending time in that

Tips and Tools

Take a look at the table on the next page and see if you fit within any of the categories. Look at the Interests, Behavior Patterns, and Personality traits. When you find a group that fits you, look at the bottom for the type of health-care career you might find interesting.

Characteristics of Specific Health-Care Professions

Organized—I	Motivational—I	Solves Practical Problems—I	Influential—I	Consistent—I	Abstract Thinker—I
Competitive—B Resourceful—P Creative—I	Team oriented—B Talkative—P Persuasive—I	Objective—B Personable—P Sees Completed Product—I	Informal—B Independent—P Outgoing—I	Systematic—B Orderly—P Careful—I	Reflective—B Plans Ideas—P Perceptive—I
Self-structured—B Practical—P	Open-minded—B Enthusiastic—P	Achievement—B Cooperative—P	Innovative—B Determined—P	Organized—B Measured—P	Conscientious—B Implements Ideas—P
Physician, Dentist, and Podiatrist	Dietitian, Pharmacist, and Registered Nurse	Clinical Laboratory Technician, Dental Assistant, and Emergency Medical Technician	Occupational Therapist, Respiratory Therapist, and Physical Therapist	Volunteer Services Director, Hospital Public Relations Director, and Admissions Director	Child Life Specialist, Health Services Manager, and Mental Health Worker

Legend: I = Interests; B = Behavior Patterns; P = Personality.

environment, if it is not a good fit for you, look elsewhere. You can think about your future career the same way that you think about buying a new pair of shoes: They may look nice, but if they don't fit you, there's no point in buying them.

SUMMARY

Finding the right career path can be both exciting and challenging. The excitement comes when we find something that feels like it fits us as individuals. The challenging part is often due to impatience and lack of knowledge about specific careers; however, with a little time and effort, you can find the right career path for you.

Glossary of Key Terms

Aptitude — refers to the natural ability or suitability for learning something new

Work values — the desire to work in certain conditions or environments

Self-assessments — instruments or evaluations used to help people understand their motives, judgments, and special skills

Work interests — preferences that help keep you motivated at work

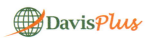 **Additional Resources are available online at www.davisplus.com**

Additional Resources

Online Resources

- O*Net Resource Center (www.onetcenter.org)—information about skills needed for various occupations

Personality Tests

- Myers-Briggs Type Indicator (MBTI)—assessment used to identify personality type
- The Big Five Personality Test—assessment used to identify personality type
- The Career Personality Test—assessment measuring your personality and career choices
- 16 Personality Factor (16pf)—assessment measuring your personality type

Career Interests

- Strong Interest Inventory—assessment measuring your career interest
- Strong High School Career Test—assessment to help high school students identify career interests

Health Career Testing

- Medical College Admission Test (MCAT)—test used for admission to medical, veterinary, and podiatry schools

- Dental Admission Test (DAT)—test used for admission to dental schools
- Optometry Admission Test (OAT)—test used for admission to optometry schools
- Pharmacy College Admission Test (PCAT)—test used for admission to pharmacy schools

Other tests that may be used for health careers

- Graduate Record Examination (GRE)—test used for graduate school admission and often used by allied health programs
- Graduate Management Admission Test (GMAT)—test used for graduate school admission and some health-care fields, such as health-care administrators
- Miller Analogies Test (MAT)—test used for graduate school admission

References

1. de Janasz SC, Dowd KO, Schneider BZ. *Interpersonal Skills in Organizations,* 4th ed. New York, NY: McGraw-Hill Irwin; 2013.

2. Dunning D. *What's Your Type of Career? Find Your Perfect Career by Using Your Personality Type* [e-book]. Boston, MA: Nicholas Brealey; 2010. eBook Collection (EBSCOhost), Ipswich, MA.

   Accessed May 15, 2013.

3. O*Net Resource Center.

   http://www.onetcenter.org.

   Accessed May 13, 2013.

4. Wischnitzer S, Wischnitzer E. *Top 100 Health-Care Careers: Your Complete Guidebook to Training and Jobs in Allied Health, Nursing, Medicine, and More* [e-book]. Indianapolis, IN: JIST Works; 2005. eBook Collection (EBSCOhost), Ipswich, MA.

   Accessed May 15, 2013.

5. Nagle, R. Medical careers for people without the structural visualization aptitudes [Johnson O'Conner Research Foundation website].

   http://www.jocrf.org/resources/OtherMedical Careers.html.

   Accessed May 14, 2013.

6. Cassel R. High school success and school accountability begin with tentative job-career plans for each student. *Education* [serial online]. Winter 98, 1998; 119(2):319. MasterFILE Complete, Ipswich, MA.

   Accessed May 15, 2013.

CHAPTER 2

The Health-Care Environment

Patricia Royal, EdD

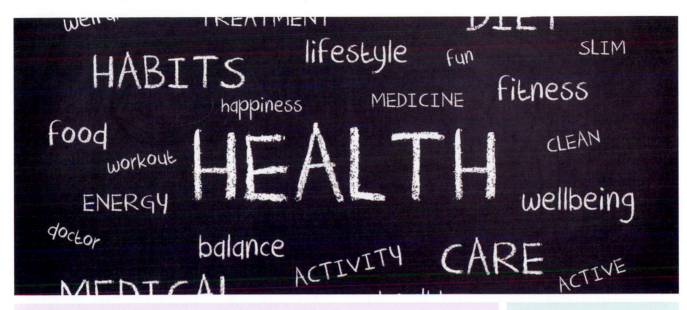

Learning Objectives

After reading this chapter, students should be able to:

- Discuss the elements of the health-care environment and their relationship to other systems
- Recognize the goals of health care
- Relate the historical events of health care to modern society
- Discuss the changes in morbidity and mortality rates over the past 100 years
- Describe some of the reasons for federal initiatives for changes in health-care issues

Key Terms

- Genetics
- Generic
- Morbidity
- Mortality
- Medicaid
- Medicare
- Health Care Education Reconciliation Act of 2010 (Obamacare)

Elements of the Health-Care Environment

Definition

The *health-care environment* can be defined as anything that affects our health status or health-care services.[1] When we think about the physical environment in which we live, we usually think about the things around us such as air, water, land, space, temperature, and weather. These environmental conditions play a major role in health status and delivery of health-care services. Unsafe water, pollutants in land and air, extreme temperatures, and weather-related conditions all contribute to health status or the delivery of health care.

To define the health-care environment, we must consider all variables that affect our health status or services—not just obvious ones such as heredity, age, and lifestyle but also less obvious ones such as the physical environment. This chapter will help you identify some of the factors affecting the health-care environment and understand the influences and relationships relevant to health care.

Heredity

Genetics is one of the most significant factors that affect health care. *Heredity* is generally defined as the genes that our parents pass on to us at conception. Within those genes are certain biological components that identify our potential for specific conditions or illnesses. If we all had perfect genes, there would be fewer or no diseases and other health problems. This would reduce the need for health-care workers, diagnostic testing, pharmaceuticals, and research. Obviously, we do not have perfect genes; therefore, we are prone to certain conditions that create the need for health-care services. We are not able to control heredity, but we are able to use knowledge to improve these conditions.

Lifestyles and Behaviors

Our behavior and lifestyle choices represent another variable in the health-care environment. If we choose to drink alcohol or smoke, we might be jeopardizing our health, the consequences of which have a direct bearing on the health-care environment. Even taking prescription medicines could potentially create the need for additional health-care services. Other lifestyle choices that affect health care include risky behaviors such as unprotected sex or reckless driving. The consequences associated with these types of behaviors include monetary expense and physical illness or injury. Obesity, which can be considered a behavioral and/or genetic condition, is one of the most costly conditions in today's society. The direct costs of obesity may include higher health-care expense and increased insurance premiums, and the nondirect costs may include associated health conditions, such as diabetes or heart disease.[2] Other behavioral and lifestyle variables include lack of exercise, criminal activity, drug use, texting while driving, dangerous work environments, seat belt usage, sunbathing, and risky sexual behaviors. All of these activities have a direct impact on the health-care environment. While recognizing the negative impact some of these activities have on health, it is important to point out the positive impact individuals can make in their overall health. Eating well-balanced meals, exercising regularly, sleeping an adequate number of hours, and maintaining routine medical examinations all contribute to positive effects on an individual's health.

Socioeconomics

Many aspects of the social environment create both direct and nondirect effects on the overall health-care environment. One aspect is economics. Economics is the complex study of the production, distribution, and use of goods and services within a given region by a specific group of people. Health care is a major component of the goods and services consumed every day in the United States. An individual's ability to pay for and use health-care services thus plays an important role in the health-care environment. If an individual cannot afford to purchase health care due to unemployment, for example, there is less money available to pay for doctors, nurses, and other health-care professionals. Less money for providers might mean layoffs, understaffed hospitals and practices, and higher medical costs. Conversely, the longer individuals go without adequate health care, the more that the risk of negative health conditions rises and the greater the need for provider care.

Another social issue is education. Educated individuals use the health-care system more than less-educated individuals. For each level of education, individuals are 12% more likely to visit their family doctor than less-educated individuals.[2] One rationale for this trend might be that education improves the likelihood of individuals having better-paying jobs that may provide health insurance or allow for the ability to pay for private insurance. Educated individuals also tend to lead healthier lifestyles. These individuals usually eat healthier meals, exercise regularly, smoke less, take medications as directed, and use preventive treatments such as vaccines, prenatal visits, and routine examinations. This means that although more-educated individuals use the system more than less-educated individuals, the cost is lower because of their lifestyle choices. Additionally, education is positively associated with lower morbidity rates and increased life expectancy.[3] Education levels and income are highly correlated, which means that less-educated individuals often seek health care only when diseases or conditions have become chronic, but the treatment costs more because of the serious nature of the health condition.[4] Therefore, socioeconomic variables play a major role in the health-care environment.

Natural and Human-made Environmental Issues

Natural occurrences affect the health-care environment greatly, even more so today than in the past. One of the reasons for the increase is weather-related conditions, which have increased greatly over the last 20 years.[5] Floods, hurricanes, earthquakes, tornados, tsunamis, and fires have created havoc for the United States and countries around the world, creating challenges for health-care systems. In addition to natural disasters, human-made disasters such as terrorist attacks (e.g., the "9/11" attacks in 2001 and subsequent attacks, such as the Boston Marathon bombing) have stepped up the need for public health systems to implement new programs and policies and increased the direct costs of dealing with the trauma itself. Other environmental issues affecting health care are water and food safety, smog control, and epidemics such as flu or virus outbreaks.

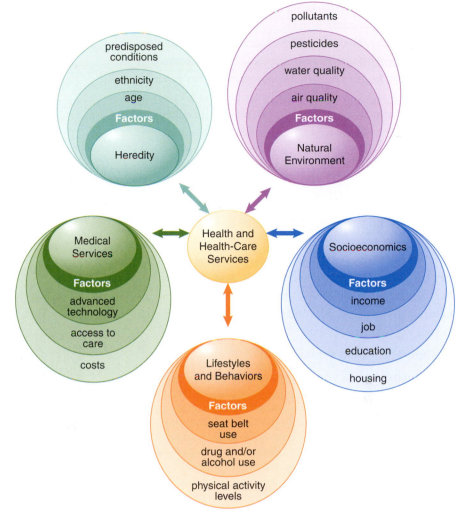

FIGURE 2-1 Determinants of health: Our health is related to many factors, such as environment and social and cultural factors.

Medical Services

Technology

Numerous factors related to medical services affect the health-care environment. One of the largest areas of impact is in technology. Advanced technology has presented medical providers with tools to better diagnose and treat more conditions than ever before; however, the costs of these new technologies have significantly increased the overall health-care budget. This increase in health-care costs has grown drastically since 1950, when the technological period was in its infancy.[1] Even with the expense of technological innovations, the diagnostic abilities and treatment options far outweigh the price paid for advanced technology.

Providers

Shortages of health-care workers have also had a major impact on the health-care environment. Although the number of patients continues to grow, the number of trained providers has not always kept up with that growth. In recent

years, severe shortages of nurses and primary-care physicians have occurred. In addition, the number of long-term care providers needed continues to escalate because of an aging population.[6] The lack of health-care providers has been a continuing problem, particularly for rural communities. Access to care and coverage is a primary issue for the United States, and the issue has become severe enough that the federal government has stepped into the situation. This growing concern is addressed later in the chapter.

Other variables in medical care services relate to the growing population's need for specialized treatments, such as preventive and long-term care. Total patient care no longer rests on the shoulders of one or two types of providers but rather on an array of individuals who specialize in specific areas. We have moved away from a society that relies on a single physician for all our ailments and now live in a society where we see several physicians or providers to handle our health-care needs. Because several providers may be involved in our care, it is imperative that all are up to date on conditions, diagnoses, and medications. Therefore, these providers must be able to communicate effectively to provide quality care to patients.

In summary, many variables affect health status and the health-care environment. This chapter lists many factors that play a role in health care, but there are many other variables as well, such as politics, gender, religion, barriers to care, and others too numerous to mention. Basically, almost everything we do or experience as humans has the potential to affect our health status or health-care services in some manner.

Goals

With a better understanding of the health-care environment, we now need to examine the goals associated with health care. Simplistically speaking, it would be logical to assume that the goals are to diagnose and treat individuals. This is true, of course, but the goals are much more complex and involved than just diagnostics and treatment. Health-care goals include the following[6]:

- Cure diseases and diminish symptoms
- Reduce discomfort during treatment
- Reduce potential disabilities
- Prolong life
- Prevent birth defects
- Prevent premature deaths
- Increase preventive medicine practices
- Improve access to care
- Provide quality care
- Provide and promote education
- Promote and enhance quality of life

As you can see, the goals of health care encompass more than just the diagnosis and treatment phases of illness. The goals provide a greater depth and understanding of the needs associated with total health care throughout the life span.

Historical Events

The practice of health care dates back thousands of years, but we will focus only on some of the major events occurring during and after the 20th century in new technologies, new lifesaving interventions or treatments, medical breakthroughs, changes in disease trends, important legislation enactments, and changes in the health-care system. These important events were the forerunners of new innovations, technologies, treatments, and legislation that occur today and will continue as driving influences that advance health care.

1900–1909:

- In 1901, Karl Landsteiner developed the classification system of blood types (Fig 2-2AB). This classification system is still used today and is credited with the first lifesaving blood transfusion in 1907.[7]

1910–1919:

- In 1910, Marie Curie coined the term *radioactivity* based on her research in radium. Her discovery in isolating radium was an important advance in the treatment of cancer.[8]

- The flu epidemic that spanned from January 1918 to December 1920 infected more than 500 million

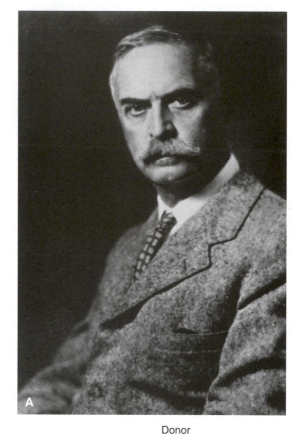

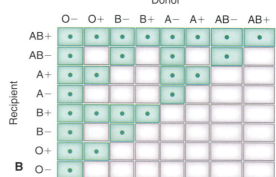

FIGURE 2-2 (A) Karl Landsteiner. (From the National Library of Medicine, History of Medicine Collection.) **(B)** Red blood cell compatibility table still in use today.

individuals worldwide. The number of deaths is estimated to be roughly 50 million people.[9]

1920–1929:

- In 1922, Frederick Banting and Charles Best discovered insulin. This lifesaving drug was first used to treat a 14-year-old diabetic boy. Insulin is still widely used today for control of diabetes.[10]

- The discovery of penicillin mold by Sir Alexander Fleming occurred in 1928; however, this discovery was not nearly as significant until about 1940 when the penicillin mold was isolated into an antibiotic for infections. Various penicillin-type antibiotics exist today and are responsible for curing many types of infections. (Fig 2-3)[10]

- In 1928, the first iron lung was used to fight respiratory failure caused by polio. The first occurrence took place at the Children's Hospital in Boston; it then was used at many other locations throughout the United States and other countries. The iron lung was a machine pressurized by vacuums to keep the lungs breathing in and out (Fig 2-4). For some individuals, the iron lung became a way of life for as long as 60 years.[10]

1930–1939:

- In 1934, group health insurance plans sponsored by Blue Cross began to appear in various locations.[10]

- The March of Dimes, formally known as the National Foundation for Infantile Paralysis, was founded by President Roosevelt and Eddie Cantor in 1938. The name March of Dimes became significant when Eddie Cantor asked his radio listeners to send in their dimes to support the foundation.[10]

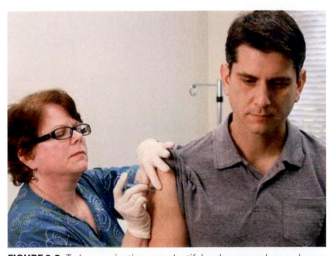

FIGURE 2-3 Today, vaccinations are plentiful and commonplace and come in several forms, such as injections. (Photo courtesy of Douglas Jordan, M.A., Centers for Disease Control and Prevention)

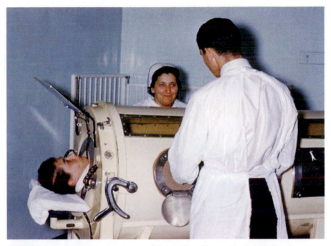

FIGURE 2-4 Iron lungs were used for polio-affected individuals who were not able to breathe on their own. Some individuals lived their entire lives inside the iron lung. This image was taken during the 1960 Rhode Island Polio Epidemic. (Photo courtesy of Centers for Disease Control and Prevention)

More about 1900–1930

During the first part of the 20th century, there was little involvement in the health care of others. Most individuals cared for family members as much as possible but did seek out other help as needed, assuming help was available. Hospitals were beginning to pop up but were still limited to specific areas, and most of them were limited to acute care. Over time, there was a shift in responsibility for health care. There was a movement from treatment in the home to treatment at medical facilities, especially in the area of acute care. Advances in medical care had started but unfortunately not in time for the great flu epidemic that killed 50 million people. After the flu epidemic, there was a great time of discovery and growth in health care. New treatments, vaccines, and experimentation with antibiotics were booming. Hospitals were being built and insurance was introduced to help pay for health-care costs. The United States was becoming a powerful country, and this newfound power became prominent in the health-care arena.

1940–1949:

- World War II caused a major shortage of health-care providers between 1941 and 1945 (Fig 2-5). In addition to the providers, many hospitals lost other workers such as maintenance staff and orderlies.

- In 1945, the Nobel Prize was awarded to Sir Alexander Fleming, Ernst Boris Chain, and Sir Howard Walter Florey for the discovery of penicillin. This particular antibiotic was especially important because of the timing of the discovery and the events of the war. Many lives were saved and the number of amputations was reduced. This antibiotic, due to its variety of forms, remains one of the most beneficial treatments even today.[10]

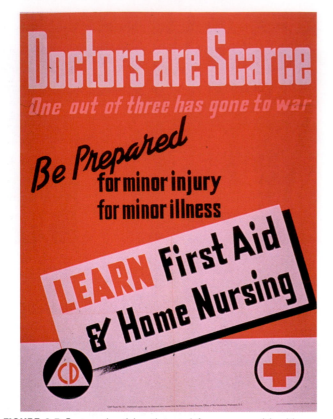

FIGURE 2-5 Poster advertising the need for nurses and health-care workers during World War II. (From the National Library of Medicine, History of Medicine Collection. Contributed by the U.S. Office of War Information)

- The first kidney dialysis machine was successfully used on a dying patient in 1945. The success of this experiment provided hope for many individuals who suffered from kidney disease. Through years of advancement, the dialysis machine is still common today and continues to be a successful way to clean and filter blood (Fig 2-6).[10]

- In 1946, the National Mental Health Act was signed by President Harry S. Truman. This act also guided the way for the creation of the National Institute of Mental Health in 1949. For the first time in history, funding was available for research into mental health issues such as causes, prevention, and treatment of mental health conditions.[10]

- The World Health Organization (WHO) was established by the United Nations in 1948. WHO is the directing authority for health-related issues within the United Nations and provides guidance and leadership on global health concerns.[10]

1950–1959:

- In 1950, the invention of the artificial femoral head made hip replacement surgery possible. The work of Dr. John Charnley and others helped make hip replacement a common surgery available to millions of Americans each year.[10]

- For the first time in history, cigarette smoking was identified as the cause of lung cancer. During this time, many individuals smoked without truly knowing the dangers until new research results were revealed in 1950 (Fig 2-7). Since this information was reported to the public, education awareness began to emerge and continues today.[10]

- In 1952, Dr. Jonas Salk tested the effectiveness of the polio vaccine on himself, his family members, and volunteers. A few years later, the vaccine was widely used across the United States and other countries, eradicating polio in North America and other developed countries (Fig 2-8).[10]

- After only a few years of using the artificial kidney, the first successful human organ (kidney) transplant occurred in 1954. The transplantation of this organ has been so successful that it continues to be the number one transplanted organ.[10]

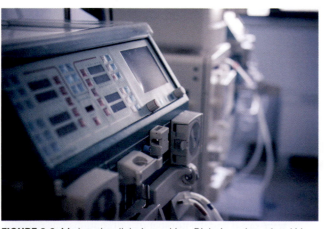

Dario Lo Presti/istock collection/Thinkstock

FIGURE 2-6 Modern-day dialysis machine. Dialysis replaces lost kidney function by artificially cleansing the blood of harmful wastes, salt, and excess fluids.

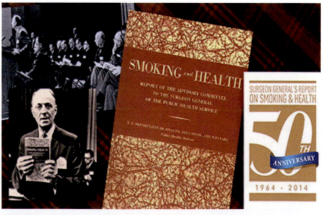

FIGURE 2-7 The year 2014 marked the 50th anniversary of the Surgeon General's report linking cigarette smoking and other tobacco uses to negative effects on health. (Photo from the Centers for Disease Control and Prevention, National Center for Chronic Disease Prevention and Health Promotion, Office on Smoking and Health)

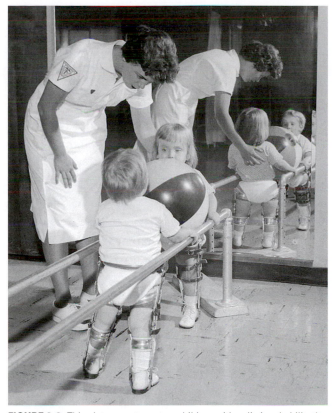

FIGURE 2-8 This picture portrays two children with polio in rehabilitative therapy. Polio, now nearly extinct in the United States, is a debilitating infectious disease caused by viruses that produce a wide array of symptoms and can cause total paralysis. (Photo from the Centers for Disease Control and Prevention)

More about 1931–1950

During the early 1930s, the United States suffered greatly from unemployment and economic woes. The Great Depression had gripped the United States, and many people were destitute. The main struggle was to feed and clothe family members, and there were few dollars left over for health care. Next came the post-Depression era, which was a time of recovery for America. This recovery period was quickly strengthened by World War II. Jobs were available and the economy was rebounding. Unfortunately, this period brought severe shortages of health-care workers. Hospitals were grossly understaffed and undersupplied as resources were diverted for military purposes. Hospitals were faced with trying to balance services and lack of personnel and supplies.

1960–1969:

- Controversy over **generic** versus brand-name drugs occurred as the American Hospital Association's (AHA's) House of Delegates supported the use of a drug formulary system in 1960. This endorsement for hospitals to begin incorporating generic drugs caused disturbances among many people due to their lack of acceptance of these "less than brand" drugs.[10]

- In 1965, **Medicare** and **Medicaid** were enacted. Both of these benefits were amendments to the original Social Security Act of 1935. In the first year alone, approximately 19 million people enrolled in Medicare. Today there are approximately 50 million Medicare recipients.[10]

1970–1979:

- In an effort to protect children from accidental poisoning, the first childproof caps were used (Fig 2-9). The enactment was titled *The Poison Prevention Packaging Act of 1970*. Two years later, aspirin became the first health product to comply with the enactment.

1980–1989:

- The first case of HIV infection in the United States was identified in 1981, which began the AIDS epidemic. Fears related to the unknown causes and prevention of

More about 1951–1970

During the early 1950s, the United States was booming again. The Great Depression had passed and so had World War II. There was renewed attention to hospitals because of federal initiatives. There was sufficient personnel to staff the hospitals and resources were plentiful. Medical breakthroughs in technology showed promise for the next generation. By the early 1960s, social change was occurring via the civil rights movement and the impending Vietnam War. By the mid-1960s, hospital costs were rising and personnel shortages, especially among nurses, resurfaced.

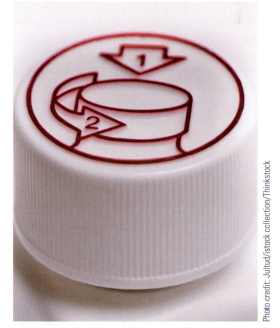

Photo credit: Jultud/istock collection/Thinkstock

FIGURE 2-9 Child-resistant packaging on a pill bottle requires the user to both push down on and twist off the cap.

HIV infection created public panic among many people, including hospital personnel (Fig 2-10).[10]

- In 1982, the first artificial heart was implanted in Barney Clark. The heart implantation took place at the Utah Medical Center, where Clark stayed for 112 days after surgery until he died.[10]

1990–1999:

- In 1991, a baboon heart was transplanted into a human. The transplantation occurred at the University of Pittsburgh Medical Center and the recipient was a 35-year-old man with hepatitis B. The transplant was a success; however, the patient died of nonrelated transplant causes 2 months later.[10]

- The first robotic surgical device was developed in 1991 and was named RoboDoc. This expensive piece of equipment had a precision accuracy rate 40 times greater than that of a human surgeon.[10]

- In 1997, the first successful cloning of two rhesus monkeys occurred at the Oregon Regional Primate Research Center. With this news, President Clinton prohibited federal funds to be used for human cloning research.[10]

2000–2013:

- On the heels of the then-recent terrorist attacks of September 11, 2001, the Public Health Security and Bioterrorism Preparedness and Response Act of 2002 was signed into law. This law provided grant money to hospitals to improve disaster preparedness.[10]

- In 2002, the Health Insurance Portability and Accountability Act (HIPAA) was implemented to protect the confidentiality of patients' health information. HIPAA compliance is required in all medical facilities where patient treatment occurs.[10]

- The battle against trans fat took a turn in 2006, when the U.S. Food and Drug Administration (FDA) started requiring food manufacturers to list information about trans fat on nutrition labels (Fig 2-11). This requirement was a result of the concern over heart disease, the number one cause of death in the United States.[10]

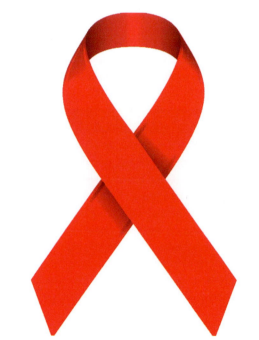

FIGURE 2-10 The first ribbon symbol ever, the red ribbon became the universal symbol of AIDS awareness and support of those living with AIDS and HIV.

More about 1971–1990

The early 1970s brought social changes and justice for equality for women and minorities. The Vietnam War was going strong despite protests from a more peace-loving generation. The economy was once again in distress because of rising costs, unemployment, and little consumer demand. Health-care *quality, delivery,* and *cost-effectiveness* were terms surfacing and being challenged by some government agencies. By the 1980s, health-care delivery needs were being met by new technologies, home health, and ambulatory care centers. Medical-care cost was still a growing concern, especially with an aging population needing services. There were more chronic diseases, and HIV/AIDS was identified. Unfortunately, more community hospitals were closing by the mid-1980s. The lack of facilities affected all citizens, especially those in rural communities where health-care disparities already existed.

FIGURE 2-11 Food nutrition labels are required to list total amounts per serving along with percent daily values.

Photo credit: Fuse/Thinkstock

- The FDA approved two important vaccines in 2006. The first vaccine was Gardasil, which is used in females to prevent cervical cancer, and can also be given to males for the prevention of anal cancer. The second vaccine approved in that year was Zostavax, which is used to prevent herpes zoster (also known as shingles).[11,12]
- The Health Care and Education Reconciliation Act was signed by President Obama in 2010 (Fig 2-12AB). This enactment contains several components that are still unresolved regarding a compliance date[13] (see Federal Initiatives later in this chapter).

These important historical events resulted in improved health-care practices, discoveries of previously unknown mysteries about the human body, increased awareness of disease-promoting practices, and many other important advances. The ultimate and most important effect has been the preservation of human life, as we can see by a study of morbidity and mortality rates throughout the years.

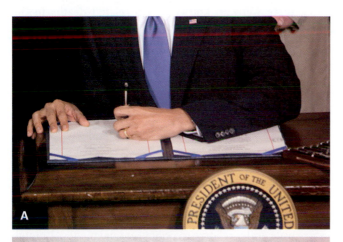

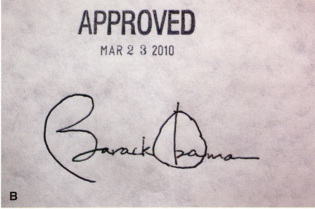

FIGURE 2-12 (A) President Barack Obama signs the *Health Care Education Reconciliation Act of 2010*. This enactment was part of the *Patient Protection and Affordable Care Act* approved by Congress in 2009. **(B)** Official Presidential seal. (Photo courtesy of Chuck Kennedy, Official White House Photographer)

More about 1991–2013

The 1990s was a time of health-care reform and legislation that addressed issues with health-care delivery systems. Legislative acts included the Family and Medical Leave Act, the Health Insurance Portability and Accountability Act, and the Balanced Budget Act. As aging baby boomers increased in numbers, the problem of caring for them grew significantly, especially considering that workforce shortages were again a returning challenge. The costs of providing health care continued to soar in the new millennium. Again, the focus was on cost containment and quality, and providers were charged with balancing these two elements of care. Electronic medical records were being pushed, and confidentiality issues were resurfacing. Thanks to the Internet, patients were more informed (and sometimes misinformed) about illness and disease. This generation was more proactive in health care and advocated more for themselves and others than any other in history. Two of the most pressing and important factors affecting Americans during this period were terrorist attacks and natural disasters. Both of these issues brought public health and disaster preparedness to the forefront, and funding was poured into these causes.

Morbidity and Mortality

To understand the changes in morbidity and mortality rates in the United States over the past 100 years, one needs to understand the terms in relationship to the historical perspective. **Morbidity** refers to the specific disease or sickness and is calculated by either numbers or rates. **Mortality** refers to actual deaths caused by the specific disease or sickness and can also be calculated in terms of numbers or rates.[6]

Looking back 100 years, you can imagine that many deaths were attributed to conditions such as tuberculosis, gastrointestinal infections, pneumonia, or influenza. The reason for these deaths was the absence of vaccines and antibiotics for treatment.[6] Additionally, the lack of health-care providers and technology needed for diagnosis played a major role. Environmental issues and concerns such as the lack of clean water and sanitary conditions created havoc for many people and caused a substantial number of deaths. Nonsterile environments in hospitals and clinics were breeding grounds for germs and contamination and increased the rates of communicable infections. Inadequate nutrition and food storage contributed to some of the conditions, particularly gastrointestinal issues. Chronic diseases such as heart disease and diabetes did exist, but people often died before the onset of these chronic conditions. During the early 1900s, the life expectancy for men was only about 47 to 49 years old. This life expectancy was roughly the same for women, whereas today, women live significantly longer than men.

The reason for women's shorter life expectancy at that time was complications of childbirth.[1]

During the mid-1900s, the life expectancy rose dramatically to between 65 and 67 years of age. During this time period, penicillin was made available to the public, and it had a significant impact on the treatment of infectious diseases. Other types of antibacterial agents were introduced that provided cures for many conditions. More hospitals were being established and preventive medicine was becoming more common, particularly in terms of vaccines. Polio remained a serious threat until the early 1960s, when the polio vaccine was licensed for public use. Chronic diseases began to become more prominent because of increased life expectancy. During this time period, the predominant causes of death were heart disease, vascular disease, and cancer. There was also a significant increase in violent deaths, particularly among males. By 1970, the mortality rate for males was 126.0 per 100,000. The reasons for the increase can be associated with wars as well as behavioral and lifestyle changes occurring during that time period. Accidents also began to increase, partly because of increased usage of vehicles and work-related causes.[14]

By the early 2000s, drastic changes had occurred in health care that created a shift in the mortality and morbidity rates. For the first time, cancer-related death rates were only marginally lower than heart disease-related death rates for men and women. However, the death rate was still significant at 597,689 per year, whereas the overall death rate for all conditions was 799.5 per 100,000 (see Fig. 2-13).[14] The decrease in heart disease can be attributed to an increase in medicines for treatment of heart disease, healthier lifestyles, and educational resources. Advanced technology also contributed to better diagnosis for all heart-related conditions. The mortality rate for violent deaths decreased during the last part of the 1990s and the beginning of this century. This change can be associated with fewer wars, safer vehicles, seat belt laws, and increased workplace safety. The infant mortality rate has also been reduced drastically from roughly 26 deaths per 1,000 live births in the 1950s to approximately 6 deaths per 1,000 live births in 2010. The decrease in infant mortality rate can be attributed to improved prenatal care, sterile environments, and advanced technology.

Even as many diseases and conditions experienced decreased mortality rates, in the early 1980s, a new condition emerged. AIDS was showing signs of becoming one of the more challenging health-care concerns of recent years. By 1995, AIDS-related deaths had reached almost 50 deaths per 100,000 males, particularly in the gay community. Before

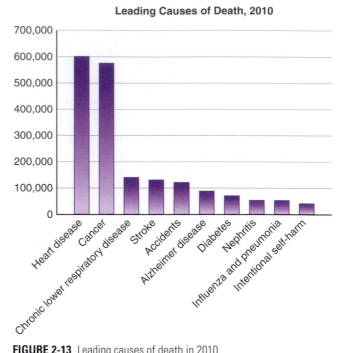

FIGURE 2-13 Leading causes of death in 2010.

1985, there were no known AIDS-related deaths in the United States, so efforts to stop the progression were established by much-needed research. Because of new treatments and education, death rates from AIDS have been declining over the last few years.

Federal Initiatives

Early Government Involvement

In the last century, many changes occurred that placed the federal government in the middle of the health-care arena. Before government involvement, health care was treated as a private entity relative to policy and payment. Although local and state governments might own the poorhouses or farms where the needy lived or worked, there was limited interaction and no accountability until around 1935. Before this, families were more or less responsible for either providing care or seeking health care for their loved ones.[1] A physician or hospital worked with the patient or family regarding payment resources. During the Great Depression in the 1930s, the economy was in such dire shape that many families were unable to provide for their families, especially for the elderly who were not physically able to work and contribute monetarily. The economic decline resulted in the *Social Security Act of 1935,* which created a shift in social welfare from personal responsibility to federal responsibility. This enactment, originally known as the

Old-Age, Survivors, Insurance Disability (OASID) program, was initiated to alleviate some of the poverty-stricken woes of American seniors, widows, fatherless children, and disabled persons. This enactment was a turning point for Americans, and although the program still exists today, there have been several amendments and adjustments to meet the demands of an increasingly aging population and dwindling funds. One of the most important amendments happened in 1950 when the federal government began providing funds for health care for individuals receiving Social Security benefits. In 1965, **Medicaid** and **Medicare** were introduced and the amendment to the Social Security Act provided federal and state funds for these programs to pay for health-care costs for the aged, disabled, and poverty stricken.[1]

After the enactment of Medicare and Medicaid programs, the government became more active in the lives of the American people, especially regarding health-care concerns. As the number of hospitals continued to increase across the United States, so did costs and the need for research. Although the growth in hospitals made a positive impact, the shortage of providers created a new problem. Therefore, in 1946, the Hill-Burton Act was passed. More than $4 billion was provided in the form of grants and loans to build new inpatient and outpatient facilities and for renovations to existing structures. To offset health-care provider shortages, the government provided funding for the education of more physicians, nurses, technicians, and managers. The National Institutes of Health (NIH) also provided funding for research initiatives, which were carried out by academic institutions, research institutes, and health organizations.[1]

War on Poverty

In late 1963, Lyndon Johnson assumed the role of president and was immediately faced with economic woes. The unemployment rate was high and job skills were low. Providing for a family on a marginal income was growing more difficult. Because of the economic depression, Johnson declared a "War on Poverty" and established the Economic Opportunity Act of 1964. Although there were many components to this act, one that was directly related to health care was the Health Center Program under the Public Health Service Act. The government provided grant funding to community health centers providing primary and preventive care to medically underserved areas (MUA) or medically underserved populations (MUP). These populations included rural communities, migrant or seasonal workers, and homeless people.[1]

Health-Care Reform

Throughout recent decades, one issue that has constantly been reviewed, evaluated, and discussed is health-care reform. As the cost of health care has risen and continues to increase, the issues of health disparities have emerged. To balance the health disparities that exist among populations, access to care must be addressed. Access to care includes having local providers as well as resources to pay for the services. Although programs exist for the aged, the disabled, and the poor, many individuals do not fit into one of these categories. These individuals are often referred to as those who "fall between the cracks," meaning that they are too young for Medicare, are not disabled, or make slightly more money than is allowed for Medicaid. However, these individuals do not make enough to buy insurance and pay co-pays for services or medicines. Even those individuals who are receiving federal assistance such as Medicare often have difficulty paying their co-pays. Others must depend on their employer-sponsored health insurance coverage. This type of coverage started in the 1930s because of the effects of the Great Depression, and it continued to grow throughout the next 7 decades. Until recent years, many working individuals depended on employers to sponsor their health insurance coverage. As insurance premiums began to rise significantly in the early 2000s, this benefit began to change by delivering either lower benefits or higher deductibles, co-pays, or premiums paid by the worker. However, having employer-sponsored insurance was still a better option than purchasing private policies because of higher premiums and limited coverage. With the continued increase in premiums, many companies had to discontinue offering insurance coverage. The other economic change that began to come into play was the unemployment rate. As the unemployment rate began to soar in 2008, many individuals lost their health insurance coverage. While the economy was falling apart due to unemployment, rising gas prices, bankruptcies, and decreased home sales, the Obama administration began to evaluate the possibility of health-care reform. In March 2010 the ***Health Care Education Reconciliation Act of 2010*** was signed by President Barack Obama. This enactment was an amendment to the previous piece of legislation signed in 2009—the *Patient Protection and Affordable Care Act,* which was passed by Congress in late 2009. This health-care reform, also known as the Affordable Care Act (Obamacare), contains many features that represent changes within the U.S. health-care system. Some of the bills have been enforced, although others continue to undergo alterations and/or have different dates for enactment. The basic premise for the health-care reform was to improve access to care, improve quality of care while lowering costs, improve the health-care delivery system, provide insurance to everyone, and hold health-care providers and insurance companies accountable.[15] While some of the original features of the health-care reform have been implemented, others are being revamped or postponed; however, some of the key features include the following[13]:

- Providing new patient bill of rights
- Providing health insurance options online
- Controlling annual limits on insurance coverage
- Reducing lifetime limits on insurance coverage
- Offering small business tax credits for health insurance
- Implementing a consumer assistance program
- Strengthening community health centers
- Reducing health-care premiums
- Providing new prescription drug discounts for seniors
- Increasing access to health-care services in the home
- Decreasing paperwork and administrative costs
- Offering more options for long-term care insurance
- Increasing Medicaid payments for primary-care providers
- Tying physician payment to quality rather than volume
- Increasing Medicaid access
- Providing free preventive care
- Increasing efforts to fight health-care fraud

As you can see from this limited list, there are many features to the Affordable Care Act, and many of these features may be revamped several times before complete implementation. Because of the length of the bill and its various features, it can be confusing for many Americans. It is safe to say that many individuals are seeking advice from experts or publications to help them understand the impact that health-care reform will have on them.

Advanced Topic

Under the Affordable Care Act, employers with 50 or more full-time employees are required to pay a penalty if they fail to provide insurance coverage to all full-time employees. This requirement began in 2014.[15] There is already some evidence that employers are cutting back on full-time employees to undermine this requirement. What effects do you think it could potentially have on businesses and the economy?

SUMMARY

Even though the goals of health care have not really changed over the past 100 years, the factors that affect the goals change on a regular basis. These changes must be addressed and kept in check to preserve the original goals of health care and those of health-care providers. The government and health-care providers must understand and stay current on trends in mortality and morbidity, health-care reform, advanced technologies, funding, and environmental threats so as to provide the best-quality care for individuals. Now that we have identified aspects of the health-care environment and the factors involved, the next chapter will focus on types of health-care structures and facilities.

Review Questions

1. Actual deaths caused by a specific disease or illness is known as:
   A. Morbidity
   B. Mortality
   C. Incident rate
   D. Death rate

2. The great flu epidemic that killed approximately 50 million people occurred in 1930.
   A. True
   B. False

3. The goals of health care include all of the following *except:*
   A. Preventing disabilities
   B. Improving quality of life
   C. Increasing the gross national product
   D. Decreasing premature deaths

4. One of the main components of the *Health Care Education Reconciliation Act of 2010* is:
   A. Affordable care
   B. HIPAA
   C. Telemedicine
   D. None of the above

5. The War on Poverty was declared by:
   A. Kennedy
   B. Eisenhower
   C. Johnson
   D. Obama

6. The direct costs of obesity include:
   A. Higher insurance premiums
   B. Fewer social activities
   C. Health conditions
   D. Social stigma

7. A federally funded program that pays health-care costs for the disabled, those with end-stage renal disease, and the older population (65 and older) is:

   A. Medicaid

   B. Obamacare

   C. Blue Cross Blue Shield

   D. Medicare

8. The Centers for Medicare and Medicaid Services was originally known as the:

   A. Health Services Organizations

   B. Bureau of Health Academies

   C. Health Care Financing Administration

   D. National Institutes of Health

9. The acronym AHA stands for:

   A. American Health Association

   B. American Hospital Association

   C. American Homeopathic Association

   D. None of the above

10. Choosing to smoke cigarettes is considered a/an:

   A. Economic issue

   B. Socioeconomic issue

   C. Lifestyle and behavioral issue

   D. Environmental issue

Glossary of Key Terms

Genetics—the biological process of parents transmitting specific characteristics to their children

Generic—a drug that is comparable to another one but is sold under a different name for a lower price

Morbidity—a specific disease or illness; usually calculated in numbers or rates

Mortality—the number of actual deaths caused by a specific disease or illness; usually calculated in numbers or rates

Medicaid—a government insurance program for lower-income individuals that assists with health-care costs; each state is able to select the eligibility criteria for its residents

Medicare—a social insurance program for individuals 65 and older, disabled, or diagnosed with end-stage renal disease or Lou Gehrig disease that pays a percentage of health-care costs

Health Care Education Reconciliation Act of 2010—the universal health-care reform under the Obama administration

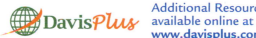

Additional Resources are available online at www.davisplus.com

Additional Resources

Morbidity and Mortality Weekly Report (MMWR)—www.cdc.gov/mmwr

This website provides information on chronic diseases and special reports on other concerning health issues, such as cigarette smoking among adults and alcohol consumption and pregnancy. There is also a weekly publication that lists the prevalence of certain diseases and illnesses such as Lyme disease or Rocky Mountain spotted fever that occur during a specific time of the year.

Centers for Medicare and Medicaid Services (CMS)—www.cms.hhs.gov

This website provides information on Medicare and Medicaid, including publications, and new policy or legislation on these government programs.

American Hospital Association (AHA)—www.aha.org

This website provides a list of hospitals and health-care organizations in the United States. It includes profiles of the facility such as size, location, type of facility, and services provided.

World Health Organization (WHO)—www.who.int

This website provides information on global health issues and statistics. The organization also publishes an annual report that includes population health indicators for specific illnesses or diseases.

Food and Drug Administration (FDA)—www.fda.org

This website provides important information regarding recalls on foods, drugs, vaccines, medical devices, and other health-related products. There is also information on regulatory issues, news releases for approval of new drugs or treatments, publications, natural disaster preparedness, and other vital reports or information on health-related matters.

The White House—www.whitehouse.gov

This website provides all types of information pertinent to health-care reform, as well as news about the economy, education, immigration, defense, technology, and many more topics of interest.

Institute of Medicine (IOM)—www.iom.edu

The IOM is an independent nonprofit organization that provides research information to the government and private sector regarding health policy issues. This website provides research study information on topics such as environmental health, education, aging population, substance abuse, and many other areas related to health care.

National Coalition on Health Care (NCHC)—www.nchc.org

This organization works to improve health care in America by promoting quality care for all citizens. Its website provides information on policy issues, research, and education regarding health trends.

References

1. Kovner A, Knickman J, eds. *Health Care Delivery in the United States.* New York: Springer Publishing; 2008.

2. Steele LS, Dewa CS, Lin E, Lee KL. Education level, income level and mental health services use in Canada: Associations and policy implications. *Healthc Policy.* 2007;3(1):96–106.

3. Health, United States, 2011, with special feature on socioeconomic status and health.
   http://www.cdc.gov/nchs/data/hus/hus11.pdf.
   Accessed October 24, 2013.

4. Crabtree S. Income, education levels combine to predict health problems. Gallup-Healthways Well-Being Index data. 2010.
   http://www.gallup.com/poll/127532/income-education-levels-combine-predict-health-problems.aspx.
   Accessed October 24, 2013.

5. Abramovitz J. Unnatural disasters. *World Watch.* 1999;12(4):30–35.

6. Longest B Jr, Darr K. *Managing Health Services Organizations and Systems,* 5th ed. Baltimore, MD: Health Professions Press; 2008.

7. Nobel Prize.
   http://www.nobelprize.org/educational/medicine/landsteiner/readmore.html.
   Accessed July 12, 2013.

8. Nobel Prize.
   http://www.nobelprize.org/educational/nobelprize_info/curie-edu.html.
   Accessed July 12, 2013.

9. Taubenberger J, Morens D. 1918 influenza: The mother of all pandemics. *Emerg Infect Dis.* 2006; 12(1):15–22.

10. Hospitals and Health Networks.
    http://www.hhnmag.com/hhnmag/index.jsp.
    Accessed July 25, 2013.

11. U.S. Department of Health and Human Services, Food and Drug Administration. June 8, 2006 approval letter—human papillomavirus quadrivalent (types 6, 11, 16, 18) vaccine, recombinant.
    http://www.fda.gov/BiologicsBloodVaccines/Vaccines/ApprovedProducts/ucm111283.htm.
    Accessed July 12, 2013.

12. U.S. Department of Health and Human Services, Food and Drug Administration. "May 25, 2006 approval letter—Zostavax."
    http://www.fda.gov/BiologicsBloodVaccines/Vaccines/ApprovedProducts/ucm132873.htm.
    Accessed July 12, 2013.

13. U.S. Department of Health and Human Services. Key features of the Affordable Care Act by year.
    http://www.hhs.gov/healthcare/facts/timeline/timeline-text.html.
    Accessed July 18, 2013.

14. Centers for Disease Control and Prevention. Deaths and mortality 2011.
    http://www.cdc.gov/nchs/fastats/deaths.htm.
    Accessed July 16, 2013.

15. The Association of Schools of Allied Health Professions. Affordable Care Act update. Trends. 2013.
    http://www.asahp.org/trends/2013/June%202013.pdf.
    Accessed July 18, 2013.

CHAPTER 3

Types of Health-Care Facilities

Patricia Royal, EdD

Learning Objectives

After reading this chapter, students should be able to:

- Understand the difference between types of hospitals
- Identify some of the services provided by hospitals
- Recognize the various health-care facilities
- Identify the populations who require the services
- Understand the historical perspective that led to the development of various health-care facilities

Key Terms

- Not for profit
- General hospitals
- Teaching hospitals
- Preceptors
- Ambulatory
- Residential care

Types of Hospitals and Health-Care Facilities

This chapter focuses on specific types of health-care facilities and the roles they play in keeping us healthy. Patients can receive treatment in many types of hospitals and facilities as an inpatient or outpatient, for skilled or unskilled needs, and at for-profit and not-for-profit facilities. This chapter explores the differences between these types of facilities and the services they provide.

Hospitals

Hospitals were established in the 18th century, and since then, the development and types of hospitals have continually changed based on needs, location, and services. Since the establishment of the first U.S. hospital, changes in population, diseases, and technology have contributed to the advancement of hospitals and services provided. The first section of this chapter explores some of the types of hospitals in existence today and the types of services they provide.

Hospital Structures

The type of hospital determines the various internal structures, such as governing board and committees; however, generally speaking, most hospitals have similar departments and services. Specialty hospitals may include additional treatment options depending on the area of expertise, but overall there is a typical organization chart for most U.S. hospitals. These areas include the following[1,2]:

- *Governing body:* Typically, the governing body is the board of directors or board of trustees. The governing body is responsible for hiring the chief executive officer (CEO) or hospital administrator and addressing the long-term goals of the hospital. The governing body is responsible for establishing a mission for the hospital, ensuring adequate performance of the CEO, and ensuring that quality care is provided, along with many other strategic operations.

- *Hospital administrator:* The hospital administrator is sometimes referred to as the CEO or president and is responsible for the day-to-day operations. The hospital administrator is directly responsible for supervision of the officers in the hospital, such as chief financial officer (CFO), chief operating officer (COO), chief information officer (CIO), and various other officers or vice presidents. The hospital administrator is responsible for risk management, development, and marketing.

- *Financial:* This department is supervised by the CFO or vice president for finance and encompasses several offices, including accounting, admitting, cashier, business, data processing, and credit and collections. The financial department maintains the accounting systems for tracking of income and expenses, development and coordination of the budget, preparation of financial reports, and internal audits, as well as many and various other responsibilities.

- *Nursing:* This department is supervised by the chief nursing officer (CNO) or vice president of nursing and encompasses several offices or departments, including inpatient units, operating rooms, outpatient clinics, emergency departments (EDs), nursing education, and central supply. The nursing department is responsible for required educational training, staffing, reports, equipment and supplies, patient care, and scheduling, along with a variety of other activities.

- *Support:* The support department is generally supervised by the COO and is divided into two groups: administrative and environment.
  - *Administrative:* The administrative division may encompass medical records, personnel and purchasing, social services, dietary, and discharge planning. The administrative division does not provide direct patient care but is involved in the care of patients. Some responsibilities include keeping medical records up to date, assessing patients' support systems, patient advocacy, meeting dietary requirements, and patient transport.

  - *Environment:* The environment division may encompass housekeeping and laundry, maintenance and plant operations, security, and safety. Some responsibilities include maintenance of building and machinery; hospital cleanliness; providing comfortable temperatures for patients and visitors; and overall safety for patients, employees, and visitors.

- *Ancillary:* The ancillary department is usually supervised by the vice president of patient care services and encompasses services such as imaging, respiratory therapy, pharmacy, clinical laboratory, physical therapy, and electrocardiography. The individuals working in this department provide direct patient care either with hands-on approaches, counseling, or testing of samples. This department is instrumental in helping the physician determine a diagnosis of disease or illness.

- *Medical staff department:* This department is supervised by the chief medical officer (CMO) or medical director and includes medicine, surgery, house staff, obstetrics/gynecology/pediatrics, and anesthesia. This department is sometimes separated from the rest of the hospital because the board of trustees appoints the medical staff. This department formulates its own medical polices and rules and is responsible for quality care to all patients.

Types

For Profit Versus Not for Profit

Hospitals are first distinguished by their profit status: for profit and **not for profit** (also known as nonprofit), that is, how the money the hospital collects as payment for services is used and distributed. For-profit hospitals can be owned by corporations, investors, individuals, or public shareholders[3] and are operated similar to any other business that makes money and pays taxes. Their profit is based on the money received for services provided minus the expenses expended to provide the services. For-profit hospitals are able to use the profit as they choose without any state and federal specifications. On the other hand, not-for-profit hospitals are usually considered charities and provide certain community benefits in agreement with state and federal guidelines. Therefore, these hospitals do not pay state, local, property, or federal income taxes because of their designation by the Internal Revenue Service. The lack of paid taxes does not mean that the hospital cannot make a profit. The hospital is entitled to make money but is required to use it in accordance with the not-for-profit specifications, such as for reinvestments or the community. This type of hospital is usually governed by a board of trustees who serve without pay. The board members are generally selected from

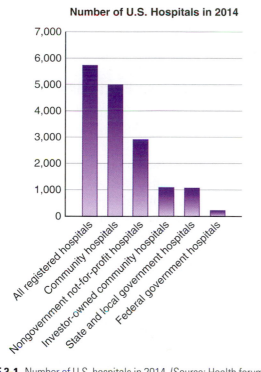

Number of U.S. Hospitals in 2014

FIGURE 3-1 Number of U.S. hospitals in 2014. (Source: Health forum, LLC, an affiliate of the American Hospital Association, 2014)

business and civic leaders who have experience in finance, administration, and management activities.[4]

Community Hospitals

Community hospitals are the most common type of hospital and are typically small in their number of beds. These hospitals are established to provide routine medical and surgical needs for a geographical location, hence the term *community*. These hospitals may also be called **general hospitals** because they are designed to meet the general acute-care needs of the local population. They are usually not-for-profit facilities and are supported by local funding, religious organizations, or cooperatives. These community hospitals went through some tough times in the 1980s, and many of the smaller ones were closed due to financial difficulties. Some of those that survived changed their tax status to become for-profit hospitals, and others joined larger hospital systems.[1,4]

Public Hospitals

Public hospitals are typically thought of as charity hospitals because of their tradition of providing services to the poor population. These hospitals are funded by federal, state, or local governments. They are generally large hospitals and serve many roles within the community. Public hospitals have EDs, which some patients use to replace the physician's office visit because this type of hospital has to treat all patients regardless of ability to pay. Some of these hospitals also provide services for prisoners and other vulnerable populations, such as individuals with AIDS, those with drug or alcohol addictions, and the uninsured and underinsured. Public hospitals also provide outreach and community education programs and serve as home bases for local 911 systems. Because public hospitals treat all patients without regard to payment source, they depend on the money received from Medicare, Medicaid, and private insurance, and often the amount paid by these sources is not sufficient to pay for the full cost of the services provided. The estimate of government support, including Medicare and Medicaid benefits, is roughly 69%; the other 31% is billed to patients in hopes of payment. The unpaid expenses are often sent to a collection agency or become a tax write-off for the hospital. Another vital role for public hospitals is the training of medical personnel. Even with budgetary constraints, public hospitals train approximately 15% of medical and dental residents.[5]

Teaching Hospitals

Teaching hospitals are usually the largest hospitals in the system and are generally located within large cities. They are affiliated with a medical school and have a commitment to graduate education to serve as **preceptors** for medical interns and residents completing their educational requirements. Some of these hospitals are private, whereas others are government supported. Many of the physicians at a teaching hospital also hold teaching positions with the affiliated university. These hospitals usually have highly qualified physicians and the most advanced technology; therefore, patients with complex conditions or difficult diagnoses benefit greatly from the medical experts and resources available. On the flip side, some patients do not like multiple examinations performed by residents and students. Providing a hands-on approach to patient care, these hospitals serve a critical role in the education of future health-care providers.

Rural Hospitals

Rural hospitals, also known as district hospitals, are located in smaller rural areas and have fewer than 100 beds. To be classified as a rural hospital, the population of the city or town typically must be under 50,000 residents. Although there has been a decline in rural hospitals over the last few years, they still account for roughly 40% of the total number of hospitals located in the United States.[5] Rural hospitals have always operated on small budgets, but with changes in demographics, the budgets for many rural hospitals have been decreasing over the past decade. The problem has resulted from younger and healthier individuals moving to larger towns or cities. The remaining members of the population are older, poorer, less healthy, and less able to pay for services. Some rural communities have had an increase in immigrant populations, who often have no health insurance or benefits to offset the costs of care. A problem in retaining skilled providers has contributed to the demise of some rural hospitals as well. For other facilities, admissions have been increasing over the past decade, and this has added to the burden of maintaining sufficient providers to care for the increase. Often, rural hospitals depend on federal grants to help alleviate some of the costs associated with attracting and retaining health-care providers.

Specialized Hospitals

Specialized hospitals are often affiliated with larger health systems, such as a children's hospital located within the main organizational structure. However, some children's hospitals are private, government funded, or religious affiliated. Other types of specialized hospitals include women's, veterans', geriatric, psychiatric, rehabilitative, and cancer hospitals.

Summary

Many types of hospitals exist, and they can be categorized by ownership, number of beds, services provided, and length of stay. Hospitals are like any other business in that they may

open and close depending on community needs, resources, and financial assets. The same occurs with other types of health-care facilities, which is addressed in the next section.

Ambulatory Care Facilities

The word **ambulatory,** in its most literal sense, means that patients are able to walk (ambulate) into the facility for services; however, the term *outpatient* is often used interchangeably with *ambulatory,* simply meaning that the patient does not stay all night. Ambulatory care can be provided by a variety of health-care facilities, including hospitals, clinics, health departments, physician offices, and many other systems. The types of procedures under the ambulatory care umbrella include same-day surgeries, emergency treatments, urgent care, diagnostic tests, rehabilitative services, and imaging. One distinction worth noting is the difference between ambulatory care facilities and freestanding ambulatory care centers. Although the same types of services are provided, a freestanding ambulatory care center must deliver the care in a facility that is not located on hospital grounds.[1] These types of facilities may be hospital sponsored or affiliated but are not directly located on the hospital grounds. Several different

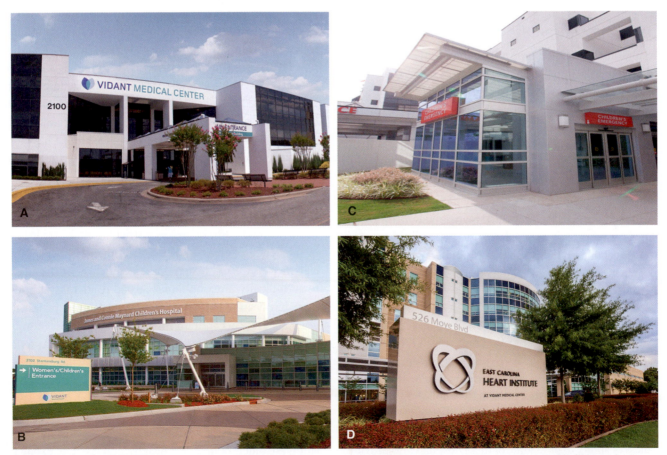

FIGURE 3-2 Vidant Medical Center in Greenville, North Carolina, is a large regional health system incorporating several types of facilities under the same umbrella. Photos illustrate **(A)** the hospital, **(B)** the children's hospital, **(C)** the children's emergency department, and **(D)** the heart institute.

types of freestanding ambulatory care centers are described after a brief history.

History

Ambulatory care centers became popular in the late 1980s and early 1990s because of the rising costs of hospital care. During the 1960s to 1980s, health-care costs increased dramatically. The challenges of delivering quality health care at lower costs were issues addressed by federal, state, and local governments as well as the governing bodies at the institutions themselves. In addition to growing concerns regarding costs, health-care delivery was also challenged. For patients, it appeared that there was only one choice for hospital-based procedures such as minor surgeries, regardless of the distance between their home and the hospital. These two forces helped to pave the way for establishments of ambulatory care centers.[5,6]

Types

Of the many types of ambulatory care facilities, one of the most popular and fastest growing is the ambulatory surgical center (ASC). The first freestanding ASC was established in 1970 by Drs. John Ford and Wallace Reed in Phoenix, Arizona. The dramatic increase in health care had not reached full intensity until around the 1980s, when others started the shift toward ambulatory centers. Although costs were an issue, the larger concern for the establishment of the ASC was based on patients' convenience and comfort.[7] The growth of ASCs has been exceptional: In 2011, there were 5,300 facilities performing more than 23 million surgeries annually.[7]

Another type of freestanding ambulatory care center is urgent care or emergency care units not affiliated with hospitals. In these facilities, patients are treated for non–life-threatening conditions such as minor cuts, broken bones, viruses, or earaches. Many individuals do not want to wait to be seen at the ED and would rather be treated at the urgent care center. Another reason for choosing these units is convenience. Criteria for classification of an urgent care center include the following[8]:

- Able to provide on-site x-rays
- Offers evening office hours Monday through Friday
- Able to suture minor lacerations
- Provides patient care primarily on a walk-in basis

Most cities and towns now have several urgent care centers within their geographical areas. Urgent care centers are common today and represent a large part of the health-care system. In 2008, there were approximately 8,000 urgent care centers in the United States.[8] Other, similar facilities that are popping up around the United States include so-called minute clinics or retail clinics, which provide services such as blood pressure, glucose, and cholesterol screenings and flu vaccines. These facilities are often found in pharmacies and retail stores.

Dialysis units are also classified as ambulatory care centers. Dialysis units treat patients who have end-stage renal disease (ESRD). People with ESRD need dialysis treatments to rid the toxins and excess fluids from their kidneys. The dialysis machine cleans the blood by filtering it through an artificial kidney. These facilities are generally open 6 days a week and have two or three shifts due to patient demand. Dialysis units have grown rapidly over the past 30 years, with approximately 4,200 centers in the United States in 2013.[9] Currently, approximately 350,000 dialysis patients are being treated in centers across the United States. This number is expected to continue to increase at a rate of 3% to 5% annually. Other types of ambulatory care or outpatient centers include substance abuse centers, radiology centers, imaging centers, blood banks, and laboratory centers.

Nursing and Residential Care Facilities

Nursing and **residential care** facilities are distinguished based on the level of skill needed for the residents. Nursing homes provide inpatient services to patients who are disabled or sick and need constant care but are not required to stay in the hospital. The services provided include nursing, personal care, and rehabilitation services to patients on a short- and long-term care basis. Residential care facilities provide some of the same types of services but offer around-the-clock services to children as well as to elderly individuals who have limited ability to care for themselves.[2] After a brief history, the various types of facilities are discussed.

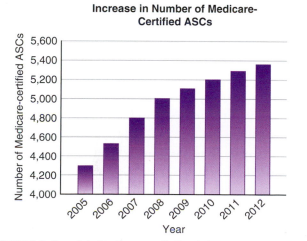

Increase in Number of Medicare-Certified ASCs

FIGURE 3-3 Growth in Medicare-certified ambulatory surgical centers. (Source: MedPAC analysis of Provider of Services files from CMS, 2012.)

History

Before the 20th century, disabled or elderly individuals needing care were sent to almshouses, which were dilapidated homes where limited care was provided. These homes were also known as poorhouses because the residents there were poor and had no money to pay for assistance. (This topic is addressed in more detail in Chapter 28.) There were no federal monies or programs established yet for this population, so those who had no family members to take care of them were placed in these facilities. With the Social Security Act in place and a growing elderly population, private old-age homes were being established by the late 1930s. Residents would live in the old-age home while collecting Social Security, which could help pay for the costs of the facility. By the mid-1950s, nursing homes were being built with federal grant money. For the next 6 decades, nursing homes' standards and compliance were improved based on legislation reform, accreditation requirements, and payer source demands, such as Medicare and Medicaid.[10]

Types

Nursing homes were established predominantly for the elderly as a place to live out their final years. Over the years, the services provided and types of patients have changed along with the demographics. Today, nursing homes still provide the sick elderly who have need for skilled care with a place to live, but in addition, nursing homes provide other services such as rehabilitative services for short-term care. Long-term residents also can receive rehabilitative services from physical, occupational, and speech therapists. There are facilities specializing in Alzheimer patients, AIDS patients, and ventilator-dependent patients. The nursing home staff consists of an administrator, nurses, registered dietitians, social workers, activity directors, nursing assistants, facility service workers, and housekeeping and laundry personnel. Nursing homes generally receive federal money (Medicare and Medicaid), in addition to private insurance or private pay. To receive federal funding the facility must achieve and maintain certain standards to be certified; approximately 80% are Medicare and Medicaid certified.[2] With an aging population, nursing home needs are expected to rise, offering ample jobs in this arena.

Assisted-living facilities are similar to nursing homes in that they are also inpatient residential facilities. The main difference between the two is that the assisted-living facility does not meet the skilled need requirements. Residents who live in assisted-living facilities must be able to complete their activities of daily living (ADLs) with limited assistance from staff. ADLs include their personal needs such as dressing, brushing their teeth or hair, and toiletry habits. There are no nurses at this type of facility; however, there are medicine technicians (med techs) who distribute residents' medications. The facility is managed by an administrator and resident coordinators manage patient medical needs such as doctor visits, medicines, supplies, and annual vaccines such as the flu and pneumonia vaccines.

Other residential care facilities include group homes, drug rehabilitation centers, and adult family homes. These facilities do not employ nursing staff, and their medical care is not the main focus. The focus is on ADLs such as bathing, dressing, and brushing of hair and teeth. Medical issues are handled by appointments to the physician's office. In these facilities, patients are grouped together according to their health conditions or ages. Some group homes house mentally disturbed youth, whereas others may provide care for disabled seniors.

Physician and Dental Offices

Another type of health-care structure is private or group physician practices and dental offices. Physician or surgeon practices can be privately owned or grouped together with the same or different specialties. Group practices can sometimes be more enticing because of the backup coverage and reduced overhead expense. These physicians see patients at their locations but may also be able to make hospital visits, depending on the individual hospital policy or privileges granted.

Dental offices are commonly found in most towns or cities. They are generally small operations with few employees; however, some larger practices are grouped together, such as many physicians' offices. Dental offices make up about 20% of health-care organizations.[9]

Home Health and Hospice

Home health agencies provide care for patients in their own homes. The services are under the indirect supervision of a medical director of the agency or the patient's own physician. The types of services provided by home health nurses and certified nursing assistants include dressing changes, medication refills, and vital sign and diabetic monitoring. Home health agencies employ nurses, nursing assistants, case managers, social workers, and administrative staff. Typically, home health agencies contract with physical and occupational therapists rather than having them on staff. Therapists help to rehabilitate the patient after some illnesses or accidents. A physician's orders dictate the service requested, but the service is usually for short-term care. Home health agencies can be for-profit or not-for-profit, hospital-based, or privately owned facilities. They must be Medicare and Medicaid certified to be reimbursed for services.

Hospices can be affiliated with a home health facility or hospital, or they can be freestanding facilities. Hospice care is provided for the terminally ill individual who has a life expectancy of 6 months or less. Similar to home health agencies, the hospice team treats patients in their home, but they can also provide services in a nursing home environment. The hospice team is made up of medical directors, administrative staff, nurses, nurse assistants, social workers, bereavement counselors, spiritual support personnel, and volunteers. Like home health agencies, they must be Medicare and Medicaid certified to receive reimbursement.

Medical and Diagnostic Laboratories

The last type of structure discussed in this chapter is medical and diagnostic laboratories. This group is one of the smaller employers in the health-care system. Their role is to provide analytic or diagnostic services based on physician orders. The types of services provided include blood analysis, x-rays, scans, and other clinical tests.[2] These facilities are common in most cities and towns, but they are often overlooked because of their small size and their small number of employees.

SUMMARY

Many types of health-care facilities provide care for patients depending on need, ability to pay, and location, among other factors. Although facilities vary greatly in size, specialization, and focus, the one thing they all have in common is their benefit of providing prevention, diagnosis, and treatment of individuals needing services.

Review Questions

1. Hospitals that make profits and reinvest the profits into the hospital or community are known as:
   A. For profit
   B. Community
   C. Not for profit
   D. Community health centers

2. A type of hospital affiliated with an academic center is known as a:
   A. Rural hospital
   B. Public hospital
   C. Teaching hospital
   D. All of the above

3. In the 19th century, elderly or disabled individuals needing care were sent to nursing homes.
   A. True
   B. False

4. Residents living in assisted-living facilities must be able to:
   A. Walk
   B. Take their own medicines
   C. Drive
   D. Take care of personal needs with limited assistance

5. Assisted-living facilities employ registered nurses, whereas nursing homes are only required to hire nursing assistants.
   A. True
   B. False

6. The facilities that employ the fewest number of workers are:
   A. Nursing homes
   B. Residential homes
   C. Medical and diagnostic laboratories
   D. Acute-care centers

7. Individuals receiving care in their own homes on a temporary basis are probably using the services of a/an:
   A. Hospital
   B. Ambulatory care center
   C. Medical and diagnostic laboratory
   D. Home health facility

8. To qualify for hospice care, a patient must be deemed:
   A. Terminally ill
   B. Mentally competent
   C. Able to complete ADLs
   D. All of the above

9. Residents with long-term diseases or conditions usually are placed in which of the following facilities?
   A. Home health
   B. Rehabilitative centers
   C. Nursing homes
   D. None of the above

10. These hospitals are sometimes thought of as charity hospitals because they provide services to the poor in their community:
    A. Private
    B. Teaching
    C. Rural
    D. Public

Glossary of Key Terms

Not for profit—a designation by the Internal Revenue Service that does not allow agencies or organizations to accrue money to be paid to an individual or private shareholders

General hospitals—hospitals that provide services to individuals on a short-term basis and for limited duration

Teaching hospitals—hospitals that are affiliated with an academic center such as a medical school

Preceptors—experienced and licensed or certified individuals who teach students in a work environment such as a hospital setting

Ambulatory—patient receiving treatment as an outpatient and not admitted to the hospital

Residential care—facility where patients live and consider the place their residence

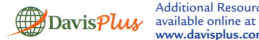 **Additional Resources are available online at www.davisplus.com**

Additional Resources

American Hospital Association—www.aha.org
The American Hospital Association publishes *The AHA Guide and Hospital Statistics.* These publications contain information on hospitals, including size, location, type, ownership, services, financial reports, and utilization.

HospitalLink—www.hospitallink.com
This website provides information on hospitals across the United States. You can click on a specific state and the link will provide you with the hospitals located there and the basic information on each one.

Centers for Medicare and Medicaid Services—www.cms. hhs.gov
This website provides information on a variety of issues related to Medicare and Medicaid. The various types of health-care facilities are also included, with information about each one. There are special topic sections that contain information on popular new items.

National Library of Medicine—www.nlm.nih.gov/databases
This website is affiliated with the National Institutes of Health and provides databases associated with health-related information, including diseases and conditions, in addition to policy and reform.

The Joint Commission—www.jointcommission.org
This website provides information on The Joint Commission accreditation for hospitals, health-care facilities, and other providers.

References

1. Griffin D. *Hospitals: What they are and how they work,* 3rd ed. Boston: Jones & Bartlett; 2006.

2. Longest B, Darr K. *Managing Health Services Organizations and Systems,* 5th ed. Baltimore: Health Professions Press; 2008.

3. Medicare News Group, August 2013.
   www.medicarenewsgroup.com/news/medicare.
   Accessed August 7, 2013.

4. Library Index, 2013.
   www.libraryindex.com.
   Accessed August 9, 2013.

5. Kovner A, Knickman J. *Health Care Delivery in the United States,* 9th ed. New York: Springer; 2008.

6. Dunn A. History of ambulatory care facilities from a roving hospital administrator's point of view. *J Ambulatory Care Manage.* 1999;22(1):8–13.

7. Ambulatory Surgical Care Association. 2013.
   www.ascassociation.org.
   Accessed August 9, 2013.

8. Weinick R, Bristol S, Marder J, DesRoches C. The search for the urgent care center. *J Urgent Care Med.* 2009;38–40.

9. First Research. 2013.
   www.firstresearch.com/Industry-Research/Kidney-Dialysis-Centers.html.
   Accessed August 12, 2013.

10. Public Broadcasting System. 2013.
    www.pbs.org/newshour/health/nursinghomes/timeline.html.
    Accessed August 12, 2013.

CHAPTER 4

Paying for Services

Patricia Royal, EdD

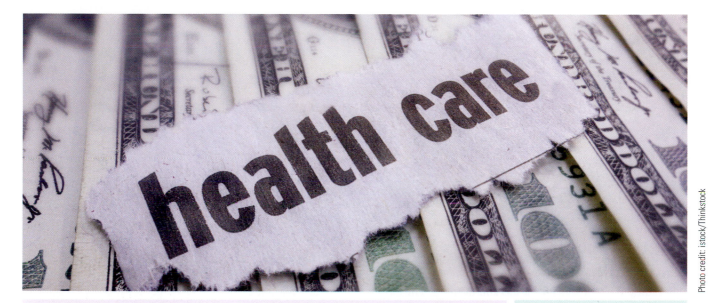

Photo credit: istock/Thinkstock

Learning Objectives

After reading this chapter, students should be able to:

- Demonstrate a basic understanding of the different health-care funding sources
- Differentiate between Medicare and Medicaid
- Identify various types of insurance
- Learn how to distinguish insurance benefits
- Discuss national health-care expenditures and revenue streams

Key Terms

- Employer-sponsored insurance
- Private-pay insurance
- Managed care
- Medigap
- Children's Health Insurance Program (CHIP)

Introduction

The way we pay for our health-care services has changed drastically in the past 100 years. We no longer use the barter system of paying the doctor with chickens or eggs. Although this system might sound absurd, the barter system was used for many years and worked well in its time. When the doctor made house calls, some people paid for the service by giving whatever products they had on hand. Such items might include chickens, eggs, sheep, cows, homemade cakes or pies, or even trading services such as yard work or helping to build houses. The patient or family member bartered with the doctor to pay for the services tendered. There was no government involvement, no patient bill of rights, no allowance regarding the time the doctor spent with the patient, no forms to be signed, no quality control, no regulations, and no certifications. Health-care decision-making was between the doctor and the patient or family member. Some people had money to pay, but others did not; therefore, a compromise occurred. During this time period, physicians received their training by the apprenticeship method rather than attending medical school. Over time, formal training, along with its associated time and costs, became the expectation for becoming a doctor. Physicians endured the expenses of education, continuing education requirements, liability insurance, and professional associations, along with many other expenses. Health care had moved away from the "country doctor" approach to a more scientific and standardized profession

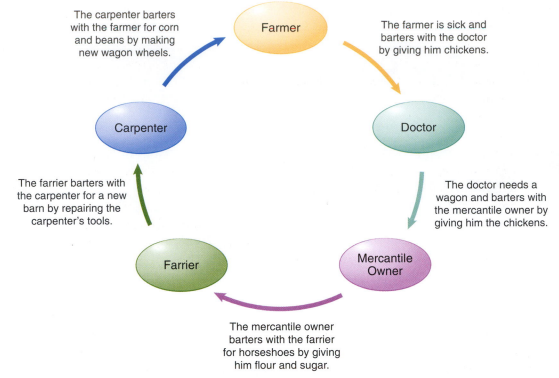

The carpenter barters with the farmer for corn and beans by making new wagon wheels.

The farmer is sick and barters with the doctor by giving him chickens.

The doctor needs a wagon and barters with the mercantile owner by giving him the chickens.

The mercantile owner barters with the farrier for horseshoes by giving him flour and sugar.

The farrier barters with the carpenter for a new barn by repairing the carpenter's tools.

FIGURE 4-1 The barter system.

that required expensive education and training. The barter system was no longer conducive to offsetting the expense of the education or the time spent in training. Therefore, new systems evolved.

This chapter examines the changes occurring in payment structures for health-care services, as well as the distribution of funds.

Funding Sources

Insurance

Most individuals understand the basic premise of health-care insurance, which is to protect against loss by assisting with medical bills. Difficulties in understanding insurance are mostly due to the various types, benefits, co-pays, deductibles, and out-of-pocket expenses. This chapter does not cover insurance plans in depth but provides a basic overview of how health insurance plans benefit the insured and health-care providers. Many types of insurance coverage exist; however, typically only health insurance covers medical expenses. Individuals purchase health insurance to be prepared should an illness or injury occur. Although insurance does not cover everything, it provides coverage for most conditions. Some of the services most insurance plans cover include routine care, major medical, dental visits, eye care, and prescription drugs. Insurance typically does not cover services such as cosmetic services, experimental procedures, or elective

surgery unless the risk of not having the procedures done can produce more harm (e.g., gastric bypass surgery). In this case, insurance will generally cover all or a portion after deductibles are met. The following section describes the various types of insurance coverage.

Insurance Types
Employer-sponsored Insurance

The first type of insurance plan we will discuss is **employer-sponsored insurance,** also known as *group insurance.* This plan is purchased through one's place of employment. Most

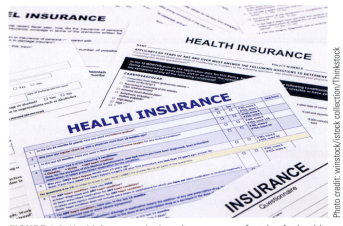

FIGURE 4-2 Health insurance is the primary means of paying for health-care expenses in the United States.

large companies have some form of health insurance available to their employees. The first major employer-sponsored insurance was started by Blue Cross Blue Shield in 1929,[1] and was supported by the American Hospital Association. The need to establish an insurance plan became clear during the Great Depression in the1930s. During this time of economic crisis many people were unable to pay their health-care bills, creating the need for some type of assistance program. Although employer-sponsored group insurance was not mandated, most employers recognized the need to offer coverage to recruit and retain employees. Purchasing group insurance through an employer has the advantage of reduced rates because the risk is spread out over all the employees (Fig. 4-3).

The employees usually select coverage based on an individual or a family basis. The amount of money paid, the *premium,* is based on the selection criteria and is deducted from the employees' salary. Some companies pay all of their employees' coverage, and the employees pay a premium for family coverage. An amount of money, the *deductible,* usually between $100 and $500, must be met before the policy pays anything. After the deductible is met the insurance policy generally pays 70% or 80% of the remaining balance. These numbers change depending on the type of coverage the employer offers and/or the coverage selected by the employee and the type of service provided. Some policies pay 100% for preventive care and routine physicals. Most policies have out-of-pocket expenses, which refer to money spent by the insured for the specific claim. For example, when a person files a claim, the deductible and the co-pay (20%–30% of the total bill) come directly from the insured, and the insurance company pays the remaining charges.

Private-pay Insurance

Private-pay insurance works the same way as employer-sponsored plans, but the premiums are generally significantly higher or the coverage has fewer benefits. Another issue related to private insurance is the extended waiting period, which means one may not be covered for preexisting conditions. Policies can be terminated by the insurer, whereas with group or employer-sponsored plans, the insurance can only be terminated by the employee or company. The primary reason individuals buy private insurance policies is that they are unemployed, they are self-employed, they work part-time, or their employer does not offer group insurance. Before the enactment of the Affordable Care Act in 2013, employers were not mandated to provide group insurance coverage.

Managed Care

The term **managed care** refers to a health-care delivery system that manages or directs the use of health-care services and the associated costs (Fig. 4-4). There are several models, such as health maintenance organizations (HMOs), provider-sponsored organizations (PSOs), and preferred-provider organizations (PPOs).[2] The degree of control and the payment methods, such as pay-per-visit or fee-for-service, are based on the model used. Managed care started in the 1980s but did not become popular until the early 1990s. This type of delivery system was a huge change in the finances of U.S. health care. The basic premise of managed care is that the health-care provider accepts a limited dollar amount for services rendered in exchange for an increased number of patients. For the patient, the cost for coverage is reduced; however, the choice of provider or hospital is limited. The patient must visit the specific provider to receive the reduced premium. Patients can be referred to specialists, but only by the managed-care provider, and they generally require prior approval unless it is an emergency situation. This type of coverage was popular until around 2000 when patients began to resent their lack of freedom in selecting their own provider. Although managed care did save money and reduce costs, patients did not like their lack of participation in their own health-care choices, so most states do not participate in it any longer.[1] Although the popularity has waned nationwide, there are a few states that still participate in managed-care

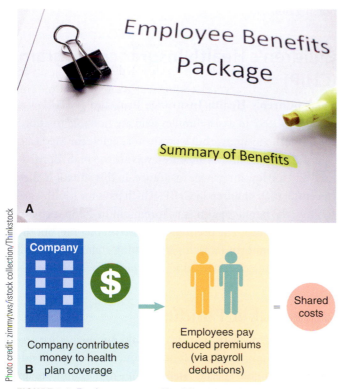

Photo credit: zimmytws/istock collection/Thinkstock

A

B Company contributes money to health plan coverage

Employees pay reduced premiums (via payroll deductions)

= Shared costs

FIGURE 4-3 Employer-sponsored health-care coverage.

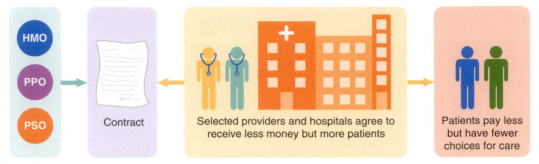

FIGURE 4-4 Managed care.

organizations. Many managed-care organizations operate under the point-of-service (POS) modality, which allows participants to select their own provider but designates in-network and out-of-network restrictions that may increase the insured's out-of-pocket expense.

Medicare

As previously defined, Medicare is a federally funded program that was established to pay for health-care costs for the older population. At the initial phase, those at least 65 years old were eligible for Medicare regardless of income. Within a few years, Medicare eligibility also included disabled individuals and individuals with end-stage renal disease regardless of age. Today Medicare is the largest payer of health-care expense in the United States.[1]

There are several parts to Medicare (Fig. 4-5). The initial coverage, Part A, covers inpatient hospital care, and all recipients eligible for Medicare receive Part A. Part B covers doctors' services and outpatient costs in addition to some costs not covered by Part A, such as physical and occupational therapy deemed medically necessary. There is a monthly premium for Part B coverage. Part C, also known as Medicare Advantage, is an alternative to the standard Medicare plan. Part C provides some additional coverage, such as prescription drug costs. The newest addition to Medicare is Part D, which pays prescription costs only. Part D, like Part B, has a monthly premium charge based on the desired coverage and is purchased by those who have not purchased Part C.[2]

Medigap

Medigap is a private supplement insurance coverage to Medicare that helps to offset expenses not covered by Part A or Part B. Medicare does not cover 100% of costs associated with health care; therefore, an individual can be stuck with a hefty bill for even a short hospital stay. Medigap helps pay the expenses, and, because it is a supplement only, it is usually reasonably priced for the benefits.

Medicaid

Medicaid, governed by Title XIX of the Social Security Act, is a federal/state/local program designed to pay for health-care costs for low-income populations[2] (Fig. 4-6). Because the program is a joint effort between the federal government and state and local governments, the plan is not necessarily the same in all states. The eligibility criteria are also different because they are based on poverty levels in each state rather than a federal poverty level. Some individuals may qualify for Medicaid at the 100% rate, which means Medicaid pays for all of their health-care needs, including prescription drugs (with a very small co-pay, usually around $3.00). Other individuals may qualify for limited Medicaid, which means they have to meet a spend-down requirement before coverage begins. (The spend-down requirement is similar to a deductible in health insurance coverage.) Medicaid is one of the key sources for funding long-term care services such as nursing homes.[2]

Children's Health Insurance Program (CHIP)

The **Children's Health Insurance Program (CHIP)** was enacted in 1997 to assist families who are not able to afford private health insurance but who are not eligible for Medicaid (Fig. 4-7). These families' income levels are too high for Medicaid and too low for private insurance. In this situation, they can enroll their children in CHIP, which pays for health-care services; the families pay a small premium in comparison to private insurance. The premium is based on income, but the coverage is uniform in each participating state. The federal government matches state funding, which offsets the costs.[3]

Other Public Funding

Some individuals with specific needs do not qualify for any of the previously discussed funding sources. These individuals may fall under special categories due to the condition or illness, ethnicity, or military experience.

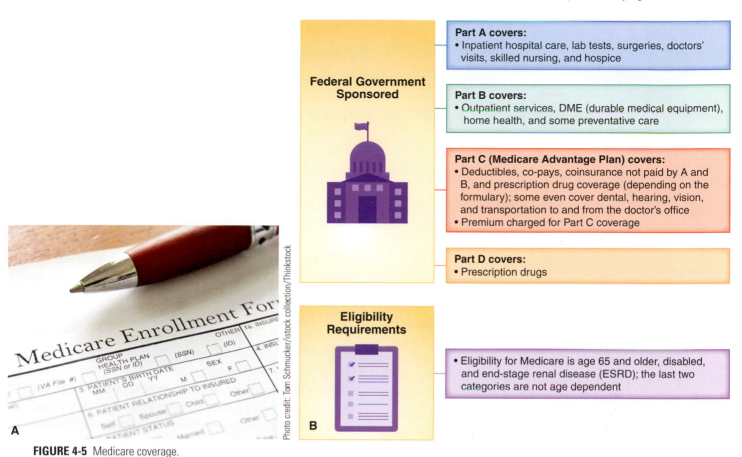

FIGURE 4-5 Medicare coverage.

Ryan White Program

The Ryan White Program is a federal program administered by the Health Resources and Services Administration (HRSA). This program was established in 1990 to provide all human immunodeficiency virus/acquired immunodeficiency syndrome (HIV/AIDS) patients with access to quality care. The namesake, Ryan White, was a teenager who contracted HIV through a blood transfusion in 1984. After his death in 1990, a federal initiative was enacted providing funding for and education about HIV/AIDS.[4]

Synder Act

The Synder Act is a federal program benefiting the Native American population. This act is now known as the Indian Health Service and is administered by the Department of Health and Human Services (DHHS). The program provides monies for health-care services in addition to other needs such as educational expenses. Eligibility for benefits requires the recipients to be members of a federally recognized Indian tribe or their descendants.[5]

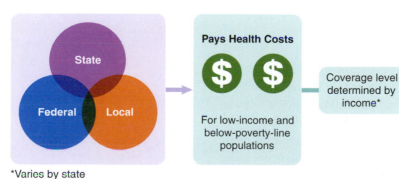

FIGURE 4-6 Medicaid.

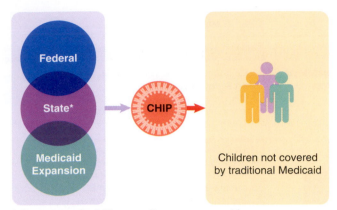

* States have flexibility regarding coverage and fees

FIGURE 4-7 The Children's Health Insurance Program (CHIP).

Retired Military

In 1966, the Civilian Health and Medical Program of the Uniformed Services (CHAMPUS) was established and administered by the Department of Defense to provide military families with health-care benefits. Active military personnel and their family members can be treated by military hospitals, but retirement can create some issues for these individuals. Some did not live close to a military base, or the wait for treatment was too long. Therefore, CHAMPUS was established to provide these families with alternatives to health-care services. In the 1990s the program was revamped, including the name, which is now TRICARE. To increase effectiveness and reduce costs, managed care was introduced to the existing plan.[6]

Workers' Compensation

Workers' compensation is an insurance-type plan that protects workers who suffer work-related illness or injury. Employers pay the premium based on the number of workers and the type of work done. The more dangerous the work setting, the higher the premiums; however, this premium allows employees to receive health-care services for events occurring on the job. Each state mandates its own legislation and policies regarding workers' compensation.

Uninsured

Even with all the various types of funding sources described in this chapter, many Americans still do not have health insurance or benefits of any kind. According to the U.S. Census Bureau, 48.6 million Americans did not have health coverage in 2011, almost 16% of the total population.[7] Part of the problem is that although costs of living continue to increase, incomes are not keeping up. Individuals have to make cuts, and, unfortunately, some of those cuts are in health insurance.

The Nation's Health Dollar

Revenues

Health-care financing is more complicated than ever. Various avenues support the health-care system by providing revenue. Each entity, whether private or public, does not systematically fund itself with equal dollars. In other words, some programs use more revenue than services produced, whereas other programs do the opposite. Funding appropriations are determined by population needs, not the generation of income. In 2011, the majority of the income (73%) was generated by health insurance. The breakdown of the health insurance category includes private health insurance, Medicare, Medicaid, and other programs such as the Veterans' Administration (VA). The remainder (27%) comes from investments, public health activities, out-of-pocket costs, and other third-party payers and programs (Fig. 4-8).[8]

Expenditures

As with revenue, various systems account for the expenditures of the health-care dollar. In 2011, the bulk of the health-care dollar expenditures were under the umbrella of personal health care. Within this category, two subcategories exist: hospital care and professional services. Professional services is further subdivided by distinct types of services, such as physician and dental services. The next largest single category of expenditures is prescription drugs, which are under the umbrella of retail outlet sales of medical products. Other types of expenditures are further delineated by specific categories (Fig. 4-9).[8]

Provider Billing

Health-care providers have different systems in place for billing. Regardless of the system used, the provider bills for services based on the type of service provided and/or the time spent with the patient. If the patient is being seen for an

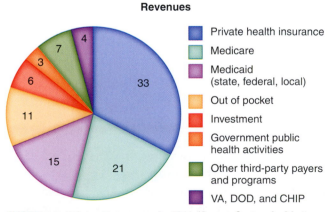

FIGURE 4-8 U.S. health revenues for 2011. (Source: Centers for Medicare & Medicaid Services, Office of the Actuary, National Health Statistics Group)

Health-Care Expenditures

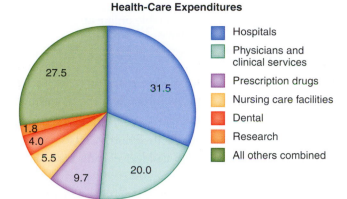

- Hospitals
- Physicians and clinical services
- Prescription drugs
- Nursing care facilities
- Dental
- Research
- All others combined

27.5 · 31.5 · 1.8 · 4.0 · 5.5 · 9.7 · 20.0

FIGURE 4-9 U.S. health expenditures for 2011. (Source: Centers for Medicare & Medicaid Services, Office of the Actuary, National Health Statistics Group)

annual physical, the billable time is usually higher because the physician is examining or inquiring about all body systems. On the other hand, a visit for a sore throat or cold will require less contact time and generally will be charged less. Once the type of visit and service have been determined, the billing coder will use a specific diagnosis code that describes the visit and procedures performed to receive reimbursement.

Health-care providers, regardless of the type, generally bill two main entities: health insurance or private pay. As discussed earlier, health insurance can encompass Medicare, Medicaid, or private insurance carriers. The other way a provider may bill for services is to uninsured individuals. Depending on income, the uninsured individual will either receive a charge for the full amount, possibly discounted if paid in advance; or, if eligible, the individual may qualify for a sliding fee amount. The sliding fee scale is based on the federal poverty level for the number of people living in the household and family annual income. If the person qualifies for the sliding fee, the fee may be reduced as much as 80% of the original charge, or the individual may pay a small co-pay. The sliding fee scale is primarily used by community health centers and public health departments where federal dollars help to offset the loss in revenue. Individuals who have Medicare are responsible for paying a deductible, if not already met, and 20% of the approved Medicare charges (unless they have a supplemental policy that pays the 20%). Medicaid recipients generally are not charged for the service or are charged a small co-pay. As mentioned earlier, private insurance companies require an annual deductible to be met, and then the insured usually pays between 10% and 30% of the allowable charges. There is a difference between charges and allowable charges. Many insurance companies and hospitals or large physician offices have already contracted a specific dollar amount that will be allowed for services. The insurance company has agreed to pay that amount, and the physician/hospital has agreed to provide the service for the designated fee.

SUMMARY

Various mechanisms are available for paying for health-care services. Age, income, health conditions, employment, and other variables help determine the way Americans pay for health care. Regardless of the choices, many Americans are still uninsured because of the high cost of health insurance. The Affordable Care Act of 2013 was implemented to help meet the needs of these uninsured individuals.

Review Questions

1. Managed care first started as a means to control health-care costs in the:
   A. 1970s
   B. 1980s
   C. 1990s
   D. 2000s

2. This type of covered is paid by employers for their employees' benefit should an on-the-job accident or certain health conditions occur:
   A. Medigap
   B. Workers' compensation
   C. Medicaid
   D. Managed care

3. The largest source of health-care expenditures occurs for:
   A. Nursing care costs
   B. Pharmaceutical costs
   C. Administrative costs
   D. Hospital costs

4. This type of coverage covers individuals who are 65 years old, are disabled, or have ESRD.
   A. Medicaid
   B. Ryan White Program
   C. Medicare
   D. Blue Cross Blue Shield

5. According to the U.S. Census Bureau, in 2011, approximately _____% of the population was uninsured.
   A. 16
   B. 21
   C. 25
   D. 29

6. The first major employer-sponsored insurance plan was started by:
   A. State Farm
   B. Blue Cross Blue Shield
   C. Progressive
   D. Prudential

7. Before any type of government-sponsored, employer-sponsored, or private insurance, physicians had to depend on the patient paying cash for services, or they used the _____ system.

    A. IOU

    B. No pay, no services

    C. Barter

    D. Free treatment

8. The Ryan White Program provides assistance to uninsured or underinsured individuals who have:

    A. AIDS

    B. COPD

    C. CVA

    D. Diabetes

9. Insurance typically covers approximately _____ of the medical bills after a deductible has been met.

    A. 40% to 50%

    B. 50% to 60%

    C. 60% to 80%

    D. 70% to 80%

10. The need to establish insurance was brought on by the:

    A. Great Depression

    B. War on Poverty

    C. World War II

    D. increased number of baby boomers

Glossary of Key Terms

Employer-sponsored insurance—insurance coverage for employees and their family members that is deducted from employees' pay; is cheaper than private insurance and usually offers greater flexibility with types of coverage

Private-pay insurance—type of insurance individuals buy when they are either unemployed or their employer does not provide coverage; typically has higher premiums and lower benefits than employer-sponsored insurance

Managed care—health-care delivery systems that manage costs and utilization of services; types include health maintenance organizations (HMOs), provider-sponsored organizations (PSOs), and preferred-provider organizations (PPOs)

Medigap—type of private insurance that supplements Medicare benefits

Children's Health Insurance Program (CHIP)—a type of insurance coverage that provides benefits to children living in families who cannot afford to buy insurance but whose income is too high for Medicaid

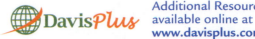

Additional Resources are available online at **www.davisplus.com**

Additional Resources

Centers for Medicare and Medicaid Services—www.cms.gov
This website provides information regarding benefits and eligibility for Medicare and Medicaid.

Children's Health Insurance Program (CHIP)—www.healthcare.gov/medicaid-chip/childrens-health-insurance-program
This website provides information regarding benefits and eligibility for the Children's Health Insurance Program (CHIP).

National Health Expenditure Data—www.cms.gov/Research-Statistics-Data-and-Systems/Statistics-Trends-and-Reports/NationalHealthExpendData/index.html
This Centers for Medicare and Medicaid Services website provides data about national health expenditures, organized by topic and dates.

Healthinsurance.org—www.healthinsurance.org/glossary
This website provides definitions for many words associated with insurance coverage and benefits.

Health Resources and Services Administration, HIV/AIDS Bureau—www.hab.hrsa.gov
This website provides information about the Ryan White Program, including benefits and information about HIV/AIDS.

References

1. Kovner A, Knickman J, eds. *Health Care Delivery in the United States.* New York: Springer Publishing; 2008.

2. U.S. Centers for Medicare and Medicaid, Medicare Program. General information.

    http://www.cms.gov/Medicare/Medicare.html.
    Accessed August 27, 2013.

3. U.S. Centers for Medicare and Medicaid, Medicaid, Children's Health Insurance Program.

    http://www.medicaid.gov/Medicaid-CHIP-Program-Information/Medicaid-and-CHIP-Program-Information.html.
    Accessed August 27, 2013.

4. U.S. Department of Health and Human Services, Health Resources and Services Administration, Health AIDS Bureau.

    http://www.hab.hrsa.gov.
    Accessed August 27, 2013.

5. U.S. Department of Health and Human Services, Indian Health Service, The Federal Health Program for American Indians and Alaska Natives.

   http://www.ihs.gov/aboutihs/indianhealthmanual.
   Accessed August 29, 2013.

6. U.S. Department of Defense, Military Health Systems, TRICARE Management Activity.

   http://www.tricare.mil.
   Accessed August 29, 2013.

7. U.S. Census Bureau, Housing and Household Economic Statistics, Health Insurance.

   http://www.census.gov/hhes/www/hlthins/data/incpovhlth/2011/highlights.html.
   Accessed August 27, 2013.

8. U.S. Centers for Medicare and Medicaid Services, Office of the Actuary, National Health Statistics Group.

   http://www.cms.gov/Research-Statistics-Data-and-Systems/Statistics-Trends-and-Reports/National-HealthExpendData/Downloads/Proj2011PDF.pdf.
   Accessed August 27, 2013.

The Divisions of Health Care

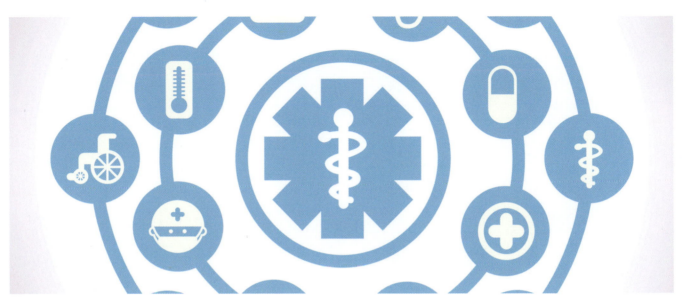

Photo credit: peterspiro/istock/images/Thinkstock

Chapter 5
Introduction to the Primary Health-Care Professions

Chapter 6
History of Allied Health Professions

Chapter 7
Interprofessional Approach to Patient Care

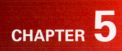

Introduction to the Primary Health-Care Professions

Patricia Royal, EdD

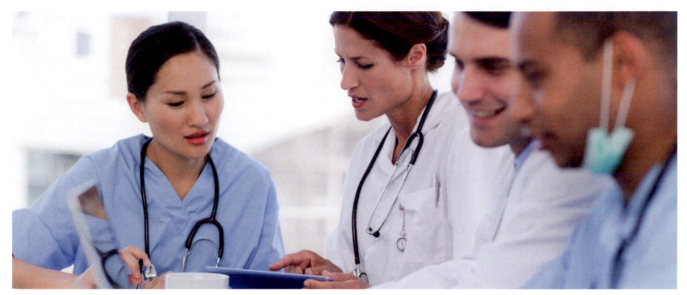

Photo credit: Wavebreak Media, LTD/Thinkstock

Learning Objectives

After reading this chapter, students should be able to:

- Explain the term *primary health-care professions*
- State the difference between primary health-care professions and other types of health-care providers
- Discuss the early significance of the primary health-care professions
- Relate the historical perspective of primary health-care professions to today's perspective
- Discuss opportunities and challenges in working in a primary health-care role

Key Terms

- Primary health-care profession
- Family medicine
- Internal medicine
- General pediatrics
- Obstetrics and gynecology
- Hippocrates
- Florence Nightingale
- Pharmaceutical
- Apothecary
- Multidisciplinary

Origin of the Primary Health-Care Professions

The definition of **primary health-care profession** can be viewed through many perspectives, including those dating back to the Hippocratic Oath (an oath taken by physicians promising to be honest in the practice of medicine) in the 5th century BC, at least in part, because it mentions medicine and pharmacology (Fig. 5-1). The more modern definition of *primary health-care profession* dates back to 1961, when the term identified those providing the care; the activities associated with the care; the level of care; and later, in 1978, the set of attributes related to the care.[1] The group of individuals originally identified as primary-care professionals

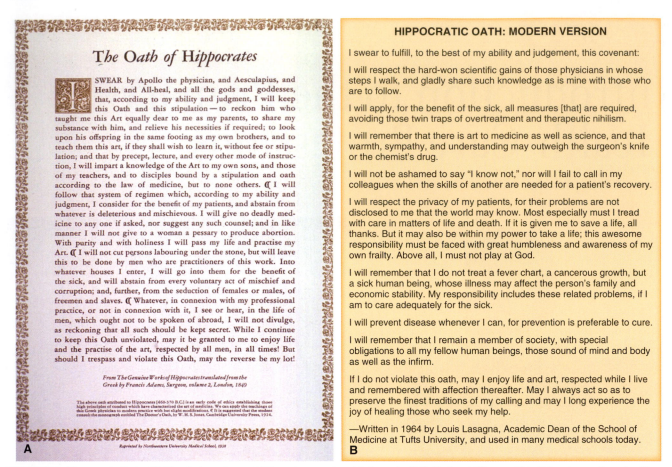

FIGURE 5-1 Hippocratic Oath. **(A)** Classical version and **(B)** modern version. (*A*, From the U.S. National Library of Medicine, Image from the History of Medicine Collection. Title: Medical Ethics, the Oath of Hippocrates.)

were physicians, pharmacists, and nurses. The physicians included **family medicine, internal medicine, general pediatrics,** and **obstetrics and gynecology.** Since then, some authorities have included physician assistants (PAs) in the group and have also made updates to include family nurse practitioners. The disciplines of medicine, nursing, and pharmacy are addressed in depth later in the book; the next section of this chapter provides a brief history of the three original health-care disciplines.

Distinction Between Primary Health-Care Profession and Primary-Care Provider

The terms *primary-care profession* and *primary-care provider* are not synonymous. The term *primary-care provider* refers to the provider acting as the principal point of contact for the patient and providing the diagnosis, treatment(s), and referrals specifically for this patient. The term *primary-care provider* is often used in reference to the patient's need to identify a primary-care physician. This is particularly important now because the Affordable Care Act passed in 2013 specifically requires patients to list a primary-care provider

for reimbursement issues related to health-care insurance, Medicare, and Medicaid. The focus of this chapter is not directed toward the last definition but rather to make the distinction between primary-care professions and allied health professions, which are discussed in the next chapter.

History of Medicine

The history of medicine can generally be dated by periods, or ages, which include the mythological, dogmatical or empirical, rational,[2] and evidence-based eras. Within each of these stages are subsets of periods that describe that time period. For instance, the primitive medicine stage, a subset of the mythological period, uses terminology such as healers, magicians, rulers, shamans, and priests to describe the physician. Treatments include magic, spells, prayers, and charms, as well as such actions as drinking the blood of a warrior to increase strength.[3]

As medicine advanced, so did treatments and their documentation. Egyptian physicians recorded case histories on sheets of papyrus, which helped to identify symptoms and suggested therapies. The physicians were still primarily priests who were assisted by other lay physicians. The treatments were crude in comparison to later years; however, some techniques developed during this time period remain in use today, such as direct compression to stop bleeding.

During the Classical Medicine period (7th century BC–5th century AD), the most famous ancient physician, **Hippocrates,** was born. The Hippocratic Oath, which is still in use today, originated with Hippocrates (see Fig. 5-1). Hippocrates was a Greek physician who influenced not only his own generation, but many generations to come. The rule of thought during this time period was the belief in imbalances among blood, phlegm, black bile, and yellow bile; their associated states, including hot, cold, moist, and dry; and the four elements of earth, air, fire, and water. When patients were sick, it was believed to be because of an imbalance in these conditions that had to be corrected to get the body back in harmony.[3]

During the Middle Ages (5th–14th centuries AD), a distinct separation between medicine and surgery began to emerge. Physicians focused on problems and conditions inside the body, and surgeons treated conditions such as fractures, dislocations, and amputations. During this period, it was recognized that medicine needed to become a more formal vocation based on an education of standardized courses and legal parameters. Some areas required the physician to pass a written examination to practice medicine.[3]

During the Renaissance period (15th–16th centuries AD), medicine became more scientific and research in the field of human anatomy became prominent. Anatomical illustrations were published and used for educating physicians and further development of the profession. In addition to advancement of medicine and education, a focus on the pain and suffering patients endured emerged. During this time, some progress was made on understanding the spread of infectious diseases.[3]

In the 17th and 18th centuries, the rational age surfaced. Although still somewhat primitive compared with the 21st century, this period of time was a turning point for medicine. Many important discoveries were made; the microscope was used to examine red blood cells and bacteria; and vaccinations were invented. Environmental issues and conditions were examined in addition to the patient's signs and symptoms. However, some of the older treatment procedures continued to be used, such as bloodletting, which was used until the end of the 19th century.[4] Some researchers refer to this time period as the *early evidence-based period.* There was a push for improvement in medical record-keeping, which could be used for research, teaching, and sharing information in journals. Professional societies began to appear, which strengthened the profession by allowing sharing of best practices. During this time period, it was expected that most, if not all, physicians would have to complete the required education to perform the duties of a physician.[3]

During the 19th and 20th centuries, radical improvements in medicine occurred. Anesthesia methods were developed to reduce or eliminate pain during surgery. The art of disinfecting surgical equipment began and prevented many infections from occurring during surgery. Antibiotics such as

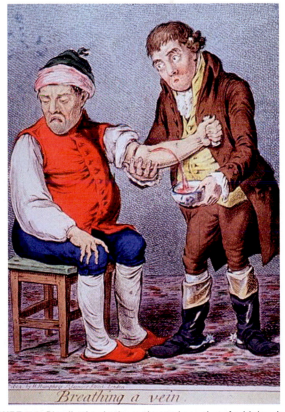

FIGURE 5-3 Bloodletting is the antiquated practice of withdrawing or leaking blood from the body to prevent or cure illness or disease. With origins dating back to ancient Egyptian and Greek cultures, bloodletting was believed to cure illness by rebalancing the "humors" of the body, that is, blood and other bodily fluids. (From the U.S. National Library of Medicine, History of Medicine Division. *Breathing a Vein,* J. Gilray, artist [1756–1815].)

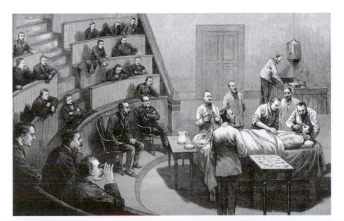

FIGURE 5-2 Surgery in the 18th century (source unknown).

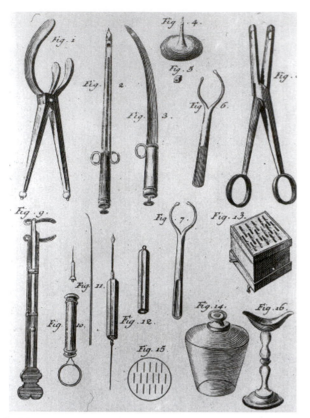

FIGURE 5-4 Bloodletting instruments. (From the U.S. National Library of Medicine, Images from the History of Medicine Collection.)

penicillin and streptomycin were developed and became routine use for many physicians. Because physicians could not possibly have advanced knowledge on all conditions and parts of the bodies, specialization became the standard for those seeking additional knowledge in a specific area.[3]

Toward the end of the 20th century, we entered the latest phase or stage of medicine, the modern evidence-based era. Evidence-based medicine uses clinical expertise and the best available outside evidence, such as clinical trials, when making decisions on a patient's plan of care. This time period focuses more on the patient and the clinical research necessary to find the best treatments for the specific patient. Patients are now advocates for their care, and the physician invites their response toward specific interventions and treatments. Other factors in the evidence-based era include random clinical trials, efficiency and effectiveness in medicine, new types of training for physicians, advanced technology in equipment and computers, and improved database software.[4]

Although the practice of medicine has been around since the beginning of time, the term *physician* was not coined until around the 13th century; however, the helping role started centuries before the official recognition of the practice. Other aspects of the history of medicine are discussed in Chapter 8. Next we examine another role that has roots in ancient times.

History of Nursing

Many people associate nursing with **Florence Nightingale,** who was a well-educated daughter of British parents. Nightingale challenged social conventions by becoming a nurse, an unrespectable profession for a well-bred woman. Nursing strangers was not appropriate behavior for someone of Nightingale's social class.[5] She tested societal limits further by leading a crusade to Crimea in1854, to provide services to British soldiers. Under Nightingale's regime, she and a small group of nurses improved the military hospital environment by using sanitation methods, preparing nutritious meals, and providing medications and treatments. Within weeks of her nursing the soldiers, infectious diseases were reduced and the death rate dropped significantly.[5]

Although not recognized as a profession, nursing, like medicine, had its early roots in the prehistoric period. Some of the earlier forms of nursing began when women acted as wet nurses for babies whose mothers were either unable to nurse or had died during childbirth.[6] Other times, wealthier women who chose not to nurse their children hired wet nurses. For centuries, nursing care was provided by religious organizations where women assumed roles of providing comfort to the sick in addition to caring for their own families.[7]

During the 16th and 17th centuries, charities were established and poorhouses were created for individuals unable to work due to disabilities or old age. During this time, the need for nursing services began to soar. Part of the reason for the increased need was due to the many epidemics, such as cholera and typhus. Before this time, nurses had typically been women; however, during the time of great epidemics, men took an active role in providing nursing services.[8]

The 18th and 19th centuries were truly turning points for nurses. In 1798, a New York physician, Valentine Seaman, planned lectures for nurses caring for maternity patients. In 1836, the Nursing Society of Philadelphia (NSP) was formed, and in 1850, schools operated by the NSP were opened for nurses. During this same time period, the British Crimean War and the American Civil War made a huge impact on the nursing profession. Both wars were significant, but for different reasons. For the Crimean War, Florence Nightingale made history by her dedication to the British military and the succession of nurse education programs in British hospitals that focused on a core set of principles to improve patient care. The Civil War made a significant impact in the United States due to the demand for nurses to assist with the sick and wounded. Approximately 20,000 nurses, both male and female, provided services for both the Northern and Southern armies. The recognition of the growing need for trained nurses helped to create training programs in larger U.S. hospitals. These training programs were forerunners to organized professional nursing education in the United States.[5]

In the 20th century, professional nursing roles became more diverse as nurses were able to select from various career choices, such as visiting nurses, private-duty nurses, public health nurses, home-care nurses, and, of course, hospital nurses. Professional nursing associations were created to set standards that would provide a distinction between professionally trained nurses and untrained ones. Additionally, the education for nurses changed during this time with the advancement of graduate education, which created another option for nurses—teaching. With the advancement in education, nurses were now able to pursue roles in management and clinical practice.[8] Additional information on the history of nursing is presented in Chapter 9.

History of Pharmacy

As with medicine and nursing, pharmacy began thousands of years ago but was not recognized as a profession requiring formal education and training for many centuries.[9] Some have argued that pharmacy itself is not a distinct discipline but rather an offshoot of medicine,[10] because physicians determined patients' need for and type of medicine (Fig. 5-7).

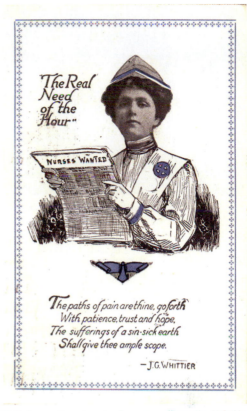

FIGURE 5-6 A recruitment poster for nurses. (From the U.S. National Library of Medicine, Images from the History of Medicine Collection. Contributed by Michael Zwerdling and the Chicago School of Nursing. Title: *The Real Need of the Hour.*)

Early historical evidence places pharmacy back to the prehistoric time period when pharmacists, also known as magicians or healers, used various potions to treat many types of conditions. Although many of them were ineffective, some were beneficial in treating diseases and conditions. Some of the recipes for them survived by being passed down through generations and are in use today. These medicines, which include morphine, quinine, ephedrine, and digitalis, are still prescribed for treatments in the 21st century but originated in the early ages of civilization.[3]

The early Egyptian pharmacists dispensed pills, ointments, and inhalants that they compounded using various herbs or potions. These pharmacists had over 800 standardized prescriptions created using mortars, mills, and sieves. It is even hypothesized that the modern-day pharmacy symbol, Rx, originated in Egypt. The symbol, known as the Egyptian Eye of Horus, was part of an illustration inscribed on the tombs of the Chihuahua Pharaohs (Fig. 5-8).[3]

Pharmacists played a huge role in Arabic medicine. As early as the 10th century, the Arabs had hospitals that housed a pharmacy in a separate room where not only compounding of medicines, but also training, took place. Arabic pharmacists used spices that we typically consider for cooking;

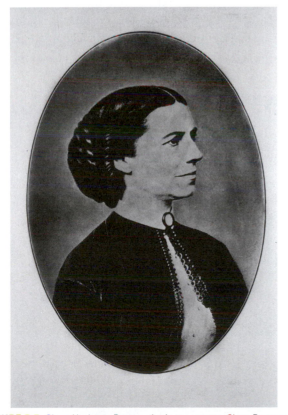

FIGURE 5-5 Clara Harlowe Barton. A pioneer nurse, Clara Barton also founded the American Red Cross in 1881. (From the U.S. National Library of Medicine, History of Medicine Division.)

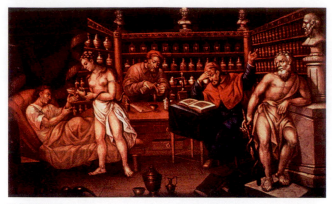

FIGURE 5-7 *Pharmacy and medicine working together. In this painting, the physician consults his medical text while the pharmacist prepares a prescription. The patient is attended by Hygeia (the patron goddess of pharmacy). Asklepios, the god of medicine, leaning against a bust of Hippocrates, observes. (From the U.S. National Library of Medicine, Images from the History of Medicine Collection. Title:* The Medical Triad of Physician-Patient-Pharmacist.)

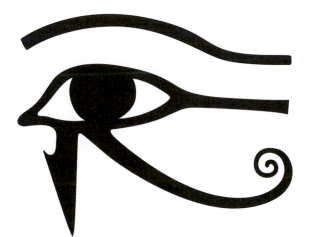

FIGURE 5-8 Egyptian Eye of Horus.

however, these spices (nutmeg, cloves, and mace) were part of the treatments for various conditions. Some of these spices are still considered to have a medicinal effect and are used today. The Arabic pharmacists were rather advanced for their time. In addition to these successful remedies, some of our modern terminology originated in the Arabic countries. These medicinal terms, such as *syrup, alcohol, drug,* and *alkali,* survived through the centuries to remain a part of the vocabulary in the Western world. The Arabic pharmacists made such an impact that even the Greek medical texts, translated into Arabic, were supplemented with the sophisticated Arabic **pharmaceutical** materials. The Arabs were so advanced that in the 10th century, they began requiring both doctors and pharmacists to pass formal tests before practicing on their own. The impact the Arabs made did not go unnoticed by other countries. During the Renaissance period, Europeans studied the Arabic pharmaceutical practices and

improved on their techniques to create a more modern practice of compounding drugs.[3]

In the early stages of pharmacy practice, those desiring to fill the role of an **apothecary** had to apprentice and study under a practicing apothecary. The student worked side-by-side with the master apothecary and observed the activities related to medication compounding. Some apprenticeships lasted for years, and often the apprentice lived in the mentor's home.[11] As the profession advanced the roles and responsibilities also changed. There was a shift from the role of compounding drugs to administering them, which meant the pharmacist would interact directly with patients rather than just providing the drugs to the doctors. The formal education process began in the 19th century when physicians started training pharmacists in an academic environment. However, there was some negative reaction to physicians training pharmacists, so within a few years, pharmacy programs were established in which pharmacists trained other pharmacists. During the 20th century, pharmacists were required to pass a licensure examination, which could only occur after a specific time spent under a practicing pharmacist. For many U.S. states, the graduating pharmacist was required to complete an internship even after passing the licensing examination.[11]

By the mid-1930s, many pharmacy schools had been established and many students were being educated in the profession. The family-owned "Mom and Pop" drugstores were part of the American culture. The drugstore filled the prescriptions, compounded as needed, and even offered a

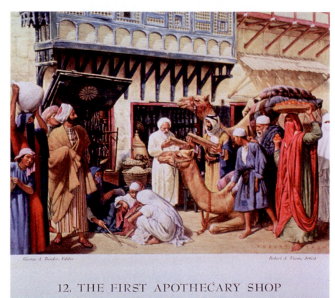

FIGURE 5-9 The first apothecary shop (about 754 AD). (From the U.S. National Library of Medicine, Images from the History of Medicine Collection. Contributed by Robert A. Thom, artist; George A. Bender, editor; and Parke, Davis and Company, publisher.)

soda fountain; however, the soda fountain was used for more than selling soda pop. The pharmacist was able to use the carbonated beverages and the flavored syrups as ingredients in some of the compounds, such as Coca-Cola, which was used for medicinal purposes.[12] The shift from compounding to administering continued, and soon there were pharmaceutical companies manufacturing ready-made drugs in various dosages. This technique was guided by clinical and laboratory science[12] and soon had government influence as the Food and Drug Administration (FDA) became an active member in the development of pharmaceuticals by ensuring the safety of certain drugs. The role of the pharmacist has changed throughout the last few centuries, but the purpose and original intent have remained constant. Additional aspects of the history of pharmacy are discussed in Chapter 10.

Bridging the Gap

The disciplines of medicine, nursing, and pharmacy date back thousands of years. These disciplines were originally responsible for providing the population's health-care needs. As the population increased and specialized needs were recognized, the shift from the three primary health-care professions to multiple disciplines occurred. Other factors that helped to fuel the drive for **multidisciplinary** care and medical specialties included access to care, health-care delivery, population health, environment health issues, mental health needs, educational resources, chronic diseases, and diverse populations. Of course, this transition did not occur overnight. It was centuries in the making. The drive to educate and train more health-care providers was met with challenges such as wars, epidemics, financial woes, and natural disasters that created even more challenges in having sufficient numbers of health-care providers to meet the population's demands.

SUMMARY

Fortunately, in today's health-care society, we have more providers, specialized medicine, and allied health disciplines, as well as technicians, who all join forces to provide holistic approaches to ensure quality care for patients. However, we still face many of the same issues that were recognized centuries ago, such as access to care, provider shortages, and delivery of health-care services. As noted in previous chapters, the aging baby boomers and increased life expectancy have created a thriving market for those who wish to work in a health-care environment. In the next chapter, we look at one of the fastest-growing trends in employment today—allied health sciences.

Review Questions

1. Hippocrates was a famous _____ during the Classical period.
   A. Nurse
   B. Pharmacist
   C. Physician
   D. Scientist

2. During the _____ period, medicine became more scientific and research was more prominent.
   A. Early Ages
   B. Renaissance
   C. Middle Ages
   D. Classical

3. During which war did Florence Nightingale support the troops by providing nursing skills?
   A. Revolutionary
   B. Civil
   C. Spanish American
   D. Crimean

4. The drug _____ was developed during the prehistoric period.
   A. Morphine
   B. Penicillin
   C. Biaxin
   D. Tylenol

5. Before the term *pharmacist* became popular, the word _____ was used to represent someone compounding medicines.
   A. Magic Man
   B. Snake Charmer
   C. Drug Maker
   D. Apothecary

6. The primitive medicine stage is a subset of the:
   A. Rational period
   B. Prehistoric period
   C. Mythological period
   D. Dogmatic period

7. Disinfecting surgical equipment became popular during the _____ centuries.
   A. 13th–14th
   B. 15th–16th
   C. 17th–18th
   D. 19th–20th

8. The term *wet nurse* refers to a nurse who:

   A. Gives baths

   B. Changes diapers

   C. Washes clothes

   D. Nurses babies

9. It is thought that the symbol for pharmacy (Rx) originated in:

   A. Israel

   B. Greece

   C. Egypt

   D. America

10. The term *primary health-care profession* refers to which of the following?

    A. Allied health science disciplines

    B. All nurses

    C. Dentists, physicians, and optometrists

    D. Physicians, nurses, and pharmacists

Glossary of Key Terms

Primary health-care profession—in this text, refers to individuals practicing in the fields of medicine, nursing, and pharmacy; physician assistants are often included as well

Family medicine—refers to physicians practicing comprehensive health care for all patients and age groups

Internal medicine—refers to physicians practicing adult comprehensive care

General pediatrics—refers to physicians who provide comprehensive health care to children (typically 0–21 years of age)

Obstetrics and gynecology—refers to specialty physicians who treat in the area of female reproductive organs in pregnant and nonpregnant patients

Hippocrates—an ancient Greek physician who is referred to as the "father of Western medicine" and is the namesake for the Hippocratic Oath that a physician pledges

Florence Nightingale—a British social reformist who is considered the founder of modern nursing

Pharmaceutical—the manufacturing of ready-made medicines for resale by pharmacies

Apothecary—the early name for one who dispenses drugs

Multidisciplinary—refers to more than one discipline in the plan of patient care

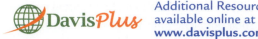

Additional Resources are available online at www.davisplus.com

Additional Resources

American Nurses Association (ANA)—www.nursingworld.org/FunctionalMenuCategories/AboutANA

American Nurses Foundation (ANF)—www.anfonline.org

American Medical Association (AMA)—www.ama-assn.org/ama

National Medical Association (NMA)—www.nmanet.org

American Pharmacists Association (APA)—www.pharmacist.com

National Community Pharmacists Association (NCPA)—www.ncpanet.org

References

1. Donaldson M, Yordy K, Lohr K, Vansclow N, eds. *Primary Care: America's Health in a New Era.* Institute of Medicine, Washington, DC: National Academy Press; 1996.

2. McWharf JM. The early history of medicine. *Trans Kans Acad Sci* 1918;29:46–49.

3. Oracle Think Quest Educational Foundation. http://www.thinkquest.org.
   Accessed September 23, 2013.

4. Claridge J, Fabian T. History and development of evidence-based medicine. *World J Surg* 2005;29:547–553.

5. Whelan J. *Nursing History and Health Care. American Nursing: An Introduction to the Past.* Penn Nursing Science, School of Nursing, University of Pennsylvania. http://www.nursing.upenn.edu/nhhc/Pages/AmericanNursingIntroduction.aspx.
   Accessed October 8, 2013.

6. National Women's History Museum (NWHM). *The Evolution of Nursing.* 2010. http://www.nwhm.org/blog/the-evolution-of-nursing.
   Accessed October 8, 2013.

7. Craven RF, Hirle CJ. *Fundamentals of Nursing: Human Health and Function,* 6th ed. Philadelphia, PA: Lippincott Williams & Wilkins; 2009.

8. Buhter-Wilkerson K, D'Antonio P. History of nursing. Britannica Academic Edition. http://www.britannica.com.
   Accessed October 8, 2013.

9. Anderson S, ed. *Making Medicines: A Brief History of Pharmacy and Pharmaceuticals.* Grayslake, IL: Pharmaceutical Press; 2005.

10. Watkins ES. From history or pharmacy to pharmaceutical history. *Pharm Hist* 2009;51(1):3–13.

11. Fink J. Pharmacy: A brief history of the profession. The Student Doctor Network Coastal Research Group. http://studentdoctor.net/2012/pharmacy-a-brief-history-of-the-profession.
   Accessed October 9, 2013.

12. Smith M. Pharmacy and radio: 1930–1960. *Pharm Hist* 1990;32(1):22–25.

CHAPTER 6

History of Allied Health Professions

Patricia Royal, EdD

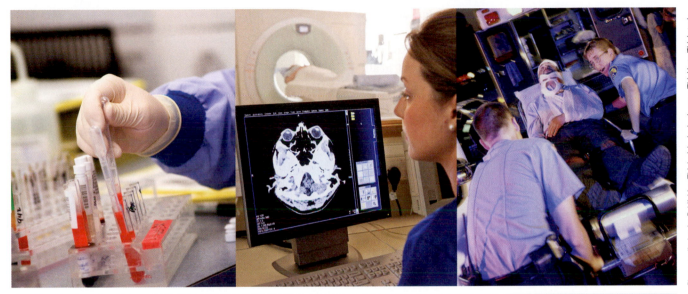

Photo credit: Ingrim Publishing/Thinkstick, Jupiterimages/Thinkbyte/Thinkstock, Purestock/Thinkstock

Learning Objectives

After reading this chapter, students should be able to:

- Define the term *allied health professions*
- Identify some of the workers classified as allied health professionals
- Discuss the importance of the evolution of allied health
- Discuss the labor trends for allied health professionals
- Identify the opportunities and challenges in working in allied health careers

Key Terms

- Allied health professions
- Osteopathy
- Podiatry
- Midlevel
- Radiographer
- EEG technician
- Histologic technician
- Cytotechnologist

Definition of Allied Health Professions

There are many different definitions to describe **allied health professions.** Some of the most commonly used refer to allied health professions as a cluster of health-care practitioners who work either directly or indirectly with patients and who are trained or credentialed by certifications, registrations, or licensure.[1,2] Allied health professionals practice independently or work in team environments and collaborate with physicians to deliver quality patient care. The American Medical Association (AMA) defines *allied health professions* as individuals assisting, facilitating, and complementing physicians and other specialists. Rather than defining allied health professions, in 1992 the Pew Advisory Panel for Allied Health defined what it is *not*—it is not medicine, nursing, **osteopathy,** dentistry, veterinary medicine, optometry, pharmacy, and **podiatry.** The Pew Advisory Panel agreed that allied health professions were **midlevel** workers who support, complement, or supplement practitioners. Regardless of definition, the field of allied health professions is diverse and offers many opportunities to work in health care. There are more than 80 different allied health professions, such as occupational and physical therapy, dietetics, dental hygiene, and health administration, to mention a few. In 2009, allied health professionals represented 60% of all health-care providers and the employment outlook indicates high growth over the next several decades.[1]

This book examines some of the allied health-care disciplines in depth by providing complete chapters dedicated to specific professions. Other allied health-care disciplines are covered to a lesser degree at the end of the text. With as many as 200 professions qualifying as allied health careers, it is not possible to include an examination of each one of them. Box 6-1 lists some professions *not* covered in this text.

Origin of Allied Health Professions

The allied health professions began before the 19th century as the Shattuck Report of 1850 established a structure for defining health workers. Before Shattuck's investigation and research into the relationship between hygiene and diseases in the United States, the focus on prevention, sanitary conditions, and public health was practically nonexistent.[3] Shattuck's framework was developed to provide parameters for organized medical education that included occupational, preventive, and public health, as well as medical health. The health-care industry was growing and more students were being trained; however, the training lacked a standard for higher admission and graduation. Abraham Flexner, noting the lack of standardization, proposed that medical schools adopt a detailed protocol to provide consistency in medical education. In 1910, the formal education was outlined in the Flexner Report and this model became the standard for providing medical education.[3] In the 1930s, the AMA, through its Council on Medical

Box 6-1 Allied Health Sciences Professions Not Identified in Textbook
Anesthesiologist assistant
Art therapist
Dance/movement therapist
Diagnostic medical sonographer
Electroneurodiagnostic technologist
Genetic counselor
Histotechnologist
Kinesiotherapist
Magnetic resonance technologist
Medical dosimetrist
Medical librarian
Medical transcriptionist
Music therapist
Nerve conduction studies technologist
Nuclear medicine technologist
Nurse aide instructor
Orthoptist
Orthotist and prosthetist
Paraoptometrician
Poetry therapist
Polysomnographic technologist
Surgical neurophysiologist
Veterinary medical technologist

Education, began an instrumental role in helping to establish accreditation for programs in occupational therapy, physical therapy, and clinical pathology. Other programs, such as health information administrator and **radiographer** programs, began the same accreditation process through the AMA in the mid 1940s as the previously mentioned professions. These professions were referred to as *paramedical education* by their accrediting organization.[4]

The initial call for more paramedical workers was made in 1952 by President Truman. The Commission on the Health Needs of the Nation recognized the need for more paramedical workers who possessed special skills needed for investigation, treatment, and prevention of disease and disability. For the next 15 years, there was tremendous growth in the number of new programs and schools for these professions, referred to as *ancillary and paramedical* workers. The growth was spurred when Congress enacted the *Allied Health Professions Personnel Training Act of 1967,* which was established to boost opportunities for training in the fields of medical technology and other allied health professions, as well as to improve the quality of education.[5,6] By 1970, a new name had emerged as the AMA House of Delegates defined *allied health professionals* as health-care workers who were able to apply independent decisions within their scope of

allied health professional One who has received professional training and credentials in an allied health field, such as clinical laboratory science, radiology, emergency medical services, physical therapy, respiratory therapy, medical assisting, athletic training, dental hygiene, or occupational therapy.

FIGURE 6-1 Allied health professionals represent a diverse and widespread population in health care.

competence, but allowing for a medical staff to have absolute accountability for patient care.[4]

Over the past century, many things have changed in allied health professions, including definitions, names, and the emergence of new specialties.[4] It is expected that many other specialties will surface as patient needs and advances in technology change. Similar to medicine, allied health will face new challenges and opportunities as the needs of an aging population dictate changes in health-care environments.

Educational Requirements

Depending on the degree or field, the allied health educational requirements vary greatly. In addition to the educational requirements, licensure and certifications differ, especially depending on state requirements. Some programs allow for on-the-job training, others require less than 1 year of education, and still others require graduate degrees. Many technology-related roles require only 1 year of training, whereas therapy-related roles typically require 4 years or more depending on the specific knowledge area and scope of practice. Following are some typical educational expectations for roles in allied health fields[7]:

- **EEG technician**—1 year
- **Histologic technician**—2 years
- Radiologist—2 years
- **Cytotechnologist**—3 years
- Occupational therapist—postgraduate
- Physical therapist—postgraduate

Educational Standards and Accreditation

Before allied health professionals became a recognized group, accreditation and educational standards were important issues for individual fields. With the help of the AMA, some programs were able to obtain accreditation that standardized curriculums. Before the establishment of an allied health accreditation organization, the AMA worked with 50 national committees and 22 review committees in preparation for accrediting 3,000 educational programs. In 1994, the Committees on Allied Health Education and Accreditation began accrediting allied health programs. The name was later changed to Commission on Accreditation of Allied Health Education Programs (CAAHEP) and it is currently the largest accreditor of programs in health-care fields with over 2,000 educational programs.[8] The accreditation process consists of six criteria: (1) evaluation and accreditation of

the programs, (2) reviewing existing educational essentials, (3) maintaining active relationships with the collaborating medical specialties and associations, (4) establishing and maintaining liaisons with technical and professional groups allied to medicine, (5) maintaining an association with institutions supporting accredited programs, and (6) working with the most directly related medical specialty when new allied health occupations are recognized by the AMA.[5]

Many of the allied health programs are accredited by CAAHEP, but many others have their own discipline-specific accreditation. In addition to university or college national accreditation, professional programs need to be competitive by meeting a standardized, nationally recognized curriculum that meets stringent educational requirements. Some of the programs and their date for adoption of educational standards include the following[4]:

- Occupational therapist: 1935
- Radiographer (previously called x-ray technician): 1944
- Rehabilitation counselor: 1971
- Ophthalmic laboratory technician: 1979
- Pharmacy technician: 1982
- Massage therapist: 1991
- Surgical assistant: 2002

Professional Associations and Relationships

Maintaining professional associations and relationships is important for both programs and students. Professional associations provide networking opportunities, conferences, internship potentials, research data, career options, and potential for continuing education credits. Professional associations that allied health programs and professionals may be involved with include the AMA, National Association for Health Professionals, Association of Schools of Allied Health Professions (publisher of *Journal of Allied Health*), and Area Health Education Centers, as well as state and local hospitals, clinics, and training sites. On an individual program level, each allied health program typically maintains some type of relationship with associations specific to that discipline. Students are usually encouraged to become a member in the professional association while still in school because the membership rates are lower for students and they transition to practitioner member after graduation.

Employment Trends

The employment projections for health professions are well above average. The health-care and social assistance category has the highest projections of growth for 2010 to 2020 compared with all categories. The health-care job market is projected to create about 28% of all new jobs in the United States, and the overall growth is expected to be around 33%. The driving factors for growth in health care are related to longer life expectances, an aging population, and advances in new treatments and technologies.[9]

The projected growth is not specific to allied health, but because allied health makes up roughly 60% of all health-care jobs, it can be assumed that the overall growth in allied health jobs will be higher than average. Following are some of the allied health disciplines and their expected percentage of growth within the next 7 years.

- Nutrition: 20%
- Physician assistant: 30%
- Respiratory therapy: 28%
- Dental hygiene: 38%
- Physical therapy: 39%
- Audiology: 37%
- Speech-language pathology: 23%
- Health services manager: 22%
- Medical and clinical laboratory: 13%

With the average growth outlook for all jobs being 14%,[9] health-care workers will have a significant advantage. Individuals training in a health-care role should feel comfortable with the job outlook and the potential for a long-term career.

Salaries and Job Settings

Salaries for allied health workers vary according to the discipline, education, training, credentials, and job settings. Common job settings include the following:

- Hospitals
- Physicians' offices
- Health-care facilities
- Schools
- Home health agencies
- Nursing homes
- Outpatient centers
- Diagnostic laboratories

Disciplines requiring a terminal degree, such as dentistry, usually have higher salaries; individuals working in private practices or clinics may earn more than those working in a state or public health-care facility. Table 6-1 provides a sampling of common allied health jobs with median salaries and male/female demographics.

Opportunities and Challenges

As with most jobs, working in allied health care has both opportunities and challenges. Most health-care jobs are exciting and fast paced, with opportunities to be on the cutting edge of technologies and lifesaving treatments. Being immersed in health care typically requires continuing education and training on new equipment, treatment, techniques, or therapies.

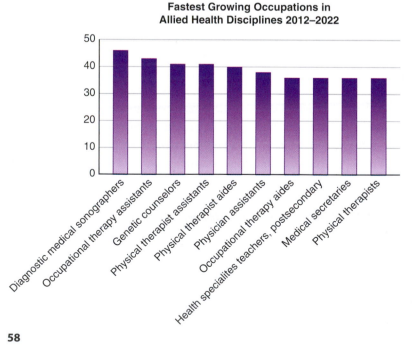

Fastest Growing Occupations in Allied Health Disciplines 2012–2022

FIGURE 6-2 Health-care professions are expected to grow steadily over the next 7 years. The occupations shown here have the fastest projection rates for all allied health fields.(Source: Monthly Labor Review, January 2012, US Bureau of Labor Statistics)

TABLE 6-1 Sampling of Allied Health Fields and Statistics

Discipline	Median Salary ($/yr)	Percent Male	Percent Female
Dentist	149,310	75.8	24.2
Nutritionist	55,240	6.7	93.3
Medical/clinical laboratory technologist	47,820	27.2	72.8
Health information technology	34,160	10.7	89.3
Occupational therapy	74,400	6.0	94.0
Physical therapy	79,860	29.3	70.7
Physician assistant	90,930	30.6	69.4
Respiratory therapy	55,870	39.6	60.4
Social work	44,200	18.4	81.6
Speech-language pathology	69,870	4.4	95.6
Health services management	47,370	27.5	72.5

Note: Salaries vary depending on credentials and job settings.

Source: Bureau of Labor Statistics, 2012.

The opportunities for new learning are higher in health care than in most other fields.

Allied health professions are growing, and with this growth come opportunities for advancement and other avenues such as specializations. As indicated, allied health fields have been around for more than 100 years; however, more than 40 new careers were born in the past 40 years.[4] As specialty areas emerge, careers will also materialize, providing more opportunities for those interested in health care.

Working in allied health can be rewarding because of opportunities for either direct or indirect patient care. Some individuals desire to have patient contact, whereas others prefer to have less direct care. Allied health professions afford individuals the opportunity for both with ample selection of disciplines. Some job choices for individuals seeking direct patient care include audiologist, physical and occupational therapists, physician assistant, and dental hygienist. Roles for individuals who prefer indirect care include nutritionist, social worker, and counselor. For individuals who prefer to work alone or with few coworkers there are some choices that satisfy that criterion. Jobs such as clinical laboratory scientist, blood bank specialist, cytotechnologist, and health information technician provide opportunities for those who prefer more solitude in their daily work activities.

Allied health-care fields can also be very rewarding. Whether you choose direct or indirect patient care, you can be assured of helping people. This internal gratification received from an allied health career often neutralizes the challenges that may come with the job. As mentioned, health-care jobs may be fast paced and demanding. There is often little down time because patients or family members are waiting for diagnosis, treatments, results, or advice in making tough decisions. Like most jobs in health care, allied health workers should have total concentration and good communication skills to interact with patients and family members. Even one misunderstanding can be potentially disastrous, and health-care professionals need to be alert and focused at all times.

Job burnout can occur in any profession; however, in health care it is more likely to occur because of job-related stress. Long hours, lack of resources, sustained concentration, and responsibility for patients' care may all contribute to work-related stress, which in turn may lead to job burnout. Understanding the potential risk for job burnout may increase the awareness of the problem and prevent it from occurring. Generally, many health-care professionals feel that the risk of job burnout and other challenges of working in health care are offset by the rewards and opportunities provided.

SUMMARY

The field of allied health is vast and still growing. Finding a suitable career as an allied health professional has never been easier because of the various opportunities available. In addition to the wide variety of choices, the employment outlook is positive with potential growth rates approaching 40% in the next 10 years. As in any job, challenges are often intense, but the opportunities often outweigh the negatives.

Review Questions

1. Before the term *allied health* was used, the term *supplement workers* was used to describe non-physician individuals working under the supervisor of a physician.

   A. True

   B. False

2. Allied health workers are _____ -level workers supporting, complementing, or supplementing the work of physicians.

   A. Upper

   B. Middle

   C. Lower

   D. None of the above

3. Allied health careers comprise roughly _____% of all health-care jobs.

   A. 30

   B. 35

   C. 50

   D. 60

4. Over the past 40 years, the number of new allied health fields created is roughly_____.

   A. 22

   B. 40

   C. 45

   D. 60

5. Individuals who prefer indirect patient care should select a role such as:

   A. Physician assistant

   B. Physical therapist

   C. Nutritionist

   D. Dental hygienist

6. One of the driving factors for increases in the allied health professions is:

   A. Aging population

   B. Higher salaries

   C. Management roles

   D. All of the above

7. Job burnout is not common in the allied health roles.

   A. True

   B. False

8. Programs in allied health are accredited for the purpose of:

   A. Creating more challenges

   B. Standardizing the curriculum

   C. Meeting the demand of the population

   D. Providing safer roles for professionals

9. The initial call for an increase in paramedical workers occurred during what presidency?

   A. Johnson

   B. Nixon

   C. Eisenhower

   D. Truman

10. The educational requirement for allied health professions varies but generally requires at least:

    A. 3 months of training

    B. 6 months of training

    C. 1 year of college

    D. 2 years of college

Glossary of Key Terms

Allied health professions—a cluster of health-care disciplines that complement and support the work of physicians and other health-care specialists

Osteopathy—alternative health care that stresses the relationship between the structure and function of the body

Podiatry—medical science area devoted to human movement, with the focus being on the foot

Midlevel—health-care professionals who are not medical doctors but have advanced education, training, and certification in their scope of practice; some (e.g., physician assistants and family nurse practitioners) may diagnose, treat, and prescribe medicine (depending on the discipline) while under the supervision of a licensed physician

Radiographer—a person with knowledge and training in the field of x-rays (previously *x-ray technician*)

EEG technician—an electroencephalogram (EEG) technician is a skilled professional trained in the operation of the EEG machine, which monitors the nervous system by analyzing brain wave activity

Histologic technician—allied health professional who performs various tissue-related procedures in the laboratory

Cytotechnologist—allied health professional trained in the microscopic interpretation of cells for detection of abnormalities

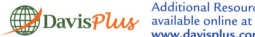 Additional Resources are available online at www.davisplus.com

Additional Resources

Association of Schools of Allied Health Professions (ASAHP)—www.asahp.org
Chartered in Washington, DC, in September 1967 as a not-for-profit national professional association for administrators, educators, and others concerned with critical issues affecting allied health education. The organization was established by the deans of 13 university-based schools of allied health professions in response to an urgent need for an interdisciplinary and interagency association to relate to improving the quality and quantity of needed workforce in

the health professions. The term *allied health* was popularized during the deliberations that led to the passage of the Allied Health Professions Personnel Training Act in 1967. The passage of this legislation brought about a new and radical concept of unifying all the various disciplines that make up allied health into academic units with a single administration.

CareerOneStop—www.careeronestop.org
Tools to help job seekers, students, businesses, and career professionals. Sponsored by the U.S. Department of Labor.

American Medical Association (AMA)—www.ama-assn. org/ama
Overview of selected allied health careers, including an overview of selected allied health career salaries.

Commission on Accreditation of Allied Health Education Programs (CAAHEP)—www.caahep.org
Provides information about accredited allied health programs.

Health Professions Network (HPN)—www.healthpronet.org
HPN is a collaborative group representing the allied health professions; organizational members include professional associations, educators, accreditors, and credentialing and licensing agencies.

Healthcare Career Connection—www.healthecareers.com
Provides information about jobs in health care.

References

1. Explore Health Careers: Allied Health Profession.
   http://www.explorehealthcareers.org.
   Accessed November 7, 2013.

2. Health Professions Network 1995–2002. Ten years of accomplishments.
   http://www.healthpronet.org/ahp_month/index.html.
   Accessed November 3, 2013.

3. Hendrix D., Charles R. Drew University of Medicine and Science. Presentation, 2006.
   http://collab.nlm.nih.gov/webcastsandvideos/drew/healthsciencecareers061.pdf.
   Accessed November 3, 2013.

4. Donini-Lenhoff FG. Coming together, moving apart: A history of the term *allied health* in education, accreditation, and practice. *J Allied Health.* 2008; 37(1):45–52.

5. Monograph # 1, Allied Health—The Past and the Future. Weber State University Website.
   http://radpacs.weber.edu/Images/R_Walker/RADT%204942/RADT%204942%20Supplemental.PDF.
   Accessed November 3, 2013.

6. The Allied Health Professions Personnel Training Act of 1966, as Amended. Report to the President and the Congress. National Institutes of Health (DHEW).
   http://eric.ed.gov/?=ED033241.
   Accessed November 7, 2013.

7. Allied health education. Medical education. Department of Allied Health Evaluation. *J Am Med Assoc.* 1978;240(26):2856–2863.

8. Commission on Accreditation of Allied Health Education Programs (CAAHEP).
   http://www.cashep.org.
   Accessed November 3, 2013.

9. Bureau of Labor Statistics, U.S. Department of Labor, Occupational Outlook Handbook, 2012–2013 Edition.
   http://www.bls.gov/ooh.
   Accessed January 14, 2014.

CHAPTER 7

Interprofessional Approach to Patient Care

Patricia Royal, EdD

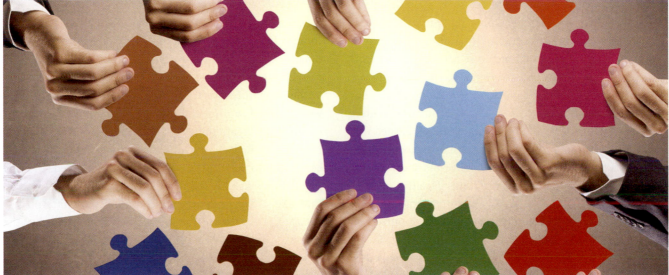

Learning Objectives

After reading this chapter, students should be able to:

- Define the term *interprofessional education*
- Explain the importance of interprofessional patient care
- Discuss some of the roles associated with interprofessional care
- Describe the different models used in interprofessional education
- Discuss interprofessional care from a historical perspective
- Describe the benefits of interprofessional care
- Discuss some of the barriers to interprofessional care

Key Terms

- Interprofessional care
- Interprofessional education
- Interdisciplinary
- Holistic approach
- Disciplines

Introduction to Interprofessional Care and Education

Definition

Interprofessional care, also known as *interprofessional collaboration* or *interprofessional practice,* is defined as two or more health-care disciplines collaborating on the care of patients. This shared experience allows the providers to view the patient holistically, rather than focusing on only one condition or ailment. Together, the team develops a patient plan of care based on the expertise of the individual team members while incorporating the team's experience, knowledge, and recommendations.

Origin

Interprofessional care is a fairly new approach to patient care. The terminology is newer than the practice. The practice of interprofessional (also called *interdisciplinary*) care in the United States began during World War II when multidisciplinary medical and surgical teams provided treatment for burns, surgery, rehabilitation, and mental health issues related to the war. More modern concepts for primary-care interprofessional teams were started at Montefiore Hospital in New York in 1948, when Martin Cherkasky developed an outreach program using teams of physicians, social workers, and nurses. Cherkasky's intent was to deliver home-care services to patients in the local community.[1] Others soon became engaged in the idea that teamwork in health care would produce better patient care. Research projects, funding, and education focusing on **interprofessional education** and care began to emerge, first at the local level and then at the state and federal levels.

Another milestone for interprofessional care occurred during President Johnson's "War on Poverty" in the 1960s. When the Office of Economic Opportunity (OEO) was created, a movement toward community health centers helped to stimulate the concept of health-care teams that would introduce training for health-care providers. The *Neighborhood Health Center Guidelines,* drafted in 1967, endorsed the need for training health-care teams. Many health-care centers responded to the drive, but others reportedly indicated that the training was too time-consuming and expensive.[1] One of the early adopters of interprofessional primary-care teams was the Martin Luther King Community Health Center in New York City. This center responded by creating eight care teams that included an internist, a pediatrician, a nurse, and a family health worker. Each team was responsible for the care of approximately 3,500 patients. This movement was led by Harold Wise, who consulted with the Sloan School of Management at Massachusetts Institute of Technology; this group produced the book *Making Health Teams Work,* one of the first books on interprofessional health-care teams.[1]

Like many other initiatives, the movement for interprofessional care and education has ebbed and flowed among providers and educators. Some individual professionals have rallied for it; others have rallied against it. The primary proponents consider the holistic patient approach as being ideal in health care, whereas the opponents have indicated time constraints as a major handicap in advocating for it. One thing that helped to keep the movement going was the creation of annual conferences where advocates of interprofessional care and education could share knowledge and the latest research. The first conference was held in Seattle, Washington, in 1979, and it has continued yearly at various locations.[1,2] In addition to a national conference, an annual international conference has been added that has heightened the awareness of interprofessional care.

Interprofessional Education

With the movement for interprofessional care continuing to grow, it became evident that there was a missing link between interprofessional practice and education. The logical question became, "How do we expect health-care providers to work together when they are educated in isolation?" The supposition was that if students were educated together, they would be more open and committed to working as a team after graduation. A major advocacy event for interprofessional education occurred in 1972 when the Institute of Medicine hosted a conference titled "Education for the Health Team" that called for interprofessional education for health science students. This level of education was termed **interdisciplinary** at both the student and faculty level, meaning that either the students were interdisciplinary or the faculty members teaching the courses were interdisciplinary.[1]

Many universities, such as the University of Kentucky, Indiana University, and the University of Minnesota, began offering courses in interprofessional education that trained medical, pharmacy, and health science students. In addition to the interprofessional education, some of these students were exposed to rural communities through outreach programs. Rural communities present a different set of complexities due to the lack of health-care providers and access to care. Additionally, the economic and social needs of rural populations increase the need for interprofessional health-care teams.[3] The push for rural community and interprofessional team experience was stressed further in 1972 when the federal government became actively involved in the creation of interprofessional training of teams for rural health care. The Institute for Health Team Development (IHTD) was established by the Robert Wood Johnson Foundation. In 1974 the Office of Interdisciplinary Programs was established, and more funding became available under the Health Manpower Education Initiative Awards (HMEIA). The purpose of these awards was to establish and support interprofessional team training of health professional students in primary care. Some of the benefactors of funding for these types of programs included medical schools located in Virginia, South Carolina, North Carolina, and Missouri.[1]

Many of the programs established during the mid-1980s to 1990s lost funding, particularly those associated with rural health. Many federal grants were cut in 2006, and unless the medical school or university was able to obtain alternative funding, the rural health programs were discontinued; however, some universities were able to continue their interprofessional education programs.

Teams, Not Groups

Often people use the words *team* and *group* interchangeably. In the case of interprofessional education and practice, however, they are not synonymous. *Team* is always used when referring to any interprofessional-related definition or activity. To further explain the difference between these words,

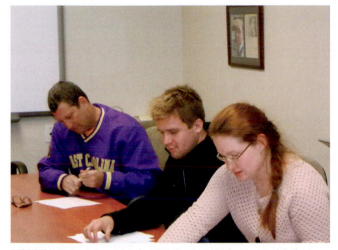

FIGURE 7-1 For interprofessional patient care to be successful, the team must work together to ensure that all needs are addressed. This group of students will ultimately work toward achieving quality care for patients, but first they must learn to work together as a team. (Photo courtesy of Dr. Michael Kennedy.)

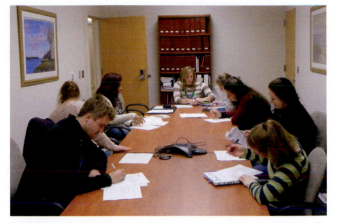

FIGURE 7-2 Professionals working together to discuss patient needs: nursing, rehabilitation, social work, nutrition, administration, and business. They are having a weekly patient care meeting where patients' needs are discussed and all disciplines contribute to the discussion.

let us look at the definitions of each. *Group* generally refers to any number of people gathered together or those who have a united relationship.[4] This word could easily describe fans at a ball game. They meet the group criteria, but they are not a team. A *team,* on the other hand, is generally made up of a smaller number of people who are dedicated to a common purpose or goal.[4] In the case of the ball game, the players would fit into the category of team. Each player has a set of skills used to accomplish the goal—winning the game. The players work toward the same goal and hold each other accountable to achieve the purpose or outcome. Interprofessional care works in the same manner. Each health-care provider has a unique set of skills that reflects the education and experience needed to enhance quality patient care. However, because each provider is limited to specific skill sets, whether by education or experience, other providers are needed to treat the patient in a holistic approach. Together the team can understand the patient's needs and discuss treatment options based on the individual patient.

Holistic Approach

Interprofessional care and education addresses the patient and family using a **holistic approach,** which means to view and analyze the patient in a manner that encompasses the whole patient rather than individual parts. The patient needs to be viewed through the eyes of physical, mental, and social conditions because these conditions may hamper recovery otherwise. For example, if a patient enters a clinic or emergency department with a broken leg, the leg (the physical part) must be treated, but the mental and social conditions should also be addressed. Understanding why and how the

break occurred may help the provider to prevent another break from occurring. Perhaps the break was due to poor living conditions, such as a rotten floor or stairs. To assist the patient and prevent another break, the provider would need to involve another discipline trained in resource management, who might be able to find resources to help the patient repair the floor or find a more suitable living environment. Another piece of this puzzle may be related to patient dietary habits. Perhaps the patient is lacking calcium due to dietary issues. A nutritionist would be able to provide the patient with a diet high in calcium that may help prevent future breaks. Other needs for this patient, depending on age and severity of the break, might be occupational or physical therapy. The provider would need to set up an appointment for a therapy consultation. As you can see, many possibilities may add to the dynamics of this patient's plan of care. Treating the patient in a holistic manner, rather than treating just the injury, will ultimately ensure overall quality care.

Disciplines

The number and types of **disciplines** used in interprofessional teams can vary depending on the models used, location of services, and other factors such as accrediting agency or payer source requirements. In certain areas, Medicare and Medicaid require specific disciplines to be involved in the patient's plan of care. For example, Medicare-certified hospice facilities require the interprofessional team to include a medical director, nurse, social worker, spiritual counselor, and certified nurse's aide, as well as a volunteer. Volunteers are individuals with or without medical expertise, who are trained by the hospice organization in accordance with Medicare requirements. This care plan team must meet on a

Working Together: A Case Study

The patient is a 70-year-old woman who slipped on ice while walking to her car. On arrival at the emergency department, the primary-care provider (PCP) ordered several sets of x-rays (radiographer). The patient was diagnosed with a fractured right hip and needs surgery. In addition to the pressing need for surgery, other health concerns include diabetes, hypertension, obesity, and three broken teeth resulting from the fall. The PCP contacts the surgeon for a consultation. After the surgeon confirms the need for surgery, she asks the nurse to schedule surgery ASAP. Before the nurse can schedule the surgery, the patient or family member must sign permission, HIPAA, and release of medical information forms, in addition to a hospital admission package. The PCP realizes that the patient will need temporary nursing home placement after surgery, so he discusses this with the social worker. The social worker begins working on finding a nursing home for the patient and gathers financial information such as insurance and Medicare coverage for the nursing home stay. The patient's surgery is successful; however, there are existing concerns that need to be addressed along with some new concerns. The patient's diabetes and hypertension are uncontrolled. The patient needs to lose at least 25 pounds. The recent fall will immobilize the patient, which will limit her ability to exercise, and her dietary needs have increased as she recovers from surgery. The PCP requests that the hospital nutritionist meet with the patient and family to discuss her dietary needs. Additionally, because there were three broken teeth, the patient may need a soft or pureed diet while in the hospital and nursing home. The PCP makes a referral for physical therapy (PT) at the nursing home and home PT when the patient returns home. The PCP also makes a referral to a local dentist regarding the three broken teeth. Although the PCP made most of the decisions regarding the patient's primary care, he needed to consult with other health-care team members to provide a holistic approach to care. Throughout the patient's stay in the hospital and nursing home, communication among the team must continue. For example, the nurse at the nursing home needs to monitor the patient's blood pressure and blood sugar levels and convey this information to the PCP and nutritionist. The PCP needs to discuss patient progress with the physical therapist to ensure that the patient is improving. The physical therapist might need to determine when the patient is able to visit the dentist for her broken teeth. Ensuring quality health care begins and ends with the team approach; therefore, until the patient is restored to her previous or better health, communication among the interprofessional team must continue.

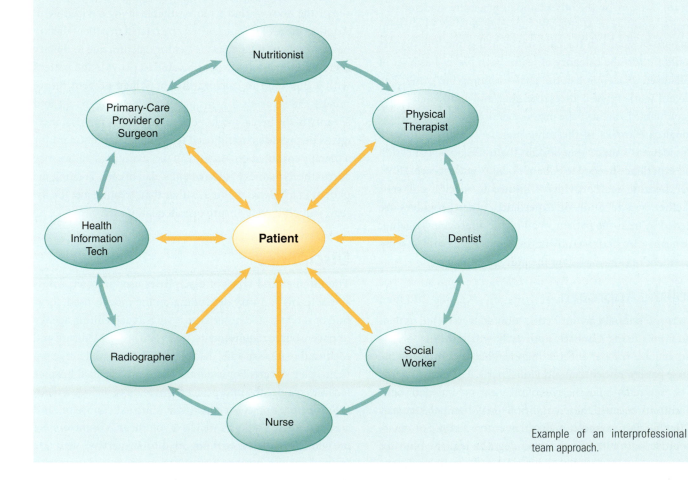

Example of an interprofessional team approach.

regular basis to discuss the patient's progress and plan of care. Other facilities such as dialysis centers require the medical director, nurse, social worker, and nutritionist to meet regularly for patient care needs. Other types of facilities may require physical or occupational therapists to be a part of the care plan team. The makeup of the team depends on the type of facility, patient needs, and other dynamics.

One such dynamic may be the determination of the interprofessional team based on roles and functions. The members may change according to the severity or complexity of the patient's condition or other variables such as age and occupation. Depending on the occupation, therapy services may be required to reintroduce the patient to the work environment. Seven key functions often help determine the team; these are the functions/roles that might be involved in the patient's plan of care[5]:

- *Entry point/referral channel*—the process of finding the appropriate health-care provider depending on the patient's problems. Generally this role involves the primary-care physician. There are times when patients can self-refer without contacting the primary-care physician. The opportunity to self-refer is usually based on the patient's health insurance.

- *Clinical director or leader/decision-maker*—the principal or primary provider treating the patient for the chief diagnosis or condition. This role typically involves the referred physician treating the patient. Other possible leaders could be the surgeon, clinical psychologist, neurologist, or other specialists, depending on the nature of the condition.

- *Consultant/technical authority*—individuals knowledgeable in certain areas. Potentially, these are experts in a specific field. Some of these roles could involve the clinical pharmacist, radiation therapist, clinical psychologist, and genetics counselor.

- *Support services provider*—services that augment primary services. The role of the support services providers is to augment the patient care provided by the other members of the team. These disciplines might include nursing, nutrition, social work, respiratory therapy, physical and occupational therapy, x-ray and laboratory, and transportation services. Again, the roles will change depending on the illness or condition and needs of the patient.

- *Coordinator of effort/point of contact*—individual who collaborates with all providers. There is not a designated individual who becomes the point of contact for patients or providers. It could be the decision-maker, but not necessarily. This individual helps coordinate the patient's appointments and retrieves medical records and test results.

- *Resource manager*—individual who assists with access to care and financial issues; may be the health services manager, billing clerk, processor, or financial manager. This individual processes the patient's insurance claims and reimbursements on the patient's behalf. Depending on the severity of the illness and the amount of time the patient will be receiving treatments or services, it is not uncommon for the patient to request one specific person for this role to minimize miscommunications.

- *Information communicator*—individual who maintains the patient's health information. This is a somewhat new position, but it has an important role in the health-care delivery system. Individuals fulfilling this duty could be health information managers, medical records specialists, or information system specialists. This function provides a means of coordination for the patient's health information. Rather than having the information spread out over various locations or providers' offices, having an information communicator can enhance coordination and resources by maintaining data in one designated location. This task is often done by implementing electronic medical records (EMRs). EMRs allow sharing of medical information with all providers involved in patient care.[5]

Interprofessional Education Models

In 2001, the Institute of Medicine Committee on Quality of Health Care in America advocated for health-care professionals to dedicate themselves to use teamwork as a method for addressing some of the complex needs of today's patients.[6] For interprofessional teams to be used effectively, health-care students must be educated in an environment conducive to sharing knowledge and resources for the common goal of better patient outcomes. Students trained in interprofessional education are more likely to collaborate with other health-care team members and advocate for the improvement of patient outcomes through the use of interprofessional care. The types of training models vary by academic institutions and include didactic, community-based, and simulation-based programs.

Didactic Programs

Academic programs teaching interprofessional education using the didactic or instructional model stress the importance of team-building skills while acquiring knowledge and understanding concepts about other health professions. This objective can be met by meeting as a group and discussing roles and scopes of practice for each discipline. Case studies

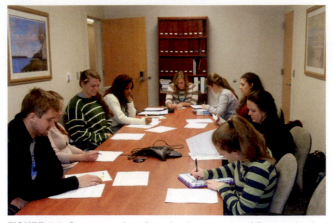

FIGURE 7-3 Representatives from the departments of Communication Sciences and Disorders, Health Services and Information Management, Addictions and Rehabilitation Studies, Occupational Therapy, Physician Assistant Studies, and Clinical Laboratory Science work together to promote allied health sciences. (Photo courtesy of Dr. Michael Kennedy.)

and role plays are also useful ways to encourage collaboration and engage students.[7]

The second part of the didactic model is service learning. Service learning allows students to interact with the community to gain a better understanding of the demographics and needs of the community. This objective can be met by developing community projects, needs assessments, and educational presentations or screenings.[7]

The last part to this model is a clinical component that gives students clinical experience working in interprofessional teams. Teams of students attend clinical sessions at community clinics, allowing students real-life patient encounters. These students often make home visits to patients with a chronic illness or condition and collaborate to develop care plans.

Cultural awareness is often part of the didactic model. Awareness of the role culture plays in health-care delivery is developed by immersing the students in community settings. Students, along with a faculty coordinator, complete patient interviews, which include questions related to the patient's culture. Understanding the patient's culture may improve communication between the patient and provider and enhance patient compliance. In some cases, the "patients" are actually volunteers who act the part of the patient; other programs encourage active communication with a real patient. Students can reflect on the manner in which cultural beliefs play a role in the patient's overall health status and gain a better understanding for future interactions.[7]

Community-Based Experience

Academic programs using the community-based experience model focus both on the accessibility of resources and the subsequent impact on health, as well as environmental issues

that might affect one's health. The other important focus for this model is the services provided to patients through the collaboration of interprofessional teams.[7]

The community-based experience uses some of the features of the didactic model, particularly the patient home visit conducted by the interprofessional students. Similar to the didactic model, students may complete several homes visits during one semester. These visits usually focus on the underserved population and the accessibility of resources for the patient and family. During the home visit the students may gather health status information and determine resources needed. Students can then complete a project to help address some of these concerns. Based on the activities done, the students gather feedback to determine if they have met their goal of improving the patient's or family's health status.[7]

Interprofessional Simulation Experience

The interprofessional simulation experience model focuses on clinical team skills training by using formative and summative simulations that allow students to participate and demonstrate their clinical skills. The simulations may be done by using standardized patients/actors who are portraying a specific type of patient, such as someone having a heart attack. It is important for the interprofessional team to develop communication and leadership skills, which can be enhanced through the use of simulation activities. Goals of the interprofessional model include learning to respect the various health-care provider roles, demonstrating consensus building, understanding how to resolve conflict while negotiating effectively, and overcoming barriers to interprofessional collaboration. Learning the effective skills for successful collaboration will ultimately enhance patient care.[7]

Elements of a Collaborative Environment

The establishment of an interprofessional team does not occur overnight, nor does it occur in isolation. It requires the entire team to be committed to working through their problems and difficult situations to become a strong, unified team for the benefit of quality patient care. Some common characteristics that indicate a collaborative, well-developed interprofessional team are described next.

Effective Communication

Effective communication is an important skill for everyone working in health care. The patient's diagnosis and prognosis may depend on the health-care provider's ability to listen and respond to what the patient has to say. Additionally, the patient must understand the provider and the instructions for taking medications appropriately, keeping all appointments, and calling the office to report changes in condition. Therefore, the provider must listen to the patient, speak clearly, and check for verbal understanding of the instructions. The same holds true for collaboration among team members. To be an effective communicator one should exhibit skills in both verbal and nonverbal communication. Nonverbal communication can be counterintuitive by producing inconsistencies between what is being said and the body language exhibited. If your body says something different than your words, confusion can occur. Therefore, one should keep both verbal and nonverbal communication consistent to prevent confusion among the group.

Support

Interprofessional teams require support from all team members. A team is a group of people who work together toward a common goal; therefore, it is imperative that the team reflect commitment and recognition of the team as one unit. Any wins or losses belong to the entire team, not to individuals. This premise is essential when involved in patient care. Because patients' lives may depend on the support of the team, team members will always need to put aside any petty differences or conflicts that may arise to enhance the team concept.[8] It is expected that all members of an interprofessional health-care team will strive for the same goal—quality patient care. However, there may be times when ego or self-interest may hinder shared goals. Therefore, team members must keep their egos in check and understand that there can be disagreements among the members, but the ultimate priority is quality care for the patient and family.[8]

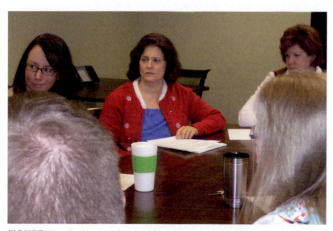

FIGURE 7-4 An interprofessional care team works in a round robin way, meaning each person has an opportunity to address issues or concerns or is able to make suggestions to problems mentioned by another discipline. In this photo, the interprofessional staff at a nursing home are holding their weekly care plan meeting.

Clear Roles

The interprofessional team members generally understand that roles vary according to scope of practice, education, and licensure of the members. There should be a clear understanding of each person's roles and responsibilities. Each team member should be accountable to the team at large and responsible for his or her own designated duties as determined by the team.[8]

Mutual Trust

Mutual trust is one of the most important parts of interprofessional teams, particularly in regard to health care. Trusting your team members to work in the best interest of the patient and share the progress with the team produces a rich team environment. Additionally, trusting in the collaborative process fosters mutual trust.

Values

Interprofessional health-care teams are made up of individual health-care professionals. For these individuals to become an effective, cohesive team, each team member must bring certain core values to the group. The five core values essential to an effective, high-functioning team are honesty, discipline, creativity, humility, and curiosity.[8]

Honesty

Honesty is one of the most important characteristics of an effective interprofessional team; therefore, each member must bring this value to the group for successful team implementation. Without individual honesty, the team itself will not grow due to the lack of trust among the members.

Discipline

Discipline can be associated with an individual team member's self-control or strong desire to improve the team's efficiency and effectiveness even during inconvenient times when members may have other things going on. The team member must carry out responsibilities as needed to enhance team functioning even in the most difficult situations. In other words, even when an individual's life may be hectic and chaotic, the commitment to the team must still be addressed and responsibilities cannot be shirked. The right amount of discipline can help push the team forward.

Creativity

Individual team members need a certain amount of creativity to help the team tackle new problems, devise new solutions, or determine alternative treatment methods.

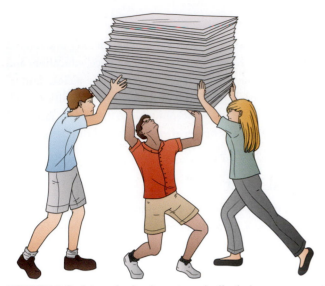

FIGURE 7-5 For interprofessional care to work effectively, everyone must be held accountable and carry his or her workload for the purpose of achieving the same goal.

Humility

To ensure team cohesion and collaboration, team members need to have an unassuming and modest attitude, recognizing that everyone has something to contribute to the team. Each member should feel that his or her opinion is worthwhile and not fear being shamed by any other member. If all members bring humility to the team, there will be an open environment that is more conducive to problem-solving.

Curiosity

Curiosity, in the interprofessional sense, refers to the team members reflecting on lessons learned in the past. These lessons should be shared with team members to improve the functioning of the team.

Benefits of Interprofessional Health-Care Practice

The benefits of interprofessional care can be viewed from four perspectives—the patient, the care team, higher education institutions, and students. There are some commonalities and overlapping of each perspective.

Tips and Tools

To learn more about health-care standards and accountability, visit the National Healthcare Skills Standards and Accountability Criteria website at www.healthscienceconsortium.org/standards.php.

The Patient

- Holistic treatment approach
- Continuity of care
- Cost-effective care due to fewer hospitalizations[1]
- Fewer prescription drugs[1]
- Higher patient satisfaction[1]
- More patient compliance

The Care Team

- Collaborative approach[9]
- Shared responsibility[9]
- Evidence-based decision-making[9]
- Team cohesion
- Expert knowledge
- Avoidance of duplication of service[9]
- Shared resources[9]

Higher Education Institutions

- Effective use of resources (faculty time and physical space)[9]
- Improved student performance and satisfaction[9]
- More grant opportunities
- Faculty buy-in
- Increased research agendas
- Increased cultural sensitivity[9]

Students

- Prepares students for future work situations[9]
- Appreciation of diversity
- Awareness of other disciplines' roles and scopes of practice
- Appreciation and acknowledgment of other disciplines[8,9]
- Improved performance
- Increased morale
- Increased development of team skills
- Empowerment
- Critical thinking skills
- Creative thinking skills

Barriers to Effective Interprofessional Teams

In addition to benefits, there are also barriers to effective interprofessional health-care teams, which can also be viewed through the same four perspectives—the patient, the care team, higher education institutions, and students. Again, there are some commonalities and overlapping of each perspective.

The Patient

- Confusion
- Uncertainty regarding primary contact
- Miscommunication
- Reluctance to allow team discussion of personal health status
- Privacy issues

The Care Team

- Lack of training in collaboration[10]
- Leadership ambiguity[10]
- Difference in levels of authority and power[10]
- Lack of commitment
- Competition among members
- Team size
- Multiple responsibilities
- Turf battles

Higher Education Institutions

- Turf battles
- Uninterested faculty for participation in interprofessional education
- Low faculty morale
- Lack of knowledge in interprofessional education[9]
- Misconception of faculty time
- Coordination with other professionals
- Changes in curriculum
- Scheduling conflicts
- Lack of clinical sites for interprofessional placements

Students

- Scheduling conflicts
- Turf battles
- Professional identity
- Unclear roles
- Lack of time
- Loss of autonomy

SUMMARY

The premise behind interprofessional health-care practice started more than half a century ago; however, for many people the concept is still foreign. The lack of knowledge of this concept may be linked to unfamiliarity. More recently, there has been a push at the federal level to encourage more participation in interprofessional care teams at both the training stage and the practice phase. However, both the education institutions and the practicing professionals continue to hesitate. Although the benefits of interprofessional health care would seem to make for much easier implementation, some consider the barriers and challenges overwhelming. With the Affordable Care Act enacted into law, accountability for health care may be the impetus that pushes interprofessional health care back into the spotlight. The relationship of financial resources to accountability of quality patient care may encourage more interprofessional team approaches.

CASE STUDY

JP is a 36-year-old man who is married and has three children. He and his wife both work to support the family. JP is a long-distance truck driver and depends on his job to help support his family. Three weeks ago, JP suffered a stroke, leaving one of his hands partially contracted. JP was not aware of his hypertension and had not visited a physician in many years due to his time on the road. Any off time JP spent with his family. JP is now facing great stress. He is concerned about his right hand because he cannot drive without the use of it. His physician advises him that in time and with some therapy his hand will probably regain strength to continue in his current occupation. Another issue JP is facing is his lack of insurance at the time of the stroke. JP had family coverage until about 6 months ago, when he had to cancel his policy because his wife was temporarily unemployed and they needed the extra money. His wife went back to work 3 months ago, but JP kept postponing the reinstatement of his insurance policy until their finances were in better shape.

Questions

1. At least five different health professionals should be consulted about JP. Can you name them and explain why you selected them?
2. Who should be a part of the interprofessional team?
3. Who is the primary decision-maker in the team?
4. What should JP's next step be?
5. Can you add one more scenario to this case that would include one more health professional?

Review Questions

1. The term *interprofessional* is a newer word for:

   A. Multidisciplinary

   B. Interdisciplinary

   C. Unidisciplinary

   D. Transdisciplinary

2. To be considered an interprofessional approach to health care, the team must be composed of five different disciplines.

   A. True

   B. False

3. The benefits of interprofessional care affect only the patient and family members.

   A. True

   B. False

4. In an interprofessional care team approach, no one assumes primary responsibility for the patient.

   A. True

   B. False

5. During _____'s presidency, the "War on Poverty" campaign helped the development of health-care teams in primary care.

   A. Nixon

   B. Roosevelt

   C. Eisenhower

   D. Johnson

6. The first primary-care health-care teams were started in:

   A. Philadelphia

   B. Los Angeles

   C. Houston

   D. New York

7. The approach to treating the whole patient rather than the physical condition only is known as:

   A. Multidisciplinary

   B. Holistic

   C. Unidisciplinary

   D. None of the above

8. There is only one model for interprofessional education.

   A. True

   B. False

9. Honesty is one of the _____ needed for an effective interprofessional team.

   A. Norms

   B. Values

   C. Barriers

   D. All of the above

10. In the interprofessional community-based model of care, the focus is on simulation activities.

    A. True

    B. False

Glossary of Key Terms

Interprofessional care—holistic health-care approach with two or more different disciplines involved in the plan of care

Interprofessional education—educational curriculum that focuses on teaching interprofessional care to students in health programs

Interdisciplinary—precursor to the term *interprofessional* care

Holistic approach—approach focusing on treating the whole patient rather than just the physical condition

Disciplines—different fields of educational or professional work; the roles within each field

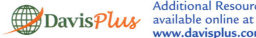

Additional Resources are available online at www.davisplus.com

Additional Resources

American Interprofessional Health Collaborative (AIHC)—www.aihc-us.org/what-is-aihc

This website provides information about the promotion of interprofessional care and the educational components for students, educators, and practitioners.

AIHC Webinar Series—www.aihc-us.org/aihc-interprofessional-webinar

This website provides information about the importance of interprofessional care and provides educational resources, such a competencies needed for practice and delivery of health care.

The Association of Interprofessional Healthcare Students (AIHS)—http://aihs.info/

This website provides information about ways to connect with other students who are interested in interprofessional education and care. Information such as conferences, presentations, new textbooks, and other resources can be found at this website.

All Together Better Health Conference VII—www. atbh7.pitt.edu

This website provides information about where the annual national conferences are held and the speakers, resources, and papers presented each year.

Interprofessional Education (IPE) Portal—www.mededportal. org/ipe

This website provides information about interprofessional education. This portal is a repository for competency-based resources such as peer-reviewed articles and cases for best practices in interprofessional care.

National Center for Interprofessional Practice and Education—http://nexusipe.org/

This website provides information about the various ways interprofessional care can improve health-care delivery and reduce costs. Students can read the latest research and practice models that enhance interprofessional care.

References

1. Baldwin D. Some historical notes on interdisciplinary and interprofessional education and practice in health care in the USA. *J Interprofessional Care.* 2007;21(81):23–37.

2. Illingworth P, Chelvanayagam S. Interprofessional education: Benefits of interprofessional education in health care. *Br J Nurs.* 2007;16(2):121–124.

3. Stamm BH. *Rural Behavioral Health Care: An Interdisciplinary Guide.* Washington, DC: American Psychological Association; 2012.

4. Weiss D, Tilin F, Morgan M. *The Interprofessional Health Care Team: Leadership and Development.* Burlington, MA: Jones & Bartlett; 2014.

5. Freshman B, Rubino L, Chassiakos YR. *Collaboration Across the Disciplines in Health Care.* Burlington, MA: Jones & Bartlett; 2010.

6. Institute of Medicine, Committee on Quality of Health Care in America. *Crossing the Quality Chasm: A New Health System for the 21st Century.* Washington, DC: National Academies Press; 2001.

7. Bridges D, Davidson R, Odegard P, Maki I, Tomkowiak J. Interprofessional collaboration: Three best practice models of interprofessional education. *Med Education Online.* 2011;16:6035.

8. Mitchell P, Wynia M, Golden R, et al. Core principles and values of effective team-based health care. *Institute of Medicine Conference Roundtable Discussion Paper: Advising the Nation—Improving Health.* October 2012.

9. Paul S, Peterson C. *Interprofessional Collaboration: Issues for Practice and Research.* Binghamton, NY: Haworth Press; 2001.

10. Grant RW, Finnocchio LJ. California Primary Care Consortium Subcommittee on Interdisciplinary Collaboration. *Interdisciplinary Collaborative Teams in Primary Care: A Model Curriculum and Resource Guide.* San Francisco, CA: Pew Health Professions Commission; 1995.

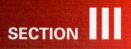
Primary-Care Professions

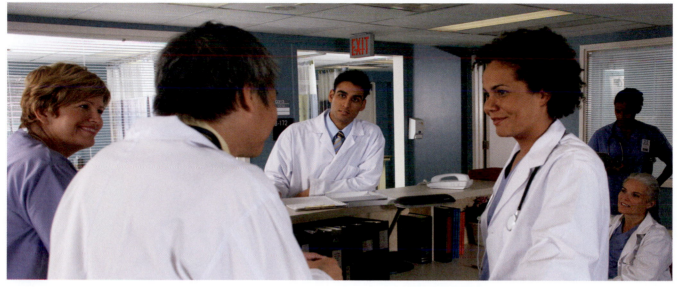

Photo credit: digitalvison/Thinkstock

Chapter 8
Medicine

Chapter 9
Nursing

Chapter 10
Pharmacy

Medicine

Thomas G. Irons, MD

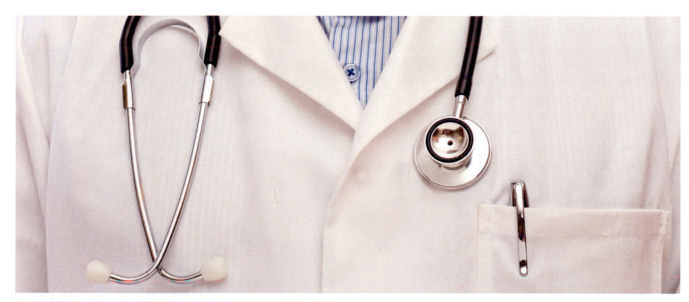

Photo credit: istock/Thinkstock

Learning Objectives

After reading this chapter, students should be able to:

- Explain in broad terms the educational, training, and licensure requirements for the profession of medicine
- Give an overview of medical specialties and practice options
- Describe in general terms the premedical education requirements for medical school application, the application process, and the layout of the 4-year medical educational curriculum
- Explain the role of the physician on the health-care team and briefly discuss the expected changes in that role in the future
- Describe the unique challenges and opportunities facing the medical profession in the United States

Key Terms

- Premedical curriculum
- Medical College Admission Test (MCAT)
- Residency
- Fellowship
- Primary care
- Capitation
- Affordable Care Act
- Electronic health records
- Integrated care
- Biopsychosocial model

 ## "A Day in the Life"

Good morning. I'm Sarah Hoyer and I am a pediatrician. I'm glad to be able to show you something of what my daily life is like. I start early because there's so much to do before I get to the office. Like most of my colleagues, I'm in a group practice. We are employed by the local hospital system. There are five of us in our office: four pediatricians and a pediatric nurse practitioner. Two of us are mothers and work 80% of the time so that we can spend more time with our children. While having my morning cup of coffee, I look over my calendar for the day. My first responsibility is to go to the hospital to see newborn babies and their mothers. We rotate this responsibility among the five of us. Then I'll drive over to the office. My first patient is scheduled for 9:30 a.m. On days when I do not have hospital duty, I arrive at the office by 7:45 a.m.

(continued)

and see my first patient at 8:30 a.m. I use those 45 minutes to complete paperwork, review test results, and look over my patient schedule.

I've now arrived at the hospital. I see most babies in the rooms with their mothers. Only those who are having lab tests or procedures done will be in the nursery. The parents of one of the boys have requested a circumcision. When I am finished with all the exams and counseling, a nurse will assist me in performing the procedure. It's a lucky day. None of our babies has complications and the circumcision goes smoothly. I am on the way to the office on time. I'll only have a few minutes to review the patient schedule. We will see about eight patients by lunchtime. If I hadn't had newborn duty, we'd have seen several more.

At midmorning, however, I see a 2-month-old infant with significant fever. This one requires careful evaluation, immediate tests, and 40 minutes of my time. The baby is not feeding well and appears somewhat listless. After reviewing the early test results and discussing them with the parents, I recommend hospitalization for further testing and antibiotic therapy pending test results. The parents are worried and need my reassurance. Although a full-time hospital-based pediatrician will be caring for the baby, I assure the parents that I will be checking on them by phone and will stop in and visit them later on my way home. One of the joys of practice is that I already know most of the patients and families so they are comfortable with me. We finish with our patients by 12:30 p.m., but before taking a lunch break I have to finish the record-keeping I was unable to get to in the morning. Lori and I order takeout and spend the break reviewing test results, making phone calls, and completing paperwork.

We finish our afternoon patients just before 5:00 p.m. and debrief with the rest of the clinical staff. We've heard that our hospitalized baby and his parents are settled into their room and the necessary tests have been performed. A social worker has stopped by to counsel them. We finish up our record-keeping and telephone calls, and I am able to leave for the hospital before 5:30 p.m. My visit with the patient and his parents is brief—things are going smoothly and a review of test results reveals nothing alarming, so I am able to start for home before 6:30 p.m.

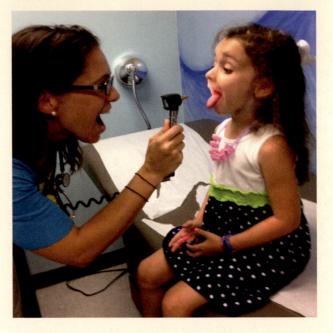

Introduction to Medicine

History

The practice of medicine in some form or another is as old as civilization. Modern medicine takes its origins from sources ranging from ancient China and the Middle East to Greco-Roman civilization, centuries before the invention of the microscope and the emergence of the germ theory. The 19th century saw the emergence of the field of bacteriology, the recognition of the importance of antisepsis in surgery, and, in 1895, the invention of the x-ray. A few women had begun to enter the profession by the turn of the century, notable among them Elizabeth Blackwell and Mary Putnam Jacobi, native-born Americans and pioneers in the field.[1]

Required Education and Licensure

By 1910, there were 155 schools of medicine operating in the United States and Canada. Abraham Flexner, a research scholar at the Carnegie Foundation for the advancement of teaching, visited every school and compiled a report, known as the Flexner Report, which was addressed to the public. In it, he recommended that all medical schools adopt a model for medical education. This is the prevailing model used today throughout the Western world. The model requires undergraduate prerequisites in science before admission and a rigorous science-based curriculum followed by clinical training in the hospital and other clinical settings. Both the American Medical Association and American Osteopathic Association endorsed the model after 1910. Many schools closed, but others modified their requirements and curricula as set forth in the report and brought themselves up to the "Flexnerian" standard.[2] Today, the material taught in medical and osteopathic medical schools is essentially the same, with the exception that osteopathic schools add a component of what is known as "osteopathic manipulative medicine."

All medical schools require **premedical curriculum** components. These include, but are not limited to, organic chemistry, physics, and advanced courses in biology. Some undergraduate institutions offer premedical majors, though no such major is required for entry as long as the prerequisites are taken. Undergraduates usually apply to medical school after their third year of college and have generally completed their prerequisite courses by this time. The **Medical College Admission Test (MCAT)** is usually taken between May and August of that year, but is offered many times throughout the year. The MCAT is a standardized, computer-administered test.[3] Competition for admission to accredited schools of medicine and osteopathic medicine is high. Strong undergraduate performance and MCAT scores are uniformly expected.

The first 2 years of medical school usually include intensive instruction in anatomy, physiology, biochemistry, pharmacology, microbiology, psychology, genetics, and epidemiology. All schools include basic clinical skills training in the first 2 years, and a majority of them include course material in medical humanities or medical ethics. The academic workload during these years is very heavy. Whereas many college students are able to work to help pay their expenses, this is impossible for medical students. The second 2 years involve more direct exposure to patient care and the practice of clinical skills in the major medical specialties. Though most of this instruction takes place in the hospital, there is also a great deal of education and training in the outpatient environment. Third-and fourth-year medical students take night call and can generally expect to work and study in the clinical setting about 80 hours a week. This model (2 years of basic science, 2 years of clinical training) is employed in the majority of schools, but a number have alternative curricula. The same material is taught, but it is distributed differently throughout the 4 years. Today there are approximately 130 accredited medical schools in the United States and Puerto Rico. As of 2013, there were 30 accredited osteopathic schools.[4]

Traditionally, medicine has been highly paternalistic and male-dominated. The emphasis on patient autonomy, which explicitly calls for shared decision-making between the patient and physician, is relatively recent. Though it has been widely adopted in the United States, it remains unusual in other parts of the world. The face of medicine has changed as well. By 2010, 47% of medical school entrants were women.[5]

> ### Tips and Tools
>
> The MCAT is changing in 2015 and will include four test sections. The sections are "Biochemical and Biological Foundations of Living Systems," "Chemical and Physical Foundations of Biological Systems," "Psychosocial and Biological Foundations of Behavior," and "Scientific Inquiry and Reasoning Skills." Visit the website for more details (https://www.aamc.org/students/applying/mcat/mcat2015/).

> ### Tips and Tools
>
> Allopathic medicine and osteopathic medicine differ primarily in their emphasis on musculoskeletal health. Osteopathic physicians are trained in a technique called osteopathic manipulative therapy and have special expertise in the treatment of musculoskeletal problems.

The cost of a medical education is very high. Public institutions are considerably less expensive than private ones. The Association of American Medical Colleges (AAMC) has developed a formula for estimating the average cost of attendance (COA) over 4 years. The estimated average 4-year COA at public schools in 2011 was $187,400 and at private schools was $264,000. Average debt at graduation from public schools was estimated at $155,000 and from private schools at $180,000. The relatively narrow debt gap between public and private schools was attributed to the much larger endowments of private schools, allowing scholarship support at those schools to be considerably more generous.[6]

Once medical school is completed, doctors require additional training, or **residency,** before they are able to practice independently. All must pass a three-phase examination before they can be licensed to practice. Step 1 is taken at the end of basic science training (usually year two), step 2 just before graduation, and step 3 during residency training. Residency duration varies greatly depending on specialty, but is at least 3 years. A high school graduate can expect a minimum of 11 years of education and training before being ready to practice. Specialties requiring a high degree of technical expertise can be much longer, and subspecialties, such as pediatric cardiology or

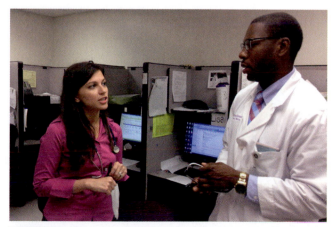

FIGURE 8-1 Although the field of medicine has been predominantly male-oriented, there has been a shift creating more women in medicine. In this photo, a male medicine student is discussing a patient with a female resident.

vascular surgery, require additional training, called a **fellowship.** Specialties with relatively few residency slots available are in high demand. Most only accept applications from students who are in the top 25% of their medical school graduating class. No matter what the specialty, every doctor who completes residency must pass a rigorous specialty board examination to become board-certified and is subject to periodic recertification examinations.

Continuing Education

All states also specify continuing medical education requirements for maintenance of licensure, usually about 50 hours per year of direct or online instruction and testing. Medical science changes rapidly, and keeping up with these changes is part of the daily life of medical doctors.

Scope of Practice

The number of ways in which one can practice medicine is very large. They vary by specialty and subspecialty, location (e.g., hospital vs. community), type of patient population served, degree of medical research activity expected, and in many other ways. For example, a pediatrician who is a member of a medical faculty may conduct research, teach students and residents in both classroom and clinical settings, and see patients in a private or public clinic. Some practices are primarily hospital based, such as cardiothoracic surgery; others may be primarily outpatient based. Some doctors, such as occupational medicine specialists, may never practice in the hospital setting. All doctors can treat patients within the scope of practice of their specialty, perform certain procedures, and prescribe medications. For example, any doctor

can stitch a laceration, but only an orthopedic surgeon can perform a hip replacement operation.

Not many students enter medical school having decided on a specialty or subspecialty. They usually choose based on their clinical experiences by the end of the third year. The American Board of Medical Specialties has 24 member specialty boards. Some, such as the American Board of Psychiatry and Neurology, certify more than one specialty. The specialties that take primary responsibility for the overall care of patients, such as pediatrics, family medicine, or general internal medicine, are collectively termed **primary care.** The specialty boards are included in Box 8-1.[7]

Salary

Physicians are generally well paid regardless of specialty, but salaries vary widely. A 2013 survey conducted by Medscape, Inc., listed average salaries ranging from $173,000 for pediatricians to $405,000 for orthopedic surgeons.[8] These are average figures. Starting salaries may be much lower. Residents or fellows in specialty training are generally paid modest salaries, starting at less than one-third of what they might make in practice and increasing as they advance through their training.

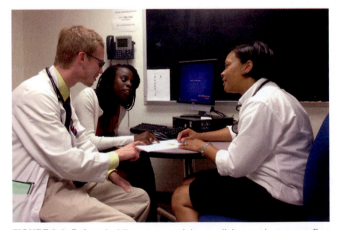

FIGURE 8-2 Before deciding on a specialty, medicine students must first complete their residency training, which is supervised by a physician. The physician allows the students to ask questions and provides recommendations for patient care.

Box 8-1   Medical Board Specialties

Allergy and immunology
Anesthesiology
Colon and rectal surgery
Dermatology
Emergency medicine
Family medicine
Internal medicine
Medical genetics
Neurological surgery
Nuclear medicine
Obstetrics and gynecology
Ophthalmology
Orthopedic surgery
Otolaryngology
Pathology
Pediatrics
Physical medicine and rehabilitation
Plastic surgery
Preventive medicine
Psychiatry and neurology
Radiology
Surgery
Thoracic surgery
Urology

Trends

The practice experience for all physicians has changed considerably over the last decade. The change for primary-care physicians, which is ongoing, is significant. Because of both public and private payment reforms, primary care is rapidly becoming a team-based process. The team varies depending on patient need. A team commonly includes physicians, midlevel providers such as nurse practitioners, physician assistants, nurses, medical assistants, nursing assistants, social workers, behavioral health professionals, and medical assistants. The team collectively assumes responsibility for a group of patients, called a *panel,* and oversees all their care. Payment for health care is moving toward a payment model called **capitation.** This means that a team is paid on a per-person or *per-capita* basis each year, to care for each patient in the team's panel. Strict quality measures are employed. Teams that deliver high-quality care at lower overall cost are rewarded accordingly.

The health-care workforce is also transforming. Most expert groups expect a marked increase in demand for primary-care doctors, nurses, and midlevel providers, to accommodate the new care models and the new patient demand resulting from federal insurance reform under the **Affordable Care Act.** Shortages already exist in all of these areas and are expected to become even more serious in the years to come. There are also shortages in other specialties, such as psychiatry and general surgery.[9]

Challenges

One of the major challenges facing physicians in the United States today is the continuous escalation in health-care costs. Recognizing that this is not sustainable over the long term, physicians have good reason to fear declining reimbursement for their services. Likewise, the transition to new models of care and **electronic health records** is likely to cause a good deal of frustration and temporary

Aptitude Profile

Many of the attributes that are well suited to the practice of medicine are the same as those for other health professions. Some are unique to medicine; others are linked to specialty choice. For example, being a physician requires a high level of stress tolerance, but one who will specialize in surgery also requires a high degree of manual dexterity. Characteristics associated with high performance in physicians include the following:

Commitment	Humility
Communication Skills	Listening skills
Compassion	Organizational skills
Dedication	Patience
Discipline	Perseverance
Emotional maturity	Self-control
Empathy	Service
Good memory	Tolerance
High ethical standards	Unselfishness
High intelligence	

loss of efficiency. These problems are much more significant for those already in practice than those entering the profession under the new models. Many doctors also believe that increasing reliance on technology threatens the doctor-patient relationship, which they value very highly. Although these threats are real, this author remains convinced that medicine is among the most rewarding of professions.

The Role of the Physician

The physician is the leader of the health-care team whether in a hospital, outpatient clinic, or office practice setting. Traditionally, this role was viewed similarly to the role of a commanding officer in the military; doctors made the decisions and gave orders, and other health professionals carried them out. In some settings, such as the operating room, this model still prevails. In many other areas of medicine, the physician leads the team in a much less hierarchical way. The team members are united in service to the patient, and every voice is respected. The physician draws on the unique expertise and experience of every other member of the team. Under the best of conditions, the voices of the patient and family are also heard and equally respected. Nevertheless, the physician remains responsible for what happens to the patient under his or her care. This is an awesome responsibility and physicians must take it very seriously.

Author Spotlight

Thomas G. Irons, MD

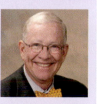

I have practiced and taught pediatrics for over 35 years, and never tire of either. I love children, love medicine, and love to teach. Both teaching and medicine can be very stressful and challenging, but I find that the rewards far outweigh the difficulties. I continually learn from my colleagues in the health professions, my students, and my patients and their families. I feel privileged to be paid for doing what I love.

Working Together

The concept of all members of the health-care team working together for the benefit of the patient has greatly increased opportunities for health professionals to learn more about each other and to freely communicate about optimal patient management. One care model that has emerged recently is that of **integrated care.** The term *integrated* has been used in many ways. In this context, it refers to the integration of biologically-based health care with behavioral health care. The evidence supporting such a model is strong. As many as 60% of all health problems presenting to the primary-care doctor have a behavioral component.[10] For example, in some community health centers in eastern North Carolina, marriage and family therapists work alongside primary-care doctors in the clinic setting. These therapists are uniquely trained to work entirely in the primary-care environment and are termed *medical family therapists.* They work alongside three or four primary-care doctors and nurse practitioners, moving from patient to patient as needed during the workday. Those working in the system on both sides find this arrangement very beneficial for the patients and satisfying for the providers. The **biopsychosocial model** of health, first described by Dr. George Engel decades ago, emphasizes the concept of illness in the context in which it occurs—patient as a *person,* family, and community.[11] It has been widely embraced today, and is one of the major drivers behind the transition to team-based care. Such a model demands that all these things be considered in the care of the patient, with team members working together to improve the likelihood of an optimal outcome for the patient. In the community health center cited in the previous example, social workers, diabetes educators, nutritionists, health educators, advanced practice nurses, nurses, medical office assistants, and the previously described medical family therapists work alongside the physicians and midlevel providers on a daily basis.

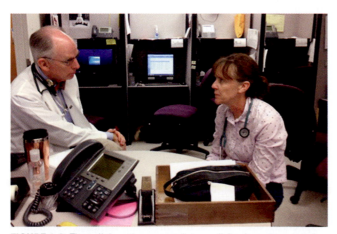

FIGURE 8-3 The collaborative approach to medicine is necessary to improve patients' care. Here, a nurse practitioner presents a case to the physician. They will discuss the best options for quality care and decide on a collaborative plan of care.

CASE STUDY

A 31-year-old immigrant woman, the divorced single parent of two children, presents to a community health center complaining of intermittent chest pain. The children's father lives out of state and provides no child support. Though her two children are insured through Medicaid, she has no health insurance. She has not seen a health-care provider since the postpartum visits after her second child 10 years ago. She works the night shift as a building custodian while a cousin takes care of her children overnight. She does not smoke or drink. She sleeps about 6 hours a day. She admits to eating a great deal of fast food. Her only exercise is her work. There is a family history of diabetes and early death from heart disease. The medical office assistant notes that the patient is moderately obese and that her blood pressure is elevated. She also assists the patient in completing a brief questionnaire designed to screen for depression. The score on the depression screen suggests the patient may have moderate to severe depression. On questioning, she admits to a high level of anxiety about a number of things, both family related and work related. She expresses feelings of loneliness and isolation.

On examination, the doctor notes the elevated blood pressure, obesity, and serious tooth decay. The heart examination is normal, as is the remainder of the general physical. Though she is having no gynecological symptoms, she has not had a Papanicolaou (Pap) smear (test for early signs of cervical cancer) in 9 years, so her physical includes obtaining a Pap smear. The doctor lists the patient's primary problems as obesity, hypertension, dental caries, social isolation, and depression.

The on-site social worker for the health center is called in to briefly interview the patient and to share in the development of a plan of action. A special appointment is made for consultation with a nutritionist, who visits the center weekly. Blood tests to screen for diabetes and elevated cholesterol are drawn. A blood pressure medication is prescribed. The patient is uninsured, so the doctor consults with the pharmacist to make sure that the prescribed medication is the most affordable and effective option.

The social worker recommends an immigrant women's support group that holds evening meetings. Because the community health center offers dental services, a dental appointment is arranged. When the patient expresses concern about cost, the social worker is able to reassure her that the dental clinic's charges are on an income-based sliding scale.

The medical assistant and social worker review the detailed plan with the patient and set a return appointment for 1 month. However, the Pap smear report is abnormal. Urgent gynecological examination and treatment are required. The doctor calls the patient personally, and the social worker follows up with her and makes sure an appointment is made. She further arranges to help the patient with transportation.

At the 1-month follow-up visit, the patient is relieved to report that she has had a successful gynecological procedure. Her blood pressure is under better control and she has been able to modestly improve her diet by eliminating sweet drinks and high-fat snacks. She will see the nutritionist every 2 weeks for weight checks and brief counseling. She has also joined the support group, and reports that she enjoyed the first two sessions. A review of her laboratory tests shows that her cholesterol level is high. The doctor prescribes a cholesterol-lowering agent. Because the medication can have significant side effects, the doctor and later the pharmacist review these with the patient. A follow-up appointment is made. In the interval, the social worker will maintain regular contact with the patient.

Questions

1. What are the factors influencing this woman's health?

2. How do the health professionals in this case work together to address these factors? Why is this important?

3. How would you describe the role of the doctor in this scenario?

4. What ongoing challenges are the patient and health-care team likely to face?

Review Questions

1. A high school graduate pursuing a medical career can expect a minimum of 8 more years of education and training before being eligible for a license to practice medicine.

   A. True
   B. False

2. An allopathic medical school graduate is required to take the three-step U.S. Medical Licensure Examination. An osteopathic medical school graduate is required to take which of the following?

   A. The three-step U.S. Osteopathic Licensure Examination
   B. A one-step osteopathic medical school examination given at the conclusion of medical school
   C. The same examination as an allopathic medical school graduate
   D. An osteopathic medical licensure examination taken after the first year of residency

3. The average 4-year cost of attendance for students at state medical schools in 2011 was estimated at about $100,000.

   A. True
   B. False

4. Which of the following is most accurate? To practice in a medical subspecialty, a medical school graduate must successfully complete:

   A. Residency and fellowship training
   B. Residency training
   C. Fellowship training
   D. Three additional years of training after medical school

5. General surgery is known as a *primary-care* specialty.

   A. True
   B. False

6. The system of payment in which physicians, hospitals, and other health professionals are paid a per-person rate to provide care for a defined population of patients is known as:

   A. Bundled payment
   B. Capitation
   C. Managed care
   D. Socialized medicine

7. A model of health on which team-based care is often based is known as the:

   A. Biological model
   B. Family-centered model
   C. Biopsychosocial model
   D. Cooperative model

8. This chapter uses the term *integrated care* to refer to the collaborative practice of medicine and behavioral health in the primary-care environment.

   A. True
   B. False

9. Most patients' problems can be successfully managed with procedures and/or medication.

   A. True
   B. False

10. Osteopathic physicians, unlike allopathic physicians, receive special training in:

    A. Osteopathic holistic therapy
    B. Osteopathic manipulative therapy
    C. Homeopathic therapy
    D. Chiropractic manipulation

Glossary of Key Terms

Premedical curriculum—the group of courses required for application to medical school

Medical College Admission Test (MCAT)—a four-part standardized, computer-administered examination required for application to medical school

Residency—the required period of graduate medical education subsequent to medical school graduation; duration is variable with a minimum of 3 years

Fellowship—a continuation of training in a subspecialty after residency, which may vary from 1 to several years

Primary care—the group of medical specialties considered to be responsible for a patient's primary medical care, including health supervision, acute illness visits, monitoring and management of chronic diseases, and coordination of specialty care and other health services

Capitation—in health care, a system of payment in which a group of providers ranging from hospitals to physicians is paid for a person's care on an annual, *per-capita* basis

Affordable Care Act—legislation passed by the U.S. Congress and signed into law in March 2012 that dictates a major overhaul in the U.S. health-care system

Electronic health records—secure health records that are entirely electronic and designed to increase consistency and quality of care while reducing medical errors

Integrated care—in the context used in this chapter, the provision of physical and mental health care simultaneously in the primary-care setting

Biopsychosocial model—a model of health care developed by Dr. George Engel that emphasizes the importance of the context in which illness occurs; patient as a *person,* family, and community

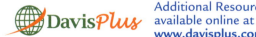 **Additional Resources are available online at www.davisplus.com**

Additional Resources

Accrediting Bodies

- Association of American Medical Colleges
- American Medical Association
- Liaison Committee on Medical Education
- American Osteopathic Association
- Accreditation Council on Graduate Medical Education

Education

- Association of American Medical Colleges
- American Osteopathic Association

State and National Regulating Bodies

- National Board of Medical Examiners
- State Boards of Medical Examiners (all states)
- American Board of Medical Specialties (24 member boards)

References

1. History of Medicine. Wikipedia, The Free Encyclopedia Website.

   http://en.wikipedia.org/wiki/History_of_medicine.
   Accessed October 15, 2013.

2. Cooke M, Irby D, Sullivan W, Ludmerer K. American Medical Education 100 Years after the Flexner Report. *N Engl J Med.* 2006; Sep 28;355(13): 1339–1344.

   http://www.nejm.org/doi/pdf/10.1056/NEJMra 055445.
   Accessed October 15, 2013.

3. Association of American Medical Colleges. Medical College Admission Test (MCAT). Association of American Medical Colleges Website.

   https://www.aamc.org/students/applying/mcat/.
   Accessed October 21, 2013.

4. American Association of Colleges of Osteopathic Medicine. U.S. Colleges of Osteopathic Medicine. American Association of Colleges of Osteopathic Medicine Website.

   http://www.aacom.org/about/colleges/Pages/default.aspx.
   Accessed October 21, 2013.

5. Brewer L, Grbic D, Matthew D. The changing gender composition of U.S. medical school applicants and matriculants. *Analysis in Brief.* 2012;12(1).

   https://www.aamc.org/download/277026/data/aibvol12_no1.pdf.
   Accessed October 21, 2013.

6. Youngclaus J, Fresne, J. Trends in costs and debt at U.S. medical schools using a new measure of medical school costs of attendance. *Analysis in Brief.* 2012;12(2).

   www.aamc.org/download/296002/data/aibvol12_no2.pdf.
   Accessed October 21, 2013.

7. Medscape. Physician compensation report.

   http://www.medscape.com/features/slideshow/compensation/2013/public.
   Accessed November 17, 2013.

8. American Board of Medical Specialties.

   http://www.abms.org/about_abms/member_boards.aspx.

   Accessed October 15, 2013.

9. U.S. Department of Health and Human Services, Health Resources and Services Administration. The physician workforce: projections and research into current issues affecting supply and demand, 2008.

   http://bhpr.hrsa.gov/healthworkforce/reports/physwfissues.pdf.

   Accessed November 18, 2013.

10. Blount A. Organizing the evidence. *Families, Systems, & Health.* 2003;21:121–134.

    http://www.2pcpcc.net/files/organizing_the_evidence_0.pdf.

    Accessed September 7, 2013.

11. Engel GL. The need for a new medical model: A challenge for biomedicine. *Science* 1977;196:129–136. doi:10.1126/science.847460

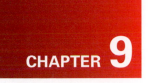

CHAPTER 9

Nursing

Annette Greer, PhD, MSN

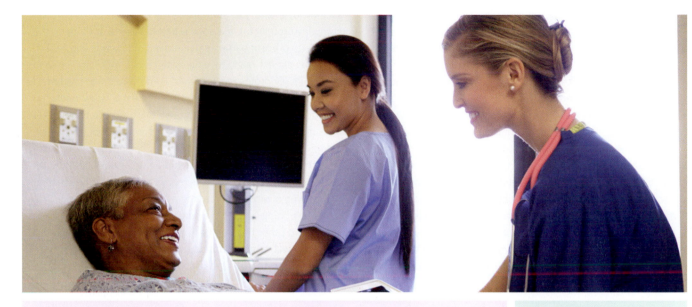

Learning Objectives

After reading this chapter, students should be able to:

- Recognize the historical role of a nurse
- Differentiate between the various types of nurses
- Describe the education and licensing process
- Explain the relationship between nurses and other members of the health-care team
- Discuss opportunities and challenges for working in the field of nursing

Key Terms

- Registered nurse
- Care
- Assessment
- Settings
- Nurse education
- Paradigm
- Nurse specialist
- Credentials

"A Day in the Life"

Hello, my name is Lillian and I am a **registered nurse.** I work in home health **care** and I am off to an interprofessional patient care plan team meeting. I will tell you all about it after the meeting. I also have to provide wound care today that includes a dressing change and a hospice admission. It's going to be a hectic day. Follow me throughout the day to learn the details.

Whew, what a day. I'm in a hurry to get to my wound care patient and hospice visit after this interprofessional team meeting. Physical therapy (PT) will follow up with the wound care; per the latest Centers for Medicaid and Medicare Services (CMS) guidelines, I must teach the family to care for the wound. Having PT assess the wound and the family's ability

to change the bandage will help the team assure quality care and prevent further hospitalization. A care plan meeting sets the process for how the interprofessional team will collaborate to deliver patient care. For the next patient, a social worker has already done an **assessment** for hospice services before hospital discharge. Based on her report, the physician ordered a nursing hospice evaluation in the home. (Hospice care is an end-of-life care service for symptom management and pain relief for those designated to have 6 months or less to live.) Family members are a vital part of the team for hospice, as are spiritual services. The nurse aide and pastoral services will meet me at the home later today, after I have completed the

(continued)

required documentation for hospice admission. Oh, and I have to contact the pharmacy to pick up and deliver the locked controlled substances transport box that secures medications used to manage pain. There is so much teaching involved for the delivery of home health and hospice care. The family really needs the interprofessional support team to manage the care provided to a patient with a complex wound or a patient at end of life.

It is dark out but the day is not done. Let's review the activity of today: (1) interprofessional care plan team conference, (2) wound care admission, (3) hospice admission . . . oh, let me tell you about that one. Well, when I got to the home the family and patient were very fearful and were refusing to go into hospice care. You see, although the social worker had thoroughly discussed hospice care with the family and patient, a well-meaning neighbor had been over to the house and led the family to believe that they were just putting their loved one out to pasture to advance the death in a shorter time period. As a nurse trained in clinical ethics consultation, I was able to help the family to decide how they wanted their family member to "live" during the time remaining based on the estimated prognosis. I started with having them tell me what they would want for their loved one; how they would want the quality of life to be for those final months and days. I explained to the family and patient that research had demonstrated hospice

patients often had a better quality of life and a longer life with a terminal illness, and I assured them that our goal was to help, not to harm. I let them know that the hospice team would be with them as the illness progressed and for a year afterward as well. The pharmacist brought the locked transit box of drugs to the home to regulate pain management for the patient and explained to the family how to use the morphine pump. He assured them that the way it was set and locked they could not kill their loved one, just help relieve the pain. The durable goods company brought out the special bed to assist with turning the patient (to prevent bed sores) and the oxygen tank and regulator. I was almost ready to leave when a daughter came in and started loudly protesting that she did not want her mother to be a "Do Not Resuscitate" (DNR). I was exhausted, thinking I did not have the energy to go through this again. But about that time our pastoral care provider walked in the door, and was I thankful. He was able to take the family aside, counsel and discuss the situation with them, and pray with them, and the resistance to the DNR order was muted. Hospice is about caring for the whole family, not just the patient, and a team approach is valuable. Well, I am home now but don't know for how long. I have two other hospice patients on my list and I am on call tonight. I will go to bed because if they call, I'll need to be rested to provide the needed care. Good night.

Introduction

Nurses in the 21st century are caring critical thinkers educated to perform the most basic tasks as well as the most skilled procedures for managing patient health on individual and population levels. Nurses are taught to approach care with consideration of the whole person—body, mind, and spirit—and to take into account the cultural role of the individual as part of a community. A nurse is educated in multiple **settings,** including hospitals, community colleges, and universities. Thus, a nurse may have various educational levels and increasing scopes of practice based on education, licensure level, practice setting, and additional certification training in a specialty area such as public health. Nurses are typically thought of as practicing in a hospital or physician's office, but they also practice in homes, in community settings, in the military, and even in mobile units used in rural areas. Nurses practice their art and science, using telemonitors to provide care for geographically dispersed patients or populations. Nurses can begin practice at the licensed practical level, advance to registered nurse, and end up in an advanced practice role as a midwife, nurse practitioner, or nurse anesthetist. The pathway to current nursing practice has been a long journey. It is helpful to explore the history of nursing to understand the nursing profession as it is today.

History of Nursing

The profession of nursing has a long and dynamic history of providing care to individuals, families, and communities in many settings, including hospitals, clinics, war zones, and homes. The history of nursing was greatly detailed by Lavinia Dock, a prominent nurse historian during the early 18th century who served as a nurse leader in the United States and on an international basis. According to Dock,[1] the documented history of nursing practice dates back to 300 BC when male priests in India, and later in other nations, cared for the infirm within their communities. In fact, the practice of nursing was historically tied to religious orders within many cultures where men and women held specific roles for care of the sick, mothers and their babies, and those injured in war, and for relief during natural disasters.[1] The association between religious orders and nursing remained strong within most cultures until the Middle Ages when changes in social and civic policies limited the roles of women, causing the decline of various nursing orders tied to religious sects. The Reformation in the 1500s and rise of the Protestant faith did little to advance the profession of nursing.[1] Previously, support for nursing had come from the wealthy monasteries, and with their demise, training for and the value placed on nursing declined. The result was reliance on the illiterate classes of women to care for those in need.[1] This sociological shift created a divide in the practice of medicine and the practice of nursing. However, the connection between the care of the sick, injured, and those in need and the church remained important to the training of physicians and nurses.

From Nurse Apprentice Training to Nurse Education

The development of nursing as a profession occurred over a period of several centuries, and education differed from century to century. Nurse training occurred largely in monastic orders for many years, and the oldest known order was the Sisters of Hotel-Dieu in Paris, whose history is documented as far back as 650 AD.[1] The Reformation closed many orders and subsequently the hospitals they operated. The Reformation then altered the level of training provided to those dedicated to a nursing order, and a culture of modesty changed the ability of nursing to serve as before. Not until St. Vincent de Paul (1576–1660) did a return to training of nurses begin. It was St. de Paul who, in 1633, recruited young women to train under the services of physicians rather than priests and assisted the development of the Sisters of Charity.[1] This movement helped to further establish an educational system for nurses as they were taught "reading, writing, and arithmetic" and were provided lectures given by physicians followed by quizzes.[1]

The revival of nursing education began with Elizabeth Fry, England prison reformist, and Amalie Sieveking, German philanthropist and hospital volunteer. They were instrumental in the formation of a nursing school in Germany known as "Kaiserswerth Motherhouse" under the direction of a young pastor, Theodor Fliedner.[2] At Kaiserswerth in 1836, church deaconesses supervised nursing training. However, theoretical and clinical training was conducted using physician teachers at the hospital and training lasted 3 years.[2] Studies included pharmacy, which required the passing of a state examination; ethics and religious doctrine, taught by Rev. Fliedner; and practical nursing, taught by Mrs. Friederike Fliedner, his wife.[2]

It was at Kaiserswerth that Florence Nightingale, known as the mother of modern nursing, received her training.

Nightingale gleaned much from the structured training of Kaiserswerth, including guidelines for ethics in nursing and practical training for nurses (framed by documentation of Friederike Fliedner). Nursing education at Kaiserswerth included training as a nurse, educator, and manager of care of the elderly and of children, and it included parish visiting that was based on religious studies. Although educated, the graduates of Kaiserswerth became deaconesses and conducted their duties without pay throughout their lives and followed the directives of physicians without question.[1] It is also important to note how the context of time and history influenced the policies for health care over time and, more important, to consider how the context of social and political action influences the practice of nursing today.

Kaiserswerth and Nightingale: Basis for Modern Nursing

Florence Nightingale is celebrated as the founder of modern nursing. The basis of that acclaim is grounded in the skills she learned at Kaiserswerth and communicated through her journal of observations and tasks. Of particular note are those completed during the Crimean War, which resulted in an 830-page report turned book, *Notes on Matters Affecting the Health, Efficiency and Hospital Administration of the British Army* (1858). Born in Italy of an influential family, and raised in England, Florence trained in Germany and served as a nurse in Russia and Turkey. Her broad education and social standing gained her access to influential government officials in Great Britain who came to respect her intelligence, service, and humility. In her book, she demonstrated a 66.7% reduction in mortality rate in the hospital where she and her nurses worked.[1,3]

Throughout her nursing career, Nightingale advocated for the use of statistical analysis based on practice observations, an important contribution to advances in nursing and public health. Nightingale instituted sanitation interventions during the war that, along with her book, resulted in the formation of the Royal Commission for the Health of the Army. For her nursing service, Nightingale was awarded £50,000, funding she used to establish the Nightingale Training School for Nurses at St. Thomas' Hospital.[1,3]

Tips and Tools

Learn more about the history of nursing from its earliest beginnings until the 1920s. *A Short History of Nursing* by Lavinia L. Dock is available online through Google Books. It is important that nurses of today study the history of nursing to appreciate the relationship of the profession to other disciplines such as clergy and medicine.

The Influence of Kaiserswerth on Nurse Education in the United States

In 1849, the Kaiserswerth influence reached the shores of the United States. The Kaiserswerth influence arrived first through the Lutheran Pastor founder Fliedner, who, at the request of Reverend William Passavant, helped to deliver

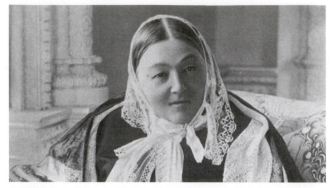

FIGURE 9-1 Florence Nightingale (photography by Lizzie Caswall Smith, 1910).

several trained nurse deaconesses to the Lutheran German Parish in Pittsburg, Pennsylvania.[4] From 1862 through 1873, several nursing schools opened in America using the Nightingale mode (enhanced and expanded from the Kaiserswerth model) and were located in Massachusetts General in Boston, Bellevue Hospital in New York, and New Haven in Connecticut. Next, through the auspices of Norway's Kaiserswerth program, Elizabeth Fedde (a Kaiserswerth graduate) opened nursing programs across the Northeast and Midwestern United States, including Brooklyn, New York, and Minneapolis, Minnesota; and she provided the impetus for hospitals in Chicago, Illinois, and Grand Forks, North Dakota. The

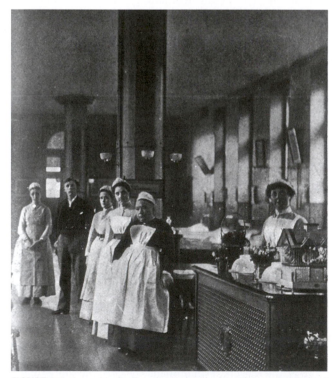

FIGURE 9-2 A ward in St. Thomas' Hospital, after the establishment of the training school. (From The National Library of Medicine, History of Medicine Collection. Created by Mary Adelaide Nutter, author. Contributed by Lavinia L. Dock.)

Mary Seacole

At the same time that Nightingale was serving in the Crimean War, a minority nurse, although less formally educated, rose to prominence. Unlike Nightingale, who was appointed by the War Office in England to be Superintendent of Hospital Nurses in the East, Jamaican-born Mary Seacole had to finance her own way to Crimea with help from friends and family.[11] Setting up a hotel near the war front, she supplied goods to the war effort and provided nursing services on the front lines. Seacole's training had come from her Jamaican-born mother, a traditional medicine healer. Seacole was known in her own country as a doctress and nurse; she became known to Crimean troops as "Mother Seacole." She received recognition after the war by commanders of the British Army, who held a benefit on her behalf to assist with debt acquired serving in war efforts. Seacole also produced a book titled *The Wonderful Adventures of Mrs. Seacole, 1857.* Learn more about Mrs. Seacole and other famous black nurses at http://www.100greatblackbritons.com/bios/mary_seacole.html.

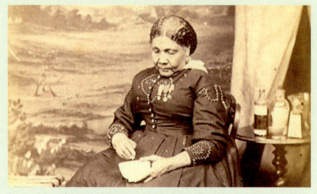

Nurse Mary Seacole (photography by Mary Evans).

movement then swept America as more women in training were recruited into a religious order, forming "deaconess orders" beckoning unmarried women of strong moral character.[5] These educated women were instrumental in similar fashion to Florence Nightingale in their influence on policies improving health conditions of the poor, women, children, and the elderly—efforts that employed the principles of sanitation, hygiene, and public health. The first black nursing graduate was Mary Mahoney, who graduated from New England Hospital in 1879. The same year, Spelman Seminary in Atlanta, Georgia, opened a nursing school specifically for black women.[3] Church influence on the development of nursing continued in the United States as orders of nursing deaconesses were created by German Protestants, Methodists, Presbyterians, and Mennonites. By 1915, a total of 62 schools of nursing had been opened in America.[1] Within this church influence a link between nursing care responsibility to the spiritual and physical/mental well-being of persons was established.

The Influence of War on Nursing

Religious affiliations had a profound influence on the development of nursing, as did war. From 1861 to 1865, the American Civil War had a profound influence on nursing practice in America.[3] Women, white and black, trained and untrained, served as nurses for troops on both sides of the Civil War. Those most notable included enlisted Army nurses such as Dorothea Dix, who served as Superintendent of Union Army nurses, and Mary Ann Bickerdyke, another Union Army nurse who focused on sanitization of Union military hospitals in the face of horrific war conditions. Some of the nurses during the era of the war became recognized for their literary works, such as Walt Whitman, male Union Army nurse who was a famous American author and poet, and Louisa May Alcott, who used humor to depict her experiences working as a hospital volunteer nurse in the Civil War.[3] Many "volunteer nurses" included individuals such as Clara Barton, the founder and first president of the American Red Cross; Harriet Tubman, a former slave who used her knowledge of herbs and home remedies to treat soldiers; and Kate Cumming, who published a journal that chronicled the practices of medicine, nursing, and Confederate hospital care. Hospitals in the United States became the leading location for **nurse education** in the late 19th century, and nursing students provided patient care as part of their education.[3] Use of nursing students to provide patient care became an economic means for hospital economic viability. Segregation in some areas of the United States affected the ability to train nurses of color because few hospitals were dedicated to the care of black Americans. Nurse training schools kept track of enrollment, and military nurses were provided identification that noted their status; however, no licensure or regulatory standards for nursing practice were yet established during the late 1800s.[3]

The Great Depression and Immigration's Influence on Nursing

As immigrants arrived at Ellis Island looking for a better life, they brought with them limited resources, settled in overcrowded cities, and demonstrated other social issues, including poverty, poor sanitation, and poor nutritional status, which were less than ideal to the support of health and well-being. In the following decades, the rapid explosion of population combined with factory employment and the population movement into cities resulted in great needs for public health care. The 19th Amendment granted women voting rights in 1920, and this signaled an increasing cultural value of the role of women in society.[3]

From 1920 through the early 1940s, women dominated nursing, with male nurses usually limited to war efforts. Feminist policies helped to move nursing education into new territories, as women served in greater organizational roles to advocate social reforms, including those meant to advance the care of women and children. These efforts, occurring within the sociopolitical context of the times, meant that nursing care started to move from the war front

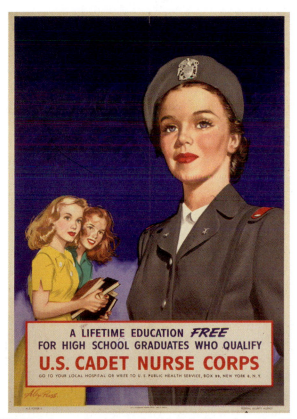

FIGURE 9-3 Poster advertising for the U.S. Cadet Nurse Corps circa World War II. (From The National Library of Medicine, History of Medicine Collection. Contributed by Ross Alexander and the U.S. Federal Security Agency.)

and hospitals to the community and to homes. Public health nursing became an emerging field pursued by practitioners known as "visiting nurses."

An organization that led in recommending changes to nursing education in the early 1900s was the American Society of Superintendents of Training Schools for Nurses, later to become the National League for Nursing. The organization consisted of Canadian and U.S. nursing training schools that were intent on advancing roles in nursing leadership. Sigma Theta Tau, the honor society of nursing, formed in 1922.[3] During this era, nursing education began to move from the hospitals into the university setting. This movement shifted the **paradigm** of the nurse, from "aid to the physician" toward a notion of nurse as researcher, educator, and essentially a more independent practitioner. The dissemination of the Flexner Report in 1912,[6] which called for more formal and structured education within medicine, provided momentum to funding of the Goldmark Report in 1923.[7] The Goldmark Report recommended that the training of nurses center on an academic education within a university setting, rather than an apprenticeship model caring for patients in a hospital. Further, it recommended that educational standards be set and that nurse educators receive advanced education. Finally, in the early 1930s, the Association of Collegiate Schools of Nursing was formed.[3] Thus, over the next century nursing education slowly moved into academic educational settings. Even so, the move has been tumultuous. In the 21st century, hospital-based education still exists at the diploma level; community college or associate degree education and university bachelor and master's degree education all provide an entry level for nursing students to qualify for the licensure examination to become a registered nurse.

Scope of Practice

The scopes of practice for nurses relate directly to the education and licensure of the individual and the requirements of the state. More than any other health profession, nursing features great variability in educational qualifications for the entrance examination for licensure.[8] Additionally, state and federal laws regulate nursing practice. These laws have the authority to place restrictions and limitations or greater expansion on scopes of practice based on certifications. In the next section of this chapter, we begin with the multiple educational entry points that allow for the initial licensure examination. Next, we discuss advanced-practice education and the additional licensure required for that level of clinical practice.

Nursing scopes of practice include the following authorized tasks allowed through licensure of registered nurses.

- Assess and record physical and mental health history of the patient.
- Provide nursing diagnoses for the care of illness, injury, disability, and end of life.
- Evaluate nursing and other team care.
- Administer medications and treatments.
- Establish nursing care plans and care management with the health team (see Fig. 9-5).
- Provide case management and quality assurance measures.
- Measure/record and trend vital signs and symptoms.
- Collaborate with the health team on delivery of needed procedures (e.g., oxygen or heart monitor).
- Consult and advocate for patients' legal and ethical rights.
- Counsel and provide patient/family education.
- Engage in policy development and revision.
- Employ private practice skills.
- Provide referral assistance.
- Supervise and lead other nursing staff or unlicensed personnel.

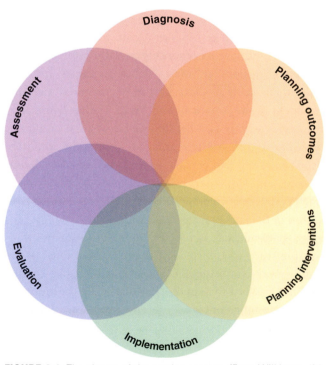

FIGURE 9-4 The phases of the nursing process. (From Wilkinson JM, Treas LS. *Fundamentals of Nursing,* vol. 1, second edition. Philadelphia: FA Davis; 2011, p. 33.)

CARE PLAN TITLE: Self-Care Deficit Dressing and Grooming

Related Factors: Neuromuscular impairment, immobility: weakness

Defining Characteristics: Unable to use hands to fasten clothing, unable to open dressers to obtain clothing, unable to stretch to get clothing on and off, unable to address hygiene needs, unable to groom.

Expected Outcomes: Demonstrate ability to cope with the necessity of having someone else assist him/her in performing the task of self-care for dressing and grooming. Allow independence in ability to conduct some level of activity as long as feasible.

Ongoing Assessment: Choose clothing that is loose fitting, with wide sleeves and pant legs, and uses elastic in waist to increase independence in doing as much as possible.
Lay clothes out in the order in which they will be needed to dress to decrease need to acquire clothing from dresser.
Assess every day and report for improvement, maintenance, or decline.

Therapeutic Interventions: Consult/refer to PT/OT for teaching how to strengthen muscle and increase ability to self-dress and groom. Make consistent dressing/grooming routine to provide a structured program to decrease confusion.

Education/Continuity of Care: Plan for person to learn and demonstrate one part of an activity before progressing further to decrease frustration and fatigue. As ability declines adjust level of assistance.

FIGURE 9-5 An example of a nursing care plan.

Required Education

As previously noted, nursing practice has tiered levels of entry into practice with some variation by state. Thus, there is variability of nursing practice that is closely tied to the education of students seeking a nursing credential. Few hospital-based diploma programs remain, and most are tied to college programs that provide seamless access to a bachelor's degree. Community colleges offer programs for licensed practical nursing and registered nursing, the latter resulting in a 2-year associate degree. Universities offer a bachelor's degree in nursing but also have alternate entry programs for registered nurses seeking advanced education. There are also university alternate entry programs that allow individuals with other bachelor's degrees in fields such as biology or nutrition to enter into a nursing program for a second bachelor's degree in nursing. Completion of these nursing education programs qualifies the student to take the National Council Licensure Examination for Registered Nurses (NCLEX-RN). Once the examination is passed, the state grants the individual a registered license to practice that in some states but not all, and it must be renewed every 2 years with evidence of continuing education units. Some states form compacts with other states allowing the endorsement of state-registered nursing licenses from one state to another.[8] For nurses employed in the military, there is a national licensure endorsement that allows them to work across state and national lines of authority.

Nurses with a registered license and a nursing bachelor's degree are eligible to enroll in a nursing master's program. Master's degrees in nursing have traditionally focused on nursing education (CNE), clinical **nurse specialist** (CNS), nurse practitioner (ANP), nurse anesthesia (CNA), or midwife (CNM). Doctoral programs have focused on doctor of nursing science, philosophy of nursing, and, most recently, the doctor of nursing practice. The acuity level of patients and the advancement of science and technologies in patient care continue to require greater advancements in nursing education. Master's degree nurses in advanced practice often have to take additional certification and/or licensure examinations to qualify for expanded practice. Advanced nursing practice examinations are administered through the Medical Board of Examiners and the Board of Pharmacy for CNA, ANP, and CNM. Accrediting agencies administer certification examinations for CNE and CNS.[8]

Professional nurses have a basic education in the sciences, including biology, organic chemistry and biochemistry, human anatomy, physiology, and microbiology. Core courses one might expect to take to qualify for the NCLEX include the following:

- Introduction to Professional Nursing
- Nursing Research (Methods and Statistics)
- Pharmacotherapeutics

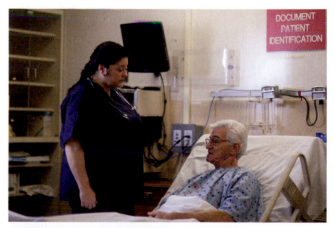

FIGURE 9-6 Some nursing programs participate in an Office of Clinical Skills and Assessment Education (OCSAE) program that uses standardized patients. This figure portrays how standardized patient rooms are set up to simulate those of a clinic. Standardized patients are actors trained to represent a character with a designated disease process. (Photo from Hull M: *Medical Language: Terminology in Context*. Philadelphia: FA Davis, 2013; p. 191.)

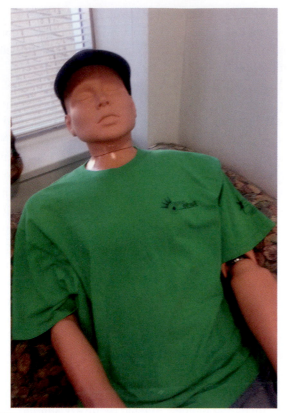

FIGURE 9-7   Modern nurse training uses simulators such as Rescue Randy to develop initial skills.

- Health Assessment
- Ethics and Sociology
- Clinical Nursing Foundations
- Pathophysiology
- Nursing Care of Populations, Children, and Older Adults
- Trends and Issues in Nursing
- Nursing Capstones and Clinical Projects

Salary

The average salary range for nurses varies according to specific area of practice, level of education, and advanced licensure status. According to the Bureau of Labor Statistics, the median annual salary range across all registered nurses regardless of education, setting, or advanced licensure status is $65,470. Nurses working in physicians' offices or in nursing/residential care homes earn less on average, between a mean range of $58,420 and $58,830. Nurses working in home health, hospital, or government settings earn a mean range of $62,090 to $68,540. Those working in settings where there are night, weekend, and shift hours often receive compensation in the form of child care, educational benefits, or shift incentives. Those working in school systems or offices

where the hours are more structured are less likely to receive the same level of incentives, and thus generally make less pay. It is important to note that women still dominate the nursing workforce and that 20% work on a part-time basis. Although the proportion of men in the nursing profession is increasing at a steady rate (from 6.6% in 2008 to 11% in 2010), female predominance in the profession since the time of Nightingale has resulted in a distinct bias that is only now being addressed. Similarly, there are efforts to recruit more minority students to nursing. A diverse nursing workforce is needed to meet the needs of a diverse population of care.

Trends

The profession of nursing is expected to grow 19% from 2012 to 2020, and nurses in advanced practice will grow 20% in numbers during the same time frame. The aging population statistics for that period of time and the technological advances for managing chronic diseases are indicators that geriatric care will represent an area of considerable growth in health care. This wave of elderly persons will comprise 17% of the total population in 2020. Elderly chronic disease has resulted in an increase in health-care costs, policy changes in terms of length of hospital stays, and transitions of care from hospital to more ambulatory settings or the home. More procedures for care will be provided in outpatient units, with discharge back to home, long-term care, or residential units. The nursing workforce will increasingly shift from hospital-based to community-based settings of practice. In addition, public health nursing and wellness promotion/illness prevention will become a primary trend for the nursing workforce.

Challenges

Moral distress is one of the most prevalent challenges in nursing today, as is nursing work fatigue. *Moral distress* is defined as a situation when there is ethical conflict and one knows the right action to take to resolve the situation but feels restrained from taking that right action. There are often multiple ethical and justifiable actions that can be taken in any given ethical conflict, but in moral distress those choices are in opposition with one another. The ethical conflict can be internal to the person. That is, opposing actions are weighed in light of the moral values of the individual. Moral distress is one of the major causes for job burnout in the nursing profession. Nurses lacking confidence in their abilities, feeling anxiety regarding actions that need to be taken, or who are fearful of a perceived need to take actions that might result in job loss may feel moral distress. The ethical conflict can be a situation between or among individuals when the values within or across professions differ regarding a health-care decision or action. In such cases, the moral distress is based on a feeling of powerlessness that might be due to health-care team power differentials, poor team communication, cost reductions and patient decisions being based on a financial rather than humanistic rationale, or fear of reprisals from legal or administrative entities.

An example of moral conflict resulting in moral distress could be when a new medical resident on night duty writes a medication order for patient care that the experienced nurse knows will result in a contraindication for an already prescribed medication. Although this is a teachable moment, if there is a cultural difference in gender or race that creates a power imbalance (e.g., the resident is an Iranian male and the nurse is a young, assertive American female), the resident may take cultural offense that the female nurse should challenge his medical authority to make a change in the order. Thus, the resident may feel conflicted in changing the order even though it is the right thing to do because he feels that making the change would cause him (relative to his culture) to lose respect in making the order change at the demand of a female nurse. The nurse, on the other hand, may know she needs to bring the change in the medication order to the resident's attention, but may hesitate, knowing that cultural and authoritative power structures may offend him, causing even greater conflict. The nurse and the resident both have justifiable opinions about what is the right action to take, the right medication to prescribe; but without interprofessional training in how to engage in open communication, moral distress may occur. Moral distress results in a threat to one's moral integrity. The outcome could be that the nurse lapses into conflict-avoidance behavior, experiences an increase in personal illness, seeks other employment to escape the environment, or becomes impersonal and uncaring in delivery of nursing duties.

Another challenge in nursing is fatigue, which involves more than mere sleepiness. Fatigue is an overwhelming feeling of tiredness that negatively affects the alertness and ability of the nurse to perform duties. Nursing work-shift patterns and hours of work within a 7-day period can be scheduled in such a manner that the nurse approaches a point of exhaustion, especially if burdened with other life roles outside of nursing duties. Insufficient sleep, extended

Aptitude Profile

A nursing career requires intellectual aptitude in math and science but also physical dexterity to use technical equipment and agility to mobilize patients. Individuals seeking to become a nurse also need emotional intelligence.[10] *Emotional intelligence* is the manner in which a nurse uses his or her feelings in a positive manner in care of the patient. Emotional intelligence nursing characteristics are listed in the accompanying table.

Emotional Intelligence Nursing Characteristics

Self-awareness	Self-confident, self-assessor, emotional awareness
Self-regulation	Self-control, trustworthiness, conscientiousness, innovativeness, and adaptability
Self-motivation	Achievement-driven, commitment, initiative, optimism
Social awareness	Empathy, service-oriented, respectful, political awareness
Social skills	Influence, collaborative, team functioning, leadership, communicating

work hours, and consecutive shifts can all impair a nurse's cognitive and physical functions, resulting in an increase in patient care errors. Geiger-Brown and colleagues[9] report that there is a direct correlation between the lack of sleep and quality of care delivered by nurses with fatigue. There is a need to increase interventions to assist in improving quality nursing care through policy provisions that would allow naps during lunch or breaks, limit work hours, and limit the number of consecutive scheduled shifts for improved work safety. Bright lighting and moderate use of caffeine stimulants during evening and night shifts are other recommended interventions.

The Role of the Licensed Practical Nurse and Nurse Aide

Nurses can have different **credentials** that provide insight into their scope of practice that varies by the level of credential and the authority providing credentials. States legislate the credentialing of nurses through a nurse practice act that is regulated by boards of nursing. Other credentials are awarded through advanced degree status from colleges or universities and from accrediting bodies that substantiate skills and knowledge. The following sections provide information regarding the various levels of credentialing across the practice of nursing.[8]

Tips and Tools

Learn more about moral distress, how to recognize it, and how to address it on YouTube: UK Moral Distress Project (https://www.youtube.com/watch?v=QdPmloh4XMk).

Nurses provide supervision to licensed practical nurses and nurse aides. The licensed practical nurse (LPN) or licensed vocational nurse (LVN) does not make independent decisions in nursing practice. Rather, the LPN is a vocational program of basic nursing skills, and the practical nurse implements the plan of nursing care designed by the registered nurse. The LPN receives education at community colleges that offer nursing programs. The LPN is authorized to supervise nurse aides and personal care assistants under the care plan prepared by the registered nurse. The nurse aide is certified by the division of facility services in some states and by nursing in other states. Regardless, the training for nurse aide care is performed and supervised by registered nurses. Nurse aides are competent to assist in taking vital signs, provide personal care, and assist the patient with activities of daily living. Boards of nursing keep registries of the individuals certified as nurse aides. Some states allow advanced training of nurse aides to perform procedures such as wound care or suctioning of patients on ventilators. Close nursing supervision and review of nurse aide documentation for patient management are required.

The Role of Registered Nurses

As indicated earlier, nurses have many pathways to become a registered nurse.[8] However, given recent policy changes, those pathways will eventually all lead to a bachelor of science degree in nursing (BSN). The role of the registered nurse with a BSN is to provide leadership in patient care. Regardless of the work environment, the registered nurse establishes a nursing plan of care and collaborates with the health-care team to ensure that care is patient-centered with unified goals to obtain or maintain the optimum health for that patient. A difference between the associate degree registered nurse (ADN) and the bachelor of science registered nurse is the level of responsibility and authority in nursing practice. Although both will direct patient care using the nursing process, the BSN will also provide care to more complex patients who have multiple diagnoses. The practice structure of the BSN is more autonomous, having a strong theoretical base that allows the BSN to apply critical thinking to the decision-making process of care. In patient interactions, the communication expectations of ADN and BSN are comparable; however, the BSN is educated to coordinate a complex communication network across the interprofessional team. Patient education is a function of the ADN and BSN registered nurse with the BSN being accountable for the design of patient education materials. In terms of nursing research, ADN and BSN nurses can interpret and apply evidence-based practice concepts to improve quality of care and both

may engage in collection of data under supervision of advanced nurses. Nevertheless, the BSN is expected to contribute ideas and resources in collaboration with the research team. The organization, management, and accountability of patient care are similar for the ADN and the BSN; again, the difference is the level of complexity, teaching of peers beyond supervision, and follow-up beyond immediate patient care that the BSN is able to provide.[8]

Registered nurses receiving additional education within their institution or through a professional accrediting organization, and who work in a specialized setting for a specified number of hours, can receive certification in that specialized area of nursing. For instance, oncology nursing, occupational nursing, maternal-child nursing, and public health nursing are all areas of specialization.[8]

The Role of the Advanced Practice Nurse

The advanced practice nurse requires a minimum of a master's degree in nursing.[8] It is the concentration of study that determines the pathway of the nurse in advanced practice. Concentrations as previously mentioned may be nurse practitioner, nurse midwife, nurse anesthetist, nurse educator, or clinical nurse specialist. The nurse practitioner, nurse midwife, and nurse anesthetist are registered licensed nurses with a master's degree level of education that use advanced assessment skills and specialized procedures for practice. Advanced practice nurses are required to pass pharmaceutical board examinations to administer and/or prescribe medications within their specialized area of training when serving as a primary-care practitioner. Further, they must be licensed with the medical board of the state of practice. Nurse practitioners can further specialize in geriatric, pediatric, adult, or family health, similar to a medical specialist. The nurse midwife provides maternal care through the delivery of the newborn for uncomplicated births. The nurse anesthetist administers and monitors medications used during surgical or other invasive procedures under the direction of a doctor of anesthesiology.[8]

The nurse educator and clinical nurse specialist also have master's degrees but do not require further license beyond registered nurse status. Rather, they get additional certification from an accrediting professional organization that administers an examination. The certified nurse educator has education in educational theory and strategies of teaching-learning that augment the ability to teach in college settings. The clinical nurse specialist is a leader in the area of specialization chosen for a practice area and is a registered nurse with experience in the particular area of concentration.[8]

The Role of the Doctorally Prepared Nurse

There is greater diversity of preparation for nursing at the doctoral level. For nurses with an existing master's degree, the career pathways at the doctoral level have typically led to research or practice. Traditionally, the doctor of philosophy (PhD) in nursing is a degree that prepares the nurse for research and/or a career in academia at the college or university level. The research could be at a theoretical level or at an applied clinical level to expand the science and art of nursing. Usually, the academic career choice is based on the specialty level of interest or practice within nursing. However, registered nurses have also obtained doctor of science in nursing (DScN) or doctor of nursing science (DNSc), which are similar in preparing the nurse for leadership roles in research and practice at the applied level. Most recently, the doctor of nursing practice (DNP) has emerged. This degree may eventually replace the nurse practitioner master's degree. Rather than taking 2 years in a master's program and then an additional 3 to 4 years for a PhD, the DNP will be a post-bachelor's professional degree. As with the medical, physical therapy, and pharmacy doctorate degrees, the focus of the DNP will be practice at the highest level of competency and independence.[8]

Author Spotlight

Annette Greer, PhD, MSN

Dr. Annette Greer began her career working the rural tobacco, corn, soybean, and other crops grown in the coastal plains of North Carolina where she was an integrated pest management scout. Greer has associate degrees in agriculture science and business and specializes in rural health, having served 10 years on the National Cancer Institutes and National Institutes of Health Agriculture Health Study Advisory Board. "Nursing is exciting and allows you to grow in many directions over a lifetime in the profession. You will never be bored!" Dr. Greer demonstrates that statement as she has worked in medical intensive care, emergency departments, rural clinics, and home health-care environments. Further, she has worked as a telehealth nurse. Dr. Greer has completed postdoctoral certificate programs in global health and in health-care ethics. She is currently employed in the Department of Bioethics and Interdisciplinary Studies and certified as an "Agrisafe Nurse." She is a faculty affiliate with the North Carolina Agromedicine Institute.

Working Together

Nurses in the hospital setting work with many disciplines and health professionals. The physician issues medical diagnoses and prescribes a medical plan of care, which the nurse and other health professionals adhere to in the delivery of comprehensive integrated care. The disciplines that the physician may include with the nurse as part of the care team are social work, physical therapy, nutrition, occupational therapy, pharmacy, health education, respiratory therapist, and radiation technician, among others. In the hospital setting these health professionals are in close proximity and work parallel to one another in most cases, each with their own plan of care but also in collaborative teams that provide care in a cohesive manner in a unified plan of care.

The nurse in the hospital setting often serves the patient at the bedside or provides direct patient care, as well as coordinating the activity of the care team. It is important for each health profession to understand the scope of practice for those who are part of the health-care team. Each health profession has unique skills that only they can do, but they also have multiple tasks that overlap. Understanding the areas of unique practice and those that overlap helps to prevent redundancy in care and reduces the cost of duplication in care. Further, clear and consistent communication across the health-care team reduces medical errors. Use of nurses to coordinate communication is often augmented by technological systems that allow for an integrated plan of care across the health professions.

In home care, the nurse still operates under the direction of physician orders but is not in close proximity to team members, so the practice is more autonomous and requires greater coordination. Technological systems help the nurse to bridge the gap of distance in collaborating with other health professions. The nurse is usually the one to report to the physician the need for other health professions to be added to the regimen of care. Regardless of setting, a relationship of trust, respect, and dependability is required among the health-care team. In advanced practice as a family, geriatric, adult, or pediatric nurse practitioner, the nurse may be the individual who writes the medical orders that provide guidance to the health-care team for care of noncomplex patient populations.

CASE STUDY

Eleanor is a 67-year-old former nursing professor living in a progressive care retirement center in California. She never married but does have family members living in Oregon and Nevada; however, she has not retained a close relationship with them. Her decision to remain in

(continued)

California was based on the relationship she shared with her academic peers within the department of nursing. Eleanor has a close female companion who has shared much of her life, but current law does not recognize the relationship as legally binding. Eleanor was diagnosed and treated 5 years ago (age 62) for breast cancer that resulted in bilateral mastectomy and removal of lymph nodes by a surgical oncologist. Her state insurance allows her to receive the best care available but has lifetime limits on expenditures, and the hospital social worker has been the case manager coordinating care with the insurance company. Eleanor decided that she wanted reconstructive breast surgery and had complications from a hospital-acquired infection that resulted in additional surgery and the need for an infectious disease consultation. Eleanor returned to work until a year ago, when she was diagnosed with brain cancer and was told that it was related to the spread of the breast cancer from lymph nodes before her first breast cancer surgery. She began aggressive radiation therapy (delivered by a radiation oncologist) followed by chemotherapy, and had complications from the port used to infuse the chemotherapy. This complication resulted in the need to move the port to another location in her left chest and to place her on outpatient infusions of high-dose antibiotics. Eleanor is asked by the palliative care nurse if she has a living will and a health-care power of attorney.

Questions

1. What are pressing ethical issues facing Eleanor?

2. What professions can you identify that have probably been involved with Eleanor's care?

3. Why is interprofessional collaboration important in this case?

4. Develop an interprofessional plan of care based on your knowledge from other chapters.

5. What are ultimately the goals for Eleanor's nursing palliative care if the doctor determines she only has 6 months to live?

6. What level of nursing care can Eleanor expect if her insurance reaches the maximum allowed and she is placed on disability insurance?

Review Questions

1. The nursing profession started in India with:

   A. Male priests

   B. Male slaves

   C. Female priestesses

   D. Female slaves

2. One of the most common challenges in the nursing profession is job burnout, and one of the causes is:

   A. Fatigue

   B. Dissatisfaction

   C. Moral distress

   D. Both A and C

3. Nurses work in the following settings:

   A. Hospitals

   B. Elementary schools

   C. Military

   D. All of the above

4. Qualifications to take the NCLEX-RN examination to become a registered nurse include education at the following levels:

   A. Diploma and associate degree

   B. Diploma, associate degree, bachelor's degree, alternate entry

   C. Diploma, associate degree, bachelor's degree

   D. Diploma, associate degree, bachelor's degree, doctoral degree

5. Nursing characteristics of emotional intelligence include:

   A. Prospective attitude

   B. Servant-centered attitude

   C. Self-awareness

   D. Math and science

6. The activity that exceeds registered nursing scope of practice is:

   A. Prescribing controlled substances for pain management

   B. Administering medications ordered for managing diabetes

   C. Assessing physical and mental status of the patient

   D. Recording vital signs and tracking trends

7. The courses required for entry into nursing programs include (select all correct answers):

   A. Biochemistry

   B. Anthropology

   C. Physiology

   D. Microbiology

8. Which of the following advanced practice nurses does not require additional state licenses to practice?

   A. Nurse practitioner

   B. Nurse midwife

   C. Nurse anesthetist

   D. Clinical nurse specialist

9. Individuals who want to conduct and teach nursing research in university settings usually hold this degree in nursing:

    A. BSN

    B. MSN

    C. PhD

    D. ADN

10. Which of the following are not a minority in nursing?

    A. White males

    B. Black males

    C. White females

    D. Hispanic females

Glossary of Key Terms

Registered nurse—nurse who is authorized by a board of nursing in a given state to function in the role of nurse and is held accountable to the nurse practice act of the given state

Care—both a verb and a noun: as a verb, care is the provision of human activity from one to another human being to acquire, sustain, or improve on health status, well-being, and safety; as a noun, care defines the manner in which the human activity is delivered (e.g., critical care, hospice care, pediatric care, home care) and is often associated with a setting of care delivery

Assessment—the activity of a nurse to determine the status of the patient's health

Settings—the locations of nurse practice or the nurse practice environment

Nurse education—refers to the educational requirements from academic and clinical settings required to meet the standards for qualifying for nursing practice as a licensed, registered, or advance practice nurse

Paradigm—way of thinking; moving from a traditional norm into a new pattern

Nurse specialist—a nurse who specializes in specific areas of nursing practice through concentrated education and clinical experience; often designated through various accrediting bodies after passing competency tests and validating hours dedicated to the specific area of practice (e.g., public health nurses, oncology nurse specialist, occupational nurse specialist)

Credentials—document or certification that signifies the level of education, knowledge, and skills needed to safely execute the duties of a nurse

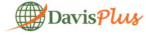

Additional Resources are available online at www.davisplus.com

Additional Resources

American Nurses Association—www.nursingworld.org

Health Resources Services Administration: Bureau of Health Professions/Nursing—http://bhpr.hrsa.gov/nursing/

National League for Nursing—www.nln.org/aboutnln/index.htm

Interagency Council on Information Resources in Nursing—www.icirn.org/default.aspx

National Student Nurse Association—www.nsna.org

National Council of Boards of Nursing—www.ncsbn.org/index.htm

References

1. Dock L. *A Short History of Nursing.* New York and London: Putnam & Sons; 1920. Retrieved from Google Books.

2. Donahue MP. *Nursing: The Finest Art,* 2nd ed. St. Louis, MO: Mosby; 1996.

3. Judd D, Sitzman K. *A History of American Nursing: Trends and Eras.* Burlington, MA: Jones & Bartlett; 2014.

4. Kinnieult E. Kaiserswerth and its founder. In *The Century Magazine,* vol 21. London: The De Vinne Press, McMillan & Co.; 1896. Retrieved from Google Books.

5. Folkedahl B. *Elizabeth Fedde's Diary.* 1888. Retrieved from Google Books.

6. Flexner A. *Medical Education in Europe: A Report to the Carnegie Foundation for the Advancement of Teaching.* New York; 1912.

7. Goodrich A, Nutting A, Wald L. *The Goldmark Report.* Rockefeller Foundation; 1923.

   http://doc.med.yale.edu/nursing/historical/images/goldmarkreport.html.

   Accessed August 18, 2014.

8. American Nurses Association. *Nursing: Scope and Standards of Practice,* 2nd ed. Washington, DC: American Nurses Association; 2010.

9. Geiger-Brown J, Rogers VE, Trinkoff AM, Kane RL, Bausell RB, Scharf, SM. Sleep, sleepiness, fatigue, and

performance of 12-hour-shift nurses. *Chronobiology Int.* 2012;29(2):211–219.

10. Mhalkar V, George LS, Nayak AK. Relationship between emotional intelligence and coping strategies among baccalaureate nursing students: An evaluative study. *Indian J Health Wellbeing.* 2014;5(11): 1291–1295.

11. Seacole M. *The Wonderful Adventures of Mrs. Seacole, 1857.* London: Thomas Herrild Printer; 1857. Retrieved from digital.library.upenn.edu.

12. McDonald L, ed. *The Collected Works of Florence Nightingale.* Waterloo, Ontario, Canada: Wilfrid Laurier University Press; 2009. Retrieved from Google Books.

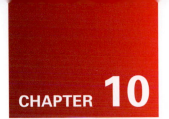

CHAPTER 10

Pharmacy

Doyle M. Cummings, PharmD, FCP, FCCP

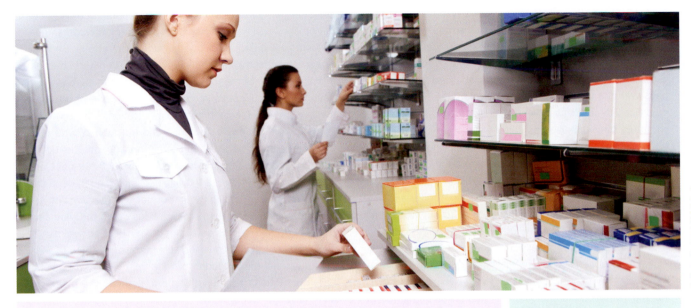

Photo credit: istock/Thinkstock

Learning Objectives

After reading this chapter, students should be able to:

- Explain the role of a pharmacist and a pharmacy technician
- Identify different work settings and responsibilities for pharmacists/technicians
- Describe the education and licensing process
- Explain the relationship between pharmacists and other members of the health-care team
- Discuss opportunities and challenges for working in the field of pharmacy

Key Terms

- Community pharmacy
- Hospital pharmacy
- Long-term care pharmacy
- Pharmaceutical industry
- Clinical pharmacy practitioner

"A Day in the Life"

Hello, my name is Crystal and I am a hospital pharmacist. I work in a large hospital next to the intensive care unit with critically ill patients who have heart disease and I am off to morning rounds with the patient care team, and then back to the pharmacy satellite. Our pharmacy is decentralized with small pharmacies called "satellite pharmacies" located next to patient care areas, allowing me more opportunity to have a direct impact on patient care. I'll tell you all about the patients in this area of the hospital and how we work to optimize their medications. It's going to be a busy day. Join me later on for details.

Welcome back. I only have a few minutes to catch you up on my day. Rounds with the patient care team in our cardiovascular unit here at the hospital went really well this morning. Our interprofessional team of health professionals spent time talking

about how each of the patients on our unit is doing, concentrating our discussion on what we can do to help those who are the sickest get well. We talked about a patient who had a heart attack and didn't come to the hospital until a day later. This patient is a 63-year-old man with diabetes and high blood pressure; he has farmed all of his life and lives a long way from the hospital. He thought his chest pain and sweating was "just some sort of chest cold" and he needed to finish his plowing anyway. By delaying coming in, he now has extensive damage to his heart muscle and he seems to have symptoms suggestive of congestive heart failure—a condition in which his heart is now not pumping enough blood to meet the demands of his body. Our doctors have ordered some additional tests to try and measure exactly how well his heart is pumping. Now, I am

(continued)

working with the doctors and nurses to get him started on some new medications that will treat both his underlying coronary artery disease that likely led to his heart attack as well as his congestive heart failure symptoms. These new medications will be in addition to the medicines he is already taking for diabetes and high blood pressure. I'll speak with the patient and family members later to find out exactly what medications he was taking at home and how he was taking them. I have already reviewed his medical chart (thankfully these are all computerized now) and have noted that he doesn't have any allergies to medications; however, his kidney function may be worsening and that might require us to reduce the dosage of certain medications for him. I already discussed treatment options with the patient's doctor and we agreed on three new medicines to start this patient on. I also talked to the doctor about the patient's diabetes control—he's not controlling his blood glucose very well and we will need to think about how to transition him back to outpatient care so that this and his other medical problems get proper attention. The doctor just wrote the orders for these medications, so I better see how my pharmacy technician is doing and get to our work. We'll catch up at the end of the day.

Wow, what a day. It's finally over. I have been at work since 7:00 a.m. It's been a long day but that is normal for my job at the hospital, where there are lots of very sick patients. After I last met with you, I completed the medication profile for the patient we discussed and worked with my pharmacy technician to get him the new medications that he needed. I also talked to the doctor about his diabetes medications. His glucose was not under good control and his worsening kidney function suggested that his previous diabetes medication needed to be changed or have the dosage reduced. I was able to chat with the doctor before he left to go to his office and he agreed that we should switch medications.

Additionally, we filled orders for medications for the other patients in the unit, one of whom we were able to wean off of intravenous medications in favor of oral medication so that she can start getting ready to go home. I have checked all of the prescription orders filled by my technician and verified that she is providing the right medication and dosage. We also had a patient admitted late this afternoon, who was transferred from another small community hospital for better evaluation and treatment here. I verified her current medications with the pharmacy staff at the other hospital so that we could immediately get her started on the right medications. She had been having abnormal heart rhythms that went undetected and unfortunately she ended up having a significant stroke. Because of her stroke, she cannot talk very well and I have had to get some of the information I needed from her husband and daughter. Also because of her stroke, she is having trouble swallowing both food and her oral medications. I have verified this with the speech pathologist and nutritionist who have been consulted to help with her care. Consequently, the doctor had to place a nasogastric tube down through her nose and into her stomach and we are giving her liquid food through that tube. We are also crushing most of her oral medications and the nurses are giving those medications down the tube also. One of her medications could not be crushed, so we have to give that medication in an injectable formulation through an intravenous catheter. Figuring out the best way to deliver the right medications at the right time to patients like these can be a challenge. Hopefully her swallowing will improve later this week and we can begin giving the patient her usual oral medications. Our team will need to monitor her carefully as she recovers to help ensure that she doesn't have a second stroke, which is a serious risk. The patient seems scared and I have talked to the nurses on our unit about giving her a little extra attention and reassurance. Our goal is to get her abnormal heart rhythms under control and stabilize her so that she can be transferred to rehabilitation to improve her abilities after her stroke. So, there you have it—another typical day in the life of a hospital-based clinical pharmacist.

Introduction to Pharmacy

Description

Pharmacy is a careful and scientifically trained profession that helps to ensure the safe and effective manufacture, dispensing, and use of medications. Pharmacists remain the only professionals who are trained in the safe compounding of medications. This skill is still frequently required for certain medications, certain dosages that are not manufactured (e.g., reduced dosages for children), certain routes of drug administration (e.g., compounding of topical creams and ointments for dermatological use), and the mixing of medications in the correct dosages into bags or bottles of sterile fluids that are administered intravenously (through a catheter directly into the patient's bloodstream) usually in hospital or emergency department settings. Because providing too little of a medicine will often not treat the illness correctly and providing too much medicine may lead to unintended adverse effects (often called "side effects"), it is the pharmacist's role to help ensure that the patient gets the right medicine, in the correct dosage, at the right time. As you might imagine, this is a tremendous responsibility, yet one that can be very exciting and fulfilling. Today's pharmacist is very well trained to accept and fulfill these advanced responsibilities. The intensive training in pharmacy school involves advanced math and science skills, combined with a thorough knowledge of diseases and medications, as well as strong interpersonal skills to communicate effectively with both the patient and the health-care team.

Pharmacist Role

Remember that the primary role of the pharmacist is to work with other members of the health-care team and with the patient to ensure that the patient gets the right medicine, in the correct dosage, at the right time, and that the patient understands how to use it properly. This means that the pharmacist frequently works with doctors, nurses, physician assistants, dentists, and patients in decisions about medication selection, dosage, frequency and timing of administration, and prevention or minimization of potential side effects from medications. This interaction is especially important in the hospital and critical care environment because patients are often very sick, are on multiple medications at the same time, and may not be able to take medications by mouth because of tubes or other problems; also, their disease state may change very rapidly. Here the pharmacists and other team members are in frequent communication about the unique needs of individual patients.

History

Medicines have been a part of treating disease for millennia. The use of medications to treat illness has been recorded by ancient Egyptians, Greeks, Romans, and Chinese, long before the birth of Christ. These treatments frequently involved the use of various plants and botanicals, which were prepared in different ways and either taken internally or applied topically to a wound. Little was known about active ingredients (the key ingredient most responsible for producing a desired effect), how they worked, or what the proper dosage and duration of treatment should be for various patients. Plants had to be located and harvested and were eventually cultivated in local gardens to ensure an adequate supply. However, important problems arose in extracting the active ingredients from plants and compounding or making them into medicines that patients consumed or used. These problems included a lack of consistency in compounding from person to person and place to place, resulting in dosages that might be too high or too low and often not the same from one day to the next. Another common problem was that many of the solvents used in extracting or delivering active ingredients were often themselves highly toxic. Challenges such as these fueled the development of the profession of pharmacy.

Regulation of Pharmaceuticals

The U.S. Food and Drug Administration (FDA) is a federal agency that is legislatively mandated to oversee that medications are both safe and effective before being made available to the public. With the exception of occasional prescriptions where the pharmacist may compound ingredients into a final dosage form for consumption or use by the patient, most medications are manufactured by the modern pharmaceutical industry. This enormous international industry now includes for-profit companies, both large and small, that comply with all of these regulations in the United States and around the world. The FDA tests medications for sale by prescription only, as well as some that are sold over the counter (i.e., without a prescription required) both in pharmacies and in a variety of other retail locations.

Pharmacists today are also supported by pharmacy technicians who assist in preparing medications and prescriptions for distribution to the patient. Pharmacy technicians are discussed later in this chapter.

Locations and Content of Practice for Pharmacists and Pharmacy Technicians

The scopes of practice for pharmacists relate directly to the education and licensure of the individual, the laws/requirements of the state, and the location of practice. Some of these roles have already been alluded to; following is a list of some of the important practice roles of pharmacists in various locations, many of which continue to evolve in the changing health-care environment.[1,2]

1. **Community pharmacy:** When people think of their pharmacist, they usually think of the person who works at a local pharmacy or drugstore. Here the pharmacist not only dispenses the right medication, he or she also answers questions about dosages and potential side effects, assists in the selection of over-the-counter medications, encourages the patient's adherence to the prescribed medication regimen, and helps patients monitor their disease. This is also a common location where pharmacy technicians work. These individuals support the work of the pharmacist by greeting patients, identifying and filling/refilling prescription medications into vials or bottles, checking with insurance companies about prescription coverage, ensuring adequate inventories of medications and supplies, and finalizing the sale of the medications to the patient and/or family member.

2. **Hospital pharmacy:** Like those in community settings, pharmacists help select the proper medications for a given patient based on an understanding of the patient's needs and past medication history. Hospital-based pharmacists assist with calculating dosages

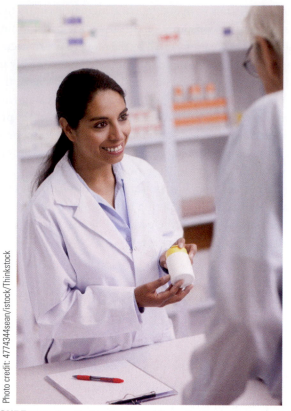

FIGURE 10-1 A patient is discussing his medications with the local pharmacist. The pharmacy may be privately owned or a chain store operated in various locations across the United States.

(especially in situations where the patient's body cannot properly metabolize or excrete the medication), prepare medications, and dispense medications for administration to the patient (although the actual administration is often done by the patient's nurses). Pharmacists also help to monitor how the medications are working to ensure optimal outcomes and to minimize adverse or side effects of the medications, as well as drug interactions (a situation in which one medication may have a change in its effects when combined with another medication). Pharmacy technicians help to support the role of the pharmacist by obtaining medication orders from the medical record system, preparing medications for delivery to the patient care unit and for ease of administration (often in single-use doses or prepared/mixed in intravenous fluids), ensuring adequate inventories of medications and supplies, and checking with nursing staff for any additional patient needs.

3. **Long-term care pharmacy:** As the population ages, more individuals are spending their final years in a system of congregate care locations for the elderly that range from assisted-living sites and rest homes

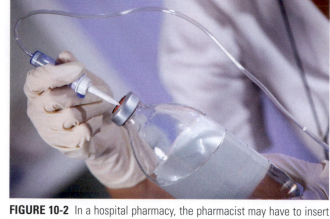

FIGURE 10-2 In a hospital pharmacy, the pharmacist may have to insert medications into intravenous (IV) fluids for patient use as directed by the physician.

to full skilled-care nursing homes with around-the-clock care. Many of these elderly patients have medical conditions and needs that prevent them from living alone in their own home. In these settings, pharmacists have multiple roles. In one role, they may work to dispense medications for these patients in a manner similar to that described for community and hospital pharmacy practice. Alternatively, as many states require regular review of the patient's medication regimen by a consulting pharmacist, they may work as *consultants*—that is, pharmacists who travel to one or more nursing homes, review medical records, discuss care with providers and/or nurses, and make formal recommendations to the provider regarding medication selection, dosing, monitoring, and patient follow-up. Much of the early consulting in nursing home settings was done by pharmacists who

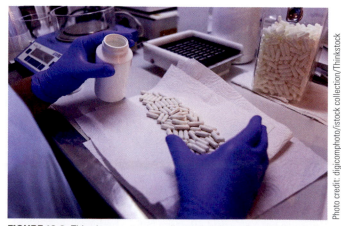

FIGURE 10-3 This photo portrays sterile preparations of medications being processed in a hospital pharmacy. The pharmacist has to order, process, and prepare the medications for patient use.

were employed by or owners of community pharmacies. This work has evolved in many locations into the development of large consulting pharmacy operations that contract with many local nursing homes to provide these services.

4. **Pharmaceutical industry:** Much of the actual manufacturing of medications into specific dosage forms (i.e., tablets, capsules, liquids, creams) is now managed by companies who then sell these products to local pharmacies for dispensing to patients. Pharmacists have important roles in this setting based on their unique knowledge of pharmaceutical compounding. In this environment, pharmacists work with medicinal chemists, chemical engineers, packaging specialists, and a variety of other individuals to ensure that the active ingredients of the medication are combined with the proper inactive ingredients or vehicles for administration to the patient, as well as the proper sterility of some final products. In this way they ensure proper dissolution of the tablet or capsule in the stomach or intestine of the patient, appropriate absorption into the bloodstream in the concentrations necessary to have a desired therapeutic effect for the patient, and consistency from batch to batch of the medication. They work with chemical engineers to take these procedures, which may work in limited quantities in the laboratory, and scale them up to produce large quantities of product that can be mass produced in advanced machinery.

5. **Clinical pharmacy practitioner:** The complexity of drug therapy and the growth in number of new medications have led to remarkable evolution in the

practice of pharmacy to the extent that some pharmacists today no longer dispense medications but work solely in clinic, hospital, or other patient care environments where they provide medication therapy consulting and management to providers and patients to optimize health-care outcomes. By working with providers such as doctors and nurse practitioners or physician assistants, these pharmacists recommend and monitor specific drug therapies to maximize disease improvement while minimizing side effects and drug interactions. Some practitioners also help patients learn how to use complex medications such as medication inhalers for asthma and insulin injections for diabetics, and many counsel patients about their medications and encourage adherence in chronic disease states. Many states have now established "collaborative practice agreements" or agreed-on relationships between clinical pharmacy practitioners and physicians that allow the pharmacist, in selected disease states such as diabetes or hypertension, to initiate medications, adjust dosages, order laboratory or other monitoring tests, and, under the oversight of the physician, manage the patient's medication regimen. This relationship is often referred to as *medication therapy management.* Medical and pharmacy boards in many states have recognized the value of this collaboration and established these agreements, but the insurance industry has been slower in recognizing pharmacists as independent practitioners that can bill insurance carriers for non–product-related services. However, this situation is changing and many health-care systems, managed-care agencies, and state Medicaid programs are employing pharmacists in these roles because overall health-care costs are often reduced, usually by optimizing medication choices that are made available and by reducing emergency department and hospital visits.

6. **Specialized areas of pharmacy practice:** Pharmacists and pharmacy technicians may find employment in a variety of other specialized areas. One of these is *radiopharmacy,* in which specific quantities and dosages of radioactive pharmaceuticals that are used in diagnosing and treating certain diseases are compounded and dispensed. Another area is working with governmental or military agencies. State and federal government agencies such as the National Institutes of Health, the FDA, the Veterans Administration, and various branches of the U.S. Armed Forces hire pharmacists for a variety of traditional and innovative roles. Another example is working in drug information and poison control

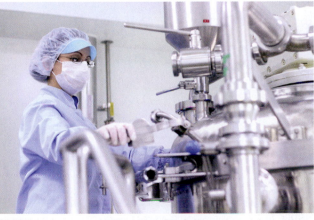

FIGURE 10-4 A person with a pharmacy degree can work in a pharmaceutical company to make and produce medications for delivery to vendors such as hospitals and health-care facilities.

centers. Large health systems frequently have a drug information center, run by pharmacists, that serves as a "help desk" or information resource about medications for health professionals throughout the health system. Similarly, there is a nationwide network of poison control centers that may employ pharmacists. These pharmacists answer questions about toxic ingestions or exposures and their acute management—usually in emergency situations—from patients, local citizens, and health-care practitioners.

Author Spotlight

Doyle M. Cummings, PharmD, FCP, FCCP

Dr. Cummings has been in academic medicine and pharmacy for many years and has helped to train countless young pharmacists, as well as physicians and other health professionals. After finishing his initial pharmacy school training, he decided that he wanted to practice in an interprofessional environment with physicians, nurses, and other health professionals. He moved to Chicago and completed a hospital pharmacy residency training program at a large university hospital system there, where he had the exciting opportunity of exploring different roles and making patient rounds with physicians. After this he matriculated into the (then) post-BS PharmD program—a 2-year program in Philadelphia where he received intensive training in pathophysiology and clinical therapeutics. After completion he went on to complete a post-PharmD training program in ambulatory care clinical pharmacy where he helped take care of patients in clinics and outpatient environments. This was a total of 9 years of education and training, and it provided him with unique and advanced skills to contribute in a changing health-care system. Since then, his career has advanced, allowing him to become a leading professor in a university health-care system that trains pharmacy students and a wide variety of other health professionals. Much of his work now focuses on patients with high blood pressure and diabetes, two important and common problems in our nation today. He has always enjoyed pharmacy because it allows the pharmacist to bring a unique knowledge and skill base—an in-depth understanding of medications and how they work—to the compelling needs of patients, both those acutely ill in the hospital and those with chronic illnesses such as hypertension and diabetes in the outpatient setting. If you do well in school, love science and math, and have a passion for helping others, pharmacy just might be right for you.

Required Education

Pharmacists

The entry-level degree for admittance into the profession of pharmacy as a pharmacist is the doctor of pharmacy (PharmD) degree. Because of a shortage of pharmacists in the late 1990s and early 2000s, there has been rapid growth in the number of pharmacy school programs. In addition to broad-based general education requirements (e.g., English, foreign language, history/humanities), admission to a pharmacy school in the United States usually requires several things[3]:

- Completion of at least 2 years of undergraduate college education at an accredited institution, although the majority of students in many programs already have an undergraduate college degree at the time of admission/matriculation.

- Completion of specific prerequisites, usually including advanced mathematics courses such as calculus and statistics, as well as advanced science courses in chemistry, organic chemistry, biology, microbiology, anatomy/physiology, and physics, all with grades of C or higher (B or higher is preferred).

- A composite grade point average (GPA) usually above 3.0. In most competitive programs, a GPA above 3.5 is preferred or required.

- Successful completion of the Pharmacy College Admissions Test (PCAT) with scores that are competitive based on the guidelines set by each college's admissions program. Many programs focus on the average PCAT composite percentile rank score. Students can take this standardized test multiple times to try to improve their score. The test is offered at a wide variety of testing centers around the United States.

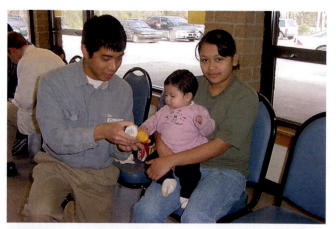

FIGURE 10-5 Pharmacy students are required to complete internships before receiving their degree. This student is working in a community-based migrant health clinic in the rural community. He is advising the mother on proper medication dosages for the baby.

- Successful completion of an in-person interview with admissions committee members from the College of Pharmacy.

Application is made through a national consolidated Web-enabled admissions process (PharmCAS) and requires submission of letters of recommendation. Supplemental application materials are also often required by each pharmacy school applied to. The admissions committees carefully review application forms, often along with a personal statement about career goals, as well as any relevant work experience and extracurricular activities. Once accepted, the traditional program of study in most schools of pharmacy is 4 years in length, the same as medical and dental schools. Demographically, many pharmacy schools have a greater percentage of females in entering classes than males. Once successfully matriculated into pharmacy school, coursework or topics include the following: biochemistry, medicinal chemistry, physiology/pathophysiology, pharmacology, pharmaceutics, pharmaceutical calculations, pharmacokinetics, pharmacotherapy, pharmacy law and ethics, pharmaceutical care delivery, drug literature analysis, and multiple clinical or applied rotations in pharmacy and medical settings similar to those described previously. Most schools require maintenance at or above a certain GPA standard and passage of all coursework to graduate.

Graduates must successfully pass a comprehensive national licensure examination to be licensed for the practice of pharmacy in a particular state. Most students take this examination right after graduation from pharmacy school and therefore passage rates are high. Once successfully licensed in a particular state, there are often reciprocity procedures (e.g., application form, personal interview, state law examination, fees) available that allow licensees to also become licensed in another state, thereby increasing job potential. Additionally, the vast majority of states require the completion of a minimum number of continuing education hours of training each year to maintain an active practice license in that state.

Pharmacy Technicians

For pharmacy technicians, there is wide variability in requirements across states. Most states do not require pharmacy technicians to have completed a pharmacy technician training program to work as a pharmacy technician; however, many students still choose to go through the training rather than simply having on-the-job experience. There is no required uniform national accreditation process for pharmacy technician training programs. Some programs are independently accredited by the American Society of Hospital Pharmacists or other pharmacy organizations; some are located in institutions that are themselves accredited even though the individual training program is not accredited; and some programs have no accreditation at all. Programs are available involving face-to-face classroom and laboratory training; others are available largely online. A voluntary certification process is now available for pharmacy technicians that involves completion of a certification examination and long-term maintenance of certification through regular continuing education. Although voluntary, this certification process can help one stand out from other applicants by demonstrating competency and commitment to the job.

Salary

The salary for pharmacists is very good and varies according to the specific area of practice and location. According to the Bureau of Labor Statistics, the median salary for a pharmacist was $113,390 per year in 2011 with the top 10% of pharmacists making approximately $144,000 a year. This median salary puts pharmacists third among health-care workers in earnings, just behind physicians and dentists. After the pharmacist shortage in the late 1990s, salaries for pharmacists have escalated and remain high.[4]

Similarly, salaries for pharmacy technicians are reasonably good and vary considerably based on responsibility, location, and experience level. According to the Bureau of Labor Statistics, in 2012 the median hourly wage for a pharmacy technician was $14.10 per hour with the top 10% of pharmacy technicians earning $20.00 per hour.[4]

Trends

As the number of older individuals in the United States has increased, so has the number of prescriptions for chronic medications and the demand for pharmacists. In addition,

Aptitude Profile

The following list includes some of the skills and characteristics required for working in the field of pharmacy:

Able to handle stress

Advanced math and science skills

Clinical skills to assess patient symptoms/findings

Critical appraisal of the medical literature

Detail oriented

Ethical

Excellent computing/database-searching skills

Excellent team member on interprofessional team

Manual dexterity for compounding/preparing

Multitasker

Responsible

there has been growth in the number and complexity of prescription medications available, the number of prescribing physicians, and the diversification of roles for advanced practice in pharmacy. As a result, there has been growth in the number of pharmacy schools, and projections now suggest an adequate supply of pharmacists, although maldistribution is still a problem in some rural or impoverished communities. Consequently, the demand for pharmacists into the future is anticipated to remain strong. Likewise, labor projections for pharmacy technicians parallel those for pharmacists and suggest a strong overall job market through 2025.

Challenges

Like most health professionals, pharmacists and pharmacy technicians face many challenges. As in many jobs, often the job requirements in contemporary pharmacy settings are to maximally produce units of work while minimizing expenses. For pharmacists or technicians, this may mean working longer shifts, filling more prescriptions, caring for more patients, or similar challenges, often without additional resources. This can result in a work environment that is stressful and constantly demanding. This is worsened by the fact that pharmacists, in particular, have tremendous responsibility to ensure accurate and high-quality work. Pharmacists are the professionals in the medication delivery process who are ultimately responsible for the calculation of proper dosages, the correct compounding of medications, the dispensing of the correct medication, and the communication of the right information to the patient. The consequences of error in any of these examples may be substantial and have the potential to result in harm for the patient. And with harm comes the potential for lawsuits against the pharmacist and against the employer/institution.

Another challenge for pharmacists in some settings is the lack of collaboration among health-care professionals. Although some health professionals have been trained to work in environments that promote interprofessional collaboration, others have not. This lack of a team approach often creates challenges, especially when the pharmacist tries to communicate information that he or she believes to be vital to the patient's well-being. It is clear that optimal patient care is often realized only when a team-based approach is consistently employed.

There are also challenges, primarily in community pharmacy settings, with some patients and their insurance companies. Challenges with patients include those who are demanding and intentionally lie or attempt to manipulate the pharmacist and/or pharmacy technician to acquire certain medications. Paramount among these challenges are patients who are attempting to purchase or acquire substances that have the potential for abuse—often painkillers or sedative-hypnotic medications. This situation requires careful action by the pharmacist and technician to ensure that there is an adequate provider-patient relationship and to ensure that the prescription the patient provides is not fake or forged in some way. Law enforcement or other individuals may need to be contacted if this problem is identified. Substance abuse is a major issue plaguing our nation, and unfortunately pharmacists and pharmacy technicians sometimes get caught in the middle. Likewise, there can be significant stress in dealing with insurance companies. Patients have a wide range of insurance plans, and many of them have different co-payment and co-insurance structures and different lists of medications (called *formularies*) that they agree to cover in their insurance plan. Along with this challenge, some patients want to pay cash for some medications and bill others to their insurance if their out-of-pocket costs are less. Pharmacists and technicians must first, at the time the prescription is filled, verify that the insurance carrier will actually pay for the prescription before it can be filled and dispensed. If the patient needs medication but no refills are authorized by the prescriber, the prescriber must first be contacted and permission to refill the medication obtained. All of these administrative hurdles can be challenging when the pharmacist and technician are trying to help the patient stay on a needed medication. Despite all of the challenges, pharmacy work has important rewards—being an integral part of the health-care team, seeing how patients are improving or have their suffering relieved, helping patients achieve their personal health-care goals, and hearing patients or their family express their gratitude for your care.

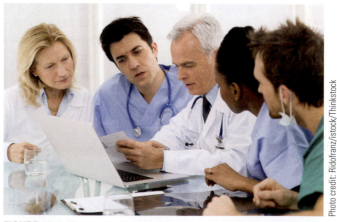

FIGURE 10-6 Pharmacists are part of the interprofessional team as seen here discussing patient care.

Photo credit: Ridofranz/istock/Thinkstock

Working Together

As you have already seen, optimal health-care delivery is a team sport, and pharmacists and technicians, depending on the setting, are often required to work with other health professionals. These include medical doctors, nurses, nutritionists, physician assistants, nurse practitioners, occupational therapists, physical therapists, social workers, speech pathologists, and rehabilitative counselors. The collaboration among these disciplines ensures that a comprehensive and holistic plan of care gets developed for the patient. All of these disciplines are part of the interprofessional care team, and the pharmacist is an important member.

CASE STUDY

Ms. R is a 49-year-old African American woman with multiple chronic problems, including diabetes mellitus, high blood pressure, high cholesterol, arthritis, nerve damage, and kidney failure. She has had diabetes since she was 19 years old and is now experiencing some of the long-term complications of this disease. She has to take many chronic (long-term) medications—currently 12 different medications—just to try to keep her conditions under reasonable control. She sometimes has trouble affording all of these medications and has not always refilled them when she was supposed to. She comes into the clinic pharmacy area today with weight gain, swollen ankles and lower legs, and weakness and tiredness. Before refilling her usual medications, you spend a few minutes talking to her. She missed her last clinic appointment and has not seen her doctor for almost 6 months. You ask about her diet, her salt intake, and whether she has talked to a nutritionist recently, because this might be contributing to her ankle swelling. She has not seen the nutritionist and you encourage her to speak to the nutritionist at her next visit. You tell her that you are also concerned that she has not refilled her medications on time and you ask if she has had trouble affording the medication costs over the last few months. She states that she has had some unexpected bills and that some months she cannot afford all of her medications and therefore only takes her medications about half the time. You ask her if she would be willing to talk to the social worker who works down the hallway in the clinic, who is sometimes able to help with medication costs. She agrees and you make a plan to take her down to the social worker's office after she is done in the pharmacy. However, she states that she ran out of medication 3 weeks ago, she has been feeling especially poorly for 2 weeks now, and her adult daughter

is worried about her. You check her blood pressure and find that it is elevated. You ask her about shortness of breath and her energy level and she states that she has been short of breath even walking around the house and frequently tired. You are concerned that she may be developing worsening heart problems, such as congestive heart failure—a condition in which the heart muscle is not able to pump enough blood to keep up with the body's demands.

Do you just refill her medications and send her home? If not, what should you do to help this woman feel better? The clinic where her doctor is located is right next door and you know the nurse and doctor, so you wonder whether it would be prudent to call them about Ms. R. What do you think you would do?

Questions

1. What factors make Ms. R's situation complex?
2. Will just refilling her current medications fix her problems?
3. What factors might cause you to send her to see her doctor before filling her usual medications?
4. Might there be a connection between not always refilling her medications and the symptoms/signs she is now experiencing?
5. Are there any medical factors that might force you to reevaluate whether she is receiving the right medications in the proper dosages?
6. Do you feel comfortable picking up the phone and talking to her doctor about how she is doing today and what your concerns are?

Review Questions

1. The Food and Drug Administration is a federal agency that is legislatively mandated to oversee that medications are both safe and effective before being distributed to the public.

   A. True

   B. False

2. Pharmacists remain the only profession that is trained in the safe compounding of medications.

   A. True

   B. False

3. In a community pharmacy setting, the pharmacist's responsibilities include(s):

   A. Dispensing the right medication

   B. Answering questions and concerns that the patient has about dosages and potential side effects

   C. Assisting in the selection of over-the-counter medications

   D. All of the above

   E. None of the above

4. In a hospital pharmacy setting, the pharmacist's responsibilities include(s):

   A. Helping select the proper medications for a given patient

   B. Assisting in calculating the dosage needed

   C. Preparing and dispensing medications for administration to the patient

   D. All of the above

   E. None of the above

5. In a long-term care pharmacy setting, the pharmacist's responsibilities include(s):

   A. Dispensing medications or ensuring that proper medications have been dispensed

   B. Reviewing medications that patients are on and suggesting alternative medications or dosages

   C. Only A

   D. Only B

   E. Both A and B

6. Clinical pharmacy practitioners recommend and monitor specific drug therapies to maximize disease improvement while minimizing side effects and drug interactions.

   A. True

   B. False

7. In a pharmaceutical industry setting, the pharmacist's responsibilities include(s):

   A. Working with others to ensure that active ingredients of the medication are combined with the proper inactive ingredients

   B. Testing to check for proper sterility of the final production of medications

   C. Only A

   D. Only B

   E. Both A and B

8. The degree necessary to become a pharmacist is a doctor of pharmacy (PharmD) degree.

   A. True

   B. False

9. Admission into a pharmacy school in the United States usually requires individuals to take the:

   A. PCAT

   B. SAT

   C. GRE

   D. MCAT

   E. None of the above

10. Challenges pharmacists and pharmacy technicians face include a decline in the number of prescriptions being filled and a slow work environment.

    A. True

    B. False

Glossary of Key Terms

Community pharmacy—type of pharmacy that provides services to the local community; the pharmacist dispenses medications and answers questions about dosages and side effects

Hospital pharmacy—type of pharmacy that is usually located within the confines of the hospital; the pharmacist provides medications for patients only and is not engaged in retail sales

Long-term care pharmacy—may or may not be located within the confines of a long-term care unit, such as a nursing home, but the focus is the medication management of long-term care patients; the pharmacist provides medications and consultations

Pharmaceutical industry—the business of developing, compounding, marketing, and selling medications; the pharmacist, along with others, helps to develop, compound, and conduct research in the area of medications

Clinical pharmacy practitioner—this type of pharmacist works with patients and providers to manage medications/therapies, promote health, and prevent future disease episodes or consequences

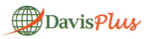 Additional Resources are available online at www.davisplus.com

Additional Resources

Accrediting Body

American Council on Pharmaceutical Education (ACPE) is the accrediting body for schools of pharmacy and for continuing education activities in pharmacy.

School Association

American Association of Colleges of Pharmacy (AACP) is a national association of colleges of pharmacy and individuals that ensures and enhances the quality of pharmacy education.

Education and Professional Resources

National Association of Boards of Pharmacy

American Pharmacists Association

American Society of Health-System Pharmacists

American College of Clinical Pharmacy

American College of Consultant Pharmacists

Journal of American Pharmacists Association

American Journal of Health-System Pharmacy

Pharmacotherapy

American Journal of Pharmaceutical Education

References

1. Posey LM, ed. *Pharmacy: An Introduction to the Profession,* 2nd ed. Washington, DC: American Pharmacists Association; 2009.

2. Schommer JC, Sogol EM, Brown LM: Career pathways for pharmacists. *J Am Pharmacists Assn.* 2007; 47:563–564.

3. University of North Carolina–Chapel Hill, Eshelman School of Pharmacy.

    https://pharmacy.unc.edu/.

    Accessed September 12, 2013.

4. Bureau of Labor Statistics, U.S. Department of Labor. Occupational outlook handbook, 2012–2013 edition, pharmacists.

    http://www.bls.gov/ooh/.

    Accessed September 11, 2013.

Allied Health Professions

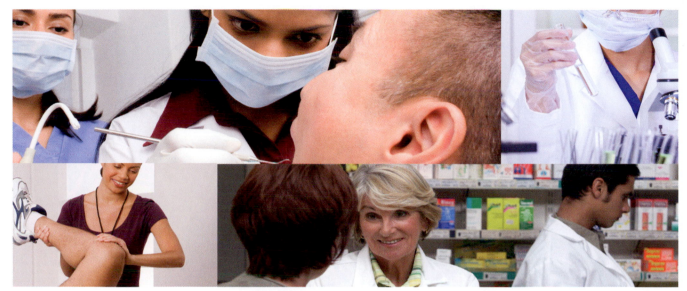

Photo credit: creatas/Thinkstock, istock/Thinkstock, Fuse/Thinkstock

Chapter 11
Athletic Training

Chapter 12
Audiology

Chapter 13
Clinical Laboratory Science

Chapter 14
Dental Professions

Chapter 15
Dietetics

Chapter 16
Emergency Medical Services

Chapter 17
Health Information
Management

Chapter 18
Health Services
Management

Chapter 19
Medical Assisting

Chapter 20
Occupational Therapy

Chapter 21
Physical Therapy

Chapter 22
Physician Assisting

Chapter 23
Radiography

Chapter 24
Radiation Therapy

Chapter 25
Recreational Therapy

Chapter 26
Rehabilitation Counseling

Chapter 27
Respiratory Care/
Cardiopulmonary

Chapter 28
Social Work

Chapter 29
Speech-Language Pathology

CHAPTER 11

Athletic Training

Katie Walsh Flanagan, EdD

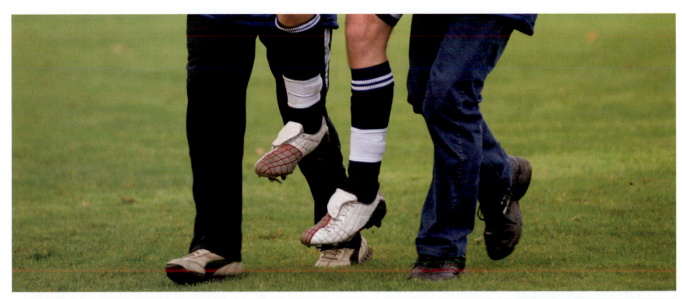

Photo credit: istock/Thinkstock

Learning Objectives

After reading this chapter, students should be able to:

- Describe the role of an athletic trainer
- Discuss the education required to take the national Board of Certification examination for athletic trainers
- Differentiate between the athletic trainer and the personal trainer (trainer)
- List different employment opportunities for the athletic trainer
- Identify characteristics of a successful athletic trainer
- Explain challenges in the profession of athletic training

Key Terms

- National certification
- Preceptor
- State regulation
- Technical Standards

 ## "A Day in the Life"

My name is Kelly, and I am a nationally certified and state-licensed athletic trainer. I work for a university that has over 25,000 students and is affiliated with National Collegiate Athletic Association (NCAA) Division I athletes. I am the assistant athletic trainer for the football team and work with the head athletic trainer, but my boss is the team physician at the student health center on campus. I also work alongside six other athletic trainers who provide medical care to our basketball, soccer, softball, baseball, and track teams. Our jobs are similar, and only differ in the types of injuries we may see and the fields or courts where we spend a lot of our time.

My day begins with setting up appointments for my athletes to see specialists: orthopedic surgeons, chiropractors, and family medicine physicians, many of whom come to our facility (the athletic training room or clinic) weekly. Some of the medical conditions require testing (x-ray, magnetic resonance imaging [MRI], bone scans, or blood work) and I make appointments for those tests around the athletes' class and practice schedules. I also update my athletes' electronic medical records (EMR), a protected Web-based program on my computer. There are always a few new athletes (all sports) who need physical examinations before participating,

(continued)

and the majority of them are done in the athletic training room with me and a physician. Besides reviewing the athlete's medical history, measuring height, weight, and visual testing, I also screen them for orthopedic laxity (looseness) in specific joints, and run an electrocardiogram to assess resting heart activity. All of our athletes also get baseline cognitive testing and Biosway postural testing. Both are tools used in concussion assessment. Athletes stand on the Biosway (it looks like a scale) and try to maintain their balance by keeping a moving dot in the center of an eye-level computer screen. Athletes do this test on both a flat and 4-inch foam surface, as well as with eyes open (watching the dot) and blinded (see accompanying figure). Both of these tests are important if an athlete sustains a concussion during the season, because we can use these baseline tests to determine if the athlete is back to preseason scores, which will assist in determining whether he or she is ready to return to participation. The rest of my morning and early afternoon are full of specialized scheduled rehabilitation appointments with my athletes. Today, I am working with different athletes who have hamstring injuries, low back spasms, a few different

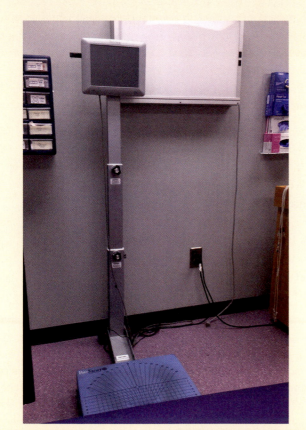

A Biosway is a machine used to establish baseline balance testing that assists in determining return to participation following a concussion.

types of postsurgical ligament knee or shoulder surgeries, and postconcussion testing. Even athletes who are on the "disabled" list and cannot fully play have rehabilitation exercises to perform daily. One example is a player who has a fractured tibia (broken lower leg); we tailored a program for him to keep in cardiovascular and core strengthening shape while he is out. The head athletic trainer does the ordering of supplies and maintenance of our expensive equipment and filing insurance claims on behalf of the athlete for medical appointments and tests, so the rest of us can just work with the athletes.

In the afternoon, athletes begin to drift in after class to the athletic training room to get prepractice attention: taping, bracing, padding of casts, or fabricating protective devices so athletes can play without further injury to that area. Specific regulations pertaining to each sport dictate what protective devices may be applied to athletes, and it can even vary by the athlete's position on the field (pitcher vs. catcher, lineman vs. receiver, etc.). My athletic training students and I are busy using therapeutic modalities, such as ultrasound treatments and electric stimulation, on our athletes who are in various stages of recovery. After we ready the team for practice, the real job begins. We bring oxygen, an automated external defibrillator (AED, which can detect an irregular heartbeat), a medical kit, splint bags, and airways to the field, and also fluids to keep the athletes hydrated. The certified athletic trainers and their students earning a degree in athletic training are the on-site medical first responders to any athletic injury/illness that may occur. Athletic trainers typically work with one or two sports at a time at a university, but typically provide care for all of the athletic teams at a high school. We do provide care for all athletes and teams representing our college, even though we may not attend all of the teams' practices or competitions. I have provided medical care on the field to athletes who have had open fractures, dislocations, concussions, and sprains; heart attacks, asthma attacks, and severe allergies; and internal bleeding and ruptured organs. All of these are scary for the injured person, but I have been well trained for this. Because we are an NCAA-regulated institution, our athletes can only practice 20 hours a week and must have 1 full day off. My athletic training friends have the same skills I do, but work in high schools, NASCAR, X-games, Broadway plays, movie studios, professional sports, dance, rodeos, clinics, military, and industry. Not everyone has a game day on TV like I do, but all of us absolutely love working with physically active, energetic, and positive athletes. Although my day can be long, I am always happy that I made a difference at the end of the day. There is not one thing I would change.

Introduction to Athletic Training

Description

Athletic training has been recognized by the American Medical Association as an allied health-care profession since 1990. According to the national organization that oversees athletic training, the National Athletic Trainers' Association (NATA),[1] "Athletic Trainers (ATs) are health-care professionals who collaborate with physicians to provide preventative services, emergency care, clinical diagnosis, therapeutic intervention and rehabilitation of injuries and medical conditions."

Athletic trainers can sometimes be confused with personal trainers (or "trainers"), who are responsible for designing and implementing a fitness program for healthy clients (Box 11-1). This chapter is about certified athletic trainers (ATs), who are allied health-care professionals. ATs are midlevel health-care providers who typically work with patients and athletes. Most people relate to the athletic trainers who run out on the fields and courts to render emergency care to fallen athletes in the scholastic, collegiate, and professional settings; but ATs also work in a variety of settings with other healthy, active individuals. In addition to preventing and diagnosing musculoskeletal and medical conditions, ATs design rehabilitation protocols and apply emergency skills in the management of injuries.[1] ATs hold the ATC credential, which indicates that a person has at least a 4-year college degree and has passed a national board examination to be a certified athletic trainer after college graduation (see discussion later in this chapter). In addition to the ATC credential, practicing athletic trainers typically hold a state license for athletic training in their state. National and state regulatory bodies oversee the medical care provided by athletic trainers, and ATs can only practice in the state in which they hold a state license, unless they are traveling to another state with their team and will only be in that state for a limited time.

Historical Perspective

Dr. S. E. Bilik first introduced athletic training in 1917 via his textbook on managing athletic injuries, *The Trainer's Bible.* Several years later the Cramer family, owners of a chemical plant in Gardner, Kansas, began to distribute a liniment that was intended to assist in treating ankle sprains. As this liniment became popular among coaches and athletes, the Cramers initiated a publication called the *First Aider* that opened communication among coaches, athletes, and ATs.[2] This historic family name is well known in athletic training today as the forefathers of the development of the field of athletic training. In the late 1930s, efforts were made to unite athletic trainers nationally via the National Athletic Trainers' Association, but it was not until 1950 that the organization formed a lasting presence. That year a group of 101 men gathered in Kansas City, Kansas, to establish professional standards for athletic trainers. The NATA has seen steady growth since then, rising from 4,500 members in 1974 to its current 41,000 active members. More than 400 of these work internationally, mainly in Japan and Canada. Preventable injuries/illnesses such as concussions and heat stroke have brought the need for qualified ATs to the attention of the media, but ATs have long been practicing safety and prevention.

Scope of Practice

All athletic trainers work under the direction and supervision of a physician licensed in the state where the AT practices. Many state AT licenses require a physician to submit a protocol or standing orders of what the AT is allowed to do in the physician's absence.

Although the majority of ATs work in athletic settings, over 40% treat patients in clinics, physicians' offices, hospitals, or recreational settings (Table 11-1).[3] Athletic trainers have the medical background, because of the classes they take and the clinical practice required to be physician

BOX 11-1 Athletic Trainer (AT) versus Personal Trainer (Trainer)

	AT	Trainer
Education	4-year college degree minimum	No minimum requirement
Precertification practice with patients	4 semesters required in college—minimum	None required
Required certification	National certification—BOC (passing examination) required	None required, but several companies offer one
Work settings	Numerous; see Box 11-2	Typically gyms/individual clients

TABLE 11-1 Industries That Employed the Most Athletic Trainers in 2012

Employer	Percentage
Colleges; universities; state, local, and private schools	25%
Health practitioner offices	15%
Hospitals (state, local, private)	13%
Fitness and recreational sports centers	13%

From http://www.bls.gov/ooh/healthcare/athletic-trainers-and-exercise-physiologists.htm#tab-3. Accessed September 9, 2014.

extenders. In this role, ATs apply orthopedic braces and casts, provide postprocedure wound care, and remove surgical staples and sutures, among other services. ATs also teach activities of daily living (ADLs) to patients. ATs are also employed as medical and surgical salespeople, who travel and teach physicians and other health-care providers about their products.

ATs work with athletes in sporting events and in health-care settings (Box 11-2). They are employed in government settings and in the military in U.S. training facilities for Navy SEALs, Camp Pendleton (Marines), and Fort Bragg (Home of Airborne and Special Operations Forces). They provide on-site medical care, prevention and rehabilitation of injuries to the physically active participants involved in performing arts, entertainment, national/international games, and industry. With their broad medical, as well as orthopedic, training, they are the primary caregivers for traveling patients (movie sets, athletics, military, etc.). ATs are unique in that they travel with the athletic teams with whom they work. Often this entails being the only medical-care provider on the road to be called on if an athlete has a cold, flu, asthma, allergies, or injury.

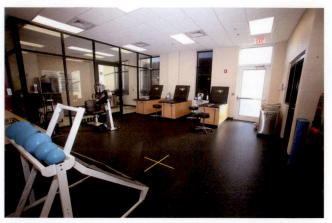

FIGURE 11-2 ATs typically work in facilities that allow athletes swift and safe return to full participation.

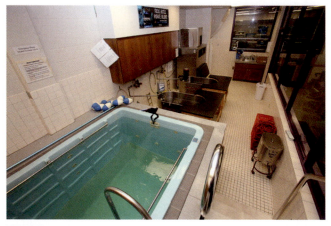

FIGURE 11-3 Hydrotherapy—therapy using water—is one type of rehabilitation tool used by ATs.

Required Education

All athletic trainers must earn a degree from a 4-year institution and then take the national Board of Certification (BOC) examination to receive **national certification.** Only students graduating with a degree in athletic training from a Commission on Accreditation of Athletic Training Education (CAATE)–accredited program are eligible to take the BOC examination. Although the majority of the country's 335 professional programs in athletic training programs offer undergraduate degrees in athletic training, several (32) offer a professional master's degree in athletic training.[4] Both cover the same general content and a minimum of four full semesters of clinical experience (college courses with credit) under a qualified **preceptor.** According to CAATE, a preceptor is "a certified/licensed professional who teaches and evaluates students in a clinical setting using an actual patient base."[5] Preceptors are typically ATs but can also be other health-care providers, including medical doctors. Usually, students log over 800 supervised hours under preceptors while attaining a degree in athletic training. These clinical experiences cover a broad variety of

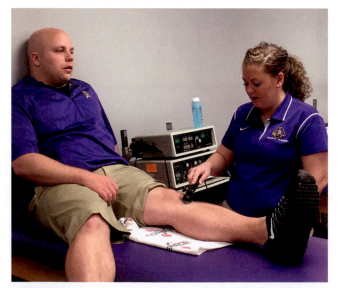

FIGURE 11-1 ATs use ultrasound therapy to assist in injury healing.

BOX 11-2 Where ATs Work

Health-Care Settings

- Hospitals
- Therapy clinics
- Rehabilitation centers
- Assisted-living centers
- Physician offices

Academic Settings

- Colleges and universities
- Junior colleges
- High schools
- Middle schools
- Boarding schools
- Researchers

Professional Sports

- National Football League (NFL)
- National Hockey League (NHL)
- Major League Baseball (MLB)
- Minor League Baseball (MiLB)
- Major League Soccer (MLS)
- Women's National Basketball Association (WNBA)
- National Basketball Association (NBA)
- Rodeo
- NASCAR
- Extreme sports (X-games)

Entertainment/Performing Arts

- Movie sets
- Television series/sets
- Cirque du Soleil
- Broadway theaters
- The National Ballet
- Disney

Industry

- Airline companies
- Automobile manufacturers
- Factories
- Manufacturing
- Independent contractors

Military

- Navy
- Navy SEALs
- Marines
- Army
- Special Forces

Government

- Federal Bureau of Investigation (FBI)
- Central Intelligence Agency (CIA)
- Drug Enforcement Agency (DEA)
- National Aeronautics and Space Administration (NASA) (private)

National/International Games

- Olympics
- Pan American Games
- Paralympics

athletes, patients, and types of venues (team and individual sports, medical facilities, working with both genders, etc.).

It is the combination of academic (classroom) and clinical (in the field) learning strategies that makes the education of ATs unique. There is no required final internship or culminating experience; students practice skills learned in the classroom and laboratories while in the clinical setting. This classroom-clinical education typically occurs concurrently, as students attend class in the mornings and usually have clinical experiences in the afternoons on the same day. This approach allows students to immediately put into practice the knowledge and skills they have learned. Most of the clinical experiences are with college and high school athletic teams, but students will also have experiences in medical practices and with nonathletic populations.

The core academic areas most often found in athletic training programs include the following:

- Human anatomy and physiology
- Kinesiology/biomechanics
- Exercise physiology
- Principles of health and fitness
- First aid and cardiopulmonary resuscitation (CPR)
- Psychology
- Nutrition
- Pharmacology
- Orthopedic evaluation
- Therapeutic rehabilitation

- Therapeutic modalities
- Medical conditions
- Evidence-based medicine
- Health-care administration

Accredited programs must adhere to the CAATE's education document *Athletic Training Education Competencies,*[1] which is currently in its fifth edition (see https://caate.net/wp-content/uploads/2014/06/5th-Edition-Competencies.pdf). This document outlines eight content areas in athletic training and a list of clinical integration proficiencies, and provides the framework for all education programs. For example, here is one of the competencies: "Establish and maintain an airway, including the use of an oro- and nasopharyngeal airways and neutral spine alignment in an athlete with a suspected spine injury who may be wearing shoulder pads, a helmet." As long as each of the competencies and clinical proficiencies is addressed in courses, and demonstrated correctly on patients (simulated or real), students should have the knowledge and skills necessary to enter into the profession.

Salary

According to the U.S. Department of Labor, the median salary for ATs was approximately $44,720 in 2013, but the range was from $26,200 in Oklahoma to $71,000 in New Jersey. The projected job growth between 2012 and 2022 is 19%, which is higher than the average occupation growth of 11% (Table 11-2).[3] The NATA website displays a 2014 salary survey of its members that yielded an average salary of $49,719 with a bachelor's degree and $54,660 with a master's degree, and a range from $38,000 to $82,180, which depends on factors such as degree level, years of experience, location, and job setting.[1] It should also be noted that 70% of certified ATs hold at least a master's degree.[1] In terms of nonmonetary benefits, many ATs working with athletic teams also get free or discounted team apparel, gear, equipment, shoes, a cell phone, housing, tuition (fees for college courses), and meals. Depending on the venue, some head ATs at large universities or professional teams also get car privileges. This means the automobile manufacturer sponsoring the team may give a complimentary car to the AT for work use. In turn, the company gets free advertising for supporting the local team.

Certification and Licensure

The BOC created a national examination in 1970 that established a means to determine if a student had the knowledge and skills necessary to enter the profession. Passing the examination informs the public that the BOC-certified individual has met the requirements of an accredited education and has the training to meet the minimum standards for an entry-level AT. The term *ATC* means *athletic trainer, certified.* It is used after a person successfully passes the BOC examination. Educational programs must post the 3-year BOC first-time pass rate on their athletic training program websites. Their most recent 3-year pass rate must be above 70% for the program to meet that specific accreditation standard of the CAATE.[5] Posting the BOC first-time pass rate on the website allows prospective students and parents to compare accredited programs.

After graduating and passing the BOC examination, students must submit official college transcripts bearing proof of a degree in athletic training and a current CPR certification card before the BOC sends out the official certification. After receiving certification, ATs can then apply for a state credential (typically a license). Texas is the only state that has a separate state license that does not first require a national BOC recognition.

Three levels of **state regulation** apply to athletic training: licensure, certification, and registration. Of these, *state licensure* is the most restrictive of all forms of regulations, as it mandates that people cannot call themselves an athletic trainer unless they have the state license. State licensure

TABLE 11-2 Athletic Trainer Employment by Industry: Percent Distribution 2012 and Projected 2022

Employer	% Employed in 2012	% Projected Employment in 2022	% Growth Change
Educational services (e.g., junior colleges, colleges, universities, and elementary and secondary schools)	8.6	9.4	10.2
Health care and social assistance (e.g., ambulatory health-care services; offices of health practitioners, offices of physicians, outpatient care; general medical and surgical hospitals)	8.7	12.0	38.2
Performing arts, spectator sports	4.5	52	14.7
Recreation and fitness industries	3.0	3.5	18.5
Government	0.3	0.4	6.7

Source: http://www.bls.gov/ooh/healthcare/athletic-trainers-and-exercise-physiologists.htm.

means only certain people have met the standards to represent themselves as ATs. Most often, a license is granted after the AT meets certain criteria, such as presenting a current BOC card, passing a state examination, and/or clearing a background check. States with licensure for ATs have practice acts that outline what ATs are allowed to do. The majority of the states have licensure for ATs. The next level of state regulation is *state certification*. Unlike the BOC certification, which is a national credential, state certification applies only to the state level. Under state certification, there may not be a restriction on who may call themselves an athletic trainer, but it does prohibit noncertified people from performing certain acts. The least restrictive regulation is the *state registration*. Under this, ATs must register with the state as an AT, but it often does not prevent others from calling themselves ATs or practicing athletic training.[2]

More about state regulation can be found under "Challenges," later in this chapter.

Trends

The majority of employed athletic trainers work with athletes in academic settings, and the remainder are nearly equally split among clinics, medical offices, hospitals, and fitness/recreation sport centers.[3] No women were recorded as athletic trainers until Dotty Cohen joined the NATA in 1966, and the first woman sat for the BOC examination in 1972. Since then, women have rapidly joined the field. The 2014 NATA membership data show that there were 47.6% male members and 52.4% female members in the athletic training profession.[1] As mentioned earlier, the projected job growth for ATs is well above the expected national average growth.

Challenges

There are three main challenges in athletic training today: state regulation, reimbursement, and professional (entry-level) education. The primary challenge in athletic training is securing state practice acts in all 50 states. Currently, 43 states have athletic training licensure, 5 have state registration (Colorado, Hawaii, Oregon, Minnesota, and West Virginia), 2 have state certification (South Carolina and New York) and 1 (California) has no athletic training regulation at all. The NATA has made great strides in securing some sort of regulation in most states, but the practice acts need to be strong enough to allow ATs to practice their specific skill set, without allowing unqualified individuals to believe they can also practice athletic training. Both the NATA and BOC websites have information about each state's regulations.

Third-party reimbursement allows an AT to charge an insurance company for services rendered. Increasing third-party reimbursement for insurances purposes is a hot topic in athletic training because it is tied to state regulation, as well as individual insurance companies' knowledge of what an AT does. There are currently medical billing codes regarding therapy, exercise, and other areas in which ATs are trained, but reimbursement for AT services is not yet widespread or as recognized as it could be. State AT organizations are working with both local and national governments to stay abreast of new insurance rules and educate involved parties to the skill set of ATs.

Professional (entry-level) education is another national challenge. Other allied health fields (physical therapists and physician assistants, as examples) have stopped offering their programs at the undergraduate (bachelor) level and have moved their entry-level education to higher degrees. There is strong debate on whether this is appropriate

Aptitude Profile/Technical Standards

As a health-care provider, ATs must have strong ethics and always consider the needs of the patient over the wants of the team, parent, coach, or game. Therefore, athletic trainers need to be unafraid to make difficult decisions, often under pressure from a coach, parent, or athlete. They need to be precise and detail-oriented, but still have empathy and good interpersonal skills.[3] Additionally, ATs need to have a strong emotional constitution, patience, and ability to explain complicated conditions or surgeries in simple language; and, of course, a good sense of humor never hurts. Because many ATs may help lift heavy patients (e.g., fallen football linemen) and stand for extended periods of time, they must be fit and healthy enough to render care without injury to themselves.

Attributes important for athletic trainers include the following[1-3]:

Strong work ethic	Physically fit
Quick thinker	Intelligent
Problem solver	Good public speaker
Leader	Fair
Maturity	Flexibility
Self-confidence	Compassion
Strong ethics	Ability to communicate effectively
Emotionally strong	
Composed in stressful situations	Confidentiality

for ATs as well. It would mean students would need an undergraduate degree in another field, and would then earn a master's degree in athletic training. Graduates would then take the BOC to be credentialed as an AT. Programs in many states offer the professional (entry-level) master's degree in athletic training, and there will be a nationwide mandate that all programs be master's degree programs in the future. However, this mandate's deadline will be 7 to 10 years away.

ATs working with athletic teams may also work some nights and weekends, as well as be available for travel with the team. Because athletic teams often practice outdoors, ATs working with some teams must be able to withstand and adapt to changing environments, including extremes in heat and cold, wind and rain.

Before admission into CAATE-accredited programs, students must sign a document termed the **Technical Standards.** This document outlines the physical and mental expectations of the athletic training degree so prospective students can determine if they need accommodations to meet the technical standards of the program.

Required Continuing Education

Continuing education (CE) is mandated for all certified athletic trainers to maintain their national credential, ATC (athletic trainer, certified). The BOC established the need for continuing education in 1974 and began to require that each certified AT earn a specific number (hours) of continuing education units (CEUs) per set time period, currently 2 years.[6] ATs must earn a minimum of 50 CEUs every 2 years, with at least 10 of the 50 CEUs from evidence-based practice–designated courses. ATs must also have evidence of ongoing and current emergency cardiac care (ECC) certification, yet no CEUs are awarded for maintaining this certification. One means of achieving the ECC is by holding current certification in "CPR/AED for the Professional Rescuer" via the American Red Cross. Athletic trainers most often earn these CEUs at BOC-approved workshops, seminars, and conferences (such as state, regional, and national meetings). Athletic trainers record their CE activity on the BOC website and maintain documentation of the education in the event they are audited. Examples of documentation include a certificate of attendance, official transcript, official letter acknowledging the AT as a speaker or panelist, copy of a publication, or title page of a book authored. Consequences for not meeting the required CEUs in a reporting period could include expiration of the BOC certification, and can lead to the need to retake the BOC examination to reinstate the certification credential.

Working Together

All athletic trainers must work under the direction of a physician, so they should be comfortable discussing medical information with other medical personnel. Just because a person has earned a medical degree (MD or DO) does not mean that he or she is well trained in specific injuries to athletes or concussion management. Another example is certain infectious skin conditions. Wrestlers may be allowed to participate after a certain time has passed if their affected skin is covered and they have been on medication for a specified time. Again, many physicians may not know this about the sport of wrestling, and the AT provides a good link to facilitate allowing the athlete to participate within the sport rules, as well as keeping the athlete and others safe. Physicians rely on the expertise of ATs to assist them with return-to-participation decisions, restrictions of the sport, and so on. For example, an athlete may be allowed to play with a cast in certain sports/playing positions. Typically, a physician would not know this and may restrict an athlete from participation until a fractured hand is out of the cast. The AT can be the link that allows the athlete to safely participate, and explain to the physician what constraints are required for the specific athlete/sport.

ATs also decide if an athlete needs to see a specialist, rather than a general physician or the team doctor. In cases where an athlete has a concussion, an orthopedic surgeon is usually not the best medical choice for management of this condition. Knowledge of the expertise of individual health-care providers is necessary for the AT to prevent unnecessary office appointments.

In schools, the nurse can be a wonderful resource. In many places, the AT is not on campus until after school is out, and the nurse may have treated athletes for their diabetes or asthma during the school day. It is critical that these two health professionals maintain good communication for the safety of the student athletes. In general, good communication is key, because ATs also must speak effectively with parents and coaches. They have to be able to calmly relay medical information to nonmedical individuals, and provide clear take-home instructions and a plan for future rehabilitation. Both parents and coaches tend to want to know exactly when their child/athlete can fully return to activity, so being able to relay a clear, focused plan in an educational manner is critical.

SUMMARY

Athletic trainers are uniquely trained to provide emergency medical care, make return-to-play decisions, and ensure safe participation for athletic activity and active people. They typically work with school, college, and professional athletes, but can also be found in clinics, the military, industry, and entertainment fields. ATs must have at least an undergraduate degree from an accredited college and pass the national BOC examination before they can practice.

Author Spotlight

Katie Walsh Flanagan, EdD

I have been so fortunate in my career as an AT. Highlights include traveling the world with the U.S. soccer teams (both men's and women's), working with men's professional soccer in Chicago, and serving the United States as an athletic trainer in international games. The best part of my career is that I have the opportunity to influence others. As a program director (one in charge of a CAATE-accredited AT program), I get to work with students and athletes every day. My research (lightning safety in sports) has made a difference in daily lives. My work is different every day, energizing, and fun. There is absolutely no other career I would choose.

CASE STUDY

Tamika was recently hired as the athletic trainer for Happy Valley High School, a private boarding school in upstate New York. She was excited to begin her career as a certified athletic trainer. Tamika grew up in Los Angeles and attended public schools and college in California, so a private school in New York was a new and exciting change for her. During a boy's lacrosse game one of the freshmen, Marco, appeared to be injured, as he was looking a bit dazed on the field. Tamika did not see if Marco was hit, or how he got injured, because she was busy talking to one of the parents who was also from California. Unsure of the lacrosse rules, she did not want to ask for a time out to evaluate Marco, so she waited until halftime to talk to him. The game had no score, and Marco appeared to be running slower than usual, and appeared to be unsure of his position on the field. Tamika did not know that Marco was highly recruited to come to Happy Valley and was among the best youth players in the East, and therefore should have known where he was supposed to be on the field. At halftime, Marco complained of being very thirsty, having a headache and being dizzy. Recalling her training, Tamika considered that maybe Marco had a concussion, because she knew that one does not have to be knocked unconscious to have a concussion, and younger athletes are even more prone to them than professional athletes. Tamika removed Marco from the game because headache and dizziness were the most common signs of a concussion. Coach Wally was upset, because Marco was his best player, and he wanted Marco to return as soon as possible. The coach told Tamika that helmets prevent concussions from getting worse, and although Tamika knew that was not completely true, she also did not want to explain this to the coach in the middle of a game. She told Coach Wally that she would reevaluate Marco in 15 minutes and decide what to do at that time. As the game progressed, both teams scored, and Tamika had to take care of other athletes, cover a wound, retape an ankle, and assist an asthmatic athlete with his inhaler. She forgot to recheck Marco, until she heard a big shout. Looking to the field to see what else might need her attention, Tamika saw Marco score a goal and collapse. As she ran on to the field, she saw the timer on the scoreboard display that the game was almost over. How did Marco get back in the game? Tamika was mentally kicking herself for spending so much time talking to the parent from her home state after Marco's injury, and taking care of the other injuries, that she forgot to recheck him. She later found out that Coach Wally substituted Marco into the game after waiting the 15 minutes Tamika mentioned. His understanding was that Marco could reenter after the short break.

Much later, Tamika found out two key things: Marco had seen his doctor—an internist—last month about his being thirsty all the time, being tired, and the headaches he was getting recently. Marco thought they were due to new glasses but learned that day that he was diabetic, like his mother. The school nurse had been involved with his care since then and was keeping his insulin and glucometer, which measured his blood sugar. Tamika was confused because she was never told about the diabetes mellitus and she did not know the school nurse was involved in Marco's care.

The next day, the school headmaster called Tamika into his office. He wanted to know if anything could have been done to prevent the situation that resulted in needing an ambulance for Marco. He, too, was unaware of Marco's newly diagnosed diabetes mellitus, and wanted to talk about how to prevent a similar situation from ever happening again.

Questions

1. What could Tamika have done to better prepare herself to be an AT for the lacrosse team?

2. What is a way to find out if New York requires athletic trainers to be state certified or not?

3. How can Tamika initiate and maintain communication with the school nurse on matters related to her athletes?

4. How can Tamika make certain that athletes inform her if they see a doctor?

(continued)

5. What sort of documentation from the internist would have helped her in this situation?

6. If you were the headmaster, whom would you talk to so this type of communication issue never happens again?

7. What questions would you have if you were Marco's coach?

8. What conversations need to be addressed with the coach and nurse? Who should be involved in the conversations?

9. How and when should athletes' medical history information be provided to the athletic trainer and coaches?

Review Questions

1. Athletic training was first organized as a profession in:
   A. 1970
   B. 1950
   C. 2003
   D. 1995

2. How many states in the United States have no state athletic training regulation?
   A. 1
   B. 4
   C. 43
   D. 50

3. The U.S. Department of Labor predicts that the job growth for athletic trainers will exceed the national occupational growth rate in 2022.
   A. True
   B. False

4. The majority of athletic trainers work in:
   A. Academics
   B. Hospitals
   C. Industry
   D. Professional sports

5. Which state regulation type is the most restrictive form of regulation?
   A. Registration
   B. Certification
   C. Licensure
   D. Exemption

6. What is the abbreviation for the organization that accredits athletic training education programs?
   A. BOC
   B. NATA
   C. NFL
   D. CAATE

7. Which is not a core academic area for athletic trainers?
   A. Chemistry
   B. Pharmacology
   C. Medical conditions
   D. Nutrition

8. What degree is required for students to sit for the BOC?
   A. Sports medicine
   B. Athletic training
   C. Kinesiology
   D. Premedicine

9. What are CEUs?
   A. Classes required in the major
   B. A certification allowing an AT to perform certain skills
   C. Continuing education after passing the BOC examination
   D. A state regulation act

10. How many semesters are students required to log hours under a preceptor?
    A. Two
    B. Four
    C. They do not log hours by semesters, only at the end in an internship
    D. Six

Glossary of Key Terms

National certification—also termed *BOC*; a national examination that is taken after students complete the degree in athletic training; only those who pass the BOC may be called *athletic trainers*

Preceptor—a certified/licensed professional who teaches and evaluates students in a clinical setting using an actual patient base

State regulation—state laws overseeing the practice of athletic training

Technical Standards—a list of attributes and skills athletic training students need to successfully complete the degree in athletic training

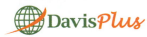 Additional Resources are available online at www.davisplus.com

Additional Resources

Commission on Accreditation of Athletic Training Education—www.caate.net
CAATE is the national association that oversees athletic training accreditation processes, and ensures that all member institutions meet the published minimum standards for accreditation.

Educational and Professional Resources
Journal of Athletic Training—http://natajournals.org
Athletic Training Education Journal—http://natajournals.org
National Athletic Trainers' Association—http://nata.org
The NATA is the national governing body of all athletic trainers, regardless of scope of practice.

Board of Certification—http://bocatc.org
The BOC is the national regulatory body of all certified athletic trainers.

National Collegiate Athletic Association—http://www.ncaa.org
National Federation of State High School Associations—www.nfhs.org
State Regulatory Boards in Athletic Training—http://members.nata.org/gov/state/regulatory-boards/map.cfm
Provides information on state regulatory acts and contact information for state regulatory boards.

References

1. National Athletic Trainers' Association. Athletic training.
   http://www.nata.org/athletic-training.
   Accessed September 7, 2014.

2. Prentice WE. *Principles of Athletic Training,* 14th ed. New York: McGraw-Hill; 2011.

3. U.S. Department of Labor, Bureau of Labor Statistics. Occupational outlook handbook.
   http://www.bls.gov/oes/current/oes299091.htm.
   Accessed September 7, 2014.

4. Commission on Accreditation of Athletic Training Education.
   http://caate.net.
   Accessed September 7, 2014.

5. Commission on Accreditation of Athletic Training Education (CAATE). Standards for the accreditation of professional athletic training programs.
   http://caate.net/wp-content/uploads/2014/07/2012-Professional-Standards.pdf.
   Accessed September 27, 2014.

6. Board of Certification.
   http://www.bocatc.org/index.php.
   Accessed September 4, 2014.

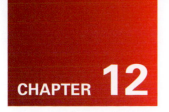

CHAPTER 12

Audiology

Ayasakanta Rout, PhD

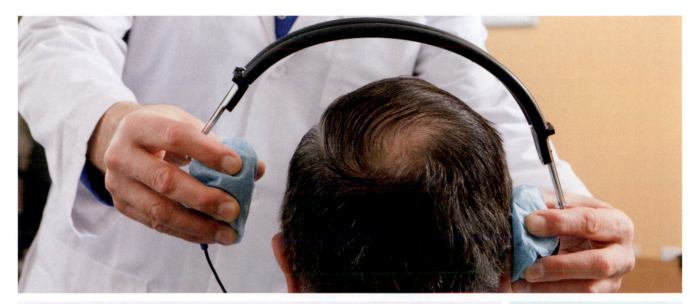

Photo credit: istock/Thinkstock

Learning Objectives

After reading this chapter, students should be able to:

- Explain the role of an audiologist
- Describe the difference between the various types of settings in which audiologists work
- Describe the education and licensing process
- Discuss opportunities and challenges for working in the rapidly growing field of audiology

Key Terms

- Audiologist
- Hearing evaluation
- Hearing aids
- Hearing loss
- Cochlear implant
- Intraoperative and neurophysiological monitoring
- Doctor of audiology (AuD)
- Psychoacoustics
- Electrophysiological evaluation

"A Day in the Life"

Hello, and welcome to my world of audiology for a day. I am a clinical **audiologist** at a university medical center. My day promises to be an exciting one today as the morning is packed with patients needing **hearing evaluation** and the afternoon has two patients who will be fitted with their **hearing aids** for the first time. One of those patients is a 6-month-old baby who was identified with **hearing loss** as a newborn.

If all goes well, he will be hearing his mother's voice for the first time.

It is 8 a.m. and I am in my office reviewing charts for the patients that are scheduled for hearing evaluation this morning. The first patient is a 62-year-old former construction worker who has gradually lost his hearing from exposure to machinery noise. His primary complaint is that he cannot understand

(continued)

what others are saying in the presence of background noise. His wife interjects and tells me that he is ignoring everyone who is trying to speak to him. Before I evaluated his hearing status, I inspected his ears to make sure there was no active ear infection or any earwax occluding the ear canal. After the visual examination we proceeded to a very quiet sound-treated room for the hearing tests. The patient was seated in a comfortable chair and listened to different sounds through specially designed earphones. After about 15 minutes we were done with his hearing test. Now it is time to explain to the patient and his wife the current status of his hearing, and reasons why he is having trouble understanding speech in noisy situations. This patient was an excellent candidate for hearing aids. I fitted him a pair of demonstration hearing aids to try out for the remainder of our appointment and he was amazed with how much more he could understand with the hearing aids. We set up another appointment in 1 week to fit a pair of custom-made hearing aids for him. Wow! One hour has just flown by and my second patient is already here in the waiting room. This patient is a 6-year-old boy who has been referred by the school because of suspected hearing problems. After the hearing evaluation was completed, we discovered that the child had partial hearing loss in one ear. The other ear was normal. That explained his inconsistent response to the teacher in the classroom. Later today, a letter will be sent to his school describing the results of the hearing test and listening strategies to overcome the partial hearing loss in one ear.

I have three more patients scheduled before lunch. All three of them are returning for their annual hearing evaluation. It is important to test one's hearing annually. If any significant changes are noticed in a patient's hearing compared with the last report, a detailed hearing evaluation will be required. It's almost lunchtime and I'm glad the three patients did not need any further evaluation. They have been taking good care of their hearing.

I am ready for the second half of the day and I am really excited about fitting hearing aids on the 6-month-old baby. The first patient of the afternoon is here. She is a retired professor who was recommended a pair of hearing aids after her hearing evaluation. She is excited about trying her new hearing aids. I programmed the hearing aids specifically for her hearing loss, and verified with special equipment that the hearing aid was programmed to maximize speech understanding.

The patient of the day is here! He did not pass his newborn hearing test and later was identified with severe hearing loss in both ears. The parents are determined to give him every opportunity to hear and speak. A team of professionals, including an audiologist, speech-language pathologist, ear-nose-throat (ENT) specialist, social worker, and psychologist have been helping the family navigate the process of learning to hear and speak. In preparation for today's appointment we had already made custom earpieces that would be coupled with his new hearing aid. The baby was sitting on his mother's lap and playing with his toys when we placed the hearing aids on his ears. When the mother called his name, he immediately turned toward the voice! It was a good first step. He is going to wear the hearing aids for 6 months while the parents decide whether to pursue **cochlear implants**. We wrapped up the appointment with lots of supporting material for the family to take home and information on care and maintenance of the hearing aid. What a nice way to end the workday with this patient!

It is time to review tomorrow's schedule. Tomorrow promises to be an exciting day with outpatient clinic in the morning and cochlear implant clinic in the afternoon. I can't wait to be back in the office tomorrow. Where else can you get to have a positive impact on so many people's lives on an individual basis?

Introduction to Audiology

Description

Audiologists work in a variety of health-care settings, including Veterans Administration (VA) medical centers, specialty hospitals, otolaryngology practices, audiology practices, hearing instrument manufacturers, research and development, universities, and schools (K–12). Audiologists are the primary health-care professionals who evaluate, diagnose, treat, and manage hearing loss and balance disorders in adults and children. The profession of audiology has seen rapid developments in its core knowledge base and scope of practice. Like many other health-care professions, audiology offers a great combination of science and art that the audiologist applies in clinical practice every day. On the scientific front, the relatively new field of audiology and hearing science sees a plethora of developments on a regular basis. The study of

hearing mechanisms and hearing loss (and its treatment) has opened up collaborative scientific efforts among audiologists, hearing scientists, physicians, biologists, physicists, biomedical engineers, and other health-care professionals. In addition to the new developments, audiologists use advanced computerized equipment to diagnose and treat hearing loss. On the artistic side, the audiologist has to apply all this knowledge to a patient population ranging from newborns to the elderly, as well as work with family members to facilitate audiological rehabilitation programs. The last part of this chapter presents a unique case study describing the role of the audiologist and other health-care professionals.

History

The profession of audiology is relatively new compared with many other health-care professions, such as medicine, nursing, and social work. Audiology has grown tremendously since its inception 70 years ago. It is reported in the literature that the term *audiology* was first coined by Raymond Carhart and Norton Canfield, in 1945, independent of each other.[1] Many veterans of World War II returned home with permanent hearing loss, resulting from exposure to excessive noise and lack of hearing protection. This huge population of service personnel entering civilian life required qualified health-care professionals to test their hearing and provide aural rehabilitation. At that time, otologists and speech pathologists had training to perform audiological testing and rehabilitation. Soon, military-based aural rehabilitation centers were started and those led to audiological services for civilians. During the early days audiologists used large, cumbersome electronic equipment to test hearing function. These tests yielded limited data about the hearing status of a patient. During a 25-year period after the war, audiologists developed many behavioral and physiological diagnostic tests to pinpoint which parts of the ear are damaged. Many of those tests are still in use today. While the diagnostic aspect of audiology was rapidly developing, important developments in electronics (miniaturization and integrated circuits) led to much smaller diagnostic equipment. Simultaneously, hearing aids became more and more powerful, capable, and, most important, smaller in size. During the past 30 years, the field of audiology has continued to grow at a rapid pace, adding new dimensions to its scope of practice, discovering new information, and moving on to a doctoral level of education as the minimum requirement to practice as an audiologist in the United States. The scope of practice and educational requirements are described next.

Scope of Practice

The American Academy of Audiology (AAA), the American Speech-Language-Hearing Association (ASHA), and the Academy of Dispensing Audiologists (ADA) are the professional organizations that represent the interests of audiologists in the United States. These professional bodies have outlined scopes of practice for audiologists in the United States. The American Academy of Audiology[2] defines an *audiologist* as a professional "who, by virtue of academic degree, clinical training, and license to practice and/or professional credential, is uniquely qualified to provide a comprehensive array of professional services related to the prevention of hearing loss and the audiologic identification, assessment, diagnosis, and treatment of persons with impairment of auditory and vestibular function, and to the prevention of impairments associated with them. Audiologists serve in a number of roles including clinician, therapist, teacher, consultant, researcher, and administrator."

The current scope of practice from the American Academy of Audiology[2] categorizes an audiologist's field of work into seven areas: (1) identification of hearing loss, (2) audiological assessment and diagnosis, (3) nonmedical treatment of hearing loss, (4) hearing conservation/prevention of hearing loss, (5) **intraoperative and neurophysiological monitoring**, (6) research and teaching, and (7) additional expertise.

Identification of Hearing Loss

Audiologists are trained to develop and oversee hearing screening programs (including universal newborn hearing screening and school screening). Audiologists may also perform speech-language screening in the pediatric population.

Audiological Assessment and Diagnosis

Audiologists apply psychoacoustic and physiological testing to accurately measure hearing sensitivity of all age groups. Psychoacoustic principles refer to hearing tests that require a response from the patient when a sound is presented to the ear. On the other hand, physiological tests measure the response from the auditory system when a sound is presented. The patient is often instructed to sit comfortably and relax during these tests. Using these advanced technologies, an audiologist can determine the degree of hearing loss and often identify which part of the ear is affected. Audiologists are also trained to evaluate and diagnose problems with the balance system (vestibular abnormality).

Nonmedical Treatment of Hearing Loss

Audiologists are trained to provide the full range of nonmedical treatment services for individuals with impairment of

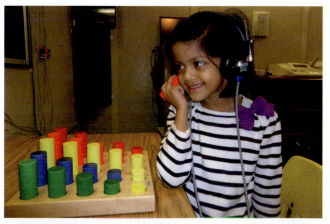

FIGURE 12-1 Hearing evaluation of a young child inside a soundproof room. The child is listening for the softest sound she could detect through the headphones.

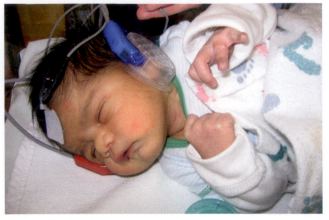

FIGURE 12-2 Hearing screening of a newborn baby using electrophysiological testing.

hearing or balance function. It must be noted that hearing loss resulting from damage to the cochlea is not medically treatable. The primary treatment option is appropriate amplification with advanced hearing aids. The audiologist is responsible for the evaluation, fitting, and verification of amplification devices, including assistive listening devices. If the ear canal is blocked with cerumen (wax), the audiologist's scope of practice allows limited cerumen removal or, in extreme cases, referral to a physician (usually an otolaryngologist, a specialist of the ear, nose, and throat).

Audiologists are also engaged in treatment of the following hearing or vestibular conditions:

- Audiologists are key members of the cochlear implant or other implantable hearing device team who determines candidacy, programs and activates the implant, provides presurgical and postsurgical counseling, implements aural rehabilitation programs, and monitors progress.
- Audiological treatment services for infants and children with hearing loss.
- Audiologists also serve as a source of information for individuals with hearing loss and their families, other professionals, and the general public.

- Full members of the team involved with treatment of persons with vestibular disorders, which may include continuous or episodic dizziness.

Hearing Conservation

Hearing loss as a result of prolonged exposure to loud noise is one of the major causes of hearing loss in adults, military personnel, and, more recently, those using personal in-ear music players (often younger persons). Considering that hearing loss resulting from noise exposure is irreversible, it is one of the most crucial roles of the audiologist to develop and oversee hearing conservation/hearing loss prevention programs in noisy environments. Audiologists also work on awareness campaigns to prevent hearing loss.

Intraoperative Neurophysiological Monitoring

Audiologists are trained to apply electrophysiological tests to monitor the vitality of auditory nerves during head and neck surgery (especially during surgeries related to the hearing and balance function). Working as a part of the surgical team, the audiologist's measurements help in differential diagnosis and presurgical and postsurgical comparison of neural function.

Basic and Applied Research

Audiologists conduct basic and applied research related to auditory and vestibular systems.

Additional Expertise

Some audiologists, by virtue of their education and additional training, work in other exciting areas such as animal audiology, telehealth service delivery, sales and marketing in the hearing industry, and many other fascinating areas.

Required Education

Most audiologists earn a **doctor of audiology (AuD)** degree. Some audiologists earn a doctor of philosophy (PhD) or

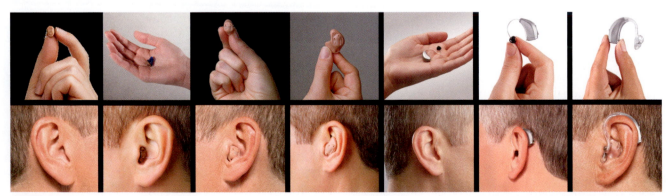

FIGURE 12-3 Different types of hearing aids. (Photo courtesy Starkey Hearing Technologies.)

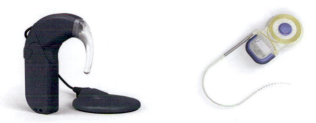

FIGURE 12-4 Cochlear implant external processor (left) and internal device (right). (Photo courtesy MED-EL Corporation).

doctor of science (ScD) degree in the hearing and balance sciences. Since 2007, the entry-level educational requirement to practice as an audiologist in the United States is a clinical doctorate in audiology (AuD). The AuD is a 4-year postbaccalaureate degree program preparing students to specialize in the area of diagnosis and treatment of hearing and balance disorders. Currently, approximately 75 universities offer AuD programs in the United States. The educational requirement to practice as an audiologist in other countries (Canada, United Kingdom, India, Australia, Brazil, South Africa, and New Zealand) is a master's degree in audiology.

Undergraduate Preparation for an AuD Degree

The majority of students pursuing an AuD degree have an undergraduate degree in communication sciences and disorders or speech pathology and audiology. However, the interdisciplinary nature of audiology works well for students with undergraduate degrees including, but not limited to, the following academic majors:

- Psychology
- Biology
- Physics

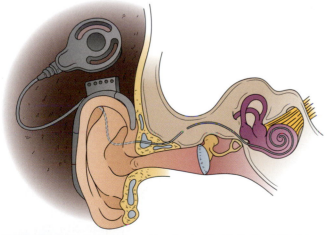

FIGURE 12-5 Illustration of a cochlear implant inside the head. The internal device is surgically implanted inside the head and a wire electrode stimulates the auditory nerves.

- Biomedical engineering
- Special education
- Music recording/audio engineering

Typical Curriculum in AuD Training Programs

A typical AuD training program comprises three educational components: (1) academic course work, (2) clinical training, and (3) research. It is worth noting that AuD programs vary in terms of these three areas. The coursework remains more or less comparable across programs, but the nature of clinical and research experience varies greatly. Core courses in an AuD program include the following:

Basic sciences:

- Anatomy and physiology
- Acoustics and electronics
- **Psychoacoustics**

Audiological evaluation, diagnosis, and identification:

- Behavioral audiological assessment (typically two to three courses)
- **Electrophysiological evaluation** of the auditory system (typically two courses)
- Vestibular evaluation

Treatment of hearing loss:

- Hearing aids (typically two to three courses)
- Cochlear implants
- Aural rehabilitation
- Counseling

Special topics:

- Pediatric audiology
- Geriatric audiology
- Tinnitus
- Pharmacological application in audiology
- Business applications in audiology
- Professional ethics

Professional tools:

- Research methods
- Statistics
- Professional communication

As one can see from this list of courses, audiologists go through a rigorous academic training. In addition, an audiology student completes a minimum of 1,850 hours of supervised clinical work during the 4-year program. Most doctor of audiology programs have an in-house clinic or are attached to a medical center where the graduate students obtain clinical experience during the first 3 years of the program. The fourth year of the AuD program is a year-long externship where students work under the supervision of licensed audiologists.

Licensure

Audiologists must be licensed or registered for practice in all states, the District of Columbia, and Puerto Rico. This requirement ensures that each licensed audiologist has obtained a certain level of academic preparation and clinical training. It is a legal requirement to maintain licensure in the state in which the audiologist practices. To obtain a license to practice audiology, a candidate must have completed both academic training and at least 1,850 hours of clinical training, and passed a standardized national examination in audiology (Praxis test).

Most audiologists maintain a certificate of clinical competence (CCC-A) from the ASHA or a board certification from the American Board of Audiology (ABA). In contrast to state licensure, certification is not a legal requirement to practice audiology. Some states also require the licensed audiologist to obtain a separate hearing aid dispensing license.

Salary

The annual salary for audiologists varies greatly depending on the type of workplace setting, years of experience, and geographical location, among other factors. The Bureau of Labor Statistics, in its 2013 database,[3] reported the median annual salary for audiologists at $69,720. A further analysis of the dataset reveals that those employed in the hearing instruments industry and in hospital settings earn significantly higher than those employed by public schools.

The ASHA 2012 salary survey of audiologists[4] reported a median salary of $73,000 across all types of employment settings. Median salary for different employment settings were reported as follows: educational audiologists ($72,000), hospital-based audiologists ($77,079), academic faculty ($72,507), hearing aid dispensing chain clinics ($60,000), nonresidential health-care facilities ($70,000), and hearing instrument industry ($79,233).

It is also worth noting that many audiologists work on a part-time or hourly basis. The median hourly wage for audiologists is $35. For a detailed report the reader is directed to the following websites:

- Bureau of labor Statistics: http://www.bls.gov/oes/current/oes291181.htm
- ASHA: http://www.asha.org/uploadedFiles/2012-Audiology-Survey-Salaries.pdf

Trends

The Bureau of Labor Statistics[3] estimates a rapid growth in the job outlook in the next decade. Employment of audiologists is projected to grow 34% from 2012 to 2022, much faster than the average for all occupations. However, because it is a small occupation, the fast growth will result in only about 4,300 new jobs over the 10-year period. Other "health diagnosing and treating" professions are projected to grow at a rate of 20% over that period.[3] Like many other health-care professions that started after World War II, many senior audiologists are reaching retirement age. A huge retiring workforce combined with changing demographics in the United States and rapid advances in technology (making hearing aids more appealing to consumers) has resulted in great demand for audiologists in the coming years.

Amid impressive developments, newer trends in the way audiologists practice are coming into the profession. Many audiologists are starting independently owned private practices; others are joining buyer groups (franchises) and operating their clinic under an umbrella. Yet another development currently underway is the training of a supporting workforce in audiology assistants. The job of the audiology assistant would be to perform basic hearing tests, troubleshoot hearing aids, and assist with complex diagnostic evaluation. This would allow the audiologist to spend more time with the patient.

Challenges

One of the greatest challenges facing the profession of audiology now is the shortage of researchers to advance the knowledge base of the profession. As noted, audiology has benefited immensely from interdisciplinary research. Many questions need to be answered. This challenge also creates a tremendous opportunity for the clinical audiologist to pursue a career in research. Some universities offer a combined

Tips and Tools

Did you know that the National and Nutrition Examination Survey (NHANES) in 2006 reported that one in every five U.S. adolescents 12 to 19 years of age demonstrated some amount of hearing loss? Compared with the 1988–1994 NHANES, this constitutes a one-third increase in the prevalence of hearing loss.[5] Exposure to loud music via personal stereo devices has been attributed as a main reason for acquired hearing loss in adolescents. This hearing loss is irreversible, and it could contribute to an increase in demand for audiologists in the near future.

AuD/PhD program to train the next level of clinical researchers.

Another challenge in the field of audiology is the lack of advancement in the profession in other countries. More recently, a new subfield of audiology has emerged that focuses on enhancing global audiology.

The third challenge facing audiology is insurance reimbursement for independent services. Currently, audiologists are not reimbursed for all of their services and most insurance companies reimburse only a small amount for hearing aids, which are expensive devices.

Role of the Audiologist

The audiologist's role varies depending on the work setting. In the scope of practice section of this chapter, the different clinical services that audiologists perform were described. Table 12-1 describes different audiology specialties and provides more information on the work setting and role. The fourth column lists different professionals an audiologist collaborates with in his or her job. The reader can get an appreciation of the interprofessional nature of the audiologist's work from Table 12-1.

TABLE 12-1 Audiology Specialties, Work Settings, and Roles

Audiology Specialty	Employment Setting	Role	Interprofessional Environment
Medical audiology	• Hospitals • Physicians' offices • Health maintenance organizations • VA medical centers	• Diagnosis and nonmedical treatment of hearing and balance disorders	• Physicians • Nurses • Physical therapy (PT), occupational therapy (OT), speech-language pathology (SLP) • Medical social worker
Cochlear implant audiologist	• Otolaryngology departments • Otolaryngology private practices • University audiology clinics	• Determine candidacy for cochlear implants • Programming the device • Counseling • Follow-up • Referral	• Otolaryngologist • Nurses • Special educators • SLP
Dispensing audiologist	• Private practices • Otolaryngology offices • VA hospitals • University clinics • Nonprofit organizations • Retail locations	• Diagnose hearing loss • Fit hearing aids according to prescription • Provide aural rehabilitation	• Physicians • Industry personnel

(continued)

TABLE 12-1 Audiology Specialties, Work Settings, and Roles—cont'd

Audiology Specialty	Employment Setting	Role	Interprofessional Environment
Pediatric audiologist	• Pediatric hospitals • Rehabilitation centers • Private practice	• Newborn hearing screening • Diagnosis of hearing loss • Family-centered aural rehabilitation	• SLP • Pediatricians • PT, OT • Special educators • Social workers
Educational audiologist	• K–12 • Schools for the deaf	• School hearing screenings • Fit hearing aid and assistive listening devices • Support services for teachers and other professionals	• Teachers • School counselors • SLP • Special educators
Industrial audiology	• Large industries • Part-time consultants	• Monitor hearing level of employees • Implement hearing conservation programs	• Administrators • Human Resources
Audiologist in the hearing instrument industry	• Hearing aid manufacturers	• Research and development • Marketing and sales	• Other audiologists • Physicians • Administrators

Author Spotlight

Ayasakanta Rout, PhD

I grew up in India with a resolute determination "not to become an engineer." Every other profession, especially health care, was particularly appealing at an early age. As it turned out, I finished high school at a much earlier age than my peers and was not eligible to enroll in an undergraduate medical program (one had to be at least 17 years of age). After a year of researching different options, I discovered the field of audiology and speech pathology, without having ever heard of it. Before I knew it, I was freshman in that major. As I was learning exciting information in many interdisciplinary areas related to speech and hearing, I was naturally leaning toward becoming an audiologist. I liked the idea of evaluating a patient's hearing, explaining what's wrong with the ear, and having a nonmedical treatment (hearing aids) available to fix the problem. I started my career working as a clinical audiologist in India. Soon I realized that audiology was a very new field and there were many questions that did not have satisfactory answers. I moved to the United States to pursue a research career in audiology. It's been nearly 20 years of learning, researching, and teaching audiology, and I can't think of one day that wasn't fun.

CASE STUDY

Baby ST, a 14-month-old girl, is being evaluated for cochlear implant candidacy. She did not pass the newborn hearing screening test after birth. Later, her hearing loss was confirmed by the pediatric audiologist at 3 months of age. She was fitted with a pair of hearing aids at 6 months of age with ear molds that were custom made for her ears. Based on the overwhelming evidence available today, this child is a good candidate for cochlear implants. However, the Food and Drug Administration (FDA) recommendations allow cochlear implant surgery to be performed only after 12 months of age unless there are any medical indications. Until then, it is recommended that a hearing aid be tried on and documented that there is not enough progress in language development. The audiologist tested baby ST's hearing status using electrophysiological measures, and then screened her speech and hearing development milestones. Based on the results it was determined that the hearing aids were not helping the child to catch up on her speech and hearing development. She was then referred to an ear, nose, and throat surgeon for medical evaluation. Cochlear implant audiologists work in a truly interprofessional model of health care. The audiologist is responsible for determining the candidacy for cochlear implants, counseling the family, programming and fine-tuning the implant device, and following up. The otolaryngologist performs the surgery, the social worker assists with finding the support system needed for networking, the speech-language pathologist works with the child on language development, and special educators work with the child in the classroom. The cochlear implant audiologist typically works in an interprofessional team, often in a medical environment.

Questions

1. Can you think of other health-care disciplines that might benefit this team?

2. How might this case be different if there were no interprofessional team members to assist in the patient's care?

3. How do the benefits of working with the other team members benefit the audiologists and the patient?

Review Questions

1. The profession of audiology in the United States started after:
   A. The Korean War
   B. The Vietnam War
   C. World War II
   D. The great recession in the 1930s

2. The Bureau of Labor Statistics predicts that job growth in the field of audiology in the next decade will be in the range of:
   A. 5%–10%
   B. 15%–20%
   C. 20%–25%
   D. 30%–35%

3. The minimum academic training required to become an audiologist in the United States is a/an:
   A. Master's degree
   B. Bachelor's degree
   C. Associate degree
   D. Clinical doctorate in audiology

4. What is the minimum academic training required to become an audiologist in Canada?
   A. Master's degree
   B. Bachelor's degree
   C. Associate degree
   D. Clinical doctorate in audiology

5. Which of the following is the most likely treatment option for a person who has hearing loss due to cochlear (inner ear) damage?
   A. Hearing aid or cochlear implant
   B. Medicine
   C. Surgery
   D. Counseling

6. Which of the following ear and/or hearing-related work do audiologists *not* perform?
   A. Cerumen (ear wax) management
   B. Hearing aid programming
   C. Diagnosing the site of lesion
   D. Surgery to fix hearing loss due to recurrent ear infection

7. With which of the following professionals does a pediatric audiologist interact on a regular basis?
   A. Otolaryngologist
   B. SLP
   C. Teacher
   D. All of the above

8. Which of the following refers to testing of vestibular evaluation?
   A. Vision
   B. Balance
   C. Smell
   D. Hearing

9. Approximately how many hours of clinical training do AuD students obtain in graduate school?
   A. 1,000
   B. 1,200
   C. 1,600
   D. 2,000

10. Which of the following pose challenges to the continued development of audiology?
    A. Shortage of researchers
    B. Lack of advanced audiology care globally
    C. Inadequate reimbursement for an audiologist's services
    D. All of the above

Glossary of Key Terms

Audiologist—a professional trained and certified to evaluate and treat disorders of hearing and balance

Hearing evaluation—a screening done to determine hearing loss and the extent of loss

Hearing aid—a miniature electronic device typically worn at ear level to compensate for a person's hearing loss

Hearing loss—the inability to hear noises or sounds; the degree of loss is dependent on the level of hearing, if any

Cochlear implant—a miniature device implanted behind the ear in the skull bone to compensate for a damaged inner ear; sometimes called a *bionic ear*

Intraoperative and neurophysiological monitoring—electrophysiological monitoring of hearing nerve status during a surgery

Doctor of Audiology (AuD)—clinical doctorate in audiology

Psychoacoustics—the study of physiological and psychological responses to sound, which includes speech and music

Electrophysiological evaluation—typically refers to hearing tests measuring nerve responses to sound; these tests do not require any voluntary response from the patient

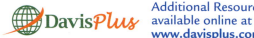

Additional Resources are available online at www.davisplus.com

Additional Resources

Accrediting Bodies

- Council of Academic Accreditation (CAA): www.asha.org/academic/accreditation/
- Accreditation Commission for Audiology Education (ACAE): acaeaccred.org/

Educational Resources

The American Speech-Language-Hearing Association (ASHA) has information available for high school students and undergraduates interested in pursuing audiology:

- High school students interested in audiology: www.asha.org/Careers/highschool/
- Undergraduate students: www.asha.org/Careers/undergrad/

Professional Organizations

- American Academy of Audiology: www.audiology.org
- Student Academy of Audiology: www.audiology.org/saa/
- American Speech-Language and Hearing Association: www.asha.org
- Council of Academic Programs in Communication Sciences and Disorders: www.capcsd.org

- American Auditory Society: www.amauditorysoc.org
- Academy of Doctors of Audiology: www.audiologist.org

Audiology News, Continuing Education, Webinars, and Jobs

- Audiology Online: www.audiologyonline.com

Hearing Instrument Manufacturers

- Oticon: www.oticon.com
- Phonak: www.phonak.com
- Resound: www.gnresound.com
- Siemens: www.siemens-hearing.com
- Starkey Hearing Technology: www.starkey.com
- Unitron: www.unitron.com
- Widex: www.widex.com

Cochlear Implant Manufacturers

- Advanced Bionics: www.advancedbionics.com
- Cochlear Americas: www.cochlear.com
- Med-El: www.medel.com

References

1. Jerger J. *Audiology in the USA*. San Diego, CA: Plural Publishing; 2009.
2. American Academy of Audiology. Scope of practice in audiology. 2004.

   http://www.audiology.org/resources/documentlibrary/Pages/ScopeofPractice.aspx.

   Accessed March 28, 2014.
3. Bureau of Labor Statistics, U.S. Department of Labor. Occupational outlook handbook, 2014–2015 edition, audiologists.

   http://www.bls.gov/ooh/healthcare/audiologists.htm.

   Accessed April 1, 2014.
4. American Speech-Language-Hearing Association. Scope of practice in audiology. 2004.

   www.asha.org/policy.

   Accessed March 28, 2014.
5. Shargorodsky J, Curhan SG, Curhan GC, Eavey R. Change in prevalence of hearing loss in US adolescents. *J Am Med Assoc*. 2010;304(7):772–778.

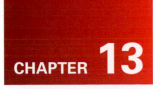

CHAPTER 13

Clinical Laboratory Science

Joan Glacken, EdD, Julie Zemplinski, MSH, and Tony Burkett, MS

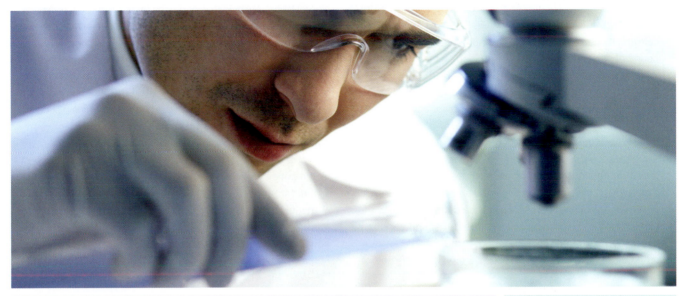

Photo credit: istock/Thinkstock

Learning Objectives

After reading this chapter, students should be able to:

- Discuss the role of a clinical laboratory scientist
- Discuss the role of a clinical laboratory technician
- Differentiate between the roles of a clinical laboratory scientist and a clinical laboratory technician
- Discuss the differences between the areas of specialization
- Discuss the differences between practice sites
- Describe the education, certification, and licensing process
- Describe the continuing education requirements
- Discuss the relationship between the clinical laboratory scientist and other members of the health-care team
- Discuss opportunities and challenges for working in the field of clinical laboratory science

Key Terms

- Clinical chemistry
- Hematology
- Immunohematology (blood bank)
- Immunology
- Microbiology
- Molecular biology
- License
- Certification
- Clinical laboratory technician
- Clinical laboratory scientist
- Continuing education

 ## "A Day in the Life"

Hi there! My name is Joe and I am a clinical laboratory scientist in the hematology laboratory. My day starts at 7:00 a.m. The first thing I do is a morning start-up for the hematology analyzer. This involves cleaning and checking all parts to make sure they are functioning properly. The analyzer has a function that cleans itself and I have to watch this process. Once this process is completed, I have to document in the maintenance log that this procedure has been performed. There is a saying in the laboratory that if it's not documented, it never happened. Therefore, it is important to document all daily maintenance, as well as extra maintenance that occurs when problems arise. Once the analyzer is cleaned and ready for daily operation,

(continued)

I have to run a series of controls to make sure my patient results will be accurate. Controls are simulated blood samples that have a set of parameters that are known values, and results must fall within the established ranges. If the results fall within these ranges, I can run my patient samples. But first I have to record the results of my controls—more documentation. If the results are outside of the established ranges, I need to further investigate why and resolve the problem. The analyzer may have to be recalibrated or some part may have to be replaced. Once the problem is resolved, I must run the controls again and make sure the values fall appropriately. I also have to document what I did to resolve the problem in the maintenance log—more documentation.

By this time it's around 8:00 a.m. and the phlebotomists (people who collect blood and urine samples) begin bringing me blood samples from the different floors of the hospital. Once I have the patients' blood samples, I can run them through the analyzer. As the analyzer prints the reports, I review them for any abnormal findings. If the results are flagged as abnormal, I have to prepare a blood smear on a glass slide. This smear is stained with special dyes so that I can view the cells under the microscope. I look for normal and abnormal white blood cells, red blood cells, and platelets. The analyzer and blood smear results are added to the patients' medical

records for physicians to review. Often, as I review the day's blood smears under the microscope, a STAT specimen arrives from the emergency department. STAT means the specimen needs to be processed as quickly as possible. So I stop what I am doing and process the STAT patient specimen and forward the results to the emergency department as quickly as possible. Once that is done, I can go back to reviewing the blood smears. While I analyze the blood specimens, another clinical laboratory scientist performs tests on urine. A urinalysis consists of a physical, chemical, and microscopic analysis. The physical characteristics are color and clarity. The chemical components include glucose, ketones, protein, blood, nitrites, leukocytes, bilirubin, pH, and specific gravity. The urine samples are placed in a test tube and centrifuged to compress the sediment to the bottom of the tube. The sediment is placed on a glass slide with a glass coverslip and viewed under the microscope. We look for white blood cells, red blood cells, epithelial cells, bacteria, crystals, and casts. The results are added to the patients' medical records for the physicians to review. Blood and urine samples come in all during the day and it is my job to process the specimens and add the results to the patients' medical records. STAT samples come in unannounced all day long. Sometimes it gets very hectic in the hematology laboratory.

Introduction to Clinical Laboratory Science

Description

Clinical laboratory science is a medical specialty that assists in diagnosing diseases through the use of laboratory tests. The laboratory tests are performed on human body fluids and tissues to detect evidence of abnormalities or diseases. Human body fluids include blood, urine, semen, sputum, feces, spinal fluid, and other body fluids. The body fluids are tested through different types of instruments, diagnostic kits, microscopic examination, and other manual methods.

The examination of human body fluids dates back to 300 BC, the time of the ancient Greek physician Hippocrates.[1] Causative agents of diseases such as diphtheria and cholera were discovered in the 1880s, which led to the development of tests for the detection of these diseases in the 1890s. The first clinical laboratory was opened in 1896 at Johns Hopkins Hospital, and at that time, testing was performed mainly by the physicians.[2] Physicians specializing in diagnosing diseases and illnesses through laboratory tests became known as *pathologists*. In the early 1900s, many physicians saw the importance of using laboratory tests as a tool to diagnose diseases, and pathologists began training

laboratory assistants. By the 1920s, standards of testing body fluids were developed for clinical laboratories.[3] Training programs were created to meet the growing need for laboratory technicians, and standards for the education of laboratory personnel were defined. By 1926, all hospital-based clinical laboratories were required to be under the direction of a physician, preferably a pathologist. In 1928, the American Society of Clinical Pathologists (ASCP) began certifying laboratory technicians. Individuals graduating from approved educational programs and passing a board examination were thereafter referred to as *medical technologists (MTs)*.[4] Over the years, the professional title of this field has changed from *medical technologist* to *clinical laboratory scientist* or *medical laboratory scientist*. Since the 1930s, other organizations have formed and some have disbanded. Educational requirements have evolved through the years along with the expansion in the scope of the field and the development of new technology. The majority of clinical laboratory scientists today work in hospital laboratories. In recent years, nonhospital opportunities have grown in areas such as reference laboratories, public health laboratories, forensics, blood and tissue banks, diagnostic industries, and pharmaceutical companies, to name a few. The employment options are numerous for those interested in a career in clinical laboratory science.

Areas of specialization within the field of clinical laboratory science include the following:

- **Clinical chemistry** uses automated and computerized instruments to analyze the chemical and hormonal contents of body fluids.

- **Hematology** uses automated and computerized instruments to analyze the cell counts of whole blood specimens and other body fluids. The microscope is used to identify and classify both normal and abnormal cells in blood and body fluids. Examination of urine specimens (urinalysis) and coagulation studies are common tests performed in hematology.

- **Immunohematology (blood bank)** collects blood samples from donors and recipients, classifies blood types and Rh factors, identifies antibodies, and prepares blood and its components for transfusions.

- **Immunology** detects antigens and antibodies to organisms or agents that pose a threat to the human immune system.

- **Microbiology** examines any body fluid or tissue for the presence of bacteria, viruses, parasites, or fungi and identifies antibiotics that will treat the infection.

- **Molecular biology** uses automated and computerized instruments to analyze complex protein and nucleic acid tests on cell samples.

The most common work setting for a clinical laboratory scientist is the hospital laboratory. Every hospital laboratory has a medical doctor, known as a pathologist, who oversees all laboratory operations. The pathologist is responsible for ensuring the quality and accuracy of results, as well as identifying normal and abnormal cells, reviewing abnormal findings, and interacting with physicians regarding patient results of laboratory tests. Each specialty area has a manager or supervisor who is a clinical laboratory scientist with many years of experience in the laboratory setting. The manager or supervisor is responsible for supervising the other clinical laboratory personnel and overseeing the administrative duties within the specialty area, such as scheduling, ordering supplies and equipment, evaluating employees, and managing budgets. The clinical laboratory scientist is responsible for performing the various laboratory tests in the specialty area and maintaining the instruments and performing quality control procedures to ensure accurate and precise testing. Clinical laboratory scientists can select an area of specialization that interests them after completing their education and clinical rotation.

According to the Bureau of Labor Statistics, clinical laboratory personnel held approximately 330,600 jobs in 2010.[5]). Here is a breakdown of where these personnel are employed:

- Hospitals (state, local, and private): 52%
- Medical and diagnostic laboratories: 16%
- Offices of physicians: 10%
- Federal government: 3%
- Other (diagnostic industry, pharmaceutical sales, forensics, etc.): 19%

Clinical laboratories currently are facing a severe workforce shortage. The U.S. Department of Labor predicts that 19,000 clinical laboratory scientists will be needed between 2010 and 2020.[5] Approximately 40% of the clinical laboratory workforce will retire within the next 10 years.[6] Clinical laboratory scientists are part of the multidisciplinary healthcare team. They provide physicians with valuable information to diagnose, monitor, and treat patients. The laboratory provides 94% of the objective data in a patient's medical record.[7] Approximately 60% to 70% of clinical decisions are influenced by laboratory test results.[7]

Scope of Practice

The scope of practice for a clinical laboratory scientist relates directly to the level of education, **license,** and **certification** required by federal and state agencies. Clinical laboratory scientists are responsible for ensuring reliable and accurate laboratory test results. This is accomplished by the following:

- Ensuring appropriate laboratory tests are ordered
- Obtaining laboratory test samples
- Producing accurate results
- Maintaining the proper function of automated instruments
- Correlating and interpreting laboratory test data
- Sending out laboratory test results to clinicians and physicians
- Assessing, designing, evaluating, and implementing new laboratory test methods
- Participating in quality control procedures and continuous process improvement for all laboratory procedures

Required Education

For anyone interested in becoming a clinical laboratory scientist, high school courses in biology, chemistry, and mathematics are recommended. The majority of states recognize two postsecondary degrees of education for clinical laboratory personnel. These degrees include the associate and the baccalaureate levels. The 2-year associate degree qualifies an individual as a **clinical laboratory technician.** The baccalaureate degree qualifies an individual as a **clinical laboratory scientist.** A technician must always work under the direct supervision of a clinical laboratory scientist. The technician cannot perform high-complexity laboratory tests and cannot assume supervisory responsibilities. Only the clinical laboratory scientist can work unsupervised, perform highly complex testing, and serve as a supervisor.

To obtain certification and/or licensure as a clinical laboratory scientist, one must have a baccalaureate degree from a program in clinical laboratory science or life sciences. Some of the core courses one might expect to take include the following:

- General biology
- Anatomy and physiology
- Microbiology
- General chemistry I and II
- Organic chemistry I and II
- Biochemistry
- Statistics
- Human genetics
- Clinical hematology
- Clinical biochemistry
- Clinical immunology
- Clinical microbiology
- Clinical immunohematology
- Body fluids
- Virology, mycology, and parasitology
- Molecular biology

Certification/License

An individual is qualified to sit for a certification or license examination after successful completion of a baccalaureate degree in clinical laboratory science. Certification is nationally recognized and offered by the American Society of Clinical Pathology (ASCP), American Medical Technologists (AMT), and American Association of Bioanalysts (AAB). Some individual states require a license to practice. As of November 2009, Puerto Rico and the following 11 states required a license for laboratory personnel: California, Florida, Hawaii, Louisiana, Montana, Nevada, New York, North Dakota, Rhode Island, Tennessee, and West Virginia. Certification is required by every state that licenses laboratory personnel to assess the initial competency of licensure candidates.[8]

Continuing Education Requirements

A certified clinical laboratory scientist is required to complete 36 continuing education units (CEUs) per 3-year cycle. **Continuing education** is a professional learning requirement that assists the clinical laboratory scientist in maintaining current knowledge and advances in the field of laboratory science. The CEUs must cover the following areas:

- Laboratory or patient safety: 1 unit
- Immunohematology (blood banking): 2 units
- Clinical chemistry: 2 units
- Clinical hematology: 2 units
- Microbiology: 2 units
- Remaining units in the areas of laboratory specialty, immunology, molecular diagnostics, management, education, or other related laboratory areas of interest

Some states also have different requirements for continuing education. It is the responsibility of the clinical laboratory scientist to check with his or her state to determine the continuing education requirements to maintain licensure.

Salary

According to the Bureau of Labor Statistics, the median annual salary for a clinical laboratory scientist was $56,130 in 2010. The lowest 10% earned more than $38,810 and the highest 10% earned more than $76,780. The median annual salary for the clinical laboratory technician was $36,280 in 2010. The lowest 10% earned more than $24,210 and the highest 10% earned more than $56,040. The average salary range for clinical laboratory scientists varies according to place of employment[5]:

- Federal government: $62,880
- Hospitals (state, local, private): $56,470
- Medical and diagnostic laboratories: $55,930
- Offices of physicians: $52,250

Trends

The workforce shortage continues to be a major problem in the field of clinical laboratory science. Employers are experiencing difficulties hiring qualified laboratory personnel due to the increased retirement of baby boomers and the shortage of licensed professionals in the field. This shortage guarantees employment and higher salaries for graduates of clinical laboratory scientist programs. According to Jobs Rated Almanac, the profession of clinical laboratory science has a 25% job growth potential and good job security.[9] As the general population ages, the demand increases for more health-care services that include laboratory testing and diagnoses. This trend is another indication of the constant need for clinical laboratory scientists. Another need is for clinical laboratory scientist educators who have continued their education in graduate school to become master's- and doctoral-prepared faculty. Qualified faculty is always needed to continue training future students as clinical laboratory scientists.

Challenges

The clinical laboratory scientist has several different challenges. Anyone employed in a clinical laboratory setting is trained to work with body fluids that may contain infectious agents. The threat of exposure to these infectious agents is a major concern to the health and well-being of the worker. An important part of the education and training of a clinical laboratory scientist is learning and practicing universal precautions for handling human samples. Personal protective equipment such as masks, gloves, and goggles are used for the safety and protection of laboratory personnel, as well as laboratory environmental equipment such as biohazard hoods and containers. Even though clinical laboratory scientists always try to follow universal precautions and use protective equipment, accidents do occur that can place them in jeopardy of contracting certain infections. It is also important that the laboratory environment be well lighted and vented for personal safety.

The laboratory environment is fast-paced and stressful. Patients' lives depend on accurate results that can be delivered in a timely manner. Physicians often order critical laboratory testing in which they need results as quickly as possible. These tests are known as STAT tests. Clinical laboratory scientists must be ready to run STAT laboratory tests on a moment's notice and relay the test results to the physician immediately. This work can be very stressful.

Another challenge is maintaining clinical laboratory scientists in the clinical laboratory setting. There is a threat of losing experienced clinical laboratory scientists to private sector jobs in the diagnostic, pharmaceutical, and biotechnology industries. These jobs usually pay much higher salaries for experienced clinical laboratory scientists that require little or no training once hired for these positions.

There is often a perceived inaccurate image of the clinical laboratory. In movies and TV shows, "the lab" is often blamed for patient medical errors. Many times other health professionals blame "the lab" for errors they themselves make. Some errors occur before the specimens reach the laboratory, such as improper labeling, collection, or handling. The clinical laboratory scientist is responsible for making sure that proper specimens are available for testing, otherwise the final results are useless.

In most settings, clinical laboratories usually operate around the clock. Clinical laboratory scientists and technicians may be expected to work evenings, weekends, and holidays.

Role of the Clinical Laboratory Scientist

There are some similarities between the baccalaureate-prepared clinical laboratory scientist (CLS) and the associate-prepared clinical laboratory technician (CLT); however, the CLT is usually supervised by the CLS. The CLS can work independently on simple or highly complex laboratory test procedures. The clinical laboratory scientist can work as a generalist in several areas of the laboratory or select a specialized area that includes one of the following: clinical chemistry, clinical hematology, immunohematology, immunology, microbiology, or molecular biology. The role of the clinical laboratory scientist is determined by his or her area of specialization.

Role of the Clinical Laboratory Scientist in Clinical Chemistry

The clinical laboratory scientist who works in clinical chemistry prepares body fluid specimens for the analysis of chemical and hormonal components. Some laboratory tests commonly performed are blood sugar levels, cholesterol,

Aptitude Profile

When deciding on a career, an individual should take into consideration the skills and abilities needed to be successful in that particular job. Many jobs in the health-care field require some of the same characteristics; however, some skills are more specific to working in clinical laboratory science. The following list includes some of the necessary skills and abilities to consider when entertaining the idea of becoming a clinical laboratory scientist. Although this list is not exhaustive, all of these characteristics are required to be effective in the field of clinical laboratory science.

Able to handle stress	Manual dexterity
Accurate and precise	Multitasker
Analytical	Organized
Detail oriented	Responsible
Emotionally mature	Stamina
Ethical	Statistical knowledge
Good communicator	Technical skills
Independent worker	Troubleshooter

Author Spotlight

Joan Glacken, EdD

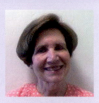

While in my junior year of high school, I was offered a job at a clinical laboratory typing laboratory reports, answering the telephone, and doing odd jobs. The laboratory director always explained all the different laboratory tests and how they were used to diagnose patient conditions and diseases. I was hooked and decided to major in the field. I worked as a clinical laboratory scientist for over 20 years and then went on to pursue a university teaching career. The clinical laboratory is a fascinating place to work—there is never a dull moment.

Julie Zemplinski, MSH

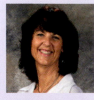

My particular career path as a clinical laboratory scientist led me from a generalist in a hospital laboratory, to a specialist in hematology and coagulation, to a specialist in microbiology and virology, to a laboratory supervisor, and to an administrative laboratory director in a hospital on one of the U.S. Virgin Islands, St. Croix. Now, I am happy to say I am making a full circle as a program director and professor for a clinical laboratory science program in Florida, training our future clinical laboratory scientists. Career choices in this field go in many directions; just follow your dreams.

Tony Burkett, MS

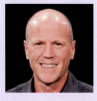

Although I am not a clinical laboratory scientist, my career as a clinical exercise physiologist working in cardiac rehabilitation could not be successful without the clinical laboratory. The laboratory scientist plays a role in confirming acute damage to the heart and in constructing a cardiac risk profile. Lipid profiles, blood glucose, hemoglobin A1C, and other tests completed by the laboratory scientist help shape the goals of the cardiac rehabilitation program. Without the clinical laboratory scientist, an individualized rehabilitation program could not have been created.

triglyceride, drug screenings, cancer markers, liver enzymes, kidney function tests, cardiac enzymes, vitamin levels, thyroid function tests, therapeutic drug monitoring, and hormone levels. Most of these laboratory tests are performed on automated analyzers. The clinical laboratory scientist is responsible for operating and maintaining highly sophisticated instrumentation, and performing quality control procedures to ensure precision and accuracy of all test results.

Role of the Clinical Laboratory Scientist in Clinical Hematology

Clinical laboratory scientists who work in clinical hematology prepare whole blood, bone marrow, and urine specimens for analysis. The components of whole blood that are analyzed include red blood cells, white blood cells, platelets, hemoglobin, hematocrit, and reticulocytes. They use microscopes, cell counters (automated and manual), and other high-tech laboratory equipment. Microscopes are used to view red blood cells, white blood cells, platelets, bone marrow, and urine sediment for normal and abnormal morphology.

Role of the Clinical Laboratory Scientist in Immunohematology

Immunohematology is also referred to as *blood banking.* Clinical laboratory scientists are responsible for collecting donor and recipient blood samples, typing and crossmatching units for transfusion, and antibody detection. They also are responsible for investigating transfusion reactions when a patient is given incompatible blood products. They detect hemolytic disease of the newborn when the newborn's blood type is not compatible with the mother's blood type.

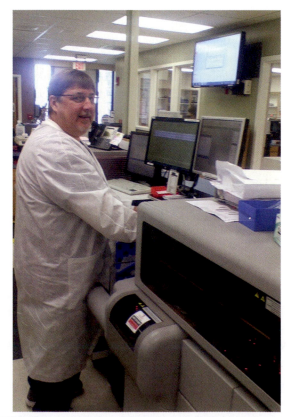

FIGURE 13-1 Clinical laboratory scientist analyzing chemistry specimens on an autoanalyzer.

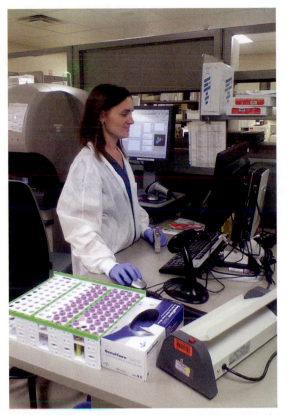

FIGURE 13-2 Clinical laboratory scientist preparing to load samples on a hematology analyzer.

Role of the Clinical Laboratory Scientist in Immunology

The clinical laboratory scientist in immunology examines elements of the human immune system and its response to foreign bodies. Common tests include the rapid plasma reagin (RPR) for syphilis, Monospot for mononucleosis, RA Latex for rheumatoid arthritis, antibodies to streptococcus, antinuclear antigens for autoimmune disease, rubella, rubeola, toxoplasmosis, cytomegalovirus, Epstein-Barr virus, herpes, chlamydia, human papillomavirus, human immunodeficiency virus, and many more. These tests are performed through manual card tests that involve latex agglutination, test tube titer assays, direct and indirect fluorescent techniques, enzyme-linked immunosorbent assay (ELISA), and more.

Role of the Clinical Laboratory Scientist in Microbiology

The clinical laboratory scientist in microbiology examines and identifies bacteria, parasites, fungi, and viruses from different body sources. Bacterial specimens include urine, throat, sputum, stool, ear, eye, wound, spinal fluid, blood, genital fluid, and other body fluids. A small sample from the specimen is plated on special agar media and allowed to grow

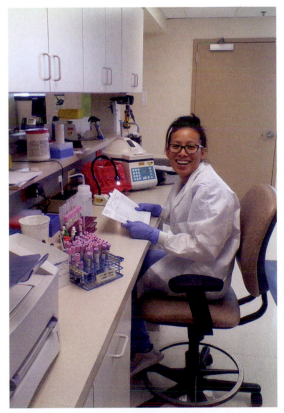

FIGURE 13-3 Clinical laboratory scientist performing blood types and crossmatches.

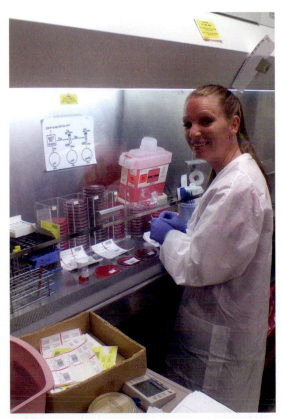

FIGURE 13-4 Clinical laboratory scientist plating microbiology specimens on agar plates.

in an incubator overnight. The next day the plates are examined for bacteria (normal and abnormal). The bacteria are identified through different chemical tests, and drug susceptibility tests are performed to determine how to treat the infection. Different procedures are used to analyze parasites, fungi, and viruses.

Role of the Clinical Laboratory Scientist in Molecular Biology

The clinical laboratory scientist in molecular biology performs complex protein and nucleic acid tests on cell samples. This is the newest field of clinical laboratory science and involves working with gene therapy, testing for cancers, genetic disease markers, histocompatibility types, and some infectious diseases.

Working Together

Clinical laboratory scientists interact with many different health professionals on a daily basis. They communicate patient results to physicians, nurses, pharmacists, dietitians, physician assistants, radiologists, and health services and information managers. The clinical laboratory scientist also is responsible for the care and maintenance of instruments. This requires interaction with diagnostic representatives, technicians, and repair services when necessary. They are responsible for reviewing and analyzing new test procedures and work with sales representatives to evaluate and purchase products.

CASE STUDY

Roger is a 16-year-old boy who was sent home from high school because of swollen glands. Roger's mother called the family physician and was told to bring him to the office as soon as possible. In his examination of Roger, Dr. Ambrosio did not detect a fever so he ordered several blood tests for Roger and requested results as soon as possible (STAT). Roger's mother drove him to the local hospital laboratory and the following blood tests were collected: complete blood count (CBC), chemistry profile, Monospot, and throat culture. The specimens were transported to the laboratory and dispersed to the appropriate departments. The CBC went to the hematology laboratory. The blood specimen was run on an automated analyzer to determine the red blood cell count, white blood cell count, hemoglobin, hematocrit, platelet count, and indices. A smear of the blood was made on a glass slide, stained, and then observed under a microscope. The clinical laboratory scientist found numerous atypical

lymphocytes on the smear. The white blood cell count was elevated and all the other results were within normal ranges. The chemistry profile was performed in the clinical chemistry laboratory on a multichannel automated analyzer. All of the results were normal except for the liver function tests. All of the liver function tests were elevated. The Monospot was performed by the immunology laboratory. The Monospot is a card test that uses latex agglutination (clumping) to determine an antigen/antibody reaction indicating infectious mononucleosis. Roger's test clumped. The throat culture was sent to the microbiology laboratory, where it was plated on agar and incubated for 24 hours. The throat culture results were normal. As soon as the clinical laboratory technologists in hematology, chemistry, and immunology completed their testing, the results were sent immediately to the physician assistant in Dr. Ambrosio's practice. The results of the throat culture were forwarded the following day. After reviewing the results of Roger's blood tests, the physician assistant consulted with Dr. Ambrosio to confirm a diagnosis of infectious mononucleosis based on the presence of atypical lymphocytes from the CBC, elevated liver function tests from the metabolic profile, and a positive Monospot test. Based on this diagnosis, the physician assistant was able to give Roger a plan of care for his illness.

Questions

1. What symptoms, or lack of symptoms, made Dr. Ambrosio order laboratory tests?

2. What areas of the laboratory assisted the physician in making the diagnosis?

3. How did the different laboratories act as a team in the diagnosis of Roger's illness?

4. How did the clinical laboratory scientists and physician act as a health-care team?

5. Was the throat culture result an important part of diagnosing Roger's condition?

Review Questions

1. What percent of clinical laboratory scientists will retire in the next 10 years?
   A. 10%
   B. 25%
   C. 40%
   D. 50%

2. The specialization area in clinical laboratory science that identifies blood types for transfusions is:

    A. Clinical chemistry

    B. Clinical hematology

    C. Immunohematology

    D. Immunology

3. The biggest concern of a clinical laboratory scientist is:

    A. Working with infectious body fluids

    B. Stress

    C. Unusual working hours

    D. Career changes

4. How many continuing education units is a certified clinical laboratory scientist required to complete?

    A. 24 CEUs per 2-year period

    B. 24 CEUs per 3-year period

    C. 36 CEUs per 2-year period

    D. 36 CEUs per 3-year period

5. When considering clinical laboratory science as a profession, it would be wise for the individual to have the following as a characteristic:

    A. Analytical

    B. Ethical

    C. Troubleshooter

    D. All of the above

6. The scope of practice for a clinical laboratory scientist includes:

    A. Accurate and reliable test results

    B. Maintain proper functioning of instruments

    C. Evaluation of new test methods

    D. All of the above

7. The individual in the clinical laboratory responsible for reviewing abnormal findings and interacting with physicians regarding patient results of laboratory tests is the:

    A. Clinical laboratory technician

    B. Clinical laboratory scientist

    C. Clinical laboratory supervisor

    D. Pathologist

8. Approximately how many medical decisions are influenced by laboratory test results?

    A. 10%–20%

    B. 30%–40%

    C. 50%–60%

    D. 60%–70%

9. Licensure for clinical laboratory scientists is required in how many states?

    A. 10

    B. 11

    C. 15

    D. No states require licensure, only certification

10. A clinical laboratory technician:

    A. Can work independently

    B. Must work under supervision of a clinical laboratory scientist

    C. Can report abnormal findings independently

    D. Can assume supervisory duties

Glossary of Key Terms

Clinical chemistry—analysis of the chemical and hormonal contents of body fluids

Hematology—analysis of the counts and morphology of whole blood specimens and other body fluids

Immunohematology (blood bank)—classification of blood types and Rh factors, and antibody identification

Immunology—detection of antigens and antibodies to organisms or agents that pose a threat to the human immune system

Microbiology—examination of body fluid or tissue for the presence of bacteria, viruses, parasites, or fungi

Molecular biology—analysis of complex protein and nucleic acid tests on cell samples

License—authorization to practice within a state

Certification—process that requires education, clinical training and experience, and successful completion of the certification examination for clinical laboratory scientists

Clinical laboratory technician—holds an associate degree, certification, and licensure (if required) to perform the various laboratory tests under the direct supervision of a clinical laboratory scientist

Clinical laboratory scientist—holds a baccalaureate degree, certification, and licensure (if required) to perform the various laboratory tests in a specialty area, maintain instruments, and perform quality control procedures to ensure accurate and precise testing

Continuing education—ongoing learning to ensure continued competency of clinical laboratory procedures

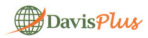

Additional Resources

Accrediting Body

National Accrediting Agency for Clinical Laboratory Science (NAACLS)—www.naacls.org

NAACLS is the accrediting body for clinical laboratory science programs at the postsecondary level.

Certification Bodies

American Association for Clinical Pathology (ASCP)—www.ascp.org

ASCP offers certification and specialization examinations for clinical laboratory technicians and clinical laboratory scientists.

American Association of Bioanalysts (AAB)—www.aab.org

AAB offers certification examinations for clinical laboratory technicians, clinical laboratory scientists, physician office laboratory technicians, and phlebotomists.

American Medical Technologists (AMT)—www.americanmedtech.org

AMT offers certification examinations for clinical laboratory scientists, clinical laboratory technicians, phlebotomy technicians, and clinical laboratory consultants.

Education and Professional Resources

American Association of Blood Banks (AABB)—www.aabb.org

AABB sets the standards and practices for blood banks in the specialty of transfusion medicine and cellular therapy to optimize patient and donor care and safety.

American Association of Clinical Chemists (AACC)—www.aacc.org

AACC is an international society comprised of medical professionals with an interest in clinical chemistry, clinical laboratory science, and laboratory medicine.

American Society for Clinical Laboratory Science (ASCLS)—www.ascls.org

ASCLS is a professional organization of clinical laboratory technicians and clinical laboratory scientists.

American Society of Hematology (ASH)—www.hematology.org

ASH furthers the understanding, diagnosis, treatment, and prevention of disorders affecting the blood, the bone marrow, and the immunological, hemostatic, and vascular systems by promoting research, clinical care, education, training, and advocacy in hematology.

American Association of Immunologists (AAI)—www.aai.org

AAI is an association of professionally trained scientists dedicated to advancing the knowledge of immunology and its related disciplines, fostering the interchange of ideas and information among investigators, and addressing the potential integration of immunological principles into clinical practice.

American Society for Microbiology (ASM)—www.asm.org

ASM advances the microbiological sciences as a vehicle for understanding life processes to improve populations' health, environmental well-being, and economic well-being worldwide.

References

1. Berger D. A brief history of medical diagnosis and the birth of the clinical laboratory. Part 1: Ancient times through the 19th century. *Med Lab Observer* 1999;31(7):32.

2. Lindberg DS, Britt MS, Fisher FW. *Williams' Introduction to the Profession of Medical Technology,* 4th ed. Philadelphia, PA: Lea & Febiger; 1984.

3. Kotlarz VR. Tracing our roots: Origins of clinical laboratory science. *Clin Lab Sci* 1998;11(1):7.

4. Kotlarz VR. Tracing our roots: The beginnings of a profession. *Clin Lab Sci* 1998;11(3):161–166.

5. Bureau of Labor Statistics, U.S. Department of Labor. Occupational outlook handbook, 2012–2013 edition, medical and clinical laboratory technologists and technicians.

   http://www.bls.gov/ooh/healthcare/medical-and-clinical-laboratory-technologists-and-technicians.htm.
   Accessed August 30, 2013.

6. American Society of Clinical Pathology. The laboratory personnel shortage.

   http://www.ascp.org/pdf/Advocacy/Workforce-Shortage-New-Strategy.aspx.
   Accessed September 26, 2013.

7. International Federation of Clinical Chemistry and Laboratory Medicine. Public relations opportunities in laboratory medicine.

   http://www.ifcc.org/media/212787/2012%2011%2019%20Labs%20are%20Vital%20-%20PRs%20Adeli-Shorter.pdf.

   Accessed September 26, 2013.

8. American Society of Clinical Pathology. State licensure of laboratory personnel.

   http://www.ascp.org/pdf/StateLicensureofLaboratory Personnel.aspx.

   Accessed September 26, 2013.

9. American Society for Clinical Laboratory Science. Career center.

   http://www.ascls.org/professional-development/career-center.

   Accessed September 26, 2013.

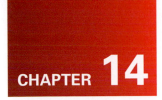

CHAPTER 14

Dental Professions

Kelley Lybrand, DDS

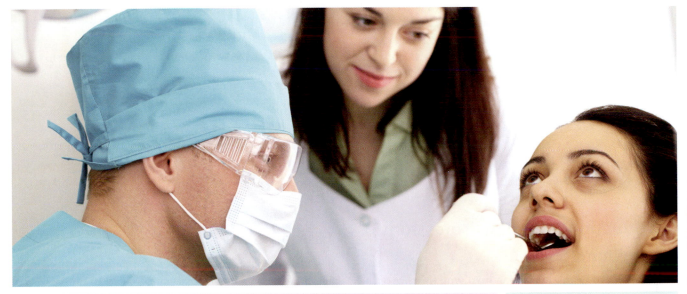

Photo credit: istock/Thinkstock

Learning Objectives

After reading this chapter, students should be able to:

- Describe the type of work dentists perform
- Discuss the talents and abilities utilized by dental professionals
- Explain the relationship between dental professionals and other members of the health-care team
- Identify the dental specialties recognized by the American Dental Association
- Describe the education and licensing process
- Discuss the opportunities and challenges present in the field of dentistry

Key Terms

- Dental hospital consultation
- Periodontal disease
- Gingival tissue
- Dental caries
- General dentist
- Dental hygienist
- Dental specialist

"A Day in the Life"

Hi, I'm Sarah and I'm a general dentist working in a clinic located within our regional medical center. My day is always full of variety with lots of different clinical challenges in several different settings. I'm going to start my day here at the hospital doing dental work on a special-needs patient with cerebral palsy. This patient is unable to sit in a traditional dental chair and cooperate with treatment so she will be treated in the hospital operating room. I also have patients to see in the hospital dental clinic, and on top of all that, I'll be responsible for providing dental consultation services for patients admitted to the hospital. Who knows what the day will bring! It's time to get changed and scrub for surgery.

Whew! Well, 2 hours later I have completed a full mouth examination, dental radiographs, dental cleaning, eight dental restorations, and a stainless steel crown on my special-needs patient while she was asleep under general anesthesia in the operating room. Patients who have special needs that prevent them from being able to sit in a normal dental chair and cooperate with treatment are often treated in the operating room setting. It is a wonderful service that keeps them pain and infection free. Now, it's on to the clinic. I have a patient coming in to have crowns placed on the four upper incisor teeth. I love these cases! The patients are so happy when I can give them a new, beautiful smile. Oh, and the dental hygienist is working

(continued)

today so there will be periodic examinations to complete. I better get moving.

Lunch was great. I ran into several friends who work in the emergency department so, the company was fantastic. On to the afternoon consultations.

I am responsible for seeing hospital patients with oral health problems today. Sometimes patients who have been admitted to the hospital have oral health concerns that require the evaluation of a dentist. In these cases, the patient's physician will request a **dental hospital consultation.** These requests for inpatient evaluation of a problem by a health-care professional with particular expertise are usually called *hospital consults.* Many of these patients are too sick to come to my dental clinic so I go to see them in their hospital rooms. It looks like I have quite a list this afternoon:

- Dental consultation requested to rule out dental infection before patient is placed on the liver transplant list
- Dental consultation requested for dental examination and treatment before cardiac valve surgery

- Dental consultation to evaluate missing teeth in a cleft lip and palate patient
- Dental consultation to evaluate spontaneous bleeding from gingiva around the teeth in a patient on active chemotherapy for lymphoma
- Dental consultation to evaluate and treat oral ulcerations in a patient undergoing induction chemotherapy for stem cell transplant
- Dental consultation to evaluate loose teeth before general anesthesia/intubation later this week
- Dental consultation in the emergency department to evaluate and treat facial swelling with associated dental infection

Time to grab my headlight and my bag of basic tools and take this show on the road! This is a great job. Where else can you see so many different types of patients in so many different settings with so many different colleagues?

Introduction to Dental Professions

Description

Dentistry is the health profession involving the care of the oral cavity, maxillofacial region, and associated structures. Dentists diagnose oral disease and promote oral health and disease prevention. They monitor proper development of the teeth and jaws. Dentists are able to diagnose and treat traumatic injuries and emergency oral/facial conditions. In addition, they perform surgical procedures of the teeth, bone, and soft tissues of the mouth and jaws. Restoration of ideal form and function of the dentition and associated structures is a major goal of dentistry. Administration of appropriate anesthetics to allow these treatments is a part of the role of the dentist.[1]

Dentists cannot do all of these things on their own. Dentistry involves a team of people who help the dentist provide quality care for patients. Members of the dental team include dental hygienists, dental assistants, and dental technicians. All of these people work with the dentist to provide excellent care. In particular, the role of the dental hygienist is discussed in greater detail later in the chapter.[1]

Dentistry also encompasses a number of dental specialists within the profession in which the doctor will limit his or her practice to a specific area of dentistry. The dental specialties vary widely in the type of procedures and treatments performed. Currently, nine dental specialties are recognized by the American Dental Association.[2]

History

For many years dentistry was not a formally recognized medical profession and no formal education and training existed. It seems incredible now, but in many cases tooth extractions were performed by the local barber.

A French physician, Pierre Fauchard, is credited with establishing many of the principles of modern dentistry in his book, *The Surgeon Dentist,* published in 1728. Eventually, dental schools were established, allowing the profession to establish more uniform standards of care and training. The first dental school in the United States was the Baltimore College of Dental Surgery established in 1840.[3] Today more than 50 dental schools in the United States are recognized by the Committee on Dental Accreditation (CODA), which is the accrediting body for U.S. dental education.[4]

Advances in technology have improved tools and materials. This technology allows dental professionals to provide sophisticated evaluation and treatment of a variety of different types of pathology. Dentists are able to diagnose and treat disease processes that degrade the structure of the teeth and gums, causing pain and loss of function. In addition to the teeth and gums, dentists are also trained to evaluate associated structures such as the tongue, salivary glands, and structures of the head and neck.

Dentists are trained to detect abnormalities in oral tissues and structures of the head and neck that can be signs of other systemic diseases of the body, such as oral cancer, infectious processes, autoimmune diseases, and systemic conditions created by problems with other organ systems in the body.[1]

Types of Diseases or Conditions

Two of the most common types of dental disease are periodontal disease and dental caries. **Periodontal disease** is a complex inflammatory disease process in which interactions between bacteria in the mouth and the body's own immune responses result in inflammation of the **gingival tissue** and eventual loss of the bone that surrounds the teeth. When teeth lose their bony support they may become loose and function poorly. Without evaluation or intervention from a dentist or dental hygienist the problem may worsen, resulting in pain and significant problems for the patient. The relationship between periodontal disease and other forms of systemic disease in the body is an area of current research. It is believed that some of the bacteria in the mouth and around the teeth can be released into the bloodstream and thus affect other areas of the body, including other organs or implanted materials such as prosthetic joints or prosthetic heart valves. In addition, the response generated by the body's immune system as a result of periodontal disease may contribute to other systemic diseases such heart disease or diabetes. Periodontal disease can be prevented and treated with regular dental cleanings by a dental hygienist and by therapy performed by periodontists, who are dentists specializing in the treatment of periodontal disease. Various pharmacological and surgical treatments are available for the disease.

Another common form of oral disease is **dental caries,** which occurs when bacteria in the mouth produce acids that degrade the structure of the teeth, resulting in eventual cavitation and loss of tooth structure. When decay reaches the nerve and blood supply of the tooth, the tooth becomes extremely painful. Left unchecked, dental caries can destroy the living tissue within the tooth. The tooth can then become infected, causing swelling, pain, and significant health problems. Dentists are able to detect dental caries and the extent of its effect on tooth structure through clinical and radiographic examination (Fig. 14-1). Treatments can then be performed to remove the decay and restore the form and function of the remaining tooth structure. These treatments vary depending on the amount of tooth structure that remains and the degree to which the nerve and blood supply of the tooth have been affected. Treatments range from the placement of restorative materials into the tooth, to the placement of a full surface crown over the tooth. If the live tissue in the tooth has been affected, it may need to be removed through an endodontic procedure known as root canal therapy. If the tooth cannot be restored it must be removed via dental extraction.

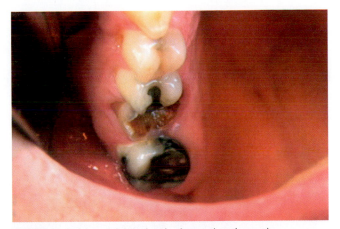

FIGURE 14-1 Advanced dental caries is seen here in a molar.

Dentists are also able to replace missing teeth through a variety of treatments, including the placement of fixed prosthodontics such as crown and bridge work. Removable tooth replacements such as partials or dentures can also be fabricated. Dental implants can be used to facilitate tooth replacement. Dental implants are titanium fixtures placed into the jaw bone that replace the root form of the tooth. These titanium fixtures provide solid supports on which various forms of tooth replacement can be built.

The design and fabrication of dental restorations require an understanding of a number of mechanical design principles, as well as an in-depth knowledge of dental materials. Dentistry involves the ability to work well with one's hands and incorporates an element of artistry. It is necessary to create tooth restorations that are both functional and esthetic. Dentists combine their knowledge and skills to diagnose and treat patients in ways that often relieve pain, improve function, and tangibly improve their patients' quality of life.

Scopes of Practice

The scope of practice of all members of the dental team, including the **general dentist, dental hygienist, dental specialist,** dental assistant, and dental technician, is legislated at the state level. Dentistry encompasses a number of specialties within the profession that vary widely in the type of procedures and treatments performed. Currently, nine dental specialties are recognized by the American Dental Association (ADA).[2] Patient cases that are particularly difficult or complex may be referred to a dental specialist for treatment. These are cases that require an expanded level of knowledge and training. Sometimes patients are referred because a general dentist would prefer that a dental specialist complete the case; other times patients may request to be treated by a specialist. Dental specialists restrict their practice to a particular area of dental diagnosis and treatment and have completed

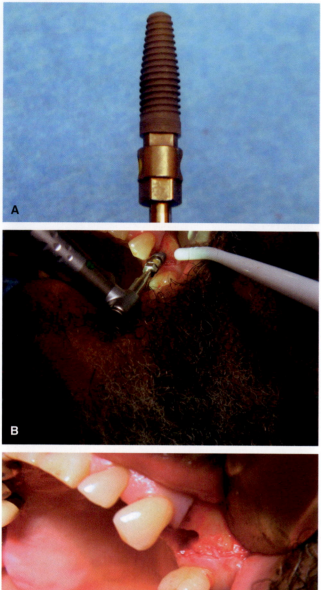

FIGURE 14-2 (A) Dental implant fixture shown affixed to placement tool. **(B)** Placement of a dental implant into a site to replace a missing tooth. **(C)** Surgical preparation of the site of a missing tooth to receive a dental implant.

additional training in this area. Following are the nine specialties recognized by the ADA[2]:

- *Public health dentistry* involves promotion of dental health through organized community efforts.
- *Prosthodontics* involves rehabilitation and maintenance of oral function through the use of biomechanical substitutes.
- *Endodontics* involves treatment of the blood vessels and nerves within teeth and their associated root structures.

- *Periodontics* involves maintenance and treatment of the hard and soft tissues surrounding and supporting the teeth.
- *Pediatric dentistry* involves preventive and therapeutic oral care for infants and children through adolescence, including those with special health-care needs.
- *Oral maxillofacial pathology* involves identification and management of diseases affecting the oral and maxillofacial regions.
- *Oral maxillofacial radiology* involves the production and interpretation of images and data gained by radiant energy to diagnose and manage conditions of the oral and maxillofacial region.
- *Oral and maxillofacial surgery* involves the surgical and adjunctive treatment of diseases, injuries, and defects of the oral and maxillofacial region.
- *Orthodontics and pediatric orthopedics* involves the diagnosis and correction of malalignment of the teeth and associated neuromuscular and skeletal abnormalities.

Required Education

To be eligible to take a licensure examination to practice general dentistry, one must complete a doctorate degree in dentistry. The degree conferred is either a doctor of dental surgery (DDS) or a doctor of dental medicine (DMD). These are equivalent degrees and the difference is essentially a matter of historical convention on the part of the particular educational institution conferring the degree.[4]

Admission to dental school requires completion of an adequate undergraduate education including several prerequisite courses. This education is commonly achieved in the form of an undergraduate college degree. Any college major is acceptable providing that the necessary courses are included. However, many of the prerequisite courses are in the fields of biology, chemistry, and physics, leading many aspiring dentists to pursue majors in the fields of science as an undergraduate major. In addition, students must take the Dental Admission Test (DAT) to be considered for admission. Students are asked to provide recommendations from their professors or mentors. In addition, experience shadowing a dentist or volunteering in a dental work environment is highly desirable.[5]

Dentists must pass written national board examinations to successfully complete their dental training. In addition, they must successfully complete a licensing examination to practice. These licensing examinations are regional in nature and currently involve didactic examination, demonstration of competence in laboratory scenarios, and demonstration of competence in clinical patient care. Several hours of continuing education are then required to maintain licensure.[1] Each of the dental specialties has its own form of board examination for that particular specialty, and some states also require additional licensure to practice as a dental specialist in that particular state.

Salary

The average salary for dentists varies according to their practice setting and region of the country. Dentists may own the practice in which they work, or they may be associates who function as employees or independent contractors for the doctor who owns the dental practice. Increasingly, large corporations are opening dental practices and hiring dentists to work as employees in these practices. Dentists also work in settings such as hospitals, dental schools/academia, dental research, industry, public health, and the military.[6]

The majority of dentists, over 90%, continue to work in the private practice setting. Traditionally, many dentists have owned the practice in which they work and essentially functioned as small business owners as well as health-care professionals. Although this arrangement may create both positive and negative consequences, it can afford significant flexibility and control of the work environment. The average income of a general dentist was $192,392 in 2011. Many factors affect the income of the practicing dentist. These include the region of the country, rural versus urban setting, gender, and employment arrangement. The most significant difference was seen between owner and employee dentists, with owner dentists making an average of $45,821 more than employee dentists when other factors were controlled. Dental specialists earned an average of $313,873 in 2011. However, the income of dental specialists can vary significantly.[7]

Trends

As the U.S. population continues to age, the demand for dental care will continue to increase. The expectation of the population is for excellent dental form and function well into their golden years. As technology continues to advance, this expectation is becoming increasingly feasible. However, this aging population will also bring accompanying medical problems. A broad medical knowledge base and interaction with other medical professionals will be increasingly important to the future dental professional. The correlations between oral and systemic health will continue to be better understood as the volume of evidence-based research in this area accumulates. Oral health will be increasingly integrated into a holistic understanding of overall wellness. The ability to interact with other health-care professionals will be of increasing importance. The need will continue for dentists to work in academia and research to develop these interprofessional collaborations and knowledge bases.

Biotechnology, in the form of genomic therapy and stem cell research, holds possibilities for even more natural restoration of oral health. Advancements in dental materials will continue to improve the care offered. Dental implants and other associated technologies are allowing restorative options for patients who previously were not candidates. Advanced imaging and the use of computer-assisted manipulation of these data will allow for more sophisticated, customized therapy that is more predictable and holds lower risk for complications. The essential role that technology and dental materials play in the practice of dentistry will no doubt substantially affect the way that dentistry is practiced in the coming years. The future of the dental profession is bright and holds the possibility of exciting and innovative therapy that can meaningfully improve patients' quality of life.

Challenges

Dentistry is a rewarding profession; however, it is also rife with challenges. Many of these challenges are similar to those

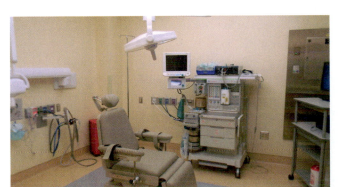

FIGURE 14-3 Dentists may work in an operating room setting.

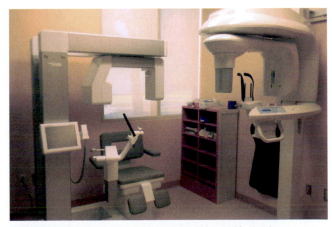

FIGURE 14-4 Advanced imaging equipment is used in dentistry.

faced by all health-care providers, but some are more specific to the field of dentistry.

Patient fear and anxiety is a problem encountered by many health-care professionals, but can be particularly acute in the dental patient population. Bad previous experiences, childhood trauma, family attitudes toward dentistry, and acute pain at the time care is sought can all contribute to the anxiety of the patient. Dental professionals must learn to help patients deal with their anxiety and manage the stress that can add to the treatment environment.

Dentistry requires a significant degree of precision, and one is required to work in a small space with minimal margin for error. This work requires significant concentration and can be highly fatiguing. In addition, patients are sometimes unwilling or unable to comply with recommended therapy or lifestyle recommendations. This noncompliance can be highly frustrating.

Dentistry is heavily influenced by changes in technology and medical and dental knowledge, and maintaining a current knowledge base and modern practice can be challenging. Dental professionals must work hard at remaining up to date with advances in the profession. Maintaining up-to-date equipment and techniques can be costly and time consuming.

Dentists often are in the position of supervising other health-care workers in their jobs, such as dental assistants, dental hygienists, and dental technicians. This added responsibility can add to workplace stress. In particular, dentists who own and operate their own practices must deal with the stress of day-to-day business management decisions on top of their responsibilities as a health-care professional.

Finally, as the cost of dental education continues to rise, recent graduates are finding that their decisions on where and how to practice are heavily influenced by their student loan debt.

Role of the General Dentist

General dentists comprise the bulk of practicing dentists in the United States. Over 80% of dentists in the United States are general practitioners; the other 20% are specialists who confine their practice to a particular area of concentration within the field.[5] General dentists provide a wide range of diagnostic, preventive, and therapeutic services to their patients. In most cases, they supervise dental hygienists, who provide oral health maintenance. Most patients receive routine dental maintenance and examinations on a regular basis to sustain their oral health. The recommended interval for these visits is based on a number of factors, including the patient's existing oral health and risk factors for the development of oral disease.

Aptitude Profile

People who work in the dental field receive extensive didactic and hands-on training to practice their profession. However, some inherent qualities and abilities are essential to the practice of dentistry. These qualities include the following:

Analytical	Good spatial judgment
Artistic	Independent
Compassionate	Intelligent
Critical thinker	Leader
Dedicated	Problem solver
Determined	Responsible
Empathetic	Organized
Ethical	Self-aware
Flexible	Self-motivated
Good communicator	
Good hand-eye coordination	

Dentists also work with dental assistants, who may perform a variety of tasks depending on their training and credentialing. These tasks may include assisting the doctor during procedures, performing sterilization of instruments, taking radiographs, and assistance in documentation.

General dentists often form long-term relationships with their patients and patients' families due to the regular, ongoing nature of dental maintenance and treatment. Many general dentists choose to see patients of all ages from children to geriatric. In fact, general dentists may see their patients more frequently than the patients see their primary-care physician. This relationship can be extremely rewarding.

Dentists monitor the overall oral health of the patient, which includes screening for oral cancer. In addition, many systemic disease processes exhibit oral manifestations that can be detected by a general dentist on routine examination. Dentists also diagnose and treat dental caries and periodontal disease, which affect the supporting bone and soft tissues around the teeth.

General dentists perform a variety of procedures to treat and restore oral disease, including dental restorations, crowns, bridges, fabrication of partial and complete dentures, and a number of other restorative procedures. They also may perform surgical procedures as needed, including removal of teeth, biopsies, and other procedures. Endodontic therapy in which the nerve and blood supply of the tooth are removed can be performed by general dentists. Cosmetic procedures such as whitening of the teeth, veneering of the surface of the incisors, and other procedures to improve the smile are also performed by many general dentists.

Although all of these functions are within the purview of the general dentist, many dentists elect to refer patients to a dental specialist for some of these treatments. This referral is usually due to the complexity of the procedure, difficulty of patient management, or the individual practitioner's comfort level with certain types of procedures.

General dentists function as the "primary-care provider" of the dental specialty as they assess and maintain patients' oral health on a regular basis, diagnose and treat basic oral disease, and refer patients for specialty care as indicated.

Role of the Dental Hygienist

Dental hygienists work alongside other dental professionals to deliver oral health care and patient education. Like dentists, they may work in a variety of settings, including hospitals, dental schools/academia, dental research, industry, public health, and the military. They examine patients for oral disease, débride and scale and root plane the teeth, and provide some preventive services. Dental hygienists play an active role in promoting good oral health through patient education. These educational activities may include counseling on oral hygiene, oral health-care aids, smoking cessation, and

Author Spotlight

Kelley Lybrand, DDS

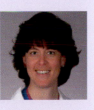

I grew up in a small town in North Carolina, where I completed high school before attending college at the University of North Carolina (UNC) at Chapel Hill. There I majored in biology and became involved with the predental student club on campus. After spending time shadowing several dentists and volunteering in the university hospital dental clinic, I decided I wanted to pursue dentistry as a career and was accepted into the UNC School of Dentistry after 3 years of college preparatory courses. After completing dental school I completed a 2-year residency in general dentistry and hospital-based practice at Carolinas Medical Center in Charlotte, North Carolina. This experience exposed me to a number of patients with oral maxillofacial surgery needs and I developed a particular interest in that specialty. I then completed an additional 4-year residency in oral and maxillofacial surgery at the Medical University of South Carolina in Charleston. After a brief stint in private practice, I returned to the Medical University of South Carolina where I currently treat patients, as well as teach dental students and oral and maxillofacial surgery residents.

nutritional counseling. Some states allow extended duties for dental hygienists with additional training and credentials. These duties include things such as the delivery of some forms of local anesthesia, placement of fluoride and sealants, and even the placement of some dental restorative materials. Most states require that dental hygienists work under the supervision of a dentist, but again this varies by state.[8]

Most dental hygienists obtain an associate degree in dental hygiene. However, certificate programs are available (though less commonly) in some areas. A bachelor's degree and master's degree in dental hygiene are also available. These advanced degrees are most often obtained by those who desire to teach or work in research. The majority of dental hygienists work in dental offices. In addition to adequate educational credentials, one must also pass a licensing examination to practice. Licensing, as well as regulations regarding the scope, location, and supervision of practice, is regulated on a state-by-state basis.[8]

Dental hygiene requires many of the same talents and abilities as dentists and other oral health-care providers. It also shares many of the same challenges and rewards. In addition, it is a highly flexible occupation. Many dental hygienists work part time or job share in multiple offices. According to the Bureau of Labor Statistics, the median salary for dental hygienists in 2010 was $68,250, or $32.81 an hour. The demand for dental hygienists is expected to grow by 38% over the next 10 years, which is much more than other occupations. The future of dental hygiene as a profession is bright, with high demand, excellent flexibility, and, in many areas, the possibility of expanded scope of practice.[8]

Role of the Dental Specialist

As mentioned, approximately 20% of dentists elect to obtain additional training to achieve specialization within a specific area of dentistry.[6] The ADA-recognized dental specialties were listed earlier in this chapter and include pediatric dentistry, oral maxillofacial radiology, orthodontics and pediatric orthopedics, endodontics, periodontics, public health dentistry, oral maxillofacial pathology, oral maxillofacial surgery, and dental prosthodontics.[2]

Dental specialists must complete residency training in their area of specialty, which includes didactic and clinical training. Acceptance into these programs is highly competitive following the completion of dental school. Length of training varies by type of specialty and between programs and can range from 2 to 6 years in length following dental school.[1] After completion of training, each specialty has a process by which individuals can become board certified. This process is often multistep and varies by specialty. In addition, many states require an additional licensing examination to practice as a specialist in that particular state.

SUMMARY

Dentistry can be a challenging and rewarding profession that affords those who work in the field an opportunity to greatly enhance the oral health and quality of life of their patients. Oral health is an integral part of overall health, and oral health-care providers must interact and communicate with other health-care professionals to provide excellent care. Many different specialties within dentistry require advanced training, and each provides advanced care for a specific area of oral health. Dental hygienists are an important part of the dental care team, and the future outlook for this profession is outstanding. Dentistry can be an excellent career choice for compassionate, dedicated individuals who enjoy integrating knowledge and artistic abilities to tangibly help patients. The future of dental professionals is bright, and their contributions will continue to be valuable and relevant to the interprofessional care of patients.

Tips and Tools

Dentists have a primary role in evaluating and treating oral health. Due to the intrinsic relationship between oral and systemic health, dentists have a key role to play on the interprofessional health-care team. Dentists interact with many other disciplines, including medicine, pharmacy, nursing, nutrition, social work, health information management, physician assistants, rehabilitation therapy/counseling, respiratory care, and speech-language pathology. Oral health is a major consideration in a variety of medical fields, including cardiology, transplant, oncology, anesthesia, emergency medicine, rehabilitative medicine, and many other fields. Excellent communication and teamwork among all of these providers is essential to quality patient care. In particular, dentists who work in medical center settings enjoy a rich interaction with a variety of health-care providers, which is both challenging and extremely rewarding.

CASE STUDY

Linda is a 76-year-old woman who is being seen in the emergency department (ED) after a fall in her kitchen earlier today. She reports that she was making sandwiches for herself and her husband when she began to feel a little lightheaded. The next thing she remembers was lying on the floor with her husband by her side. She immediately noted pain in her mouth and blood on her shirt, as well as pain in her left wrist and hand. Her husband called

911 and she was transported to the ED for evaluation. The ED physician is evaluating Linda's condition. She currently has stable vital signs; however, she is a little short of breath with mild wheezing. She reports a history of heart problems and is on a number of medications, including blood thinners. Her left hand continues to give her pain, but her most pressing complaint is the pain and bleeding she is having from her mouth. She is spitting blood into a cup by her bedside and is beginning to panic now that she sees the blood on her shirt and face. She can tell that at least one tooth is loose and it does not feel like her teeth meet properly when she bites down. Her husband is at her bedside and extremely upset. He continues to rifle through his wallet looking for insurance cards while repeatedly mumbling, "I have no idea about any of this. Linda always takes care of all these things." The ED physician has called several different health-care providers, including a physician assistant, ED nurse, radiology technician, respiratory therapist, and social worker, to assist in providing care to this patient. Should a dentist be part of the team taking care of Linda? If so, how?

Questions

1. What are the indications to get a dentist involved in Linda's care?

2. What disciplines should be involved with Linda's care?

3. Why is interprofessional collaboration important in this case?

4. What are barriers facing interprofessional collaboration?

5. Develop an interprofessional plan of care based on your knowledge from other chapters.

Review Questions

1. The first dental school was established in:
   A. 1492
   B. 1776
   C. 1812
   D. 1840

2. General dentists diagnose the following:
   A. Gum disease
   B. Abnormalities of development of the teeth and jaws
   C. Trauma to the teeth and gums
   D. All of the above

3. How many ADA-recognized dental specialties are there?

    A. 7

    B. 9

    C. 10

    D. 12

4. Requirements for admission to dental school include all of the following *except:*

    A. Completion of prerequisite courses

    B. Completion of the Dental Admission Test (DAT)

    C. Recommendations from professors/mentors

    D. Completion of health profession personality test

5. The following must be completed before beginning the practice of dentistry:

    A. Passage of the specialty board examination in pediatric dentistry

    B. Passage of Part I of the United States Medical Licensing Examination

    C. Successful completion of a dental licensing examination

    D. Completion of an IQ test

6. The following characteristics are helpful in pursuing a career in dentistry:

    A. Inattention to detail

    B. Unsympathetic attitude

    C. Good hand-eye coordination

    D. Impatience

7. A general dentist may consider referral to a dental specialist for the following reasons:

    A. The case is extremely complex.

    B. The general dentist does not feel comfortable completing the case himself or herself.

    C. The patient requests to see a specialist.

    D. All of the above.

8. Which of the following works in a dental office under the supervision of a dentist?

    A. Dental assistant

    B. Pharmaceutical sales representative

    C. Insurance claims processor

    D. Dental litigator

9. Most dentists in the United States practice in what setting?

    A. Military

    B. Teaching institution

    C. Private practice

    D. Industry

10. Which of the following is the greatest factor in a dentist's income?

    A. Employment arrangement (owner vs. employee)

    B. Practice logo design

    C. Marketing plan

    D. Laboratory technician selection

Glossary of Key Terms

Dental hospital consultation—request for evaluation of the oral health or condition of a patient who is being treated in a hospital setting

Periodontal disease—inflammatory disease process in which interactions between bacteria and the body's immune responses result in loss of soft and hard tissue support of the dentition

Gingival tissue—soft tissue surrounding the teeth and covering the upper and lower jawbones

Dental caries—oral disease in which bacteria produce acids that degrade tooth structure, resulting in eventual cavitation and loss of tooth structure

General dentist—health-care provider involved in diagnosis and treatment of oral disease and pathology of associated structures, and restoration of form and function of the dentition and maxillofacial region

Dental hygienist—health-care provider involved in examination and cleaning of the dentition and oral cavity, as well as patient education and some preventive services

Dental specialist—dentist who limits his or her practice to a specific area of dentistry

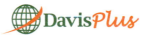 Additional Resources are available online at www.davisplus.com

Additional Resources

American Dental Association—www.ada.org

The American Dental Association is the largest national organization of dentists in the country and advocates for dentists and the oral health of their patients. It is an excellent source of oral health–related information.

***Journal of the American Dental Association* (JADA)— http://jada.ada.org/**

The *Journal of the American Dental Association* is a peer-reviewed dental journal concerned with current issues in dentistry and is one of the most widely read dental journals in the United States.

American Dental Education Association—www.access. adea.org

This organization is devoted to the quality of dental education and provides resources for dental students and educators to accomplish this goal.

References

1. American Dental Association. Dentists: Doctors of oral health.

    http://www.ada.org/4504.aspx.

    Accessed November 6, 2013.

2. American Dental Association. Education/careers: Specialty definitions.

    http://www.ada.org/en/education-careers/careers-in-dentistry/dental-specialties/specialty-definitions.

    Accessed September 29, 2014.

3. Encyclopedia Britannica. Dentistry.

    http://www.britannica.com/EBchecked/topic/158069/dentistry.

    Accessed November 9, 2013.

4. American Dental Association. Current and future students.

    http://www.ada.org/students.aspx.

    Accessed November 6, 2013.

5. American Dental Association. Current and future students: College students.

    http://www.ada.org/2195.aspx.

    Accessed November 6, 2013.

6. American Dental Association. Current and future students, dentistry_fact.pdf.

    http://ada.org/beadentist.aspx.

    Accessed November 6, 2013.

7. Vujicic M, Wall T, et al. Research brief: Dentist income levels slow to recover. American Dental Association, Health Policy Resources Center; 2013.

    http://www.ada.org/~/media/ADA/Science%20 and%20Research/HPI/Files/HPIBrief_0213_1.ashx.

    Accessed November 6, 2013.

8. U.S. Bureau of Labor Statistics. Dental hygiene: Occupational outlook handbook.

    http://www.bls.gov/ooh/Healthcare/Dental-hygienists.htm.

    Accessed November 9, 2013.

CHAPTER 15

Dietetics

Michelle Hesse (Battista), PhD, RD; Tonya Orchard, PhD, RDN, LD; and Julie Kennel, PhD, RDN, LD

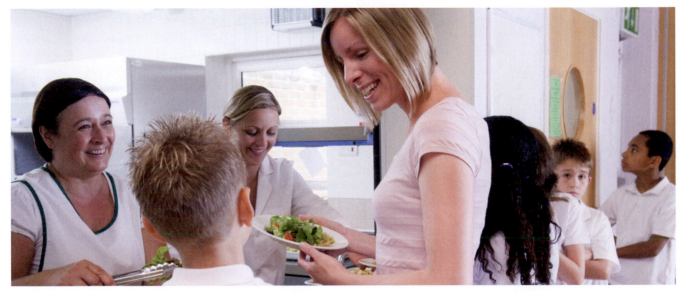

Photo credit: istock/Thinkstock

Learning Objectives

After reading this chapter, students should be able to:

- Understand the role of a registered dietitian (RD)/registered dietitian nutritionist (RDN)
- Describe the education and credentialing process
- Understand the various settings in which RDs/RDNs practice
- Understand the relationship between RDs/RDNs and medical, food-service, and community professionals
- Discuss trends, opportunities, and challenges for working in the field of dietetics

Key Terms

- Registered dietitians
- Registered dietitian nutritionists
- Didactic program in dietetics
- Coordinated dietetics program
- Dietetic internship program
- Assessment, diagnosis, intervention, monitoring, and evaluation (ADIME)
- Food-service systems management
- Community nutrition
- Board-certified specialist in dietetics

"A Day in the Life"

8:00 a.m.: Hello, my name is Emily and I am a registered dietitian nutritionist. I work at a local hospital in a unit that cares for patients with diabetes. I am starting my day with a staff meeting to review the patients currently admitted into the hospital and all of the new patients we will be seeing today. Right now on the schedule there are 15 patients, so it is going to be one busy day!

12:00 noon: I only have a few minutes to catch you up on my day. Our staff meeting went well today and I just completed rounding with the patients on my morning schedule. I mostly saw patients who were admitted into the hospital to help them manage and care for their diabetes. When a patient stays in the hospital, we call this *inpatient*. One of my patients, a 65-year-old woman, had difficulty managing her blood glucose (sugar) and has been feeling very ill for the last several days. After conducting a dietary assessment on this patient, this is what I learned about her dietary habits:

- She has a limited access to healthy food items like fresh fruits and vegetables.
- She was not counting how many carbohydrate foods she was consuming at each meal.
- She was forgetting to take her insulin shots at dinnertime.

Based on this assessment, I educated the patient on how to count carbohydrates and how to monitor and record her blood glucose levels before and after meals. A nurse and I also educated the patient on how to use her carbohydrate counts and her blood glucose readings to determine how much insulin to give herself during a meal. I'm still working on a way to determine how we can get this patient more access to fresh fruits and vegetables when she leaves the hospital, but I will have to update you on that later because it's time for me to see my afternoon patients!

5:00 p.m.: What a day! I referred the 65-year-old female patient with diabetes to a program that can help her gain access to fresh fruits and vegetables. Based on her income she was eligible for the federal food stamp program, better known as the Supplemental Nutrition Assistance Program (SNAP). The hospital social worker and I worked together to help her complete the SNAP benefits application. In addition to helping this patient, I also saw eight additional patients this afternoon. Two patients were newly diagnosed with diabetes and had to be admitted to the hospital and six patients were in the outpatient clinic for a follow-up appointment. For the patients who were admitted into the hospital, I had to review their blood work and the formal medical diagnosis, perform a complete nutritional assessment including measuring their weight, and complete a diet history. Finally, I established an intervention plan along with a system to monitor the patients' progress while in the hospital. Part of the intervention plan includes making sure the food they eat is in compliance with a carbohydrate-controlled diet (appropriate for patients with diabetes). I accomplish this by working with the hospital's food-service director to establish the patient's diet orders. Diet orders specify what the patient can and cannot have at each meal. For the patients who returned to the outpatient clinic for follow-up, a diet history is always conducted to determine how well the patients are progressing/following their prescribed diet at home. I also use other assessment tools such as weight status or change in laboratory values to monitor their progress. The nutrition intervention and education that I conduct is all based on these assessments. I find that when patients return to our outpatient clinic they usually need education on the types of foods compliant with a carbohydrate-controlled diet, how to count carbohydrates, and how to schedule their medication with meals and snacks.

Well, I have to go now to catch up on my charting and documentation. This includes recording all of the assessments I performed on the patient, the nutritional diagnosis made, any intervention or education provided to the patient, and future plans to monitor the progress of the patient. I have to document each patient's record that I saw today. Although I have been at work since 7:30 this morning, I will probably need to work until about 5:30 p.m. This long day is typical for my job. Hope to see you soon!

Introduction to Dietetics

Description

Dietetics, the use of diet to promote health, has been practiced since ancient times. In the 5th century BC, Hippocrates, the most eminent Greek physician, wrote a treatise on the role of diet in disease treatment. The Greek philosopher Plato frequently included dietary recommendations in his writings and advocated a "healthy diet" consisting of cereals, legumes, fruits, milk, honey, and fish, with only moderate quantities of meat, confectioneries, and wine.[1] With the discovery of the major nutrients in foods during the 19th and 20th centuries, scientific bases for many dietary recommendations were found. In 1917, dietitians were officially recognized as the food and nutrition experts.[2]

Today, **registered dietitians** (RDs), also known as **registered dietitian nutritionists** (RDNs), are the professionals who translate the science of nutrition into practical solutions for healthy living. RDs/RDNs typically are involved in educating the public, specific groups, or individuals on topics related to food and nutrition, providing medical nutrition therapy for those with health conditions, and managing meal

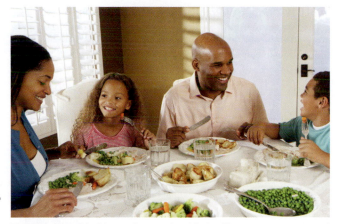

FIGURE 15-1 Dietitians often work with families to encourage good nutrition habits from young age to old age.

TABLE 15-1 Core Courses in a Didactic or Coordinated Dietetics Program

Anatomy	Advanced nutrition and metabolism	Medical nutrition therapy
Biology	Food safety	Nutrition assessment
Chemistry	Food science	Nutrition education and counseling
	Food-service management	
Microbiology	Fundamental nutrition	Nutrition across the life span
Physiology		Public health nutrition

programs or food-service operations. Dietitians are a vital part of the health-care team and frequently work in health-care settings. However, these are just a few examples of the career opportunities for individuals in this profession.

According to the U.S. Bureau of Labor Statistics, the job outlook for RDs/RDNs is expected to increase faster than the average for all occupations through 2020.[3] Currently, about one third of all RDs/RDNs work in hospitals. This number is expected to remain fairly stable in the near future, but employment in other health-care settings such as long-term care facilities and clinics is expected to grow over the next decade due to an aging population and increased emphasis on disease prevention.[4] Other workplace settings for RDs/RDNs include food and nutrition-related industries, educational institutions, corporate wellness and sports nutrition programs, research facilities, community and public health arenas, and private practice. In fact, nearly 15% of RDs/RDNs are self-employed.[3] Many RDs/RDNs have certifications in specialized areas such as renal nutrition, pediatric nutrition, sports dietetics, gerontological nutrition, and oncology nutrition. These areas of specialized dietetics practice are discussed in more detail later in this chapter.

Required Education

RDs/RDNs have a minimum of a bachelor's degree in nutrition, dietetics, public health, or a related field that includes an accredited dietetic course of study; have completed a specialized, accredited internship; and have passed an examination to obtain registration status.[5] The registration status is required for state licensure. Currently, 46 states require state licensure and certification in the United States.[6] Some of the core courses one might expect to take in a **didactic program in dietetics** (DPD) or **coordinated dietetics program** (CP) are listed in Table 15-1.

By 2024, the minimum education requirement for RDs/RDNs will elevate to an advanced, master's-level degree. With the increase demand in health-care fields, many agencies and organizations already require RDs/RDNs to possess an advanced degree. Additionally, RDs/RDNs comply with continuing education requirements to maintain their professional skills and to stay abreast of new knowledge in the field.

There is sometimes confusion about the difference between a nutritionist and a registered dietitian. Only individuals who have met the educational and professional requirements can use the RD/RDN credential. In contrast, the term *nutritionist* is not a legally protected term in many states and can be used by individuals without any formal training. All RDs/RDNs are nutritionists, but not all nutritionists are RDs/RDNs.[7]

Individuals interested in becoming an RD/RDN can choose between two options to meet educational requirements (see Fig. 15-2). The first option is to complete a DPD that is typically part of a bachelor's or master's degree program, followed by an accredited **dietetic internship program** (DI). In this supervised practice, students learn to prepare for and perform specific responsibilities under the guidance and supervision of a qualified preceptor. Acceptance into a DI is very competitive due to the large number of qualified applicants compared with the number of available internship openings. Approximately 52% to 53% of students who applied for internships in spring 2012 and 2013 were accepted or "matched" during the initial application process.[8] Because of this relatively low acceptance rate, the Academy of Nutrition and Dietetics, the national organization of food and nutrition professionals, is working to increase the number of preceptors and internship placements available to students. The second option for those desiring to become an RD/RDN is to complete a coordinated dietetics program (CP) that combines degree-granting didactic coursework with supervised practice. There were 225 didactic and 53 coordinated programs in dietetics in the United States in 2013.[8] Either route prepares graduates to take the national registration examination and enter the dietetics profession. There are advantages to both types of programs.

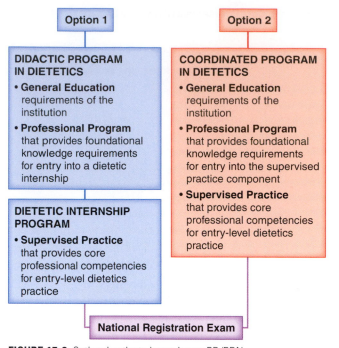

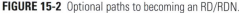

FIGURE 15-2 Optional paths to becoming an RD/RDN.

TABLE 15-2 Scope of Practice Areas for RDs/RDNs[8]

Tests and Measures	Interventions
Perform nutrition-related assessments	Advocate for nutrition access and care for patients, community groups, and special-needs populations
Assign nutrition-related diagnoses	Provide food and nutrition education to the public (in settings such as schools, community centers, government-funded nutrition programs, supermarkets, social media outlets)
Recommend appropriate nutrition interventions based on nutritional diagnosis	Supervise or manage food-service operations (e.g., food and equipment purchasing, assurance of quality and safe food for consumers, budgeting and payroll)
Provide nutrition counseling	Develop recipes and menus
Monitor patient progress during nutrition intervention phase	Analyze recipes for nutrient content and menus for nutritional adequacy
Evaluate the outcome of nutrition interventions and treatment	Conduct food and nutrition research
Coordinate patient nutrition care	Educate dietetics students, interns, and other allied health professionals
Develop nutrition policy recommendations	

A DPD usually offers more flexibility with scheduling and entry into the program, as well as the ability to apply to a dietetic internship that suits the student's specific area of interest in nutrition. A primary disadvantage of this pathway to becoming an RD/RDN is that not all students who complete a DPD will be matched to an accredited dietetic internship. A CP offers a less flexible but a more streamlined path toward the RD/RDN credential. Similar to a dietetic internship, admittance into a CP is very competitive, but once accepted, students do not need to apply to a separate dietetic internship program; they complete supervised practice as part of the CP.

The supervised practice component (through either a DI or as part of a CP program) requires that interns meet competencies in clinical nutrition, community nutrition, and food-service management. Each program has a designated concentration designed to prepare for future proficiency in a particular area (e.g., medical nutrition therapy, health disparities, research, or public health nutrition). Interns must demonstrate proficiency in about 40 competencies and document at least 1,200 supervised practice hours to complete the supervised practice component. On completion, individuals are eligible to take the Registration Examination for Dietitians.

Scope of Practice

The scopes of practice in the dietetics profession directly relate to the education, licensure of the individual, and credentialing requirements of the state. Examples of general areas included in the RD's/RDN's scope of practice are given in Table 15-2. Because RDs/RDNs have a wide array of career options,

including jobs in health care, food-service management, community and public health, and private practice, among others, standards of practice specific to those unique settings will also differ. However, despite the area in which dietetics is practiced, RDs/RDNs are expected to reflect the Academy's core values, which include "optimizing the nations' health and advancing the profession of nutrition and dietetics through safe, person centered, culturally competent, quality food and nutrition services."[9]

Salary

A recent survey conducted by the Academy of Nutrition and Dietetics estimates a salary range of $43,000 to $92,700 for all RDs/RDNs, in all areas.[10] Salary ranges for RDs/RDNs reflect the number of years in the field, highest dietetics degree received, and geographical location. In general, dietitians were better compensated the longer they were employed in the field and if they possessed a doctoral or master's degree in addition to their clinical designation. Salary ranges are also dependent on the area of practice. RDs/RDNs employed in food and

Author Spotlight

Michelle Hesse (Battista), PhD, RD

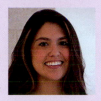

Dr. Hesse is a registered dietitian with experience in community nutrition, food-service systems, and teaching. She is currently an Assistant Professor of Health Sciences, Dietetics Program, at James Madison University, where she teaches a basic human nutrition course, life cycle nutrition, and laboratory-based food science courses. Dr. Hesse states: "From very early in my undergraduate career I knew that I wanted to become a registered dietitian (RD). What I did not anticipate was becoming a researcher and professor. It was not until my senior year in college where I had the opportunity to conduct an undergraduate research project. It was the ability to answer my own questions through research that drove me further into this career path and motivated me to receive my doctorate in nutrition. After receiving my PhD and RD, I worked in a variety of settings in the community as well as in food-service operations. Working as an RD requires a great deal of interpersonal skills and interacting with others. This is the best part of my job, watching individuals I work with reach their goal. My love of working with others grew into a passion for teaching. Now, I am able to teach my students all that I have learned as an RD to help them achieve their own goals and passions!"

Tonya Orchard, PhD, RDN, LD

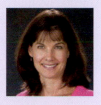

Dr. Orchard is a registered dietitian with over 20 years of experience in clinical nutrition, nutrition counseling, and consulting. She is currently the Director of the Didactic Program in Dietetics and an Assistant Professor of Human Nutrition at The Ohio State University.

Dr. Orchard states: "I have always loved science, so majoring in chemistry in college was a natural choice for me. But, as I progressed through my education I was drawn to more work outside of the laboratory. I began researching nutrition careers and found that dietetics allowed me to combine my love of people, applied science, physiology, health, and of course food, in one profession. I changed my major to medical dietetics and after completing my degree, worked in health care for 18 years before returning to graduate school. I have found that a career in nutrition and dietetics is never stagnant, which makes it both exciting and challenging. It's a great career for those interested in lifelong learning."

Julie Kennel, PhD, RDN, LD

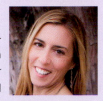

Dr. Kennel is a registered dietitian nutritionist with over 10 years of experience in sports nutrition and nutrition counseling for prevention and wellness. She is a Clinical Assistant Professor and Director of the Human Nutrition Dietetic Internship Program in the Department of Human Sciences at The Ohio State University. She teaches medical nutrition therapy to senior-level dietetics students. Dr. Kennel states: "4-H was a big part of my childhood. I began experimenting with food and nutrition through 4-H project books at 9 years old. The projects were an easy and fun way to integrate the linkages between food, nutrition, and health and wellness. When I started college, someone said to me, 'Follow your passion.' So I enrolled in an introductory nutrition course. It wasn't until I took a 'careers in nutrition' course that I began to see how I could make food and nutrition (my passion) a career by becoming a registered dietitian nutritionist. I have never regretted my decision."

nutrition management, consultation and business, and education and research practice areas received the highest compensation. Practice areas reported to have the least compensation included community dietetics and inpatient and outpatient care.

Trends

The profession of nutrition and dietetics is projected to expand, with great opportunity and demand for professionals in this health-care field. A study of the dietetics profession revealed several factors that will contribute to its expansion and growth in future years.[11,12] Shortages in the supply of dietetics professionals are anticipated due to an increase of retirement-age dietetics professionals, as well as demand for such professionals to care for the aging U.S. population. Several other changes are also expected to drive an increase in demand for dietetics professionals. For one, as the American population grows, so will the rates of chronic health risks. Many of these diseases such as obesity, heart disease, and cancers will require some form of nutritional treatment and management.[11] Furthermore, an increased focus on the prevention of such diseases will require health professionals such as dietitians to educate the public on the link between good nutrition and good health. Across all health sectors, the need for teaming up with other health-care providers to coordinate patient care has resulted in an interprofessional health-care model. Dietitians are an important part of the health-care team and provide expertise to help solve complex nutritional concerns. Overall, jobs in nutrition and dietetics are expected to increase 20% over the next decade (2010–2020).[12] The projected increase in job demand is faster than the growth rate for all other occupations. These statistics are promising not only for the growth of the profession, but also for job stability.

Challenges

Although job prospects for RDs/RDNs are expected to grow, those working in the dietetics profession face several challenges. Despite the high consumer interest in food and nutrition, and the recognition of RDs/RDNs as the most credible source of nutrition information, RDs/RDNs are not named as primary sources of nutrition information by the public. One reason for this may be the exploding amount of nutrition-related information available on electronic media. The Internet, cooking shows, and television are all named as sources of nutrition information much more commonly than RDs/RDNs, even though consumers recognize that electronic media are fraught with misinformation.[13] This may be related to lack of Medicare and insurance reimbursement for preventive nutrition counseling and most medical nutrition therapy, which prevents direct access to nutrition services provided by RDs/RDNs.

RDs/RDNs are able to bill directly for services such as diabetes management, renal disease, and weight management. Yet reimbursement is not provided for medical nutrition therapy of other conditions. Often, RDs/RDNs see patients with diagnoses that are not reimbursable in the outpatient setting, unless the individual is willing to pay for nutrition services "out of pocket." It is uncertain how changes in health-care policy resulting from the Affordable Care Act will affect this situation.

Dietetic professionals are challenged to stay abreast of current advances in the field and communicate these accurately to clients and the public. One of the primary roles of the RD/RDN is to translate scientific findings into easy-to-understand, actionable advice for consumers.[13] To fulfill this responsibility, RDs/RDNs must find reliable resources that compile nutrition information into a useable format easily accessed by professionals with a busy schedule. The Academy of Nutrition and Dietetics offers resources such as the online Evidence Analysis Library and *Daily News* e-mail updates, as well as a scientific journal to help keep members current with scholarly literature and its interpretation. However, even with access to accurate information, RDs/RDNs must recognize that science-based conclusions may differ between professionals, which makes clearly communicating food and nutrition information to the public even more challenging.

The Role of Registered Dietitians in Clinical Settings

As mentioned previously, about one third of all RDs/RDNs work in acute-care settings such as hospitals, and another 12% work in clinics. Individuals working as RDs/RDNs hold jobs in outpatient or inpatient settings, or a combination of these two areas. In both settings, clinical RDs/RDNs use the nutrition care process to perform nutrition **assessment, diagnosis, intervention, monitoring, and evaluation (ADIME).** The ADIME approach facilitates documentation of the nutrition care process. The RD/RDN promotes optimal nutrition status through a range of treatment strategies, including nutrition education, nutrition counseling, food and nutrient delivery, and coordination of nutrition care through collaboration with other medical providers. RDs/RDNs develop nutrition prescriptions that describe a patient's energy, fluid, and nutrient requirements. Prescriptions address meals, snacks, and supplements, as well as enteral (tube feed; refer to Figure 15-4 for example of Enteral Order.) and parenteral (intravenous) nutrition when the patient is not able to meet nutrient needs by mouth. Clinical dietitians treat patient/clients in hospitals (inpatient, acute care), primary-care and ambulatory clinics, home care, or private practice.

The Role of Registered Dietitians in Long-Term Care

RDs/RDNs working in long-term care facilities also practice clinical nutrition, but in an environment that differs from the often fast-paced acute-care setting. Long-term care facilities include traditional nursing homes, rehabilitation centers, mental health residential facilities, and other assisted-living centers. The RD/RDN may be employed by the facility, be an independent consultant, or be part of a company that contracts to provide dietetic services. No matter which type of working arrangement the RD/RDN has with the facility, he or she is required to provide nutrition expertise across a range of topics. The RD/RDN works with an interdisciplinary team that includes physicians, nurses, speech therapists, physical and occupational therapists, and social workers to develop an individual plan of care for each resident (Fig. 15-5). The nutrition care process is used to address nutrition problems, just as in the acute-care setting, with the primary difference being the ongoing interaction between the resident and the RD/RDN that often occurs over a period of weeks, months, or even years. This interaction allows for building of relationships and follow-up, whereas in acute care these relationships are not always possible because patients are only seen one or two times for a brief period. RDs/RDNs in this setting often work closely with the health-care team to treat residents who are nutritionally compromised. Many residents have poor food intake due to chronic diseases, congenital disorders, and terminal illnesses, putting them at high risk for malnutrition and its consequences. The RD/RDN, in collaboration with the health-care team, is responsible for developing a plan of care to improve outcomes in residents with nutrition-related problems. Besides direct nutrition care, the RD/RDN may provide expertise in

Client: HS					Date: 11/12/2014

Assessment: Nutritional Assessment   **Age:** 65   **Gender:** F   **Reason/concerns:** Uncontrolled diabetes

Height: 5′5″   **Weight:** 165   **Ideal Weight:** 140   **Preferred Weight:** Not assessed   **Weight HX:** Weight stable for the last 5 years

Personal Medical HX: T2DM, high cholesterol, hypertension
Family Medical HX: Grandparent had T2DM and many complications—amputation, blindness

Activity Level: Limited to activities of daily living—shopping, cleaning, occasional walk to the neighbor's house

Alcohol Consumption: None   **Smoker?** No

Medical/Supplements: Insulin regimen reviewed and noted. She forgets to take her insulin shots at dinnertime. Pravastatin 20 mg/day. Amlodipine 10 mg/day. Prescribed a daily calcium + vitamin D supplement; she takes at least 5 days/week.

Previous diet efforts: Struggled with her weight after having three children in her late 20s and early 30s. "I try to limit the candy and cookies I eat."

Behavior: 24-hour intake vs. carbohydrate-controlled goals

	Calories	Grains	Vegetables	Fruits	Dairy	Protein	Discretionary
Recommended	1,500	5 oz	2 cups	1.5 cups	2.5 cups	5 ounces	120/day
Actual	1,600	4 oz	0	1 cup	2 cups	7 ounces	300–400/day

Describe food habits/patterns here:
Eats three meals and one snack a day. Mostly packaged foods or ones that are easy to make (Pop Tarts, granola bars, yogurt). Lunch: sandwich, chips. Dinner: frozen meal. Drinks coffee at breakfast and at lunch.

Attitude:
Says that fruits and vegetables are expensive. She prioritizes food dollars for meat (protein) and starchy grains because those are the foods that fill her up. She is not counting carbohydrates at meals and snacks.

Knowledge:
The patient received education about carbohydrate-containing foods when she was diagnosed 3 years ago with T2DM. Today, she had trouble identifying foods that contain carbohydrates. She knows she should stay away from sugar, so she buys low-sugar ice cream, cookies, and candy instead of traditional products.

Diagnosis:
PES1: Fiber intake related to limited access to fiber-containing foods like fruits and vegetables as evidenced by T2DM and estimated intake of fiber that is insufficient compared to desired amount (25 g/day).
PES2: Food- and nutrition-related knowledge deficit related to insufficient prior nutrition-related education as evidenced by verbalizing inaccurate/incomplete information and inability to apply food- and nutrition-related information—specifically carbohydrate-controlled meal pattern.

Intervention:
Nutrition education for carbohydrate-containing foods and amounts. Nutrition education for the role of fiber in the diet (specific to diabetes) and sources of fiber in the diet. Nutrition education (with nursing staff) on how to use carbohydrate counts and blood glucose readings to determine insulin dose during meals. Referral to social work for resources to stretch the patient's food budget.

M/E Monitoring and Evaluation:
Fruit, vegetable, and total fiber intake from self-reported food recalls
Self-report for CHO counting at meals
Blood glucose readings, HbA1c

Dietitian's Signature: *Emily Dietitian*   **Date and Time:** 11/12/2014 3:45pm

FIGURE 15-3 Client progress note using the ADIME process.

the areas of food safety, food-service management, and menu development, often working closely with dietetic technicians, registered (DTRs), dietary managers, and food-service supervisors. RDs/RDNs who work in long-term care are often involved in teaching staff members of the dietary and nursing departments about food and nutrition for their specific resident population along with applicable health and food safety rules and regulations.

The Role of the Dietitian in Food-Service Systems Management

RDs/RDNs who choose employment in food-service management work in a variety of settings such as hospitals, long-term care facilities, universities, school systems, and even the hospitality industry, such as hotels and restaurants. Similar to dietitians working in long-term care, RDs/RDNs in food-service

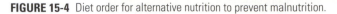

Enteral Nutrition Order

Jevity® 1.5 @ 85 mL/hr for 16 hours per day via G-tube. Flush tube with 180 mL water q6h. Check residuals q6h. Hold tube feeding if residuals >200 mL.

Date: 2/4/2015   **Signature:** *Amanda S. Dietitian, RD, LD*

FIGURE 15-4 Diet order for alternative nutrition to prevent malnutrition.

Problem	Goals	Interventions	Monitoring/Discipline
Inadequate oral intake related to prolonged catabolic illness, as evidenced by calorie intake of <75% of estimated energy requirement and weight loss of >5% in last 30 days.	A. Increase calorie intake to meet estimated needs of 1,700-1,800 kcal/day B. Prevent further weight loss	1. Regular diet with calorie-dense meal plan 2. Provide nutrient-dense liquid supplement at medication pass 3. Refer to MD for evaluation for appetite stimulant	1. Three times a day/ Dietary 2. Twice a day/Nursing 3. Initial Eval/ Medical Director

Signature: *Eric R. Dietitian, RDN*   **Date:** 1/15/2015

FIGURE 15-5 Sample long-term care facility nutrition plan of care.

management may be employed by the facility or part of a company that contracts to provide dietetic services. RDs/RDNs are responsible for providing leadership and management of the dining facility, its operation, and its staff. Besides being proficient in menu development, food safety, and food management, RDs/RDNs in management roles must have a working background of business and management principles including budgeting, staffing, and employee law.

RDs/RDNs in food-service management often work collaboratively with chefs and the food industry to ensure that high-quality and safe food are provided to consumers, as well as designing menus and meal plans that meet specific nutritional needs of the consumer. Depending on the setting, dietitians working in **food-service systems management** can also work with clinical dietitians, medical doctors, and nurse practitioners to execute nutrition care procedures. This area of dietetics differs from RDs/RDNs who work in clinical or long-term care settings, as interactions are usually with staff and health-care professionals rather than with the consumer. Yet, as part of their scope of practice, RDs/RDNs in food-service management should perform assessments of consumer satisfaction and use this information to adjust how services are delivered.

The Role of Registered Dietitians in Community Settings

Community nutrition includes any nutrition program or intervention that targets the community. Settings include government agencies (e.g., federal, state, local), day-care

centers, clinics, nonprofit health organizations, and consultants for companies providing nutrition programs/services. Practitioners working in community/public health nutrition settings work directly with individuals, families, groups, populations, programs, and grants. They also participate in food and nutrition policy development and evaluation based on community needs and resources.[14] RDs/RDNs establish strategic partnerships within the community and act to identify, solve, and prevent health problems.

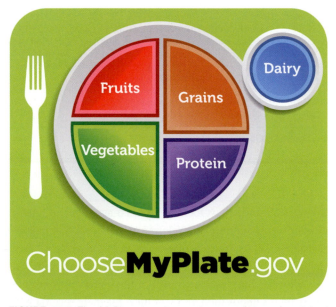

FIGURE 15-6 The MyPlate Icon (www.choosemyplate.gov) and food models are two of the tools that dietitians use to educate individuals and populations on food and nutrition.

Many of the organizations and programs a community RD/RDN might work for target financially disadvantaged populations who may have limited access to food resources. RDs/RDNs in community-based settings are required to have a large knowledge base over an array of nutrition-related topics. Community dietitians work with numerous populations, from infancy to the elderly, so a deep understanding of life span nutrition is also expected. For example, community dietitians employed with the Women, Infants, and Children (WIC) program perform nutrition-based assessments and counseling and monitor the nutrition-related health status of infants, children up to 5 years of age, and their mothers. RDs/RDNs in this setting make health-care referrals if serious health concerns are made evident.

RDs/RDNs employed by food pantries or community advocacy programs and even the federally sponsored Expanded Food and Nutrition Education Program (EFNEP) and Supplemental Nutrition Assistance Program Education (SNAP-Ed) programs promote access to nutritionally sound foods. RDs/RDNs in this setting often deliver skill-based nutrition education in small-group settings that cover topics such as meal planning, feeding a family on a budget, and even basic cooking and food preparation skills. The development of these skills can help financially disadvantaged populations have the opportunity to meet nutrition and health goals.

Emerging Areas of Practice for the Dietitian

Over the past several decades, the breadth of the RD's/RDN's work has extended beyond the setting of health care, community nutrition, and food-service management. The role of RDs/RDNs in food and nutrition-related businesses varies widely but may include participating in marketing, sales, product development, consumer affairs, media communications, and public relations. Some RDs/RDNs who are board certified in sports dietetics work with individual athletes or teams at the college or professional level, providing nutrition recommendations to enhance athletic performance. RDs/RDNs may work in corporate wellness programs, educating clients about the connection between food, fitness, and health. RDs/RDNs with advanced degrees (e.g., master's or doctoral degree in nutrition, food science, and public health) may work as scientists in university or industry settings, identifying nutritional involvement in diseases, improving nutritional values in foods, exploring causes of nutrient deficiencies, addressing world hunger issues, and so on. Nutrition touches countless areas of society, and there are many opportunities for creative, entrepreneurial dietetic professionals to carve out their own unique niche.

The Role of the Board-Certified Specialist in Dietetics

Many RDs/RDNs hold additional certifications in specialized areas of practice, including pediatric nutrition, renal nutrition, gerontological nutrition, oncology nutrition, and sports dietetics (all granted by the Commission on Dietetic Registration). Often, dietitians are eligible for other credentialing programs, such as the Certified Nutrition Support Clinician (National Board of Nutrition Support Certification, Inc.), Certified Diabetes Educator (National Certification Board for Diabetes Educators), and International Board Certified Lactation Consultant (International Board of Lactation Consultant Examiners). The certifications are earned in recognition of an applicant's documented practice experience and successful completion of an examination in the specialty area.[15] Certifications can be a way to advance the RD's/RDN's career, add competitiveness for career placement, and provide unique benefits to clients and employers.

Personality Traits and Characteristics

A career in nutrition and dietetics often means working independently as well as with a team of people to make decisions and manage programs. RDs/RDNs who are involved in education and counseling must have good listening skills and demonstrate empathy toward patients and clients. They excel at teaching both individuals and groups, using a variety of instructional methods.

Working Together

RDs/RDNs work closely with a variety of professionals depending on the employment setting. Clinical dietitians collaborate with multiple disciplines in the course of providing nutrition care to patients and clients. These RDs/RDNs frequently communicate with doctors and nurses about the patient's medical condition, review medications and dietary supplements with pharmacists, discuss issues involving swallowing difficulties and texture modification with speech therapists/pathologists, gather information from social workers regarding family circumstances and dietary services needed for discharge, and talk with physical and occupational therapists about the patient's ability to perform activities of daily living or exercise. From these collaborations, the interdisciplinary team works together to develop a plan of care that promotes the best possible 9outcome for the patient.

RDs/RDNs who work in a food-service setting collaborate with a variety of professionals, including chefs and food

(continued)

167

industry personnel. Collaborating with such professionals helps ensure that consumers receive the highest quality safe foods for consumption and that menus designed to meet the needs of the consumer are nutritionally sound. In a hospital setting, the RDs/RDNs work with teams of doctors, clinical dietitians, nurses, dietetic technicians, and dietary managers. Communication among these professionals is important to the food-service operation in the event that accommodations need to be made to meet specific nutritional needs of the patient.

RDs/RDNs employed in the community setting often collaborate with or make referrals to not-for-profit organizations, including food pantries, hospitals/doctors' offices, social workers, and government-sponsored food assistance programs such as WIC, EFNEP, and SNAP. Collaboration in the community is important so that populations with nutritional needs are able to access nutritious foods and utilize these foods in a way to enhance health and well-being. Community RDs/RDNs can also work alongside local, state, or federal politicians, schools, and nonprofit organizations to develop policies and best practices that will enhance availability and access to nutritionally sound foods for any population.

CASE STUDY

VC is a 46-year-old man of Asian (Cambodian) descent. He presents today with a nurse practitioner at a primary-care clinic to be checked for diabetes and address right knee pain. VC works as a technician for a cable company. He lives with his wife and two young children. VC states he was at urgent care last week and was told he had sugar in his urine. The patient reports polyuria (frequent urination), polydipsia (excessive thirst), and a red rash on his right shin for 1 month. He reports blurred vision for about 6 years; he does not wear glasses. Also, VC complains of feeling chronically tired for 2 years.

VC plays tennis three times a week for 2 hours at a time. His usual foods include donuts, cakes, or pastries with coffee for breakfast, rice with vegetables and meat with brown sauce and water for lunch, and three pieces of pizza and green salad with medium soda for dinner. He drinks 100% apple juice throughout the day. At the visit, he shares concerns that the salt in his diet is causing his current symptoms.

Height 1.65 meters (5 feet 5 inches), weight 78.7 kilograms (173 pounds, 10 ounces), body mass index (BMI) 28.9. VC reports an 8- to 10-pound weight loss in the last 2 to 3 weeks. His usual body weight (UBW) is 180 pounds.

Blood pressure 100/70 mm Hg, pulse 76, temperature 97.3°F, respiratory rate 16.

Blood sugar 523 (random, nonfasting); HbA1c 14; urinalysis: no ketones.

VC is alert with no distress or edema. He has visible central adiposity.

The nurse practitioner diagnoses him with uncontrolled type 2 diabetes mellitus. The treatment plan includes home glucose monitoring, hypoglycemia education, referral to the pharmacist for use of medications (metformin), and referral to RD/RDN for carbohydrate-controlled diet education and counseling.

Questions

1. VC has questions about how much metformin to take and if he should go on insulin. What health professional would be ideal to refer him to for assistance with medications?

2. VC may change jobs soon and is worried about his prescription drug coverage during his transition. What health professional would be best for VC to speak with about health insurance options and prescription drug assistance programs?

3. VC has been having some pain in his right knee. Physical activity can help mediate uncontrolled diabetes. What health professional is best suited to evaluate his knee pain?

Review Questions

1. RDs/RDNs are typically engaged in which of the following career opportunities?

   A. Food-service management

   B. Community dietetics

   C. Medical nutrition therapy

   D. All of the above

2. All RDs/RDNs are nutritionists, but not all nutritionists are RDs/RDNs.

   A. True

   B. False

3. Which of the following courses are the core requirements of a didactics or coordinated didactics program? Choose all that apply.

   A. Exercise science

   B. Anatomy

   C. Medical nutrition therapy

   D. American history

   E. Food-service management

   F. Chemistry

4. One of the most common challenges in the dietetics profession is:

   A. Time pressure

   B. Lack of reimbursement for medical nutrition therapy services

   C. Lack of information made available to the public

   D. Inability to collaborate or work with other health professionals

5. The scope of practice for the RD/RDN includes all of the following except:

   A. Perform nutrition-related assessments

   B. Develop nutrition policy recommendations

   C. Develop recipes and menus

   D. Prescribe medications

6. A dietitian who works in a community-based setting would likely interact with which of the following professionals?

   A. The director of a local food pantry

   B. An emergency department doctor

   C. A speech therapist

   D. A chef

7. A dietitian who works in a food-service setting would likely interact with which of the following professionals?

   A. A dietitian from Women, Infants, and Children (WIC)

   B. A physical therapist

   C. A medical doctor

   D. A professional athlete

8. The general term for an RD/RDN who has received certification in a specialized area of dietetics practice is:

   A. Specialty dietitian, certified

   B. Board-certified specialist in dietetics

   C. Expert dietitian

   D. Registered dietitian

9. Community-based settings for dietitians include:

   A. Hospitals

   B. Day-care centers

   C. Long-term care facilities

   D. Dialysis units

10. Eligibility to take the Registration Examination for Dietitians includes at least _____ hours of supervised practice.

    A. 700

    B. 900

    C. 1,200

    D. 1,500

Glossary of Key Terms

Registered dietitians/registered dietitian nutritionists—credentialed experts in the field of food and nutrition who translate scientific research into practical guidance for individuals and populations

Didactic program in dietetics—an accredited undergraduate academic program that provides introductory knowledge for the field of food and nutrition

Coordinated dietetics program—an accredited undergraduate or graduate academic program that provides introductory knowledge for the field of food and nutrition, as well as supervised practice in food and nutrition

Dietetic internship program—an accredited postbaccalaureate program that integrates introductory knowledge with supervised practice in food and nutrition

Assessment, diagnosis, intervention, monitoring, evaluation (ADIME)—a series of steps that aid in the identification of nutrition-related health concerns and the planning of appropriate nutrition interventions to address those concerns

Food-service systems management—describes an area of food and nutrition that directs the management and operational procedures of food-service establishments

Community nutrition—encompasses individual and interpersonal-level interventions focused on creating changes in knowledge, attitudes, behavior, and health outcomes either individually or in small groups within a community setting[16]

Board-certified specialist in dietetics—an advanced area of specialization where the RD/RDN has met specific competencies and successfully passed a secondary examination

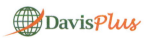 Additional Resources are available online at www.davisplus.com

Additional Resources

Websites

Academy of Nutrition and Dietetics—www.eatright.org

Accreditation Council for Education in Nutrition and Dietetics—www.eatright.org/ACEND/content.aspx?id=146

Academy of Nutrition and Dietetics, Dietetics Practice Groups (DPG)—www.eatright.org/About/Content.aspx?id=8767

Commission on Dietetic Registration—http://cdrnet.org/

Blogs

The Makings of a Registered Dietitian—www.katheats. com/kathrd/the-makings-of-a-registered-dietitian
Questions for the Registered Dietitians—www. preventionrd.com/rd-qa/
The Candid RD—http://candidrd.com/

References

1. Skiadas PK, Lascaratos JG. Dietetics in ancient Greek philosophy: Plato's concepts of healthy diet. *Eur J Clin Nutr.* 2001;55:532–537.

2. Winterfeldt EA, Bogle ML, Ebro LL. *Dietetics: Practice and Future Trends,* 2nd ed. Sudbury, MA: Jones & Bartlett; 2005.

3. Bureau of Labor Statistics. U.S. Department of Labor, Occupational outlook handbook.

   http://www.bls.gov/ooh/healthcare/dietitians-and-nutritionists.htm.

   Accessed August 16, 2013.

4. Academy of Nutrition and Dietetics. ACEND educational and professional requirements.

   http://www.eatright.org/ACEND/content.aspx?id=7980.

   Accessed August 14, 2013.

5. Academy of Nutrition and Dietetics. What are the qualifications of a registered dietitian?

   http://www.eatright.org/Public/content.aspx?id=6713.

   Accessed November 15, 2013.

6. Commission on Dietetic Registration. State licensure.

   http://cdrnet.org/state-licensure.

   Accessed November 8, 2013.

7. Academy of Nutrition and Dietetics. What is an RDN?

   http://www.eatright.org/Public/landing.aspx?TaxID=6442452104.

   Accessed August 14, 2013.

8. Accreditation Council for Education in Nutrition and Dietetics. ACEND update (May 2013).

   http://www.eatright.org/ACEND.

   Accessed August 14, 2014.

9. Academy Quality Management Committee and Scope of Practice Subcommittee of the Quality Management Committee. Academy of Nutrition and Dietetics: Scope of practice for the registered dietitian. *J Acad Nutr Diet.* 2013;113:s17–s28.

10. Academy of Nutrition and Dietetics. Compensation and benefits survey of the dietetics profession.

    http://www.eatright.org/shop/product.aspx?id=6442478272.

    Accessed November 12, 2014.

11. Haughton B, Stang J. Population risk factors and trends in health care and public policy. *J Acad Nutr Diet.* 2012;112:s35–s46.

12. Rhea M, Bettles C. Future changes driving dietetics workforce supply: Future scan 2012–2022. *J Acad Nutr Diet.* 112:s10–s24, 2012.

13. Quagliani D, Hermann M. Practice paper of the Academy of Nutrition and Dietetics. Abstract: Communicating accurate food and nutrition information. *J Acad Nutr Diet.* 2012;112:759–760.

14. Gilmore CJ, Maillet JO, Mitchell BE. Determining educational preparation based on job competencies of entry-level dietetics practitioners. *J Am Diet Assoc.* 1997;97(3):306–316.

15. Commission on Dietetic Registration. Board-certified specialist home.

    http://cdrnet.org/certifications/board-certified-specialist.

    Accessed November 15, 2013.

16. *Public Health Nutrition and Community Nutrition Definitions.* Public Health Task Force, Academy of Nutrition and Dietetics; 2012.

CHAPTER 16

Emergency Medical Services

Keith Monosky, PhD

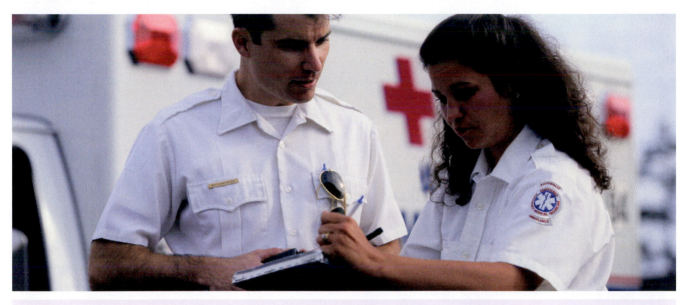

Photo credit: Photodisc/Thinkstock

Learning Objectives

After reading this chapter, students should be able to:

- Describe the role of the emergency medical technician (EMT) and the paramedic
- Explain the origin and history of the discipline of emergency medical services
- Describe the differences in the required education and provider roles of the EMT and the paramedic
- Explain the typical certification and credentialing process associated with providers of emergency medical services
- Discuss the developing future of emergency medical services and its emerging contribution to health care in general

Key Terms

- Paramedic
- Electrocardiogram (ECG)
- Emergency medical services (EMS)
- Emergency medical technicians (EMTs)
- Advanced EMTs (AEMTs)
- Endotracheal intubation
- Protocols
- Standing orders
- Community paramedicine
- Mobile Integrated Health care (MIH)
- Ambulance volantes

- National Highway Transportation Safety Administration (NHTSA)
- Cardiopulmonary resuscitation (CPR)
- Ambulance technicians
- Medical first responders
- National Registry of EMTs (NREMT)
- Committee on Accreditation of Educational Programs for EMS Professions
- Commission on Accreditation of Allied Health Education Programs

- Cardioscope/defibrillator
- Pulse oximeter
- Capnography
- *National EMS Education Standards*
- Personal Protection and Affordable Care Act
- Department of Health and Human Services (HHS)
- Laryngoscopy
- Continuing medical education (CME)

"A Day in the Life"

My name is Gregg and I am a **paramedic** for a moderate-sized city that has about 35,000 emergency medical calls each year. My colleagues and I work an unusual schedule that is unique to fire departments and emergency medical service (EMS) agencies. We work 24 hours on-duty, followed by 48 hours off-duty. This enables us to be available at all times to the community while practically living at our station where the ambulances are kept. I am beginning my shift so I am in the process of checking all of my equipment on the ambulance. I check the medications to make sure they are not expired or damaged in any way and I check the supplies to make sure they are well stocked. I examine the heart monitor (cardioscope/defibrillator) to make sure it is working properly and the batteries are well charged. I also ensure that the oxygen supply is full and systematically reconcile a long list of medical equipment and materials. My partner, John (an emergency medical technician), and I also check the ambulance to make sure it is fueled, that the tires are properly inflated, and that the oil and engine fluid levels are satisfactory. We then wash the outside of the ambulance and disinfect the inside. We do all of this in our ambulance bay because it is a cold winter day and the water would freeze onto our ambulance.

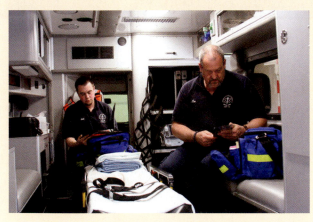

Soon after we've finished our equipment checks, we are summoned to respond to a middle-aged man with chest pain. Based on the dispatch information, we suspect he's having a heart attack. To expedite our response, we use the loud siren and flashing lights to help us maneuver through traffic. Despite the nature of this emergency, we must always abide by the traffic laws. Operating an emergency vehicle takes a lot of training and vigilance. We arrive at the patient's home and find him sitting in his living room chair. He is sweating, is having some difficulty in breathing, is nauseated, and reports severe chest pain. While my partner connects the patient to the heart monitor, obtains vital signs (pulse rate, breathing rate, and blood pressure), and places him on oxygen, I am obtaining a medical history and conducting a physical examination. I learn about his symptoms, what medications he takes, and what medical problems he's had in the past. I listen to his lung sounds and heart sounds with my stethoscope and I then examine the **electrocardiogram (ECG)** tracing closely. It appears that he is having a heart attack. My partner assembles the intravenous (IV) equipment and assists me in starting his IV line. I then administer a medication to help relieve his pain and another medication to control the chaotic activity in his heart. Once he's stabilized, we will transport him to the hospital where he'll have his coronary blood vessels opened inside of a catheterization laboratory. He will have a good chance of a full recovery.

Now it's 3:00 o'clock in the morning and my partner and I are called to respond to an automobile accident on the interstate highway. The weather has turned to snow with a cold, blowing wind. We arrive to find a car that has rolled over onto its roof. There are two patients inside, each with serious injuries and uncontrolled bleeding. The rescue personnel have already arrived on the scene and have gained access to the passenger compartment of the vehicle. After donning our protective gear, we climb inside the overturned vehicle to begin assessing the victims and start emergency treatment. One of the passengers has a severe head injury and must be taken at once to a trauma center. We call for a medical helicopter to fly the patient directly to the trauma room. Within 15 minutes, the helicopter is making its final approach to the landing zone on the highway. We load the patient into the helicopter while the rotors are still turning (we call that a "hot load") and the flight crew takes over the treatment. The other victim has superficial cuts and bruises with a broken arm and possible abdominal trauma. My partner and I will transport this patient to the local hospital via our ambulance.

After we deliver the patient to the hospital, my partner cleans the back of the ambulance and restocks our supplies while I write the patient care report. This report will become a permanent part of the patient's medical records. It will detail all of the medical information we discovered and what treatments we rendered. We can't wait to get back to the station to enjoy a hot cup of soup and warm up after our early-morning call. We have to get warmed and nourished because who knows when the next call will come in?

Introduction to Emergency Medical Services

Description

The discipline of **emergency medical services (EMS)** is the profession that provides critical care to the sick and injured in the community and provides transportation of those patients to hospitals and similar health-care facilities. Transportation of the patients is provided in ambulances (sometimes referred to as *mobile intensive care units*), as well as helicopters and fixed-wing aircraft in select circumstances. The personnel that deliver the emergency care are often **emergency medical technicians (EMTs), advanced EMTs (AEMTs),** and **paramedics.** The distinction between each of these is the level of care that can be provided. The EMT level has basic education as an emergency provider, the AEMT level has some additional advanced skills, and the paramedic has the greatest amount of basic and advanced education.

EMTs must currently undergo between 150 and 190 hours of training in basic emergency care.[1] This training consists of lectures, practice sessions in laboratories, and some clinical experience in hospital emergency departments. Advanced EMTs receive extended education that includes starting IV lines and inserting certain advanced airway devices (these devices help to ensure adequate breathing in unconscious victims). By comparison, paramedics undergo considerably more education that enables them to deliver advanced medical care. Such advanced care often includes not just IV lines and advanced airway devices, but even more specialized airway procedures (e.g., **endotracheal intubation**), ECG monitoring of the heart, medication administration, electrical shocks to the heart (defibrillation), and other highly advanced skills. The paramedic possesses an expanded scope of skills and cognitive knowledge. Most paramedic programs provide education exceeding 1,200 hours, and some offer associate and even bachelor's degrees in paramedicine.[2]

Many describe the role of EMTs and paramedics as the "eyes and hands" of the physician outside of the hospital. While performing their duties, EMS providers are caring for patients under the medical authority and direction of a physician. They provide emergency medical care based on prescriptive orders from a physician called **protocols**. These protocols direct the care to patients based on the nature of their illness or injury. In select cases of dire conditions, these protocols are supplemented with **standing orders** that provide the paramedic with the ability to treat emergencies without the need to consult with physicians beforehand. Paramedics and EMTs typically wear uniforms to distinguish them from the public. About half of the EMS organizations throughout the United States are fire-based, meaning that they are firefighters as well as EMS providers.[3]

Over the years, the education of EMTs and, in particular, paramedics has become increasingly comprehensive and expansive. This has led to greater professional recognition as health-care providers and greater relevance to the overall health-care system. In some communities, paramedics and EMTs deliver preventive and simple primary care to residents in their homes—a new role within EMS called **community paramedicine** or **mobile integrated health care (MIH).**[4] As the profession of EMS grows, the educational requirements have also grown. At present, approximately 30 paramedic programs throughout the United States offer a bachelor's degree associated with paramedicine.[5] Some have a greater focus on the management of EMS systems, whereas others have an emphasis on the clinical practice of paramedicine. More and more colleges and universities are offering paramedic education programs, and some offer graduate programs in EMS as well. The future is bright for careers in EMS.

Historical Perspective

By comparison with other allied health careers, EMS is one of the youngest health professions. The origin of EMS is often attributed to the practices of Napoleon Bonaparte's chief surgeon, Baron Dominique Jean Larrey[6-8] (Fig. 16-1).

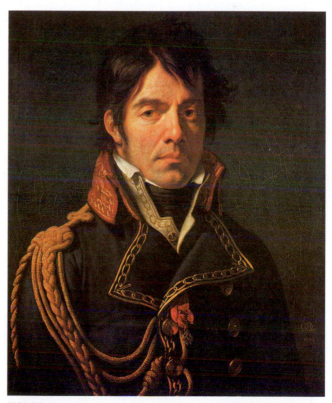

FIGURE 16-1 Baron Dominique Jean Larrey was the chief surgeon for Napoleon Bonaparte and is often credited with the origin of the ambulance. (Portrait by Anne-Louis Girodet de Roussy-Trioson, Musée du Louvre ambulance)

In 1792, Larrey attempted to improve injured soldiers' survival by bringing medical equipment to their side and removing them from the battlefield in horse-drawn carriages, called "**ambulance volantes**" or "flying ambulances" (Fig. 16-2). Over the years, this practice evolved and became a standard in many areas outside of military campaigns. For example, the Knights of the Order of Saint John (also known as the Knights Hospitaller) was a religious military order that provided aid to wounded soldiers in Mediterranean and European theaters. This military practice transformed into civilian medical aid throughout Europe, resulting in the formation of an ambulance service in London in 1877, the St. John's ambulance service, which remains in service to this day. While EMS continued to grow and spread throughout Europe, similar practices were developing in the United States, where New York's Bellevue Hospital initiated the first American civilian EMS in the late 1860s.[8] After that, ambulance services began to emerge throughout the United States, often using modified hearses operated by funeral directors. The use of modified hearses eventually transformed into using station wagons and specialized emergency vehicles operated by fire departments and independent ambulance services in the mid-1960s (Fig. 16-3).

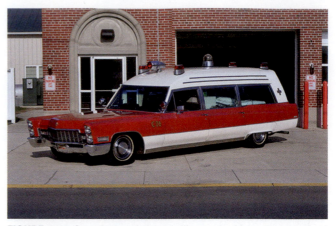

FIGURE 16-3 Over time, ambulances, like most vehicles, have changed to represent modern times. This ambulance was a 1968 Cadillac/Miller-Meteor ambulance owned by the Frankford, Delaware, Volunteer Fire Company. (Reprinted with permission of the Frankford, DE Volunteer Fire company.)

Modern-day EMS was motivated by a revolutionary report from the National Academy of Sciences and the National Research Council in 1966 that compared the life expectancy of soldiers wounded on the battlefields of Vietnam with victims of motor vehicle crashes on the highways of America. The report confirmed that soldiers wounded in combat were more likely to survive than the civilian traffic accident victims. This report, *Accidental Death and Disability: The Neglected Disease of Modern Society,* became known as the "White Paper" and drew public and Congressional attention to the need to develop a unified system of emergency care in the United States.[9] This need is largely the reason why EMS still receives federal oversight from the **National Highway Transportation Safety Administration (NHTSA)** in the Department of Transportation (DOT).

The first modern-day ambulance service to feature paramedics is often disputed. Nonetheless, by the late 1960s, several major metropolitan areas such as Cincinnati, Pittsburgh, Seattle, Miami, and a few others began services utilizing paramedics.[10] Since that time, ambulance services have become a critical part of public safety, along with fire and police protection, within the responsibilities of municipal governments.

Initial providers of emergency care had little more than first-aid and **cardiopulmonary resuscitation (CPR)** training, with little regulation or standardization. From that time of inception, a variety of instructional programs emerged, including courses that enabled certifications as **ambulance technicians**, emergency medical service technicians (EMTs), advanced EMTs, intermediate paramedics, paramedics, critical-care paramedics, and advanced-practice paramedics. Currently, most states recognize four levels of EMS education: emergency

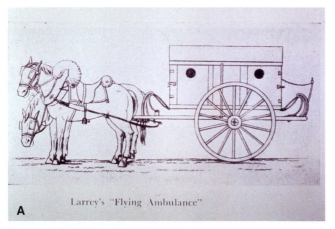

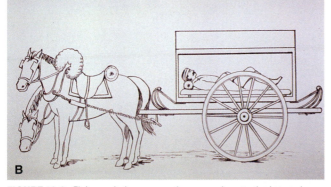

FIGURE 16-2 *Flying ambulances* was the name given to the horse-drawn carriages used to remove injured soldiers from the battlefield in the late 18th century. (From the National Library of Medicine, History of Medicine Collection.)

medical responder (EMR), EMT, advanced EMT (AEMT), and paramedic.[11-13]

Most **medical first responders** are affiliated with public safety organizations such as police departments, fire departments, recreational safety associations (lifeguards or ski patrols), or similar agencies. EMTs and AEMTs are often affiliated with ambulance services (more commonly referred to as EMS agencies), as are paramedics. As a career option, some paramedics also deliver emergency care in air ambulances (helicopters or fixed-winged aircraft) (Fig. 16-4). All EMS providers must be certified or licensed by a state authorizing entity or the **National Registry of EMTs (NREMT)** in accordance with standardized competency requirements. Educational programs that deliver EMT and paramedic training must be accredited by a national EMS education accrediting organization, specifically the **Committee on Accreditation of Educational Programs for EMS Professions** under the auspices of the **Commission on Accreditation of Allied Health Education Professions,** and must have physicians serve as medical directors.[14]

With the development of education and certifications in EMS came advances in technology and equipment. Early ambulance personnel worked with basic tools such as bandages, splints, mechanical resuscitators, and stretchers. Today, EMTs and paramedics use a range of advanced equipment and technology to provide the most effective care possible and ensure the best possible outcomes. Cardiac monitoring with a **cardioscope/defibrillator** (Fig. 16-5), measurement of oxygen in the blood with a **pulse oximeter,** determination of carbon dioxide in exhaled breath with **capnography,** video-assisted endotracheal intubation devices, and even portable ultrasound devices are now being used in some EMS systems.

EMS is on the verge of new beginnings with the advent of mobile integrated health-care (MIH) teams (sometimes

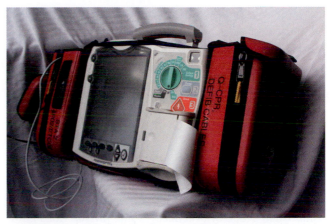

FIGURE 16-5 Cardioscope/defibrillators, which are used to restart the heart, are standard equipment in EMS vehicles.

referred to as community paramedicine), which have grown rapidly nationwide. For more information on MIH, see Current Trends later in this chapter.

Scope of Practice

There are two levels of care in EMS: basic life support and advanced life support. Basic life support care is provided by both EMTs and paramedics, whereas advanced life support is provided by paramedics (and, to a limited extent, AEMTs). The scope of practice for each is presented here.

Basic life support entails the delivery of care that meets all of the emergency care needs of a patient without invasive or sophisticated procedures, knowledge, or skills. All paramedics must be trained to the basic life support level as EMTs before they can undergo paramedic education. The scope of practice among EMTs includes, but is not limited to, each of the following:

- Establishing and ensuring safety at the scene of an accident.

- Lifting and moving patients.

- Assisting patients with certain prescribed medications.

- Managing the airway of a patient using manual techniques and various basic devices; assisting respiration; and administering oxygen.

- CPR and use of an automated external defibrillator.

- Assessing patients of acute medical illness or injury and obtaining vital signs (i.e., pulse, respirations, temperature, and blood pressure).

- Managing the emergency care for patients of acute medical illnesses and trauma (EMTs can manage all emergencies to a basic life support level, including respiratory,

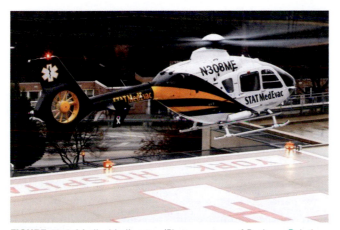

FIGURE 16-4 Medical helicopter. (Photo courtesy of Business Relations and Development Manager of STAT MedEvac.)

cardiovascular, neurological, psychiatric, gastrointestinal, musculoskeletal, infectious and immunologic, endocrine, toxicological, hematological, genitourinary, geriatric, pediatric, and gynecological and obstetric emergencies, as well as all forms of trauma).

- Providing basic emergency incident management in rescues, trauma, hazardous material incidents, and similar public safety threats.

The skills and abilities of EMTs may vary somewhat from state to state and among EMS systems, but a national standard ensures that all EMTs can perform a minimally established scope of practice.[15] Some jurisdictions allow EMTs to perform select skills at an advanced life support level.

Advanced life support includes all of the skills of the basic life support provider and an additional set of skills that involve invasive interventions, use of medications and therapeutic technologies, comprehensive patient assessment abilities, and other advanced procedures and techniques.[16] Paramedics, as providers of advanced life support, are expected to serve as a critical member of the emergency health-care team and to develop critical thinking skills, problem-solving skills, and leadership skills. The scope of practice for paramedics is extensive and may include, but not be limited to, each of the following:

- The knowledge and skill of an EMT with enhancement of many cognitive areas, such as anatomy and physiology, pathophysiology, public health, pharmacology, and many others.

- Comprehensive patient assessment, including extensive history-taking, physical examination techniques, and the use of modern technology to aid in the assessment process.

- Advanced airway management, including all forms of endotracheal intubation (placement of a breathing tube into the airway of the patient).

- Use of assistive devices to aid in respiratory and cardiovascular diagnostics and therapeutic interventions.

- Starting IV lines and the administration of a multitude of emergency medications through IV and alternative routes of administration.

- Managing the emergency care for patients of acute medical illnesses and trauma (the paramedic can manage all instances of emergencies to an advanced life support level, including respiratory, cardiovascular, neurological, psychiatric, gastrointestinal, musculoskeletal, infectious and immunologic, endocrine, toxicological, hematological, genitourinary, geriatric, pediatric, and gynecological and obstetric emergencies, as well as all forms of trauma).

- Initial delivery of preventive and primary care under strict guidelines that facilitate an integration of health-care delivery (see Current Trends later in this chapter for more information).

The paramedic is considered the terminal level of credentialed provider in prehospital emergency care. Paramedics have an extensive interaction with physicians and other health-care professionals to oversee patient care and ensure a continuity of care from the prehospital setting to the hospital setting.

In most EMS systems, paramedics and EMTs work together. Usually, teams consist of one paramedic and one EMT. In some EMS systems, only EMTs provide care and teams consist of two EMTs. And in even fewer EMS systems, teams consist of two paramedics. In EMS systems that are referred to as "two-tiered," a team of EMTs will render care to the patient and a team of paramedics can be summoned if the EMTs deem it necessary.

Required Education

EMTs and paramedics are trained in accordance with published national educational standards.[1] These **National EMS Education Standards** establish minimum educational objectives with which all EMT and paramedic training programs must comply. Training for EMTs and paramedics can occur in a variety of settings. Some programs are provided by local fire departments, technical schools, or independent and private training organizations; some are provided by community colleges; and some are provided by 4-year colleges and universities. As the profession continues to grow, more and more colleges and universities are offering paramedic education programs. Currently, approximately 30 universities

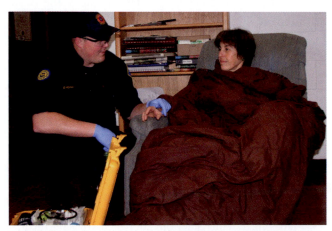

FIGURE 16-6 This emergency medical technician is providing care to a patient.

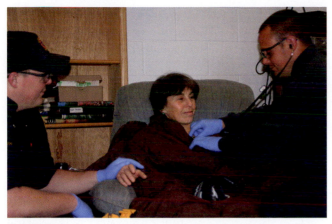

FIGURE 16-7 A paramedic is providing advanced life support care to a patient.

provide paramedic education and award bachelor's degrees across the United States.[5]

Some of these universities provide additional levels of education for degree-seeking paramedics that advance and expand the knowledge of emergency medical services. Sample topics include courses in EMS management, leadership, advanced pathophysiology, health policy, principles

of research, analysis of EMS systems, and many others. Educational content that extends beyond standard paramedic education usually focuses on either management practices common to EMS systems or advanced clinical practice of paramedic providers.

EMT education typically consists of a single course in basic life support. These courses often have durations of 9 to 10 months and consist of both lectures and practical laboratory sessions.[15] Most EMT programs also provide students with a brief opportunity for actual clinical observation in hospital emergency departments. At the conclusion of the EMT training, students are afforded an opportunity to become certified either through a state certification examination or through the National Registry of EMTs.[17] These certifications are necessary to enable EMTs to practice emergency care.

Paramedics, by comparison, undergo much more extensive educational instruction than do EMTs. The *National EMS Education Standards: Paramedic Instructional Guidelines* establishes the minimum content necessary for all paramedic education programs.[16] Most programs that teach paramedic education provide between 1,200 and 1,600 hours of instruction. Like the EMT courses, paramedic education also includes lecture and practical laboratory sessions. These educational components are much more extensive than the EMT curricula and also include a comprehensive clinical education component. In addition to attending lectures and participating in practical laboratory sessions, paramedic students must also participate in clinical education in hospitals and with EMS agencies to learn the profession. Hospital clinical experience may include specialized areas such as the emergency department, operating room, intensive care units, respiratory care departments, psychiatric units, labor and delivery, and many other clinical units. The field experience that paramedic students attain at EMS agencies enables them to learn the practices of the profession and helps develop the skills necessary to lead EMS crews.

Paramedic education programs must be accredited to provide these services. The accrediting organization is the Commission on Accreditation of Allied Health Education Programs (CAAHEP) in conjunction with the Committee on Accreditation of Educational Programs for the Emergency Medical Services Professions (CoAEMSP).[2,14] Each year, the paramedic education program must demonstrate compliance with the educational standards and evidence of educational success by submitting reports to the CoAEMSP organization. In addition, approximately every 5 years the CoAEMSP sends representatives to conduct site visits to ensure compliance to standards and delivery of effective paramedic education.

Author Spotlight

Keith Monosky, PhD

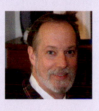

I began my career in EMS just before graduating high school. I was intrigued by the opportunity to help others in the time of crisis and impressed by the collegiality among EMS providers. Training was very basic back then—I was trained to be an ambulance attendant, then an EMT, and finally a paramedic. There were no role models as there were not many paramedics back in the late 1970s and early 1980s. Without realizing it at the time, we were setting the stage for future paramedics. As I practiced as a paramedic, I came to realize that there was a need to educate more people to become EMTs and paramedics and to lead EMS organizations. I went to school to earn my bachelor's degree in behavioral neuroscience and continued to earn a master's degree in the management of health systems, all while working either as a paramedic or as a coordinator of EMS systems (overseeing the administration of EMS delivery). Eventually, I became a director of an EMS education program and earned my doctorate in health policy. Since beginning in EMS, I've been a provider of emergency care, an educator of EMS, a researcher, an author, and an administrator of university paramedic programs that award bachelor's degrees. I have had the great fortune of experiencing and participating in the growth and development of EMS over the years.

These practices help to ensure a standardized delivery of educational content and effective paramedic education across the nation.

Paramedic education is experiencing a developing trend of university-based education with the opportunity for students to earn a bachelor's degree. This process is being motivated by a growing recognition of EMS as a genuine health-care profession, as well as the identified need for well-educated EMS professionals to take on greater roles in leadership, policy development, and profession advocacy. This trend is evidenced by the fact that paramedic program directors must now possess a bachelor's degree at a minimum and the proposal that lead paramedic instructors must also hold a bachelor's degree in the near future.[14] More and more EMS administrators, educators, and managers are attaining college degrees that are relevant to the profession of EMS. Some of these 4-year degrees deliver education in an online format and even award degrees specific to paramedicine. Some are incorporating mobile integrated health-care practices (community paramedicine) into their educational curriculum.

Salaries and Career Opportunities

For years, the *Journal of Emergency Medical Services (JEMS)* has been surveying the current salaries and benefits of EMTs and paramedics from across the country. Although salaries and benefits have steadily increased over the years, the profession of EMS is only recently receiving compensation with parity to other allied health professions. For example, according to the *JEMS* survey, the average salary for a paramedic in the United States in 2012 was $37,909; in 2013 it was $39,749; and in 2014 it was $41,084.[18-21] This steady growth reflects increasing recognition of EMS as a true health profession among leaders and policymakers. Growth of the profession has been more rapid in certain geographical regions than in others. In some regions of the United States, salaries of paramedics after several years of employment reach over $70,000 annually.[20]

As health-care opportunities expand, so do career opportunities in EMS. With the development of new trends in EMS, particularly its new role as a mobile integrated health-care delivery component within a larger system of coordinated community health care, new career options will likely become more plentiful. EMS providers will begin playing a larger role in preventive and primary care for people in their communities. This, coupled with a more cooperative and integrative network of health-care delivery, will enhance access to health care, reduce costs, and improve the overall quality of care. It is expected that this expanded role of EMS will play a critical part in achieving those goals.

In the meantime, there will remain many opportunities for EMTs and paramedics to provide traditional emergency medical care to citizens within the community. Across the nation, municipalities have an inherent obligation to provide public safety to the citizens of their communities. Much like police and fire protection, EMS is also considered a public safety need. Individuals will always become sick or injured and will often require the services of EMS. Every geographical sector of the United States has some level of EMS provision.[11] Fortunately for U.S. citizens, most of those areas have a rapid response from EMS agencies—often within 8 minutes from the time of the call for help.

EMS delivery systems may vary in structure, design, and operation, but all have a shared purpose of providing the most expedient emergency medical care to the community. For these reasons, career opportunities will always exist for EMS providers. The question that remains is, "To what extent will EMS providers become part of a larger health-care delivery system?" The extent to which mobile integrated health-care delivery expands the traditional role of EMS will determine what additional future career opportunities will exist.

Current Trends

With the evolution of EMS and the recent adoption of the **Personal Protection and Affordable Care Act** of 2010 (also known as the Affordable Care Act or "ObamaCare"), a pivotal change is occurring in the role of EMS within the context of total health care in the United States.[22,23]

There is a widespread effort among EMS leadership and policymakers to utilize EMTs and paramedics in new and exciting ways. EMTs and paramedics will always be the

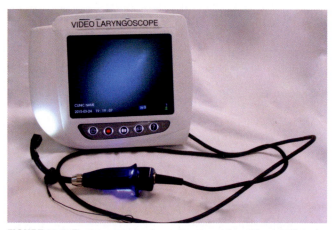

FIGURE 16-8 The laryngoscope is used to place a breathing tube into the trachea of the patient. In patients that present difficulties, the video-guided laryngoscope aids in the insertion with fiber-optic views of the trachea during insertion.

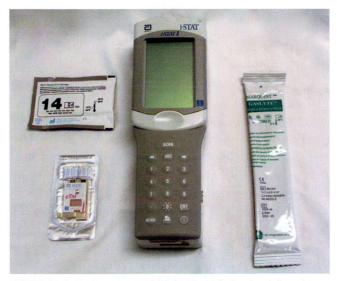

FIGURE 16-9 The i-stat is a portable handheld device that delivers immediate laboratory test results, including blood gases, glucose, hematology, coagulation, and many other tests.

principal providers of emergency care outside of the hospital, but another role is rapidly emerging. This new role involves providing early primary and preventive care to individuals while in their homes. Enhancing access to health care by having EMS providers visit individuals who are homebound or who were recently discharged from the hospital is one of the major goals of this new initiative. In this role, EMS providers will not only provide care, but will also enable referrals to other health-care professionals, navigate available resources to meet the needs of patients, and facilitate the integration of all health-care services. It is projected that this integration into a patient-centered, multidisciplinary approach will enhance access, improve the quality of care, and reduce overall health-care costs substantially. The national agency that oversees health care in the United States and is facilitating this integration is the **Department of Health and Human Services (HHS).**

This new role has been called *community paramedicine*, but a newer and more descriptive term, *mobile integrated health care*, is rapidly gaining preference. The reason for the newer term is that it is more representative of what this new role does. The paramedics and EMTs are already in the community and commonly travel from home to home, thus they are mobile. Furthermore, they facilitate the integration of health care from many different professionals on behalf of the patient. This role serves as a facilitator of rapid access to appropriate health care.

Trends in the delivery of emergency care capitalize on advances in knowledge through evidence-based practice (where interventions are justified through research and evidence of improved outcomes) and technology. In some EMS systems, paramedics are taking advantage of improved portability of devices such as handheld ultrasonography to gather additional clinical information from the patient and video-guided **laryngoscopy** to facilitate the placement of a breathing tube into the lungs. Current trends in paramedicine are largely influenced by policymakers and evolving events in the economy, general health care, and emerging political agendas. It is a dynamic process that changes with public need.

Role of EMTs and Paramedics

Most EMTs receive their training through community colleges or universities, trade schools, or fire departments. An EMT can function independently as an emergency medical care provider, as an employee of an ambulance service, or as a firefighter/EMT for a fire service that combines fire-fighting with initial EMS response. In these roles, the EMT provides emergency care for the acutely sick or injured in the community, at accident scenes, or in industry.

An increasing number of paramedic education programs are taking place in universities across the United States. This educational platform will enable a greater foundation of knowledge for practicing paramedics in the near future. Paramedics that graduate from these university-based programs will have earned a bachelor's degree, which will advance their careers into areas of more advanced clinical practices, management, and administrative roles within EMS.

 Aptitude Profile

Someone choosing a profession within emergency medical services must have a passion for helping others, have the ability to think independently and critically, and have the ability to perform under pressure in urgent situations. This person must also be willing to sacrifice opportunities to sleep, eat, or socialize while on duty. As the EMS professions continue to grow and develop, the demands on cognitive abilities, psychomotor skills (ability to use one's hands to perform interventions), and affective control (ability to manage one's own fears, anxiety, and other emotions and behaviors) also increase with this development.

Even though many who enter the field of EMS adapt to its emotional challenges early in their career, a significant percentage of individuals suffer from "burnout" or a lessening ability to manage their on-the-job responsibilities. Burnout is common among EMTs and paramedics, and in some EMS systems there are strategies and supportive services in place to help EMS providers cope with the many emotional challenges of their profession.

Both EMTs and paramedics may work outside of traditional EMS delivery in emergency departments, critical-care units, urgent-care centers, insurance agencies for health assessments, and many other allied health roles. As the concept of mobile integrated health-care delivery emerges, there will likely be increasing roles for the EMT and paramedic in the future.

Role of Bachelor's Degree–Prepared Paramedics

Paramedics from degree-awarding institutions will be able to perform in all of the roles that a nondegree paramedic can hold, but there are some opportunities for bachelor's degree–prepared paramedics that require this level of credential. As an example, directors of programs that deliver paramedic education must currently possess a bachelor's degree at a minimum. More and more specialized or high-level positions in EMS (administration, directorship, education, etc.) are requiring bachelor's degrees or higher for employment. In time, it is likely that a bachelor's degree will become the standard minimum requirement for all paramedics.

Required Continuing Education

All certified paramedics and some EMTs are required to participate in **continuing medical education (CME)** on an annual basis.[17] This standard exists to ensure that all EMS providers maintain their proficiencies in the skills they perform and the knowledge they possess, as well as to provide opportunities to learn new information.

CME typically is of two forms: reeducation and continuing (or new) education. The reeducation component focuses on relearning skills and concepts that are prone to deterioration or imprecision over time. Skills such as endotracheal intubation or the placement of IV catheters into the subclavian vein are complex and require considerable practice to maintain proficiency. Reeducation helps to maintain a high level of proficiency.

Continuing education that introduces new content is important to enable the EMS provider to grow within the profession. New ideas, concepts, and knowledge are introduced into medicine daily. Much of that information has applicability to EMS. For example, if a new drug has been introduced that reduces the complications from a heart attack, it is important that paramedics learn the characteristics, side effects, dosage, and indications for that drug's use in the prehospital setting. Continuing medical education is an integral element in paramedical practice.

Working Together

EMTs and paramedics traditionally work closely with emergency department nurses and physicians. As the profession has grown, there has been an expansion of interaction with physician specialties such as cardiologists, trauma surgeons, and family practice physicians. In addition, EMS has greater interaction with dialysis units, primary-care clinics, geriatric centers, skilled nursing and extended-care facilities, pediatric centers, and mental health facilities. With the advent of mobile integrated health care, there is an even greater extension of EMS into preventive and public health, social services, pharmaceutical services, case management, outpatient support services, and community support agencies. As the duties of the EMS provider expand into a greater facilitative role on behalf of the patient, there are increasing opportunities to engage with multiple health-care disciplines.

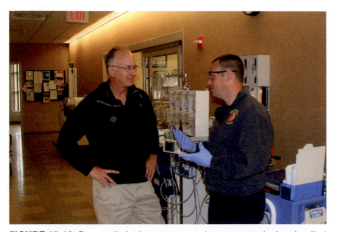

FIGURE 16-10 Paramedic in the emergency department relaying detailed patient information as needed.

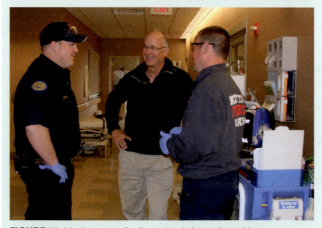

FIGURE 16-11 A paramedic discussing information with an emergency department physician.

CASE STUDY

Mr. Rockwell is a 70-year-old retired farmer who suddenly developed chest pain while cutting firewood. His wife, 68-year-old Joan, summons the ambulance by calling 911. Within 8 minutes the paramedics arrive to find Mr. Rockwell in severe distress due to chest pain and difficulty breathing. After a thorough history and physical examination, the paramedics obtain a 12-lead ECG that confirms their suspicion of a heart attack. They start an IV line and begin drug therapy to stabilize the heart and prevent further damage to the heart muscle. They transport him promptly to a hospital for cardiac catheterization and lifesaving clot-dissolving intervention. He recovers a week later with some resultant heart failure.

The paramedics return Mr. Rockwell from the hospital to his home 10 days after his heart attack. They arrange for the mobile integrated health-care paramedic to check on him the next day. After several days of home visits, the community paramedics determine that Mr. Rockwell is having some difficulty with fluid retention and recurrent heart failure. They start some specialized therapy at home and make arrangements for Mr. Rockwell to visit his cardiologist at his office. In addition, the community paramedics provide transportation to a cardiac rehabilitation center where Mr. Rockwell begins his recovery therapy. The community paramedics also collect a new prescription for him from the pharmacy and continue to visit with Mr. Rockwell three times a week to ensure his full recovery and to adjust his new medication regimen. Additional services through the local home health nursing agency have been established to supplement the community paramedicine visits. The two disciplines interact with each other to share information and provide updates on Mr. Rockwell's condition.

Through this integration of emergency services with cardiology, pharmacy services, home health care, in-home monitoring, and cardiac rehabilitation, Mr. Rockwell is assured of his best chances for a full recovery.

Questions

1. How important is calling 911 to summon EMS for Mr. Rockwell?

2. How were the paramedics able to determine the nature of Mr. Rockwell's illness?

3. How was the integration of EMS and cardiovascular care important in saving Mr. Rockwell's life?

4. Once Mr. Rockwell was discharged from the hospital, what services was the EMS system able to provide him through integrated health-care delivery?

5. What would have been Mr. Rockwell's likely outcome following the complications that developed after coming home from the hospital had the community paramedics not been checking in on him?

Review Questions

1. What professions are the three main providers of prehospital emergency care in EMS?

   A. Paramedics, nurses, and physicians

   B. EMTs, paramedics, and nurses

   C. EMTs, AEMTs, and paramedics

   D. AEMTs, paramedics, and nurses

2. Which of the following providers of EMS delivers only basic life support?

   A. EMTs

   B. AEMTs

   C. Paramedics

   D. Nurses

3. What did Baron Dominique Jean Larrey, Napoleon's personal surgeon, introduce to medical care?

   A. The tourniquet

   B. Bandaging wounds

   C. IV lines

   D. Ambulances

4. What did the "White Paper" of 1966 establish?

   A. That survival of trauma victims was better in military theaters than it was on the streets of America

   B. That ambulances were not adequately equipped to treat all victims of car crashes

   C. That EMS should be under the federal direction of the Department of Health and Human Services

   D. That EMS should include not only basic life support, but also advanced life support

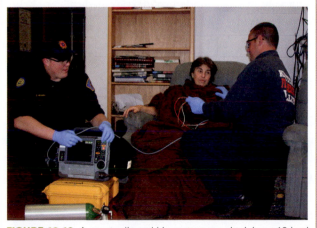

FIGURE 16-12 A paramedic and his partner are obtaining a 12-lead electrocardiogram (ECG) on a patient. An ECG detects the heart's activity.

5. What organization accredits paramedic educational programs in the United States?

   A. CoAEMSP through the CAAHEP

   B. NHTSA through the DOT

   C. NREMT

   D. PPACA

6. What does a cardioscope/defibrillator do?

   A. Enables the paramedic to view the vocal cords to insert a breathing tube

   B. Enables the paramedic to determine the concentration of carbon dioxide in the exhaled breath of a patient

   C. Enables the paramedic to view the electrical activity of the heart and deliver electrical therapy if necessary

   D. Enables the paramedic to determine how much hemoglobin is saturated with the oxygen molecule

7. Which of the following interventions would be considered to be an advanced life support procedure?

   A. Cardiopulmonary resuscitation

   B. Starting an IV line

   C. Administering oxygen

   D. Assisting the patient with prescribed medications

8. Approximately how many colleges or universities currently award bachelor's degrees for EMS in the United States?

   A. 5

   B. 30

   C. 50

   D. More than 100

9. In 2014, what was the reported average salary of a paramedic in the United States?

   A. About $37,000

   B. About $41,000

   C. About $60,000

   D. About $90,000

10. What societal benefits are mobile integrated health-care (community) paramedics expected to provide in the near future?

    A. The replacement of home care by nurses

    B. Reducing the need to visit the family physician

    C. Improvement in the scope of care that patients can receive in clinics, hospitals, and doctors' offices

    D. Improved access to care, enhanced quality of care, and a reduction of overall health-care costs

Glossary of Key Terms

Paramedic—the standard advanced life support provider for EMS

Electrocardiogram (ECG)—a mechanical tracing onto heat-sensitive paper that represents the electrical activity in the heart

Emergency medical services (EMS)—the profession of EMTs, Advanced EMTs, and paramedics that provide emergency care to individuals in the prehospital setting

Emergency medical technicians (EMTs)—providers of emergency care at the basic life support level

Advanced EMTs (AEMTs)—level of EMS providers who administer basic life support care and some limited advanced life support interventions

Endotracheal intubation—the process of placing a breathing tube into the trachea of a patient; performed by paramedics, emergency medicine physicians, nurse anesthetists, and anesthesiologists

Protocols—written directives for paramedics and EMTs that prescribe what actions should be taken in the care of patients given a specific set of circumstances

Standing orders—protocols that enable the paramedic to initiate treatment for patients in dire emergencies without consulting with physicians beforehand

Community paramedicine—a new role for paramedics that enables them to facilitate preventive, primary, and follow-up care of patients

Mobile integrated health care (MIH)—a new role for paramedics and EMTs that enables the delivery of preventive, primary, and follow-up care to patients in an integrated manner with other health-care entities and professions

Ambulance volantes—literally means "flying ambulances"; a concept of Napoleon's personal physician, employed during war to bring wounded soldiers to medical care behind the battle lines

National Highway Transportation Safety Administration (NHTSA)—the federal agency that oversees and directs EMS across the nation; an agency under the Department of Transportation

Cardiopulmonary resuscitation (CPR)—the manual application of artificial function of the heart and lungs in an effort to revive a victim

Ambulance technicians—a previous level of EMS provider training (typically 27 hours in duration) that included only essential procedures of emergency care

Medical first responders—the most basic level of emergency care provider recognized in EMS; typically associated with public safety providers

National Registry of EMTs (NREMT)—an organization that delivers skill and knowledge assessment for EMTs, AEMTs, and paramedics and provides a nationally recognized certification

Committee on Accreditation of Educational Programs for EMS Professions (CoAEMSP)—the accreditation organization for all paramedic education programs nationwide under the auspices of CAAHEP

Commission on Accreditation of Allied Health Education Programs (CAAHEP)—the accreditation organization for most allied health profession education programs nationwide; provides the accreditation to EMS education through CoAEMSP

Cardioscope/defibrillator—a medical device that is used to monitor the electrical activity of the heart and to deliver electrical energy to reset the heart rhythm

Pulse oximeter—a medical device that indirectly measures the amount of hemoglobin in the blood that is saturated with oxygen molecules; an assistive means of determining how well a person is oxygenating his or her blood

Capnography—a diagnostic medical device that measures the amount of carbon dioxide in the exhaled breath

National EMS Education Standards—the detailed description of the minimum educational objectives for each level of EMS provider

Personal Protection and Affordable Care Act—a law enacted in 2010 that promotes innovative methods of improving access to health care, improved quality of care, and an overall reduction of health-care costs, among many other provisions

Department of Health and Human Services (HHS)—the federal department that oversees the administration of health care throughout the United States

Laryngoscopy—the process of visualizing the vocal cords to place a breathing tube into the trachea of a patient

Continuing medical education (CME)—education for health-care providers that promotes ongoing knowledge and skill development throughout their professional careers

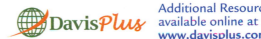

Additional Resources are available online at www.davisplus.com

Additional Resources

Accrediting Bodies

Committee on Accreditation of Educational Programs for EMS Professions (CoAEMSP)—www.coaemsp.org

CoAEMSP is the principal accrediting organization for educational programs of the EMS professions.

Commission on Accreditation of Allied Health Education Programs (CAAHEP)—www.caahep.org

CAAHEP is the principal accrediting organization for all allied health education programs. It is the main EMS accrediting institution in concert with CoAEMSP

Federal Oversight Agencies

U.S. Department of Health and Human Services (HHS)—www.hhs.gov

The U.S. Department of Health and Human Services is the government's principal agency for protecting the health of all Americans and providing essential human services, especially for those who are least able to help themselves. It is responsible for almost a quarter of all federal outlays and administers more grant dollars than all other federal agencies combined.

National Highway Transportation Safety Administration (NHTSA)—www.nhtsa.gov

NHTSA was established by the Highway Safety Act of 1970 and is dedicated to achieving the highest standards of excellence in motor vehicle and highway safety. It works daily to help prevent crashes and their attendant costs, both human and financial.

National EMS Education Standards—www.ems.gov

These standards represent the minimum expected educational objectives for all EMS professions in the United States. The educational standards and other EMS-related information can be found on the national EMS website.

EMS Organizations

National Association of EMTs (NAEMT)—www.naemt.org

Formed in 1975, NAEMT is the principal national EMS organization that represents the professional interests of EMS practitioners, with a membership of more than 50,000.

National Registry of EMTs (NREMT)—www.nremt.org
The NREMT serves as the national EMS certification organization by providing a valid, uniform process to assess the knowledge and skills required for competent practice by EMS professionals throughout their careers, and by maintaining a registry of certification status.

Mobile Integrated Health Care and Community Paramedicine—www.communityparamedic.org
The Community Paramedic of the North Central EMS Institute of Minnesota is one of the first organizations to introduce, promote, and support the growing concept of community paramedicine.

***Mobile Integrated Healthcare: Approach to Implementation,* Matt Zavadsky and Douglas Hooten (MedStar Mobile Healthcare)**
Mobile Integrated Healthcare: Approach to Implementation is the first all-inclusive textbook that describes, guides, and promotes the development of a community-based mobile integrated health-care delivery system.

References

1. National Highway Traffic Safety Administration, EMS Office. *National EMS Education Standards.*
    http://www.ems.gov/pdf/811077a.pdf.
    Accessed October 17, 2014.

2. Commission on Accreditation of Allied Health Education Programs.
    http://www.caahep.org/Content.aspx?ID=39.
    Accessed October 18, 2014.

3. National EMS Assessment, National Highway Traffic Safety Administration, in conjunction with the Federal Interagency Committee on EMS.
    http://www.ems.gov/pdf/2011/national_ems_assessment_final_draft_12202011.pdf.
    Accessed October 18, 2014.

4. National Association of EMTs. What is mobile integrated healthcare and community paramedicine?
    http://www.naemt.org/MIH-CP/WhatisMIH-CP.aspx.
    Accessed October 24, 2014.

5. Consortium of Academic Programs in EMS.
    http://www.capems.org/.
    Accessed October 24, 2014.

6. Skankdalakis PN, Lainas P, Zoras O, Skandalakis JE, Mirilas P. To afford wounded speedy assistance: Dominique Jean Larrey and Napoleon. *World J Surg.* 2006;30(8):1392–1399.
    http://www.ncbi.nlm.nih.gov/pubmed/16850154.
    Accessed October 31, 2014.

7. History of trauma: Dominique-Jean Larrey.
    http://www.trauma.org/archive/history/larrey.html.
    Accessed October 31, 2014.

8. Edgerly D. Birth of EMS: The history of the paramedic. *JEMS.* 2013; October.
    http://www.jems.com/article/administration-and-leadership/birth-ems-history-paramedic.
    Accessed October 31, 2014.

9. National Academies Press. *Accidental Death and Disability: The Neglected Disease of Modern Society.* September 1966.
    http://www.nap.edu/openbook.php?record_id=9978.
    Accessed October 31, 2014.

10. Haller JS. The beginnings of urban ambulance service in the United States and England. *J Emerg Med.* 1990;8(6):743–755.
    http://www.jem-journal.com/article/0736-4679%2890%2990289-8/pdf.
    Accessed October 31, 2014.

11. Delbridge TR, Bailey B, Chew JL Jr, et al. EMS agenda for the future: Where we are . . . where we want to be. *Ann Emerg Med.* 1998;31(2):251–263.
    http://www.sciencedirect.com/science/article/pii/S0196064498703166.
    Accessed November 1, 2014.

12. Monosky KA. Perceived effectiveness and utility of various EMS credentials. *ProQuest.* Dissertation. The George Washington University; 2010.
    http://gradworks.umi.com/34/11/3411938.html.
    Accessed November 2, 2014.

13. National Association of EMTs. About EMS.
    http://www.naemt.org/about_ems/about_ems_home.aspx.
    Accessed November 2, 2014.

14. Committee on Accreditation of Educational Programs for the EMS Professions.
    http://www.coaemsp.org/.
    Accessed November 6, 2014.

15. National Highway Traffic Safety Administration. *The National EMS Education Standards: Emergency Medical Technician Instructional Guidelines.*

    http://www.ems.gov/pdf/811077c.pdf.

    Accessed November 9, 2014.

16. National Highway Traffic Safety Administration. *National EMS Education Standards: Paramedic Instructional Guidelines.*

    http://www.ems.gov/pdf/811077e.pdf.

    Accessed November 9, 2014.

17. National Registry of EMTs.

    https://www.nremt.org/.

    Accessed November 8, 2014.

18. Greene M. JEMS 2012 salary and workplace survey. *JEMS.* 2012;October.

    http://www.jems.com/articles/print/volume-37/issue-10/administration-and-leadership/jems-2012-salary-workplace-survey.html.

    Accessed November 20, 2014.

19. Greene M. JEMS 2013 salary and workplace survey. *JEMS.* 2013;October.

    http://www.jems.com/article/surveys/2013-jems-salary-workplace-survey.

    Accessed November 21, 2014.

20. Greene M. JEMS 2014 salary and workplace survey. *JEMS.* 2014;October.

    http://www.jems.com/article/surveys/2014-jems-salary-workplace-survey.

    Accessed November 21, 2014.

21. Bureau of Labor Statistics, U.S. Department of Labor. Occupational outlook handbook 2012–2013 edition, EMTs and paramedics.

    http://www.bls.gov/ooh/healthcare/emts-and-paramedics.htm.

    Accessed November 22, 2014.

22. U.S. House of Representatives, U.S. Congress, Office of the Legislative Council. Compilation of the Personal Protection and Affordable Care Act, May 2010.

    http://housedocs.house.gov/energycommerce/ppacacon.pdf.

    Accessed December 5, 2014.

23. Rosenbaum S. The Patient Protection and Affordable Care Act: Implications for public health policy and practice. *Public Health Rep.* 2011;126:Jan–Feb.

    http://www.ncbi.nlm.nih.gov/pmc/articles/PMC3001814/pdf/phr126000130a.pdf.

    Accessed December 6, 2014.

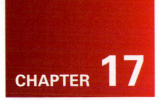

CHAPTER 17

Health Information Management

Patricia Royal, EdD

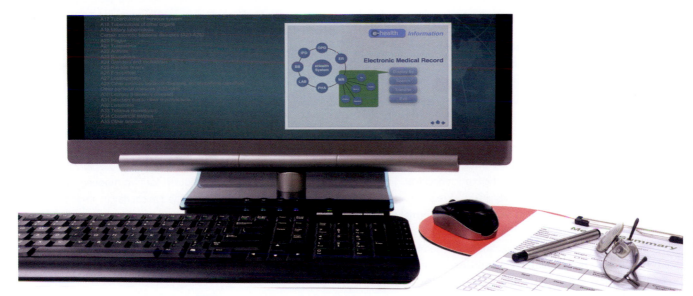

Photo credit: istock/Thinkstock

Learning Objectives

After reading this chapter, students should be able to:

- Discuss the role of a health information manager
- Discuss the various employment opportunities for health information managers
- Explain the educational requirements/levels as appropriate for working in a variety of roles
- Understand the historical perspective related to the origin of health information managers
- Recognize the personal characteristics deemed appropriate for working as a health information manager
- Discuss the difference between program accreditation and program certification
- Describe the relationship between health information managers and other members of the health-care team
- Discuss opportunities and challenges for working in the field of health information management

Key Terms

- Electronic health records
- Accrediting
- Health information management
- American Health Information Management Association (AHIMA)
- Health Insurance Portability and Accountability Act (HIPAA)
- Certification
- Commission on Accreditation for Health Information and Informatics Management Education (CAHIIM)
- Health information technician

"A Day in the Life"

Hello, my name is Justine and I am a health information manager for a public hospital in a large city. This is my first experience in a managerial position and since I have only been in this role for 1 year I still have a lot to learn. My responsibilities are many and I must always be cognizant of the happenings in my department, as well as the overall fundamental operations within the hospital environment. Although the job is rewarding and often exciting, I usually work long hours and am always called for emergency issues. Before I even reached my desk this morning, I received a phone call from the hospital administrator. When I receive phone calls before I get to work, I know there must be an urgent situation. I was informed that a breach of confidentiality regarding a patient's medical records occurred and my department is responsible for assisting with the investigation. It's true that my department is responsible for electronic medical records, but other departments often play roles in the breach, so I have to dig through the evidence to see where the breach occurred. I must also notify the patient due to liability issues. I really do not like having to tell patients that their personal health information has been divulged, but as manager this task rests on my shoulders. In addition to this crisis, we have recently switched from partial to complete **electronic health records (EHRs)** and have run into

some glitches with the transition. While in the process, we are creating a system for patients to log in to a secure site and review their own tests results; therefore, the breach has to be addressed immediately before we go live with this new system.

As I am in the middle of trying to resolve the confidentiality breach, I am made aware of another issue that is under my direct supervision. Our risk manager has been out sick for a couple of days and I was just now informed that he is in the hospital with a serious infection and expected to be out of work for at least another week. His absence presents a problem because he is responsible for identifying the potential risk associated with any type of confidentiality breach. I am not sure if there is anyone here who can assist with this concern. I am beginning to wonder what more can happen when I find out that our **accrediting** body representative just walked through the front doors. This cannot be happening today! It is already past lunch, which I didn't eat yet, and I am scheduled for two meeting this afternoon and now—this happens. The typical day in a health information manager's life is exciting and busy; however, today is a little busier than usual, but I have it all under control. The positive about this job and most jobs in health care is that there is always something going on—never a dull moment.

Introduction to Health Information Management

Description

Health information managers are professionals who work in a variety of health-care settings. The professional title is based on the **health information management** (HIM) definition, which refers to the management of health-care information such as patient demographics, diagnostics, results, provider notes, and insurance and reimbursement information. This management includes acquiring, analyzing, and protecting electronic and traditional medical information, which is essential for quality care. This information includes data such as patient visits, health status, medical history, diagnoses and treatment plans, symptoms, and laboratory or other test results. For payment to occur to the provider, all of these data must be captured, analyzed, and then billed to the appropriate source. The health information manager helps bridge the gaps between the clinicians, administrators, and technologists.[1] There are many settings and a variety of roles for individuals interested in health information management.

History

The original title for HIM was *medical records,* a term still used today by many individuals; however, as a career, HIM

is rather young in comparison to other health-care disciplines. HIM standards date back to the introduction of the **American Health Information Management Association (AHIMA),** formerly known as the Association of Record Librarians, in 1928.[2,3] Although some form of medical records was used before 1928, the professional association of AHIMA was established when the American College of Surgeons (ACOS) wanted to increase and improve the standards of medical records created in the clinical setting, which included the diagnosis and treatment of patients. These records were written on paper, which helped to establish the name "record librarians." These records detailed information about the patient's demographics (name, address, etc.), symptoms, any complications of previous treatments, diagnosis, and outcomes. Having the ability to refer back to the last visit and access this information helped the physician to better treat the patient. In recognition of the need for training, the first baccalaureate degree program in medical record science was started in1934.[2,3] These records were kept in paper format until the 1960s and 1970s when some universities began to merge computer technology and medical records. The expense of computers, the challenges of various users, and lack of consistency halted the process for some facilities. However, as overall interest in computers boomed and the application in health care began to take hold, individual departments in larger facilities, such as patient registration, forged ahead with computerized processing of patient information.[2]

In the 1980s, computer software packages (programs that enable computers to perform certain tasks) became more plentiful, and more departments in health-care facilities began using computerized medical records. During this time patients were also realizing some benefits of computerized medical records (e.g., the ease of computerized check-in). However, the benefit of the master patient index, which includes all patient names and information, was enjoyed mostly by the medical record department personnel because not all departments had this type of access.[2]

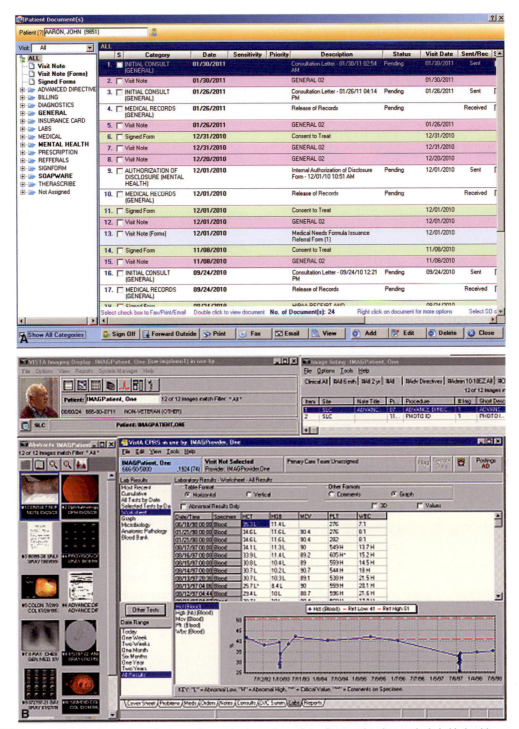

FIGURE 17-1 (A) This mental health electronic medical records sample shows the variety of categories that are included in health-care visits. Patients are often able to access some of this information via an online portal. **(B)** Electronic health records are popular today. There are many advantages for facilities to change from paper to electronic records. One primary reason is security. In this electronic health record the patient's photo is included, which enhances security. (Courtesy of the United States Department of Veterans Affairs)

The 1990s were an important time for the profession of health information management. Advancements made in software and computer applications provided hospital ancillary departments, such as laboratory and radiology, a means to enter patient data and view it on various computers; however, the connection between the computers was the key issue. Only employees within these departments were able to view the results. In other words, the information was restricted to the original department. While other businesses and industries seemed to be thriving with advancements and were able to achieve novel results in this area of computerization, the medical field lagged behind due to factors such as the need for confidentiality and patient-protected rights.[2]

By the millennial period, electronic health records (EHRs) were touted as the method for reducing patient deaths and injuries caused by health-care providers. In his state-of-the-union address, President George W. Bush advocated for the implementation of EHRs to avoid medical errors, reduce costs, and improve care.[2] The popularity of EHRs has continued to flourish, especially at the federal level. In 2009, the American Recovery and Reinvestment Act (ARRA) was introduced to create a stimulus in a lagging economy. Part of the incentive focused on supporting health-care providers in the selection and implementation of EHRs with the establishment of regional extension centers (RECs). These organizations received federal funding under the Health Information Technology for Economic and Clinical Health (HITECH) Act to support 100,000 primary-care providers with a particular emphasis on those treating the uninsured, underinsured, and medically underserved populations. The funding has allowed the RECs to provide training and support, information and guidance, and technical assistance in the adoption of EHRs for many health-care facilities that would otherwise be unaffordable.[2]

Job Environment

The number of jobs held in health services management in 2012 was approximately 315,500, with the majority (60%) located in hospitals and integrated delivery systems[3] (networks of health-care organizations under one parent company). Other employment opportunities for HIM personnel include ambulatory health-care services, health departments, nursing and residential care facilities, physicians' offices, laboratories, outpatient facilities, cancer registries, correctional facilities, medical software companies, pharmaceutical companies, health insurance providers, medical record-keeping facilities, and federal, state, and local agencies.[4] A small percentage of health services managers work in higher education systems as teachers. There are many options for someone interested in becoming a health services manager, and jobs are typically abundant with continued growth expectations (see later in the chapter).

Scope of Practice

The scope of practice of health information managers relates directly to the education level, employment location, and individual state requirements. Federal guidelines may also restrict the activities associated with health information managers. Often, health-care facilities require clinical managers to supervise clinical departments. The scope of practice for clinical health information managers will also vary. However, the following scopes of practice or job-related activities provide a general overview associated with health information managers.[5,6]

- Review medical documentation and assign medical codes
- Complete chart audits and complete reports
- Implement and maintain EHRs
- Provide expert knowledge within health law areas of the **Health Insurance Portability and Accountability Act (HIPAA)**
- Manage projects, staff, and patient records
- Investigate patient records to determine admission criteria
- Maintain databases with provider information
- Accountable for patient admission and insurance verification
- Maintain budgets and responsibility for operations of hospital/medical departments

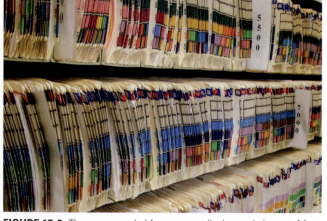

Photo credit: inkaone/istock/Thinkstock

FIGURE 17-2 The space needed for paper medical records is vast. Many facilities still use this type of filing system, but most have replaced this system for EHRs.

- Evaluate requests for release of information
- Develop policies and procedures for medical releases
- Transcribe medical reports
- Collect and evaluate data regarding workers' compensation
- Responsible for strategic planning
- Analyze data for research purposes

Required Education

The majority of health-care organizations require health information managers to have at least a bachelor's degree in HIM or administration. Other organizations, depending on the type, may require an advanced degree in health information or health-care informatics. For individuals interested in academics, a doctorate degree in health information management or informatics may be required for teaching purposes. The required education of individuals working in health services management is often reflective of the standards set forth by the accreditation or licensure agency.

Before acceptance into an HIM program, prerequisites such as medical terminology, anatomy and physiology, math, statistics, information systems, and health professional roles may be required in addition to the general education courses. After acceptance into the program, courses such as research, professional writing, coding, practice management, quality management, legal environment, human resources, leadership, data management, personnel management, health-care delivery systems, and finance are typical courses that will be required before graduating with a bachelor's degree. Advanced degrees require some of the same courses, such as finance, management, legal, research, and statistics, but require a deeper level in addition to courses focusing on current health-care laws and global initiatives.[7]

Accreditation and Certification

Accreditation and **certification** can be achieved at different levels. The entire university can be accredited by a national and regional accreditation council. One example of national accreditation is the Council for Higher Education Accreditation, which is the largest organization in the United States and accredits approximately 3,000 universities and colleges.[4] Regional accreditations are broken down by geographical areas across the United States. There are six different regional accreditations[8]:

- Middle States Association of Colleges and Schools
- New England Association of Schools and Colleges
- North Central Association of Colleges and Schools
- Northwest Commission on Colleges and Universities
- Southern Association of Colleges and Schools
- Western Association of Schools and Colleges

Individual programs within each school or college may have additional accreditations based on the type of program and applicable accreditation associations. The bachelor's and master's degree in HIM might be accredited by the **Commission on Accreditation for Health Information and Informatics Management Education** (CAHIIM), which sets forth standards that must be met by the program.[9]

Certifications work much the same way accreditation associations work in that they ensure the certified programs have met the approved standards set by the certification board. Like accreditations, certification processes include a defined external peer review process that ensures the programs have met all criteria needed to be deemed "certified." Students graduating from certified programs are eligible to take a state board examination that signifies competencies have been met. A common certification for HIM programs across the United States is the American Health Information Management Association (AHIMA).[6,9]

Salary

Like many occupations, the average salary for health services managers varies from state to state, between health-care organizations, and with educational levels. Some individuals work as midlevel managers whereas others are administrators or specialize in other areas; therefore, the salary ranges vary greatly. In 2012, salary ranges for individuals possessing a health information technician degree ranged from $22,250 to $56,200 with the median wage set at $34,160. Individuals holding a health information manager degree can expect a salary range from $32,000 to $84,000 depending on registration and certification.[10]

Trends

An aging population and longevity have helped create a positive outlook for health information managers. Additionally,

What Is Informatics?

The term *informatics* refers to information processing; however, there are many types of informatics. Health informatics combines information science, computer technology, and health care to create tools and resources that ensure delivery, planning, and management of health care. One such tool is electronic health records (EHRs).

Tips and Tools

To better understand the current and emerging trends and education needed for each, visit the following website: http://www.hicareers.com/CareerMap/.

Author Spotlight

Patricia Royal, EdD

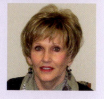

If you love health care and technology, you will love working in health information management. This field is exciting and always changing because you are dealing with technology. Working in health information management assures you many opportunities for continuing education because of the advancements in technology. There are many concentration areas that you can work in depending on your preferences. Having so many opportunities for work is one of the reasons I like this career.

Aptitude Profile

When deciding on a career, one should consider the specific knowledge and skill set needed for that job. Many health-care careers have some of the same characteristics, but certain skills may be more specific to management than direct practice care. Below is a list of characteristics one should probably have before deciding on a career as a health information manager. This list is not exhaustive but provides a general overview of some of the knowledge or skills needed when working in HIM[5,10]:

- Ability to motivate others
- Active listener
- Adaptability/flexibility
- Analytical skills
- Critical thinking ability
- Data analysis skills
- Delegation skills
- Detailed oriented
- Emotional maturity and intelligence
- Good communication skills
- Good judgment and decision-making skills
- Good interpersonal skills
- Good organization skills
- Inductive and deductive reasoning skills
- Mathematical skills
- Time management skills

the technological advances in health care have created more patient data, which results in more privacy and confidentiality issues. The transition from paper medical health records to EHRs will continue to drive the job market for those working in HIM. The job outlook for this occupation is projected to grow 21% between now and 2020. Some areas will grow faster than others, but the overall projection indicates faster than average growth.[10]

Challenges

Working in the field of health information management can offer many rewards and opportunities, but like many careers in health care, one of the biggest challenges is the changes in the health-care environment. Although the changes may be exciting for most individuals, being knowledgeable and up to date on medical practice management, software programs, and medical coding requires frequent training or educational workshops. These educational endeavors take individuals away from their daily activities, which often creates the need for overtime to complete job requirements. Health information managers must also stay abreast of changes in reimbursement schedules for payers such as Medicare, Medicaid, and private insurance. Changes in compensation require diligence in staying up to date to prevent potential loss of income due to errors or denied claims. Patient privacy and confidentiality concerns require much attention for health information managers. Those working in these areas are often

expected to train and update others for the protection and liability of the facility. Recruiting, hiring, and retaining qualified individuals may be a challenge because some of the roles in HIM require advanced education or registration (e.g., medical coders). The aging population creates other challenges for health information managers, such as increased demand in services without sufficient resources to handle the demand. As more patients are treated, more patient data are created that must be analyzed, stored, and protected, but also must be accessible to authorized personnel as needed. Although the challenges can be intimidating at times, working in HIM can be exciting and can provide individuals with a meaningful and rewarding career.

Role of the Associate Degree-Prepared Health Information Technician

Individuals who possess an associate degree are typically referred to as **health information technicians (HITs)** as opposed to health information managers. The difference in the designation is typically used to refer to educational status, not necessarily job roles or functions. There are some specializations for individuals with an HIT degree, such as medical coders and cancer registrars; however, these specialty areas require additional education such as certificates and/or registrations. One of the registrations that associate-prepared HITs can sit for is the registered health information technician (RHIT).[5] Some of the roles and responsibilities may overlap with individuals possessing a baccalaureate degree in HIM. Often the difference in roles may be due to the size of the organization or department, the level of the administration, the practice experience of the employee, any legal/licensing requirements, or the responsibilities assigned by the employing agency.

- Organize and maintain data
- Review patient records for accuracy, timeliness, and appropriateness of data
- Retrieve patient records
- Monitor patient results for quality assurance
- Assign classification codes for reimbursement and data analysis
- Protect patients' health information for confidentiality
- Ensure authorized access for appropriate personnel
- Analyze, evaluate, and compile patient information for research purposes

Role of the Baccalaureate-Prepared Health Information Manager

Individuals who possess a baccalaureate degree in HIM are eligible to sit for the national registry examination, the registered health information administrator (RHIA). On successful completion of the examination, students are credentialed as RHIAs and have many more options than those who receive the associate degree. Many hospital and medical facilities require personnel to be credentialed either before employment or soon afterward. Once credentialed, the individual may seek employment in a variety of settings and perform tasks related to education, business, administrative tasks, and legal tasks. The roles may vary depending on the size of the organization or department, the level of the administration, the practice experience of the employee, any legal/licensing requirements, or the responsibilities assigned by the employing agency. There may be some overlapping between roles for the associate- and baccalaureate-prepared degrees.[5]

- Supervise employees
- Manage day-to-day operations of a hospital department or physician office
- Work with consulting firms to provide expert knowledge in HIM

- Work with law firms to provide expertise in areas of health law and HIPAA
- Design software and provide training to end-user personnel
- Conduct quality care audits in compliance with an accrediting agency
- Maintain databases with physician information to provide physician accreditation
- Work in utilization review of patient records to determine admission criteria
- Review medical documentation and assign codes for billing purposes (Fig. 17-3)

Role of the Master's-Prepared Health Information Manager

As mentioned, some of the roles listed may overlap with those already presented. Individuals who have master's degrees usually are in upper-level management, and their scope of practice will typically increase with each level of management. These individuals are often the administrator of large departments, clinics, organizations, or hospitals. Often graduates may perform research to advance the body of knowledge and standards associated with HIM, particularly in the area of EHRs (AHIMA). There is some overlap between master's-prepared and doctoral-prepared individuals when addressing roles and responsibilities.[5,10]

- Identify potential areas of compliance vulnerability and risk
- Monitor and coordinate compliance activities of other departments
- Teach in academic environments
- Develop health information applications

Tonsillitis Example

► Acute tonsillitis expanded at the fourth character (to indicate organism) and fifth character (to indicate acute and recurrent) levels in ICD-10-CM

J03	Acute tonsillitis	
	J03.0	Streptococcal tonsillitis
		J03.00 Acute streptococcal tonsillitis, unspecified
		J03.01 Acute recurrent streptococcal tonsillitis

FIGURE 17-3 Example of ICD-10 coding.

What Is Credentialing?

Credentialing is a term used to describe the process of verifying information on medical staff and providers. The verified information can include education, training, residency, current license, certifications, and practice history. This information is used for evaluation and liability purposes to ensure quality patient care.

- Develop policies and procedures
- Establish strategic plans based on the organization's mission and vision
- Serve as a consultant for specialized practice management
- Analyze data
- Conduct research

Role of the Doctoral-Prepared Health Information Manager

Due to the limited number of doctoral programs in HIM, many individuals pursue a doctorate in other related areas such as informatics or health-care administration. Individuals obtaining a doctoral degree in health information management typically have a specific reason for the degree and

Working Together

Like most careers in health care, there is constant contact with other disciplines for those working as health information managers. Although not directly involved in patient care, health-care managers are in the midst of care provided by the medical facilities. Health-care managers may address quality issues and therefore must have constant contact with those who work in patient care, such as physicians, nurses, and other providers. Health-care managers are often responsible for credentialing of the direct patient care providers, which again aligns them with the direct providers. Because health information managers often handle reimbursements from Medicare, Medicaid, and private insurance, they must verify the diagnosis and treatment for patients and know the allowable amount specified by these payers. Sometimes, the verification requires direct questions to and answers by the practicing providers. Health information managers may decide that research is their interest and join a research team in various disciplines, such as medicine, pharmacy, health science, and audiology. Compliance monitoring and chart auditing are both roles that place health information managers in the center of activity surrounding interprofessional care. The manager must meet and address any deficiencies with appropriate personnel to safeguard the agency's legal ramifications.

A few types of interprofessional interactions have been described. There are many more that incorporate both health information managers and other disciplines in an interprofessional approach to health care. Patient care does not begin and end with only one discipline. There are many others who may not be publicly seen but are just as important in the interprofessional approach.

are able to select from several concentrations to emphasize their unique area. Some reasons for seeking a doctoral degree in HIM include teaching in academic centers, consulting, conducting health-care research, or becoming a CEO/president of a large hospital, organization, or federal agency. Others may pursue the degree to enter into the political arena as special-interest lobbyists. Their roles will vary depending on their chosen path.

CASE STUDY

Sarah is a 29-year-old woman who is visiting her physician today to confirm her suspicions of pregnancy. Sarah and her husband have been trying to have a baby for some time and she is hopeful that her pregnancy will be confirmed today. The facility she visits is in the process of transitioning from paper to electronic health records so things seem a little chaotic, but Sarah's excitement about her pregnancy takes center stage. At the check-in window, Sarah provides her information, including her name and birth date, and also provides an insurance card. She sits down and waits to be called. While waiting, she thinks she hears another patient come to the window who shares the same name as Sarah, but she dismisses the thought because she is so preoccupied. When the nurse steps out to call the patient in, she calls Sarah's name, and another woman stands up as well. They both stare at each other, and then the other woman, who appears to be about 10 years older, sits down while Sarah heads to the examination room. After visiting with her physician, Sarah's pregnancy is confirmed by a urine test. The physician also orders a complete blood panel to be done and provides information to Sarah about prenatal care. The physician then asks her to step down the hall to the nutritionist's office to learn about the diet that should be followed during pregnancy. Additionally, the physician states that the nurse will bring in a prescription for prenatal vitamins. After Sarah visits the nutritionist, the nurse sees her and hands the prescription to her. Sarah then proceeds to the check-out window to pay her deductible and make her next appointment. As she arrives at the window, she notices that the same woman from the lobby is leaving the check-out window but does not dwell much on it because her mind is swirling with thoughts. The insurance clerk states that there is no co-pay and Sarah finds that strange because her insurance has always required a co-pay of $15. Sarah heads off to the pharmacy to pick up her vitamins. As she hands the prescription to the pharmacist, she notices that he looks a little puzzled. Sarah had not paid much attention to the prescription because she was not sure of the name of the medicine anyway. The pharmacist verifies the demographic information with Sarah and fills the prescription as directed. He confirms that she has never taken this medicine before. Sarah picks up the medicine and heads home after a visit to the grocery store for some healthy food as advised by the nutritionist. After dinner that night, Sarah picks up her medicine bottle to take her pill as indicated on the bottle. Just as she starts to open the bottle she receives a call from the clinic, and the person on the other end of the phone tells her to not take the medicine. The health information manager explains that there was a mix-up with patient charts. Both patients had the same names and the same birth date. The only difference was the year of birth. As it happened, the coder was assigning a code to Sarah's chart and the code indicated hormone replacement therapy, while the "other Sarah" was receiving prenatal vitamins. The coder realized that the other Sarah had previously had a hysterectomy so she could not possibly need prenatal vitamins. She then notified her supervisor, who immediately contacted the pharmacy to determine if the medicine had been picked up. The health information manager then examined the charts, reviewing the diagnosis, treatment, medicines, and billing; realized what had occurred; and placed the call to Sarah.

How could electronic medical records prevent the problem that occurred in this case?

Questions

1. If the health information manager had not realized the error, what do you think would have happened next? When might the error have been found?

2. What other way do you think this situation could have been handled to prevent the mistake?

3. What disciplines were involved in the plan of care for Sarah?

4. What other disciplines should be included in the plan of care but were not?

Review Questions

1. Before the 1960s and 1970s, all medical records were kept on:
   A. Paper
   B. Microfilm
   C. Electronically
   D. Compact disc

2. The acronym HIPAA stands for:
   A. Hospital Information and Patient Account Act
   B. Health Informatics Paper Accounting Agency
   C. Human Information and Protection Affordability Act
   D. Health Insurance Portability and Accountability Act

3. President _____ was the first presidential proponent for electronic health records.
   A. Carter
   B. Bush
   C. Obama
   D. Reagan

4. The occupational outlook projection for the health information management professions is that they are expected to grow at a/an _____ rate:
   A. Average
   B. Slightly below average
   C. Faster than average
   D. Stay the same

5. The career of health information management is _____ in comparison to other health professions.
   A. Young
   B. Old
   C. Nonexistent
   D. Just starting

6. The American Recovery and Reinvestment Act was established due to:
   A. A booming economy
   B. A stagnant economy
   C. A lagging economy
   D. A political agenda

7. Individuals who complete the required education in health information management can sit for the _____ examination.
   A. HIM
   B. RHIA
   C. HITT
   D. COTA

8. The standards for health information management began with the establishment of the American Health Information Management Association in:

   A. 1940

   B. 1925

   C. 1961

   D. 1928

9. The majority of health information managers work in _____.

   A. Hospitals and integrated delivery systems

   B. Long-term care facilities

   C. Ambulatory care centers

   D. University settings

10. _____ is the accrediting organization that enforces standards for health information management educational programs.

   A. AHIMA

   B. CAHIIM

   C. HIIM

   D. HIIT

Glossary of Key Terms

Electronic health records (EHRs)—computerized records of patient information and data such as medical history, symptoms, and test results

Accrediting—process whereby a program is peer reviewed by experts in that field who ensure that the appropriate standards have been met; in addition to the specific criteria by the accrediting organization, integrity and quality must be addressed

Health information management—study and practice of maintenance and care of health records involving aspects of security, privacy, and confidentiality

American Health Information Management Association (AHIMA)—professional membership association for health information management professionals

Health Insurance Portability and Accountability Act (HIPAA)—represents many aspects of health; some are related to health insurance, and others are related to patient privacy and confidentiality

Certification—process whereby peer reviewers confirm that the characteristics and qualities of a particular program have been met

Commission on Accreditation for Health Information and Informatics Management Education (CAHIIM)—accreditation organization for education programs in health information management

Health information technician (HIT)—practice of organizing and managing health information data

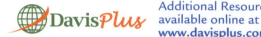

Additional Resources are available online at www.davisplus.com

Additional Resources

Occupational Outlook Handbook, Medical and Health Services Managers—www.bls.gov/ooh/management/medical-and-health-services-managers.htm

- The Bureau of Labor website provides information on labor market activity and working conditions for those seeking jobs in this occupation.

- Provides information on what health services managers do, work environment, how to become a health services manager, pay, and job outlook.

Managers Who Lead: A Handbook for Improving Health Services—https://www.msh.org/resources/managers-who-lead-a-handbook-for-improving-health-services

- Provides information to health managers on becoming a leader and empowering others to accept the challenges as well.

Journal of the American Health Information Management Association (AHIMA)—http://journal.ahima.org/

- The official publication of the American Health Information Management Association, delivering best practices in health information management and keeping readers current on emerging issues that affect the accuracy, timeliness, privacy, and security of patient health information.

Healthcare Information and Management Systems Society (HIMSS)—www.himss.org

- HIMSS is a not-for-profit organization focused on better health through information technology. HIMSS leads efforts to optimize health engagements and care outcomes using information technology.

- *Vision:* Better health through information technology.

- *Mission:* Globally, lead endeavors optimizing health engagements and care outcomes through information technology.

U.S. Department of Health and Human Services, Health Resources and Services Administration (HRSA)—www.hrsa.gov/index.html

- This website provides information about the roles this agency plays and the people affected by them.

- *Goals:* Goal I: Improve Access to Quality Care and Services. Goal II: Strengthen the Health Workforce. Goal

III: Build Healthy Communities. Goal IV: Improve Health Equity.

The Health Manager's Website—www.who.int/management/en

- Provided by World Health Organization (WHO).

- Directs and coordinates authority for health within the United Nations system.

- Some of the concepts, guidance, and tools available to help you make the best use of resources or solve problems include topics such as budgeting and monitoring expenditures; collecting and using information; maintaining equipment, vehicles, and buildings; and interacting with the community and other partners.

AHIMA's Engage Online Communities—http://engage.ahima.org/home

- The communities contain strategically aligned content and forums focused on areas of importance to HIM professionals.

- These areas include the following domains: Coding, Classification, and Reimbursement; Confidentiality, Privacy, and Security; Consumer Engagement and Personal Health Information; Health Informatics; Health Information Technologies and Processes; Health-Care Leadership and Innovation; and Information Governance and Standards.

References

1. Health Information Management, Kansas University Medical School, School of Health Professions.

   http://www.kumc.edu/school-of-health-professions/health-information-management/what-is-a-health-information-manager.html.
   Accessed May 5, 2014.

2. Van Fleet D. *Health Information Management (HIM) History: Past to Current Day.* Rasmussen College; December 12, 2010.

   http://www.rasmussen.edu/degrees/health-sciences/blog/health-information-management-history/.
   Accessed May 11, 2014.

3. Dixon-Lee, C. A health information profession with a long history. Chicago Hospital News. February 2010. http://www.chicagohospitalnews.com.
   Accessed May 10, 2014.

4. Georgia CTAE Resource Network. *Health Information Management—Student Information Guide.* Instructional Resources Office; 2010.

5. Summary Report for Medical Records and Health Information Technicians. O*Net Online.

   http://www.onetonline.org/link/summary/29-2071.00.
   Accessed May 5, 2014.

6. American Health Information Management Association (AHIMA).

   http://www.ahima.org/topics/psc?tabid=role.
   Accessed May 11, 2014.

7. Bureau of Labor Statistics, U.S. Department of Labor. *Occupational outlook handbook, 2014–2015 Edition, Medical Records and Health Information Technicians.*

   http://www.bls.gov/ooh/healthcare/medical-records-and-health-information-technicians.htm.
   Accessed May 5, 2014.

8. Database of Institutions and Programs Accredited by Recognized United States Accrediting Organizations. Council for Higher Education Accreditation.

   http://www.chea.org/search/default.asp.
   Accessed May 11, 2014.

9. Commission on Accreditation for Health Informatics and Information Management Education (CAHIIM). *Program Approval Manual.* 2006.

   http://bok.ahima.org/PdfView?oid=67035.
   Accessed May 5, 2014.

10. Health Information Manager. Explorehealthcareergs.org.

    http://www.explorehealthcareers.org/en/Career/33/Health_Information_Manager.
    Accessed May 5, 2014.

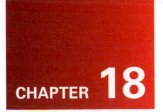

CHAPTER 18

Health Services Management

Patricia Royal, EdD

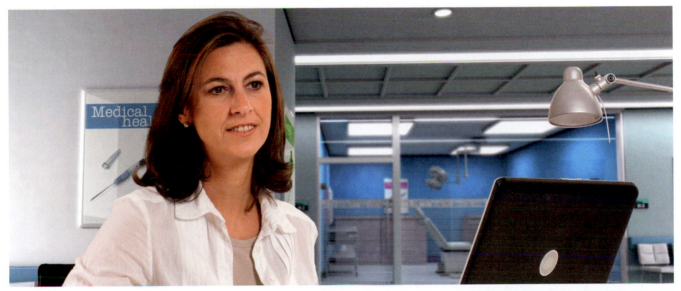

Photo credit: istock/Thinkstock

Learning Objectives

After reading this chapter, students should be able to:

- Describe the role of a health services manager
- Discuss the various employment opportunities for health services managers
- Describe the educational requirements/levels as appropriate for working in a variety of roles
- Discuss the historical perspective related to the origin of health-care managers
- Recognize the personal characteristics deemed appropriate for working as a health services manager
- Describe the difference between program accreditation and program certification
- Understand the relationship between health services managers and other members of the health-care team
- Discuss opportunities and challenges for working in the field of health-care management

Key Terms

- ICD-10 codes
- Health Insurance Portability and Accountability Act (HIPAA)
- Health services managers
- Health-care administrators
- Superintendents
- Internship
- Accreditation
- Certification

"A Day in the Life"

Hello, my name is Andy and I am the health services manager for a rural health clinic. I am responsible for several aspects of management of the entire clinic. My supervisor is the CEO of the clinic and handles management issues when I am unavailable. I received a telephone call on my way to work stating that one of our employees would miss work today. Unfortunately, this employee is a direct patient provider. This employee's supervisor, the medical director, is not in the clinic today; therefore I must find a replacement or patient visits will have to be canceled for the day. As I am entering the clinic, one of the family members of a long-time patient asks to see me regarding the attitude of our patient representative. I can tell by Mrs. Brown's face that she is extremely upset, so I ask her to step into my office and tell her I'll be with her in a moment. In

(continued)

the meantime, I ask one of our administrative assistants to provide me with a list of possible providers whom I can call regarding working today. One bit of good news is that the first patient was not scheduled until 9:00 a.m., so I do have some time (about an hour) to find another provider. While I'm waiting for the names and numbers of possible providers, I go to my office to see Mrs. Brown. She informs me that her mother was here for a scheduled visit at 8:00 a.m. and when the patient representative tried to check her in, she was told her appointment was for tomorrow. The family member stated that this was not a problem in itself, but the attitude the representative displayed was inappropriate. Mrs. Brown stated that her mother has dementia and may have confused the appointment, but the patient representative made a snide remark about her mother's memory and how she was always confusing her appointments. I promised Mrs. Brown I would handle this issue as soon as possible. I apologized for the behavior of our staff and assured her it would not happen again.

After Mrs. Brown left, I returned to the problem of finding a replacement provider, and after making several calls, I was able to locate someone. However, even at best, she cannot get to the clinic until after 10:00 a.m.; therefore, I need to talk with the patients out front to explain the long wait. As I head to get my daily cup of coffee, I'm stopped by one of our coders regarding the new **ICD-10 codes.** She stated that until she was trained in their use, the clinic would probably lose money because the insurance companies, Medicare, and Medicaid were all using the updated codes and it was necessary for us to file our patients' reimbursement forms using the new system. I asked if her supervisor had addressed this issue, but she stated that she had asked her supervisor about it months ago and nothing has been done. Therefore, the next item on the agenda is searching for upcoming training for the employee and a discussion with the supervisor, who should have handled this situation months ago. It is only 10:30 a.m. and it is turning out to be a busy day. I am already exhausted. I still have to complete an activity report that's due at 5:00 p.m., a telephone conference scheduled for noon, a budgeting meeting at 2:00 p.m. to discuss the upcoming insurance hikes for our employees, and an in-service at 3:30 p.m. regarding the new **Health Insurance Portability and Accountability Act (HIPAA)** and confidentiality forms that all of our patients must complete at their next visits. Luckily for me, I brought my lunch and dinner with me because it appears this will be a long day!

Introduction to Health Services Management

Description

Health services managers are professionals who work in a variety of health-care settings. Sometimes they are referred to as **health-care administrators,** health-care executives, or health-care managers. The title often changes depending on the individual's work environment. Health services managers are often viewed as working behind the scenes. Not typically in direct patient care, these managers provide an important function in health-care organizations. Health services managers run health-care facilities in whole or in part depending on experience, education, and the organization's size. They are responsible for the overall management functions of the facility.

History

The term *health services manager* did not come into existence until after hospitals and other medical facilities began to emerge nationwide and the need for management of them became apparent. The first groups of health-care managers were called **superintendents.** Individuals working in this role were typically nurses who were trained as clinicians but not administrators. Others who also assumed the superintendent role at times included physicians, laypersons, and Catholic sisters. These individuals received on-the-job training because no formal education for administrators was available. In 1900, Columbia Teachers College in New York became the first formal hospital administration educational program.[1] In the early 1920s, Marquette University in Wisconsin started the first hospital administration degree-granting program, but unfortunately the program had dissolved by 1928 due to lack of students.[1] In 1929, author Michael Davis strongly argued for a graduate program that would train students in hospital administration. His book, *Hospital Administration: A Career; The Need of Trained Executives for a Billion Dollar Business, and How They May Be Trained*, proposed a 2-year curriculum centered around core courses such as accounting and statistics in the first year followed by practical work (**internship**) in the second year. Within 3 years after the publication of Davis's book, the Committee on the Costs of Medical Care suggested that universities begin to incorporate a curriculum focusing on hospital administration. In 1933, the American College of Hospital Administrators was established by practicing administrators. This organization became the first professional association of hospital administrators; however, the name was later changed to American College of Healthcare Executives to include a wider range of health-care facilities.[1]

In 1934, the University of Chicago established the first graduate program for hospital administrators. Not surprisingly, Michael Davis was asked to head the program. The 1940s to 1960s became a time of growth for graduate programs in hospital administration. During this period, more than 32 programs were established across the United States. In 1958, the Sloan program at Cornell University established a program requiring 2 years of formal study, which is the dominant educational structure used today.[1]

Job Environment

The number of jobs in health services management in 2012 was approximately 315,500 with the majority of them in hospital settings[2] (Fig. 18-1). Other employment opportunities for health services managers include ambulatory health-care services, health departments, nursing and residential care facilities, physicians' offices, laboratories, outpatient facilities, pharmaceutical companies, health insurance providers, medical record-keeping facilities, and federal, state, and local agencies. Nonprofit organizations such as the Red Cross or Salvation Army, as well as medical

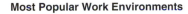

Most Popular Work Environments

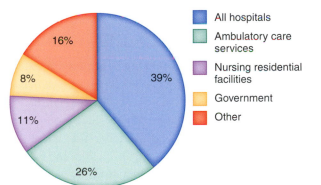

- All hospitals
- Ambulatory care services
- Nursing residential facilities
- Government
- Other

FIGURE 18-1 This chart shows the facilities that employed the majority of health services managers in 2012. (Source: Bureau of Labor Statistics, 2014.)

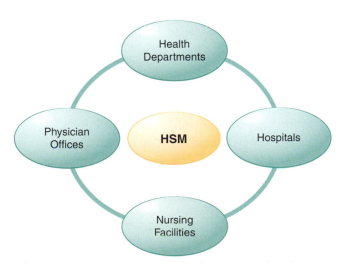

FIGURE 18-2 Health services managers have many options for career choices. The ones listed here are some popular choices.

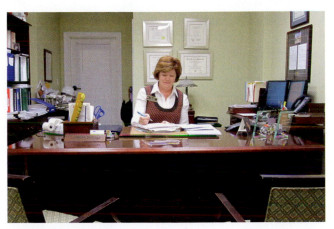

FIGURE 18-3 A popular role for individuals educated in health services management is working as the executive director for residential nursing facilities, as seen here.

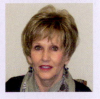

Author Spotlight

Patricia Royal, EdD

I have been teaching in health services management for 9 years and love it. I was lucky that my experience in health care and my education allowed me the opportunity to teach in health services management. One of the best things about teaching in this field is the variety of job choices that are available to our students. Sometimes, students start out in an entry-level position but advance quickly within the health-care organization. When I hear their stories about being promoted, it makes me enjoy my job even more. If you like health care, but not necessarily direct patient care, health services management may be a great choice for you!

supply agencies, also employ health services managers. A small percentage of health services managers work in higher education systems as teachers or within the school's health-care facility. There are many options for someone interested in becoming a health services manager, and jobs are typically abundant.

Scope of Practice

The scope of practice of health services managers relates directly to the education level, employment location, and individual state requirements. Federal guidelines may also restrict the activities associated with health services managers. Often, health-care facilities require clinical managers to supervise clinical departments. The scopes of practice for clinical health services managers will also vary.

However, the scope of practice and job-related activities provide a general overview associated with health services managers.[2,3]

- Supervise and evaluate work-related activities of medical, clerical, and service personnel
- Responsible for fiscal operations such as accounting and budgeting
- Responsible for implementation and administration of programs/services
- Responsible for activity reports related to programs/ services
- Institute objectives and evaluative standards for managed units
- Responsible for recruitment and hiring of personnel
- Develop training programs for personnel
- Monitor resources to ensure effective use
- Keep current with health-care laws and regulations affecting the organization
- Communicate regularly with medical personnel and department heads
- Establish organizational policies and procedures

Required Education

The majority of health-care organizations require health services managers to have at least a bachelor's degree in health services management or administration. Other organizations, depending on the type, may require an advanced degree in health services or health-care administration. For individuals interested in academics, a doctorate in health services management or administration may be required for teaching purposes. For individuals already working in health care, a certificate in health services

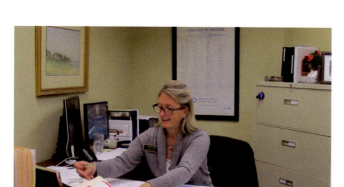

FIGURE 18-4 The administrative staff shown here is preparing for the day in a nursing home setting.

management or administration may present an opportunity for advancement in the organization. The required education of individuals working in health services management is often reflective of the standards set forth by the accreditation or licensure agency.

The core courses for either health services management or health-care administration are basically the same because the titles are interchangeable. Before acceptance into the program, prerequisites such as medical terminology, biology, math, statistics, information systems, and health professional roles may be required in addition to the general education courses. After acceptance into the program, courses such as research, professional writing, practice management, quality management, legal environment, human resources, leadership, data management, health-care delivery systems, and finance are typical courses that will be required before graduating with a bachelor's degree. Advanced degrees require some of the same courses, such as finance, management, legal, research, and statistics, but require a deeper level in addition to courses focusing on current health-care laws and global initiatives.

Accreditation and Certification

Accreditation and **certification** can be achieved at different levels. The entire university can be accredited by a national or regional accreditation council. One example of national accreditation is the Council for Higher Education Accreditation, which is the largest organization in the United States and accredits approximately 3,000 universities and colleges.[4] Regional accreditations are broken down by geographical areas across the United States. There are six different regional accreditations[4]:

- Middle States Association of Colleges and Schools
- New England Association of Schools and Colleges
- North Central Association of Colleges and Schools
- Northwest Commission on Colleges and Universities
- Southern Association of Colleges and Schools
- Western Association of Schools and Colleges

Individual programs within each school or college may have additional accreditations based on the type of program and applicable accreditation associations. The master's degree in health services management might be accredited by the Commission on Accreditation of Healthcare Management Education (CAHME), which ensures integrity within that program.[5]

Certifications work much the same way accreditation associations work in that they ensure the certified programs have met the approved standards set by the certification board. Like accreditations, certification processes include a defined external peer review process that ensures the programs have met all criteria needed to be deemed "certified." A common certification for health services management programs across the Unites States is the Association of University Programs in Health Administration (AUPHA). AUPHA, a nonprofit body, represents more than 400 colleges and universities at the undergraduate and graduate level.[6]

Salary

Like many occupations, the average salary for health services managers varies from state to state, between health-care organizations, and with educational levels. Some individuals work as midlevel managers whereas others are administrators; therefore, the salary ranges vary greatly. The median salary for 2012 was $88,580 per year, averaging between $40,000 and $110,000 per year. Health services managers working in hospitals tend to be at the higher range; those working in nursing homes or personal care services tend to be closer to the bottom range.[3]

Trends

An aging population and career longevity have helped create a positive outlook for health services managers. The job outlook for this occupation is projected to grow 23% between now and 2022.[3] Some areas will grow faster than others, but the overall projection indicates faster than average growth. Facilities treating or housing senior populations will likely be among the higher growth areas.

Challenges

As with many health-care careers, the rewards of the job may be many, but the challenges can be overwhelming at times. Because the health services management role typically includes some form of supervision, whether entire departments or a few individuals, there are always challenges in supervising employees. These challenges come in the form of personality clashes, differences in opinions, employee conflicts, and creating evaluations that are fair and equal for all. Long hours are common for managers in all types of business but even more so when health care is involved, given the 24-hour operation of facilities such as hospitals and urgent-care centers. Although health services managers are not typically involved in direct patient care, they face the challenges of ensuring quality patient care and safety. Employee recruitment and retention may be challenging at times due to shortages of nurses and other

Aptitude Profile

When deciding on a career, one should consider the specific knowledge and skill set needed for that job. Many health-care careers have some of the same characteristics, but certain skills may be more specific to management than direct practice care. Below is a list of characteristics one should probably have before deciding on a career as a health services manager. This list is not exhaustive but provides a general overview of some of the knowledge or skills needed when working as a health services manager.

Ability to motivate others	Good interpersonal skills
Active listener	Good judgment and decision-making skills
Adaptability/flexibility	
Analytical skills	Good negotiation skills
Critical thinking ability	Good organization skills
Data analysis skills	Inductive and deductive reasoning skills
Emotional maturity and intelligence	Mathematical skills
Good delegation skills	Time management skills
Good communication skills	

health-care providers. The aging population creates other challenges, such as increased demand for services despite a lack of sufficient resources. Trying to juggle the rising cost of care against the allowable dollar amount by Medicare or other insurance programs can also be discouraging at times. Other challenges include staying current with new medical technology,[1] as well as policy changes at the federal or state levels affecting health care in general. Although the challenges may seem daunting, the rewards of being part of a health-care team outweigh the challenges.

Role of the Baccalaureate-Prepared Health Services Manager

To be recognized as a health services manager, the minimum degree is usually the baccalaureate degree in health services management. The baccalaureate-prepared health services manager's role will have some similarity to one who is master's prepared. Often the difference in roles may be due to the size of the organization or department, the level of the administration, the practice experience of the employee, any legal/licensing requirements, or the responsibilities assigned by employing agency.

- Develop, revise, and implement policies
- Create work schedules and assignments

- Supervise and evaluate personnel
- Conduct and administer fiscal operations
- Develop budgets and justify allowances
- Develop instructional materials
- Attend educational trainings/conferences
- Attend meetings and disseminate information to personnel
- Produce activity reports on status of programs
- Recruit, hire, and train personnel
- Monitor the use of resources and assess the need for additional personnel, equipment, and services
- Marketing, sales, and distribution of medical equipment

Role of the Master's-Prepared Health Services Manager

As mentioned, some of the roles listed below overlap with those already presented. Individuals who have master's degrees usually are in upper-level management, and their scopes of practice will typically increase with each level of management. These individuals are often the administrators

of large departments, clinics, organizations, or hospitals. Some of them may have specific scopes of practice due to requirements mandated by state or federal requirements (e.g., nursing home administrator). Therefore, the following scopes of practice incorporate any individual working in an upper management or administrative role regardless of the organization.

- Represent the agency/organization at all meetings/functions and communicate necessary information to personnel
- Supervise, direct, and evaluate all personnel (some restrictions may apply to certain medical personnel)
- Establish objectives for operational criteria for managed units
- Inspect facilities and recommend building or equipment modifications
- Ensure emergency readiness and compliance for safety
- Manage all changes within the integrated health-care delivery system
- Develop/approve budgets for all departments
- Ensure credentialing of personnel
- Authorize expenditures and establish rates for services
- Assess need for additional personnel or services

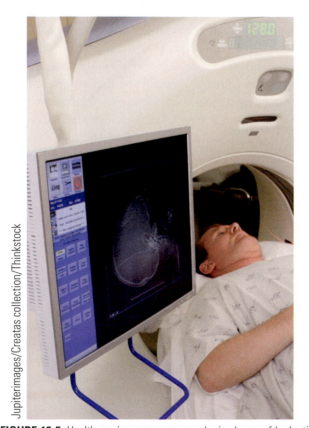

Jupiterimages/Creatas collection/Thinkstock

FIGURE 18-5 Health services managers may be in charge of budgeting for hospital equipment, such as this magnetic resonance imaging (MRI) scanner.

Role of the Medical Health Services Manager

In some cases, supervising personnel of a clinical department are required to have a degree in a medical field and a degree in health services management. Due to state licensing requirements, some health professions require supervision by personnel licensed in the same degree. Therefore, clinical managers may supervise a specific department such as nursing or physical therapy and have responsibilities based on that specialty.[3] Again, some of the roles and responsibilities overlap with those already mentioned. Following are roles associated with medical health services managers.

- Supervise and evaluate personnel
- Ensure efficiency and quality in health-care delivery systems
- Manage patient fees and billing
- Establish policies and procedures
- Create reports and budgets
- Ensure credentialing and training of medical personnel
- Monitor and assess the need for additional resources such as staff or inpatient beds
- Establish quality assurance programs
- Conduct in-services for personnel

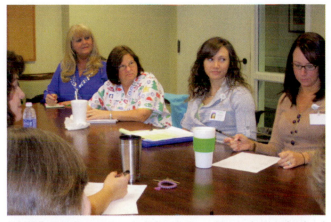

FIGURE 18-6 Patient care is being discussed by an interprofessional team. Disciplines represented include administration, nursing, social work, rehabilitation, nutrition, activities director, and finance.

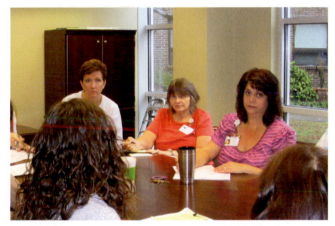

FIGURE 18-7 Regardless of the health-care career taken, individuals working in health care must work together to ensure quality care.

- Keep abreast of new innovations and technologies for patient care
- Stay current with accreditation requirements for the organization/department

Role of the Doctoral-Prepared Health Services Manager

Individuals obtaining a doctoral degree in health services management typically have a specific reason for the degree and are able to select from several concentrations to emphasize their unique area. Reasons for seeking a doctoral degree in health services management include teaching in academic centers, consulting, conducting health-care research, or becoming a CEO/president of a large hospital, organization, or federal agency. Others may pursue the degree to enter into the political arena as special-interest lobbyists. Their roles will vary depending on their chosen path.

Working Together

Health services managers do not usually perform clinical procedures or deal directly with patient care; however, they are in constant contact with disciplines who are actively involved in the clinical aspects of patient care. As noted, one of their roles is management, which places them in the middle of activities surrounding patient care. Health services managers may complete necessary justification of budget requests for the necessity of new equipment. for special equipment for better-quality care. The equipment may be needed by physical therapists, occupational therapists, physician assistants, or other types of direct providers. However, before the request can be made, collaboration between the provider and the health services manager must take place. Some health services managers recruit and hire direct-care providers such as nurses. However, to understand the staffing needs, the health services manager will need to meet with the nursing supervisor to inquire about the number and type of nurses needed. Some health services managers are responsible for credentialing of the clinical staff and must maintain contact with them regarding continuing education requirements. Considering the many ways that health services managers collaborate with other disciplines, it is understandable why they are part of the interprofessional care team. In fact, most health-care organizations have regular interprofessional meetings and health services managers are generally an expected team member. Individuals desiring to be educated as a health services manager must also understand the need to collaborate across disciplines and be prepared for this interaction.

SUMMARY

Health services management can be a rewarding occupation. One of the most exciting elements of working in this discipline is the diversity in jobs and roles. One can easily find an appropriate fit based on education level, location, and one's personal characteristics. The overall job projection expects faster than average growth, which provides job stability and opportunities.

CASE STUDY

Jeffrey K. is the licensed administrator for a skilled nursing home. Jeffrey has many good employees working in the nursing home, and over the years he has developed a good rapport with most of them. He is responsible for supervision of all departments, which include the business office, nursing, physical and speech therapy, social work, admissions, food services, laundry, and maintenance. Although the role of an administrator is sometimes hectic,

(continued)

overall he has been pleased with his staff and has really enjoyed his job. However, recently some issues have arisen that have created tension for Jeffrey. It seemed that many patient concerns were arising, quality care was questioned, and recruiting and retaining staff was difficult as well. Staff morale was low and collegiality was almost nonexistent. The following case is only one of the patient issues that occurred during this time that began to jeopardize patient safety and family satisfaction, in addition to the viability of the facility.

About 9 months ago, a dementia patient was admitted to the unit. On admission, the patient, Ms. L, was cognizant of self and family, and to some degree her surroundings. She was able to feed herself, go to the bathroom, and walk unattended for short distances. Her daughter visited daily and was active in her mother's plan of care. Over the next 3 or 4 months, the patient's health deteriorated to the point that a wheelchair was needed for any type of mobility. However, Ms. L's dementia kept her from remembering that she was supposed to use a wheelchair, so she would try to walk unassisted and would fall. She also tried to get up during the night to go to the bathroom, but again, without assistance, she would fall. These falls became more frequent and serious and always required emergency department visits. There was a broken nose once, sterile strips for her arm another time, and a couple of times sutures were required for her forehead. The falls were happening so frequently that the daughter requested a meeting with the staff to try a different approach to care. One of the emergency department's physicians had seen Ms. L and her daughter so often that he began to question the falls. Additionally, Ms. L's weight dropped quickly and she could no longer chew her food well enough to support the calories needed to maintain her present weight. On top of everything else, the state facility surveyors had made a surprise visit and asked to review patient charts. Three charts were selected for in-depth review, one of which was Ms. L's chart. One of the surveyors asked to meet with the daughter because Ms. L was no longer able to answer questions or converse in any logical manner. At the end of the surveyors' review they asked to meet with Jeffrey and expressed their concern for this patient's safety and quality of care. Jeffrey was expected to find creative ways to reduce patient falls, keep the patient dry, implement a restorative feeding program, and increase communication measures with the daughter. Jeffrey knew he needed his interprofessional team to brainstorm ways to meet all of these patient needs. Obviously, Jeffrey needs to gather his team. Who should be a part of this team?

Questions

1. Does Jeffrey need to seek external sources to aid in this scenario?

2. Can you think of anything that might help with the patient's care?

3. What can be done to improve the overall morale in the facility?

4. Are there other issues pertaining to this case that need addressing?

Review Questions

1. The first groups of health-care managers were called:
   A. Nurses
   B. Physicians
   C. Superintendents
   D. Physical therapists

2. Health services managers are able to perform clinical duties.
   A. True
   B. False

3. A health services manager working as an administrator in a/n_____ is required to have a license.
   A. Hospital
   B. Nursing home
   C. Ambulatory care center
   D. All of the above

4. Health services manager is a good career choice for someone who desires to work alone.
   A. True
   B. False

5. The first state to have a hospital administration education program was_____.
   A. Illinois
   B. North Carolina
   C. Wisconsin
   D. New York

6. There is no difference in the scopes of practice in the educational level of health services managers.
   A. True
   B. False

7. Health services managers working in _____ typically have the highest salaries.
   A. Nursing homes
   B. Hospitals
   C. Physicians' offices
   D. Dentists' offices

8. The projected employment growth for health services managers is around _____%.

   A. 15

   B. 18

   C. 23

   D. 39

9. The first professional organization for hospital administrators was established in___.

   A. 1933

   B. 1941

   C. 2001

   D. 2010

10. Clinical health services managers are those who have _____.

   A. Completed a clinical course

   B. A degree in a clinical area plus the management degree

   C. Taken first aid safety courses

   D. Read the clinical training book

Glossary of Key Terms

ICD-10 codes—International Classification of Disease codes used when classifying data related to health-care illness or diseases; are recognized worldwide and are instrumental to patient medical records

Health Insurance Portability and Accountability Act (HIPAA)—represents many aspects of health; some are related to health insurance, and others are related to patient privacy and confidentiality

Health services managers—individuals who manage a health-care organization or department of a health-care facility

Health-care administrators—see health services managers (the terms are interchangeable)

Superintendents—individuals who act as the lead administrator of a system, whether health care or education; oversee the hospital, organization, or school; manage the work of the employees; and direct the establishment based on mission and vision statements

Internship—real-world experience in the educational process that allows the student to see the inner workings of an organization/health-care environment while still in school; typically are not paid positions but are required by specific degree programs

Accreditation—process whereby a program is peer reviewed by experts in that field who ensure that the appropriate standards have been met; in addition to the specific criteria by the accrediting organization, integrity and quality must be addressed

Certification—process whereby peer reviewers confirm that the characteristics and qualities of a particular program have been met

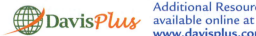

Additional Resources

Occupational Outlook Handbook, Medical and Health Services Managers—www.bls.gov/ooh/management/medical-and-health-services-managers.htm

The Bureau of Labor website provides information on labor market activity and working conditions for those seeking jobs in this occupation. Provides information on what health services managers do, work environment, how to become a health services manager, pay, and job outlook.

American College of Health Care Administrators (ACHCA)—www.achca.org/index.php/about-achca

This website provides information about professional membership association, programming, certification, and career opportunities for members.

Health Services Management Research—http://hsm.sagepub.com

Health Services Management Research is a research-based journal that examines issues related to health policy, systems, and evidence-based research.

Association of University Programs in Health Administration (AUPHA)—www.aupha.org

AUPHA is one of the certification bodies for both undergraduate and graduate programs in health services management.

Journal of Health Administration Education

This journal, published by AUPHA, is a peer-reviewed journal that chronicles research, case studies, and essays written by health-care administration educators. It can be accessed at www.aupha.org.

Managers Who Lead: A Handbook for Improving Health Services—https://www.msh.org/resources/managers-who-lead-a-handbook-for-improving-health-services

Provides information to health managers on becoming a leader and empowering others to accept the challenges as well.

Health Management Associates—www.healthmanagement.com

Health Management Associates (HMA) is an independent, national research and consulting firm that provides services to individuals in health-care management. Services include finance and reimbursement strategies; procurements, proposals, and applications; HMA community strategies; system development and restructuring; and regulatory compliance.

U.S. Department of Health and Human Services, Health Resources and Services Administration (HRSA)—www.hrsa.gov/index.html

This website provides information about the roles this agency plays and the people affected by them. Goal I: Improve Access to Quality Care and Services. Goal II: Strengthen the Health Workforce. Goal III: Build Healthy Communities. Goal IV: Improve Health Equity.

The Health Manager's Website—www.who.int/management/en

Provided by World Health Organization (WHO). Directs and coordinates authority for health within the United Nations system. Some of the concepts, guidance, and tools available to help you make the best use of resources or solve problems include topics such as budgeting and monitoring expenditures; collecting and using information; maintaining equipment, vehicles, and buildings; and interacting with the community and other partners.

References

1. Haddock CC, McLean RA, and Chapman RC. *Careers in Healthcare Management: How to Find Your Path and Follow It.* Chicago, IL: Health Administration Press; 2002.

2. Bureau of Labor Statistics, U.S. Department of Labor. *Occupational outlook handbook, 2014–2015 edition.*

   http://www.bls.gov/ooh/management/medical-and-helath-services-managers.htm.

   Accessed February 12, 2014.

3. O*Net Resource Center. Summary report for medical and health services managers.

   http://www.onetonline.org/link/summary/11-9111.00.

   Accessed March 14, 2014.

4. Council for Higher Education Accreditation.

   http://www.chea.org/default.asp.

   Accessed February 12, 2014.

5. Commission on Accreditation of Healthcare Management Education.

   http://www.cahme.org.

   Accessed February 12, 2014.

6. Association of University Programs in Health Administration. About AUPHA.

   http://www.aupha.org/about.

   Accessed February 12, 2014.

CHAPTER 19

Medical Assisting

Laura Melendez, BS, and Patricia Royal, EdD

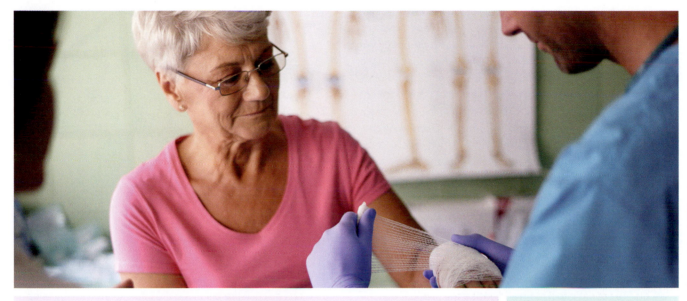

Photo credit: istock/Thinkstock

Learning Objectives

After reading this chapter, students should be able to:

- Describe the role of a medical assistant in today's health-care system
- Discuss the different clinical and administrative duties of medical assistants
- Describe the education, accrediting, and certification processes
- Explain the relationship between medical assistants and other members of the health-care team
- Discuss career opportunities and career laddering of medical assistants
- Discuss the importance of continuing education and learning new skills for medical assistants

Key Terms

- Providers
- American Registry of Medical Assistants (ARMA)
- American Medical Technologists (AMT)
- American Association of Medical Assistants (AAMA)
- Certified Medical Assistant (CMA)
- Registered Medical Assistant (RMA)
- Accrediting Bureau of Health Education Schools (ABHES)
- Commission on Accreditation of Allied Health Education Programs (CAAHEP)
- Externship

"A Day in the Life"

Hello, my name is Belkis and I am a lead medical assistant. I work in an urgent-care practice with 10 different **providers,** so we are always on the go, go, go! We see everything from seasonal allergies, to urinary tract infections, to fractured toes. The beginning of my day is a morning meeting to boost morale and productivity. Occasionally, I have in-services on certain procedures and protocols in the office according to the needs of the practice. Last week I demonstrated how to correctly use a bladder scan and this week we have a new electrocardiography (ECG) machine that is linked to the patient's record through the EMR, which is an electronic medical record system we use to document patient visits. First, the patients check in with the administrative medical assistant at the front desk by completing forms and providing demographic and insurance information. Then, I take the patient back into a triage room to assess the patient's immediate concern while being personable yet professional. I've been in the profession for several years, and I can anticipate the doctor's needs based on the patient's symptoms and complaints.

I complete a review of the patient's history, chief complaint, and vital signs. If any further testing is needed before I take the patient to the provider room, I ensure that it is done. I then escort the patient into a room and advise the provider that the patient is ready to be seen via the EMR tracking system. I ensure the rest of the medical assistant team is on schedule and delegate any miscellaneous duties such as inventory and our famous "2-day callbacks." Essentially, our 2-day callbacks are a way of making sure the patient is feeling better and is content with the level of service we provided. I have the best team of multitasking superheroes as staff and I appreciate their genuine concern for the health of others.

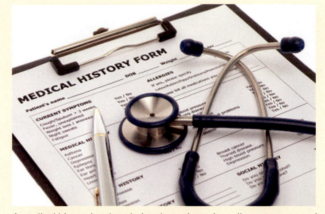

A medical history is taken during the patient triage. (Image courtesy of pasingphoto at FreeDigitalPhotos.net)

Now that my patient is ready to be discharged, I print out the discharge forms, prescriptions, and education related to the visit. I discuss the plan with the patient, answer any questions, and end the encounter by walking the patient to the check-out desk. Finally, we have our closing duties for the day.

Introduction to Medical Assisting

Description

Medical assisting comprises the administrative and clinical tasks performed in physician offices, urgent-care centers, clinics, hospital outpatient centers, and, more recently, home health.[1] Many individuals perform a variety of tasks in collaboration with a team of allied health-care professionals to reach a common goal of optimal patient health.

Within the medical office, it is common for medical assistants to assume a variety of roles. Some medical assistants answer the phone, manage insurance claims, and print bills; some lean toward office management, while others remain purely clinical. There are many other specialties and subspecialties in health care in which a medical assistant might work, but whatever the practice area, all medical assistants share in the mission to deliver efficient patient care.

History

Medical assistants work beside physicians, primarily in outpatient or ambulatory-care facilities, such as medical offices and clinics. The first medical assistant positions came about in the early 20th century specifically to assist nurses who had become overwhelmed with their duties and responsibilities, which had increased greatly because of World Wars I and II. Doctors and nurses needed more assistance to care for sick and wounded soldiers. Around that time, more physicians began to practice in clinics and open medical offices. These physicians hired medical assistants to perform noninvasive clinical procedures such as taking weight and vital signs. The addition of this allied health member enabled the nurses and physicians to focus more on patient care. In the 1950s, the **American Registry of Medical Assistants (ARMA)** began holding meetings to further professionalize the field and was incorporated to accommodate for the need of medical assistants in physician practices. The ARMA provides continuing education and serves as an ethical guideline for the profession. Its members own the title of "registered" primarily just for being a member and showing interest in keeping up with the latest trends in health care. The term *registered medical assistant* stems from registered nurses, who trained and worked with medical assistants in medical offices. This is not to be confused with the "registered medical assistant" credential that can be acquired from passing the **American Medical Technologists (AMT)** examination.[2]

In 1956 the **American Association of Medical Assistants (AAMA)** began its operations to establish cohesiveness and competencies in medical assisting.[3] The AAMA created competences for safe practice that would establish the need for individuals to become certified in those competencies. Until 2014, it was not a requirement to be certified as a medical assistant. Centers for Medicare and Medicaid Services implemented a "Meaningful Use" incentive program that would evolve the nation's health-care system to become more cost efficient and improve clinical outcomes. One of the Meaningful Use criteria is to migrate health records into an electronic format known as an electronic medical record (EMR). In the meantime, keeping paper medical records in addition to EMRs is optional. Another criterion specifies a requirement of certification and/or licensure for the individual who enters patient information into the EMR.

Scope of Practice

The scopes of practice for medical assistants vary immensely and are a product of the education, certifications, and specific laws of the state. Universally, medical assistants hold the responsibilities of understanding the administrative competencies that pertain to the following areas:

- Anatomy and physiology
- Medical terminology
- Medical law and ethics
- Registration, certification, and professional development
- Human relations and interpersonal skills
- Patient education
- Insurance—plans, claim forms, coding, and financial applications of medical insurance
- Bookkeeping, billing, collection, medical office accounting procedures, office banking, payroll, financial calculations

Tips and Tools

The term *providers* refers to physicians, nurse practitioners, and physician assistants because they "provide" the patient with medical services. They may also be called *clinicians*. Medical assistants provide support services alongside providers. A proficient medical assistant is able to anticipate the provider's noninvasive needs of a patient through education and experience.

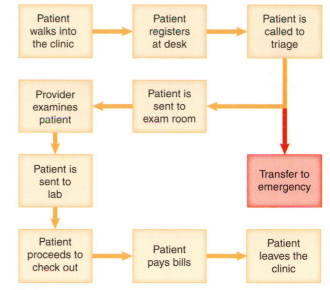

FIGURE 19-1 During the course of a single patient visit, medical assistants may occupy a variety of important roles and execute many tasks.

- Receptionist duties, handling phone calls, scheduling, records management, charting guidelines, transcription of dictation, inventory, office computer applications

Depending on the state and its scope of practice for the medical assistant, clinically the medical assistant is able to perform the following procedures:

- Demonstrate and apply medical and surgical asepsis
- Sterilize, identify, and use surgical instruments and assist in minor surgeries
- Obtain vital signs/mensurations, recognize normal and abnormal results, obtain patient histories, perform ancillary testing
- Administer medications through various routes and handle prescription requests

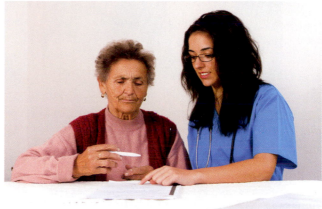

FIGURE 19-2 A medical assistant assists an elderly patient with filling out forms.

Photo credit: Lighthaunter/iStock collection/Thinkstock

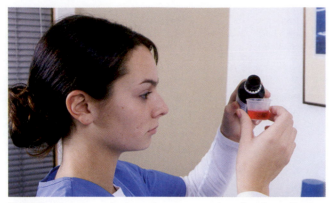

FIGURE 19-3 A medical assistant measuring liquid medication. (From Eagle S, Brassington C, Dailey C, Goretti C. *The Professional Medical Assistant: An Integrative, Team-Based Approach.* Philadelphia, PA: F.A. Davis; 2009.)

- Demonstrate positioning; perform electrocardiograms, venipunctures, and various laboratory specimen collections; administer first aid; suture removal and wound care

- Position and prepare patients for various radiographic examinations

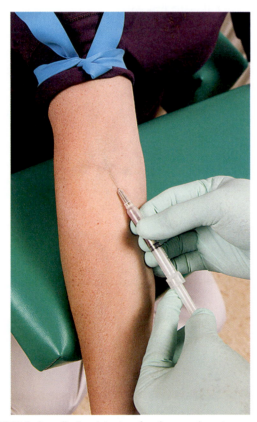

FIGURE 19-4 A medical assistant performing a venipuncture procedure. (From Eagle S, Brassington C, Dailey C, Goretti C. *The Professional Medical Assistant: An Integrative, Team-Based Approach.* Philadelphia, PA: F.A. Davis; 2009.)

Required Education

In the early stages of the profession, no educational requirements were necessary. Whatever tasks could be trained on the job were the responsibilities that the medical assistants performed as learned. Perhaps that is why the field encompasses many different proficiencies and areas of specialization. For this particular field, the two main certifications are the **Certified Medical Assistant (CMA),** certified by the AAMA, and the **Registered Medical Assistant (RMA),** certified by the AMT.[3]

Both technical schools and career colleges offer medical assisting programs with the curriculum varying from 8 to 12 months for a medical assistant diploma/certificate to 18 to 24 months for an associate degree in medical assisting. To be eligible to take the CMA, one must pursue a curriculum accredited by the **Accrediting Bureau of Health Education Schools (ABHES)** or the **Commission on Accreditation of Allied Health Education Programs (CAAHEP).** An RMA may either be accredited by these two agencies, or may challenge (sit for) the examination after being employed as a medical assistant for 5 consecutive years. However, the challenge method has a very low pass rate because foundational knowledge is not always learned on the job. After failing a second attempt, the applicant must enroll in a suitable educational program before qualifying to take the examination again. Within the curriculum, a clinical practicum or **externship** serves as an extension of schooling. An externship is mainly an opportunity to learn and observe by shadowing a professional on the job and is unpaid. An internship, conversely, may be compensated and is an opportunity to learn by performing actual job-related duties. The core courses differ across educational institutions, and some training is required to be employed (whether obtained in school or on employee orientation). Some of these certifications may include the following[3]:

- Cardiopulmonary resuscitation and basic life support

- Four-hour HIV/blood-borne pathogens training

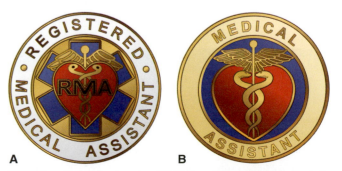

A   **B**

FIGURE 19-5 Certification pins. **(A)** RMA and **(B)** CMA. (From Eagle S, Brassington C, Dailey C, Goretti C. *The Professional Medical Assistant: An Integrative, Team-Based Approach.* Philadelphia, PA: F.A. Davis; 2009.)

- Health Insurance Portability and Accountability Act (HIPAA)
- Standard and universal precautions
- Occupational Safety and Health Administration (OSHA)

Salary

The salary range for medical assistants varies with location. According to the Bureau of Labor Statistics, in 2012, the median salary was $29,370.[4] This figure may deviate in either direction by approximately $10,000 depending on experience, educational level, and specialty.

Trends

The Bureau of Labor Statistics cites that medical assistant employment is expected to increase by 29% through 2022,[4] which is much higher than the average for all occupations. According to federal health legislation the need for medical assistants will continue to increase. Part of the increase is due to the expansion in the number of individuals who have access to care. Another factor that contributes to the demand is the increase in the numbers of older adults who will need health care. With an aging population, the rise in overall health-care needs is expected to create new opportunities for those working in health care.

Challenges

There are many challenges in the field of medical assisting. One issue in particular is the difficulty of classifying medical assisting as a profession, given its relative newness. The general public classifies clinical medical assistants as nurses, and although it is an extension of the profession, it is not the same because they do not perform all of the same functions as nurses. Currently, the medical assistant profession has disassociated with the nursing profession because vocational nurses are considered more parallel to registered nurses and are therefore considered a related profession; however, some medical assistants carry out some responsibilities that nurses may not necessarily carry out, and vice versa.

Another challenge is that because there were no educational requirements before 2014, it made more business sense to hire someone without credentials, apply on-the-job-training, and pay the minimal salary. It is hoped that new legislation will place an added emphasis on the importance of credentialed allied health professionals and set the tone for salary accordingly.

Yet another challenge facing medical assistants is that the field remains nonspecific. For example, a provider may have two medical assistants where one is clinical and the other is administrative. Sometimes, there is only one clinical medical assistant and the administration carries the brunt of insurance denials and appeals, referrals, prior authorization, precertifications, surgical scheduling, and so forth. The specifics vary by practice, clinic, city, and state. Therefore, it is difficult to assign duties at an accurate productivity rate that is realistic because circumstances change depending on many factors.

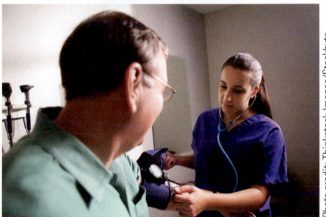

FIGURE 19-6 Taking a patient's vital signs is part of a clinical medical assistant's duties.

Photo credit: Thinkstock Images/Stockbyte collection/Thinkstock

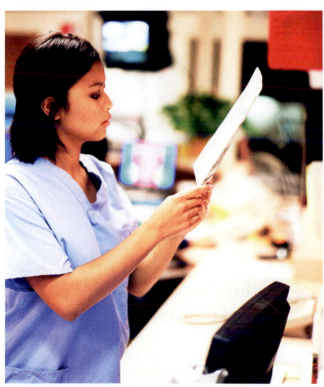

FIGURE 19-7 Patient record-keeping and completing referrals are often part of an administrative medical assistant's duties.

Photo credit: Jupiterimages/Photos.com/Thinkstock

Aptitude Profile

When deciding on a career, the individual should take into consideration the skills and abilities needed to be successful in a particular job. Many jobs in the health-care fields require some of the same characteristics; however, there are some skills that are more specific to working in medical assisting. Listed below are some of the necessary skills and abilities to consider when deciding whether to become a medical assistant. Although this list is not definitive, most of these characteristics are required to be a resourceful medical assistant.

Able to handle stress	Multitasker
Assertive	Nonjudgmental
Compassionate	Objective
Emotionally mature	Responsible
Empathetic	Resourceful
Ethical	Self-aware
Emotionally mature	Sensitive
Good communicator	Skillful in interviewing
Independent worker	

Author Spotlight

Laura Melendez, BS

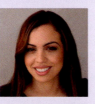

I've been in the field for approximately 14 years in multiple facets. When I started, it was a relatively new profession and many were unable to understand the title of medical assistant. It was also slightly daunting because you have a direct effect on patients' lives. It is and will remain a fast-paced and very rewarding career. It was exciting, but confusing since the scope of practice did not have conformity throughout the different states.

Diversifying myself was the best attribute for me personally. You can do so much and find what you love to do on your journey. I went from clinical, to administrative, then to manager, and now to instructor/program coordinator. The possibilities are endless.

Role of the Medical Assistant as a Clinical Assistant

Many begin in the field performing clinical duties such as measuring vital signs, assisting in surgeries and procedures, and collecting/processing laboratory specimens. Generally, it is advantageous to be initially employed at an internal medicine, family, or urgent-care practice to strengthen and broaden skills learned in school. However, some medical assistants have a natural preference for one field over another. For example, if a medical assistant specializes in dermatology, he or she would likely be more proficient in Mohs surgeries, topical applications, and esthetic procedures than one who specializes in cardiology. Mohs is a surgery set in a highly controlled environment where a skin growth or abnormal mole is removed, is reviewed immediately by a pathologist, and directions are instantaneously given on where to remove the next piece of tissue to ensure no cancerous cells are left in the skin. If the cancerous tissue is left behind, the patient may be at risk.

In the area of specialization, the nonspecific nature of the medical assisting profession may actually serve as a benefit. A medical assistant might specialize in a field, such as dermatology, but may change his or her path at any given time to specialize in another field, such as gastroenterology, without extra training or credentials. Hence, a medical assistant need not be "locked in" to one field, nor fear regressing to, or starting over in, general medical assisting. At times, a medical assistant may be given the title of *lead medical assistant* and the responsibility of managing the rest of the team and ultimately make the decisions that influence quality care and efficiency.

Role of Medical Assistants as Office Managers

Because physicians and other midlevel providers are busy focusing on medicine, medical assistants may be asked to take on the role of an office manager. The role of an office manager may be different from specialty to specialty, but for the most part the job duties are similar. Some of the responsibilities include, but are not limited to, the following: payroll, reviews and reprimands of employees, maintenance and preparation of the providers' schedules and itineraries, accounts payable, accounts receivable, coordination of continuing education for providers, management of complaints (both internal and external), negotiation of insurance contracts, and research for trends and marketing opportunities. The job of office manager can be challenging because there are many checks and balances that must be mastered in terms of rapport, respect, and continual growth and improvement of patient care and finances.

Role of Medical Assistants as Support Staff

Medical assistants may take on many roles, and some medical assistants thrive best as support staff. These job titles may include referrals coordinator, medical records clerk, front desk receptionist, check-out receptionist, and billing clerk. Traditionally, some of these jobs have been occupied by on-the-job-trained candidates; however, there has been more of a desire to hire someone with experience or education so that mistakes are kept to a minimum. Each of the roles listed as support staff requires patience and a willingness to learn the job of medical assistants despite continuously changing policies, both in-house and legislatively. In time, medical assistants become experts in that particular trade, and a clinical education background helps create a seamless transition in patient care.

Role of Medical Assistants in Other Settings

Recently, due to increased technology and the need for convenience, there has been an increasing trend in medical assistants employed for traveling assignments. These traveling assignments include, but are not limited to, the following: traveling phlebotomists, home health aides, insurance collections technicians, and concierge medical assistants. Job duties include assistance with dialysis, wound care, medical equipment training, home collection of specimens, and patient histories/follow-ups. In addition, there are electrocardiogram (ECG) technicians, patient care technicians, and other hospital-created roles that fall under the medical assistant task list that can be performed by a certified (and registered through examination) individual. The National Healthcare Association (NHA) provides continuing education and various specialized certifications such as the following:

- Certified phlebotomy technician (CPT)
- Certified ECG technician (CET)
- Certified electronic health records specialist (CEHRS)
- Certified clinical medical assistant (CCMA)

- Certified medical administrative assistant (CMAA)
- Patient care technician/patient care assistant (CPCT/CPCA)
- Billing and coding specialist

Evolving Role of Medical Assistants

The medical assisting profession offers many possible employment opportunities, so why not venture into different roles? A multiskilled background increases marketability and improves morale. Although the title of medical assistant was previously generalized to refer to one who offered noninvasive types of assistance to a medical professional, it has become more commonplace for a medical assistant's responsibilities to become more distinct and identifiable. Hence, there are more programs specified to surgical technology, medical records and health information technology, billing and coding, and office management.

Working Together

Because of the many responsibilities bestowed on medical assistants, it is imperative to understand interprofessional collaboration. At times, a medical assistant may need to discuss patient care with a physician, pharmacist, nurse, physical therapist, diagnostic imaging specialist, behavioral health technician, home health aide, office administrator, pharmaceutical representative, network administrator, attorney, and insurance company representative. To ensure optimal patient health, the interpersonal skills utilized with these professional members are as important as the information exchanged.

CASE STUDY

Russell is a 56-year-old white man with a previous medical history that includes a car accident, which consequently resulted in back surgery. As a result, he was put on two different pain medications: Percocet and OxyContin. He works in the mortgage industry as a loan officer, and has made a decent salary. Recently, the housing market has slowly plummeted and he has had a dramatic change in lifestyle. His wife divorced him over financial struggles and moved to a different state with their children, and Russell has become depressed over it. This morning's encounter is his follow-up visit. He states that he was just in another accident on his way into the medical building parking lot and may need an x-ray. He also admits that he has an addiction problem with the pain medication and needs counseling to help him cope with

(continued)

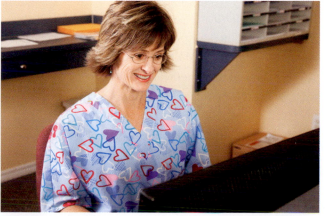

FIGURE 19-8 Medical assistants often work in reception, billing, and other support staff roles.

Photo credit: Lisa F. Young/iStock collection/Thinkstock

his recent divorce and job instability. As the medical assistant, you decipher his story for documentation, which will take place after measuring vital signs. He has high blood pressure and an increased heart rate. On the way out of the patient room, police officers greet you in the lobby and ask to be taken back to the patient who just caused an accident in the parking lot. The police officers also state that there were victims and that they would like to press charges on the person who caused the accident.

Questions

1. What are the medical issues that Russell is experiencing?

2. What plans of treatment should be involved with Russell's care?

3. Why is interprofessional collaboration important in this case?

4. Develop an interprofessional plan of care based on your knowledge from other chapters.

5. What are ultimately the goals for Russell's care?

6. What are some barriers facing interprofessional collaboration?

Review Questions

1. Approximately when did medical assistants become a profession?
   A. 18th century
   B. 20th century
   C. 19th century
   D. 21st century

2. What is the rate of job growth for medical assistants?
   A. Undetermined
   B. Slower than average
   C. Average
   D. Faster than average

3. The American Registry of Medical Assistants (ARMA) began in the:
   A. 1950s
   B. 1960s
   C. 1970s
   D. 1980s

4. Which agency grants the registered medical assistant title after passing its examination?
   A. National Healthcare Association (NHA)
   B. Medical Assistants of America (MAA)
   C. American Association of Medical Assistants (AAMA)
   D. American Registry of Medical Assistants (ARMA)

5. Students must complete an extension of schooling on site called:
   A. Volunteering
   B. Mentorship
   C. Internship
   D. Externship

6. Medical assisting careers are expected to increase by _____ through 2022.
   A. 25%
   B. 29%
   C. 33%
   D. 36%

7. A recent trend in medical assisting has created the opportunity for _____ assignments.
   A. Flexible
   B. Stay-at-home
   C. Traveling
   D. Bonus hours

8. Sometimes a medical assistant has to take on the role of:
   A. A nurse
   B. A physician assistant
   C. An office manager
   D. A dietitian

9. A ___ medical assistant manages the rest of the team.
   A. Lead
   B. Supervising
   C. Managing
   D. Directing

10. The acronym CCMA stands for:
   A. Clinical care medical assistant
   B. Certified clinical medical assistant
   C. Critical care medical assistant
   D. Continuing care medical assistant

Glossary of Key Terms

Providers—professionals who are licensed to diagnose and treat patients and bill for services

American Registry of Medical Assistants (ARMA)—a chartered nonprofit that advances the professionalism of qualified medical assistants

American Medical Technologists (AMT)—a national and international certification agency and membership association for specific medical assisting professions

American Association of Medical Assistants (AAMA)—an organization that provides medical assistant professionals with education, certification, and credential acknowledgment, along with many other resources

Certified medical assistant (CMA)—Medical assistants who have met the standards of certification proposed by a certifying board

Registered medical assistant (RMA)—Medical assistants who have successfully passed the registry exam

Accrediting Bureau of Health Education Schools (ABHES)—a private, nonprofit, independent accrediting agency

Commission on Accreditation of Allied Health Education Programs (CAAHEP)—the largest programmatic accreditor in the health sciences field

Externship—an experiential learning opportunity that is similar to an internship but is shorter in duration and generally at the community college level

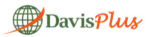 Additional Resources are available online at **www.davisplus.com**

Additional Resources

Accrediting Bodies Recognized by the U.S. Department of Education

Accrediting Bureau of Health Education Schools (ABHES)—www.abhes.org

The purpose of ABHES is to raise the professional standards and aptitudes of education and training to health education schools. ABHES also encourages institutional and programmatic responsibility through methodical and consistent program evaluation.

Commission on Accreditation of Allied Health Education Programs (CAAHEP)—www.caahep.org/default.aspx

CAAHEP is the largest programmatic postsecondary education accreditor of health science occupations.

Education and Professional Resources

CMA Today—www.aama-ntl.org/cma-today/about

CMA Today is a professional journal dedicated to the professional advancement within the medical assisting profession and deals with topics such as continuing education, AAMA news, issues surrounding the profession, and other subjects relevant to medical assisting professionals.

Journal of Continuing Education Topics & Issues—www.americanmedtech.org/default.aspx

The *Journal of Continuing Education Topics & Issues* deals with multiple facets of allied health, including medical assisting. The journal includes continuing education articles, legislative updates, trends in the field, and nuances in the profession.

References

1. American Registry of Medical Assistants. About ARMA.

   http://arma-cert.org/aboutarma.

   Accessed June 25, 2014.

2. American Association of Medical Assistants. 2013 medical assisting compensation and benefits report.

   http://www.aama-ntl.org/docs/default-source/about-the-profession-and-credential/cb-survey.pdf?sfvrsn=6.

   Accessed June 25, 2014.

3. American Association of Medical Assistants. History.

   http://www.aama-ntl.org/about/history.

   Accessed August 26, 2015.

4. Bureau of Labor Statistics, U.S. Department of Labor. Occupational outlook handbook, 2014–2015 edition, medical assistants.

   http://www.bls.gov/ooh/healthcare/medical-assistants.htm.

   Accessed February, 2015.

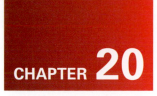

CHAPTER 20

Occupational Therapy

Gregory Wintz, PhD OTR/L

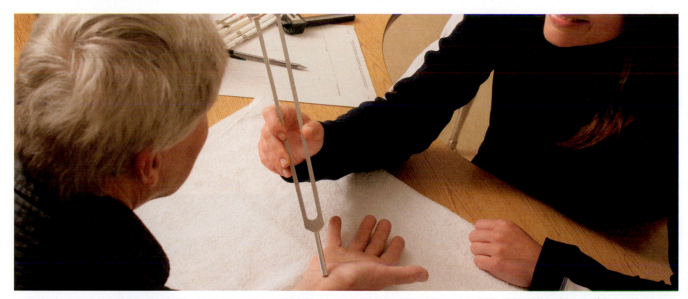

Photo credit: Design Pics/Thinkstock

Learning Objectives

After reading this chapter, students should be able to:

- Describe the role of an occupational therapist and an occupational therapy assistant in the health-care system
- Describe the education and licensing process for occupational therapy practitioners
- Explain the relationship between the occupational therapist and other members of the health-care team
- Discuss opportunities and challenges for working in the field of occupational therapy

Key Terms

- Occupational Therapist
- Individuals with Disabilities Education Improvement Act (IDEA) of 2004
- Individual education plan
- Affordable Care Act of 2010
- Occupations
- Activities of daily living (ADL)
- Moral treatment
- Occupational performance
- Americans with Disabilities Act of 1990 (ADA)
- Occupational therapy assistant

"A Day in the Life"

Hello, my name is Camille and I am an **occupational therapist.** I work in a rural school district, and I am planning to meet with a young girl who has a developmental disability. Jody is an 8-year-old girl born at 31 weeks of gestation, and her birth history includes an interventricular subdural hemorrhage, infant respiratory distress syndrome, bronchopulmonary dysplasia, and mechanical ventilation. She is diagnosed with spastic quadriplegia cerebral palsy. As an occupational therapist working in the schools, my role is to support the student in important learning and school-related activities that are covered under the **Individuals with Disabilities Education Improvement Act (IDEA) of 2004.** I am planning her yearly **individual educational plan program (IEP)** conference with Jody, her parents, her classroom teacher, the resource room assistant, the school psychologist, and her legal advocate. An IEP guides the delivery of special education supports and services for a student with a disability, as defined in the public law referred to as IDEA. To develop an IEP, the student, parents, teacher, and interprofessional team members meet and examine the student's individual needs. When we meet as a team, I'll report on Jody's current status, discuss her progress in the last year, and make recommendations on goals and objectives for the next year.

Hi, my name is Joe and I am an occupational therapist who works in a skilled nursing facility. I'm scheduled to meet with a resident for an evaluation to determine how he might benefit from a reminiscence group at the skilled nursing facility. Richard, a 65-year-old man, was recently admitted to our nursing home by his wife of 35 years for two primary concerns: memory problems, such as forgetting to turn off the stove after cooking, and a tendency to wander the neighborhood during the evening hours. His wife fears that her husband might injure himself, get lost, or accidentally set the house on fire. Richard has been diagnosed with dementia and atherosclerosis (a type of artery disease). The occupational therapy documentation indicates that Richard has twice seen therapists for initial evaluations, but both times refused to participate in occupational therapy. He is pleasant during our interview, responds to my questions, but once again dismisses the need for occupational therapy, despite my suggestion that it could be beneficial. During the assessment, he could not copy the picture of a house, a two-dimensional figure. In fact, his efforts resulted in disconnected lines. Richard requests and is given a ruler, which he uses to draw a series of parallel lines, but is unable to draw a house. He

explains that he had "never been able to draw freehand." I then began administering a cognitive assessment by asking Richard to perform a variety of leather-lacing stitches as an initial estimate of cognitive function, but he has difficulty following directions on the test and quickly loses focus. Richard has functional range of motion and muscle strength, but is unsteady rising from a seated position to standing. He requires the support of furniture or another person. Richard used to enjoy gardening, bicycling, travel, and visiting art museums. Listening to operas and classical music was also a favorite pastime. I suggest Richard's participation in a reminiscence group in the skilled nursing facility. Reminiscence groups use photographs, recordings, and other familiar objects to trigger personal memories. Mrs. Miller is receptive to this idea and our meeting seems somewhat fruitful.

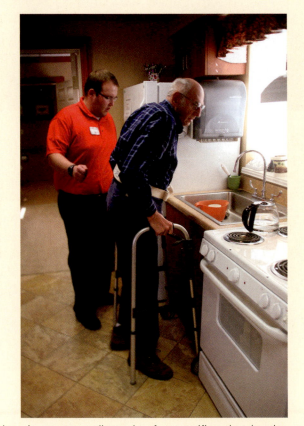

Learning to use a walker and perform specific tasks takes time and practice. In this photo, the occupational therapy student is demonstrating the proper instructions for filling a coffee pot while using the walker.

Introduction to Occupational Therapy

Description

In 2008, baby boomers began to reach age 62; that and the **Affordable Care Act of 2010** are expected causes for increased need of occupational therapists, particularly in the area of health, wellness, and prevention of illness and accidents. It is less expensive to assist persons living independently and functionally at home, at work, and in their communities than at a care facility. Occupational therapists are vital to the health and human services team and provide clients and family members with the skills, knowledge, and adaptations to live independently and stay engaged in those meaningful, purposeful, and goal-directed activities called **"occupations."** Occupations are activities that offer meaning to clients, and occupational therapists are charged with adapting a client's environment and educating the client and the client's family to facilitate enhanced performance of daily activities (Fig. 20-1). Treatments to maintain and improve daily living of clients with a physical, mental, or developmental condition vary from client to client. The

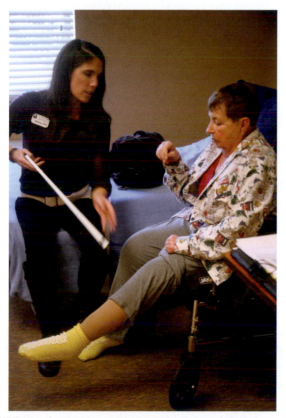

FIGURE 20-1 Continuing your activities of daily living (ADLs) can be challenging at times. In this photo, the occupational therapist is demonstrating how to use the reacher for donning socks.

American Occupational Therapy Association in the Model Practice Act defines *occupational therapy* as the following:

> The therapeutic use of everyday life activities (occupations) with individuals or groups for the purpose of participation in roles and situations in home, school, workplace, community, and other settings. Occupational therapy services are provided for the purpose of promoting health and wellness to those who have or are at risk for developing an illness, injury, disease, disorder, condition, impairment, disability, activity limitation, or participation restriction. Occupational therapy addresses the physical, cognitive, psychosocial, and sensory aspects of performance in a variety of contexts to support engagement in everyday life activities that affect health, well being, and quality of life.[1]

Brief History

The concept of using **activities of daily living (ADL)** or "occupations" to promote recovery from disease, injury, congenital disability, and mental illness dates back to ancient Greece. Asclepiades of Bithynia, a Greek physician, used music to treat mentally ill clients. His medical beliefs focused on regaining harmony in the body when pores or fluids became constricted. In addition to music, he used diet, bathing, and exercise to restore one's equilibrium. Asclepiades of Bithynia noted this connection between health and daily life activities over 2,000 years ago, and current research continues to affirm this early notion.[2]

In the late 18th century, a movement titled **Moral Treatment** emerged. Moral Treatment created a therapeutic community and provided clients a stable, disciplined routine. The work chores and leisure activities offered clients a sense of contribution to the common good.[3] Kindness and respect were promoted over the use of restraints such as chains. Bockoven[4] describes Moral Treatment as an endeavor to awaken feelings of communality (a sense of belonging to a social group) and explains that it was achieved through occupation, which required the client to "invest interest in something outside himself in cooperation with others." Moral Treatment became the preeminent institutional therapy for the mentally ill in the 19th century.[5] It and the therapeutic milieu movement, which also utilized therapeutic communities, provide the historical roots for occupational therapy.

The occupational therapy profession shares similar thoughts about the importance of health in the design and construction of living environments with the Arts and Crafts movement. Founders of the Arts and Crafts movement, such as William Morris and Charles Robert Ashbee, saw value in creating healthy utopian-like communities through the engagement of skilled and creative workers. In this environment, whole items were made and assembled by individuals or small groups; art objects, houses, furniture, book covers, and household utensils are examples of this craft production.

In the early 1900s, American physician Dr. Herbert Hall encouraged a therapeutic practice representative of the Arts and Crafts movement. As the Arts and Crafts movement encouraged a return to a simpler lifestyle, favoring manual labor over machines and factory work, so too did Dr. Hall's practice. He believed that factory work limited happiness.[6] Industrialization and its many methods of creating efficacies by way of assembly-line work were thought to have had deleterious effects on the human condition and cultivating one's community.

In March 1917, the Society for the Promotion of Occupational Therapy met for the first time. Members of the Society actively engaged mentally and physically ill clients in arts and crafts and observed reduced or eliminated symptoms of physical illnesses with tuberculosis, nervous disorders, and polio. During this time, the United States was thrust into a world conflict resulting in millions of World War I soldiers being wounded in battle. Their permanent disabilities required rehabilitation and vocational training; this training was called "reconstruction aid." Schools to train occupational workers, nurses, or those serving the mentally ill began surfacing. The occupational worker or "reconstruction aid" used handicrafts to retrain those with orthopedic injuries, limb loss, and psychiatric problems.

"Reconstruction aid" resurfaced almost 30 years later in World War II; however, this time, occupational therapy shifted from the traditional use of arts and crafts to more scientific treatments, such as prosthetic training that encouraged the use of adaptive devices to engage in daily life activities.[7] Thus began the 60-year evolution of the occupational therapy one recognizes today. From the 1940s through the 1960s, during the "Rehabilitation Movement," the demand for occupational therapists surged. Thousands of injured soldiers (physically and mentally) were returning home from war and needed rehabilitation from spinal cord injuries, amputations, traumatic brain injuries, and many others. To meet the rising demand for occupational therapy services, the certified occupational therapy assistant (COTA) position was created in 1956. Occupational therapists began to specialize in pediatrics and developmental disabilities. In 1965, under amendments to the Social Security Acts, Medicare began covering inpatient occupational therapy services. Occupational therapists

were needed to assist in the shift to deinstitutionalize the mentally ill and physically infirm. In 1975, the Education of the Handicapped Act was passed and occupational therapy was included in the schools as a "related service." During the 1980s and 1990s, occupational therapy began to focus on one's quality of life, thus assuming greater responsibility in prevention, screenings, and health maintenance. Today, occupation-based intervention is the main focus of occupational therapy. This entails the skilled process of improving a client's capacities to participate in daily life activities, particularly in roles meaningful to the client.[7] Those with a physical, emotional, or developmental deficit can be referred for service by a physician, school, or parent for prematurity, birth defect, spina bifida, attention-deficit disorder, developmental disabilities, cerebral palsy, sensory dysfunction, autism, hyperactivity, Down syndrome, amputation, stroke, arthritis, burns, head injury, dementia, diabetes, or cardiac conditions.

Philosophy

The philosophy of occupational therapy includes five key beliefs: (1) value human life; (2) recognize human capacity for growth and self-understanding; (3) understand the power of occupation; (4) understand that the influences of the social and physical environment are shared values and beliefs from medicine, psychology, anthropology, sociology, art, and architecture; and (5) the ability to develop a therapeutic rapport with a client, termed *client-centeredness*. Occupational therapy provides a broad and holistic approach to health; its origins and foundations come from a variety of disciplines.

A primary tenet of occupational therapy is that individuals possess vast resources for personal growth, development, and self-understanding. The role of the occupational therapist is to help one discover these resources and provide opportunities for daily life activities and encourage the client to reach optimum performance. Occupational therapy values the human capacity and drive for growth and self-understanding.

The occupational therapist shows clients how intrinsically motivating activities can improve their health and environment. Occupational therapy is a process that promotes personal growth, meaning, and self-identity by engaging or reengaging a person in productive self-care and leisure activities and by teaching new skills, redesigning familiar activities, or changing the contextual environment.

Humans seek balance by complementing meaningful and goal-directed occupations with activities that support and enhance one's daily life. As a result, daily life activities within social and cultural contexts become meaningful.[8]

Author Spotlight

Gregory Wintz, PhD, OTR/L

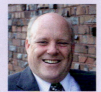

My primary interests in high school and college included drawing and painting. To accurately draw the human body, an art professor encouraged his students to take an anatomy course. I did, and an interest in understanding and attending to the human body was born. During my university studies, I worked in a group home where I taught and supported developmentally disabled adults to live independently. After graduation, I worked with developmentally disabled adults in both residential and vocational aspects of training programs. Our objectives were to teach adults skills to enable them to live more independently and integrate themselves successfully into their communities. Then, for 2 years I lived and worked in a therapeutic community titled *L'Arche*, French for "the Ark." L'Arche is an international federation of communities where people who are developmentally disabled live, work, and cultivate their skills and talents alongside non-handicapped persons. Those at L'Arche community where I lived were charged with providing the residents a permanent home and meaningful work, such as woodworking, candle making, and gardening. At L'Arche, I witnessed the powerful influence environment can have on individuals living in community and thus grew interested in community-based treatment environments.[9,10] This stint in L'Arche sparked my desire to become an occupational therapist.

On completion of a master's of occupational therapy degree from Texas Woman's University, I relocated to the Northwest. One particularly formative post was program director at Spokane's Shriners Children's Hospital. The children and families came to us with abundantly different pediatric orthopedic needs and, as occupational therapists, we listened to their concerns and facilitated solutions. I was rarely bored as each concern required creative and individual solutions.

Scope of Practice

The scope of practice for occupational therapists and occupational therapy assistants, as well as most health-care providers, is determined by eight factors: (1) professional associations, (2) professional education accreditation standards, (3) continuing education and specialty training, (4) state licensure, (5) reimbursement, (6) health-care organizations and context, (7) professional ethics, and (8) mutual accommodations, which is the sharing and respectful relationship that exists among team members. The American Occupational Therapy Association (AOTA) is a national voluntary, professional association that represents the concerns and interests of occupational therapists and endeavors to improve the quality of occupational therapy services. In addition, AOTA partners with state occupational therapy organizations to lobby state legislators for expanded practice and increased funding. Education standards are established and reinforced by the association's educational accreditation process to ensure that each practitioner has the necessary knowledge, skills, and attitudes to become a licensed therapist.

Occupational therapists must earn an entry-level master's or doctorate degree. In 2004, the Accreditation Council for Occupational Therapy Education determined that all entry-level occupational therapy education must be completed at a master's or doctorate level rather than the bachelor's degree.[11]

The scope of practice for an occupational therapist is based on evaluation and intervention focused on three areas: (1) improved human capacity in the area of neuromotor, cognitive, visual-perceptual, and psychosocial skills and abilities; (2) engagement in all daily life activities by the adaption and modification of how the activity is done; and (3) modifications in the environment where daily life activities occur (see Fig. 20-2). The process of evaluation and interventions with the client may involve the following strategies and methods [12,13]:

- Assess the development of human capacities including motor, cognition, perception and communication/interaction skills that are undeveloped or have been impaired
- Assess human capacities (e.g., neuromuscular, sensory, visual, perceptual, cognitive) including body systems and structures (e.g., cardiovascular, digestive, integumentary, genitourinary systems)
- Support skills to develop or redevelop habits, routines, roles, and behavior patterns
- Maintain and augment human capacity in everyday life activities
- Prevent barriers to skilled development and human performance
- Promote health and wellness to improve performance in daily life activities
- Support adaptation of physical, cognitive, neuromuscular, sensory functions, and behavioral skills
- Encourage skilled use of self in the therapeutic process
- Offer instructions to individuals and caregivers

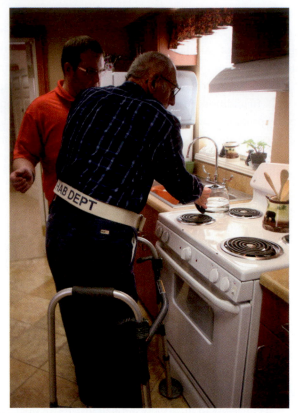

FIGURE 20-2 Therapy student is teaching the patient how to safely make a cup of coffee while using a walker.

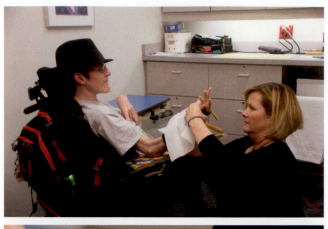

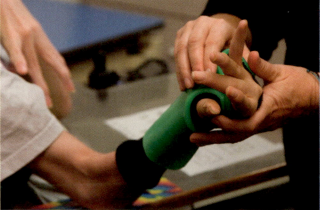

FIGURE 20-3 One of the roles of an occupational therapist is helping to create assistive devices such as splints. In these photos, the occupational therapist is creating and fitting a client with a splint to enhance hand movement and coordination.

- Coordinate and manage care

- Consult

- Assess, design, fabricate, and instruct in the use of assistive technologies and adaptive, orthotic, and prosthetic devices (Fig. 20-3)

- Use physical agent modalities to enhance performance skills

The process of evaluation and interventions using skilled application of daily life activities may involve the following strategies and methods [12,13]:

- Skilled use of exercise, daily life tasks, and occupations

- Skills training in self-care, home management, leisure, and work tasks

- Use of daily life tasks and activities to enhance daily life skills

- Assessment, recommendations, and training in techniques to ensure mobility and wheelchair use

- Skills training with driving and community mobility

- Skills training with feeding, eating, and swallowing to ensure nutritional demands

The process of interventions for modifying or adapting environments to support daily activities may involve the following strategies and methods [12,13]:

- Evaluate social, cultural, physical, and spiritual contexts and environments that affect engagement in daily life activities

- Modify environment and use ergonomic principles in home, work, school, and community settings

The AOTA Practice Framework outlines these general areas and helps to guide the occupational therapist and occupational therapy assistant in their practice by describing core concepts that are foundational to occupational therapy practice and enacting the profession's vision.[1]

Required Education

Most state licensure boards recognize four degrees of education for occupational therapists: an entry-level baccalaureate degree (this level of training was discontinued in 2004), an entry-level master's of occupational therapy degree (MOT, MSOT, etc.), an entry-level occupational therapy doctorate (OTD, DOT, etc.), and a 2-year associate degree to practice as an occupational therapy assistant (Fig. 20-4) (OTA). All states require completion of an occupational therapy or occupational therapy assistant program accredited by the Accreditation Council for Occupational Therapy Education (ACOTE).[11] Fieldwork requirement averages 24 weeks for those studying occupational therapy and 20 weeks for the occupational therapy assistant program. After successfully completing the academic curriculum and fieldwork education, graduates must pass a national certification examination administered by the National Board for Certification in Occupational Therapy (NBCOT).

Core courses in either the master's or doctoral entry-level programs include the following[11,12,13]:

- Anatomy
- Physiology
- Neuroscience
- Abnormal psychology/psychopathology
- Life span development
- Foundation of occupational therapy
- Activity analysis
- Theories of occupation or **occupational performance**
- Group process
- Environmental adaptation
- Health and wellness
- Research and methods
- Management of occupational therapy services

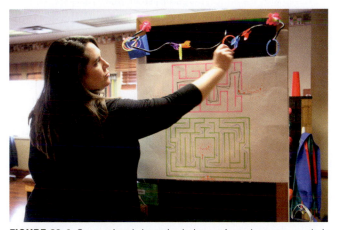

FIGURE 20-4 Occupational therapist helps patients learn to use their motor skills more effectively. This occupational therapy assistant is teaching a patient about gross and fine motor skills and the best strategies for effective use.

- Evaluation and treatment of occupation dysfunction
- Fieldwork education experience and licensure

Specific licensure requirements vary from state to state. Most states require occupational therapists to successfully complete an accredited program and fieldwork experience, pass the NBCOT examination, and pay a state licensing fee. Some states also require first-time license applicants to take a test on the rules and regulations specific to that state. Likewise, maintenance of one's license varies according to the state. Most states require the therapist to renew his or her license every 1 to 2 years. License renewal usually mandates the occupational therapist to complete a certain number of professional development units (PDUs) early. These PDUs can be earned by such activities as attending conferences, workshops, and classes; performing professional services, such as mentoring an occupational therapy colleague or volunteering for an organization; and presenting or publishing professionally.

Salary

The average annual income for occupational therapists is $65,000, and the average salary for occupational therapy assistants is $44,000.[14] Entry-level salaries average $52,000 for occupational therapists and $34,298 for occupational therapy assistants. Salaries vary according to the chosen field of practice, employment shortage, geographical location, and years of experience. Those working in long-term care facilities earn more than those in the school system. Competition among employers to hire qualified, licensed occupational therapists sometimes results in sign-on bonuses, generous coverage of moving expenses, and/or tuition reimbursement programs. Occupational therapy and occupational therapy assistant services are often supported by federal laws and programs such as the Affordable Care Act, **Americans with Disabilities Act,** IDEA, Medicare/Medicaid, and many others. It is important for occupational therapy practitioners to understand how federal laws can affect reimbursement for their services.

Trends

According to the most recent Workforce Trends in Occupational Therapy, the largest employers of occupational therapists and occupational therapy assistants are hospitals (26%), school systems (22%), and nursing facilities (20%).[14] The other 32% of occupational therapists work in outpatient clinics (9%), home health (6%), academia (5%), early intervention (5%), community health programs (4%), and mental health (3%). Hospital employment is expected to be the highest-need area of occupational therapy services because of the increasing needs of aging baby boomers. Within the hospital system, new service areas such as low-vision rehabilitation, treatment of dementia and Alzheimer disease, and older driver safety and rehabilitation have developed to meet the needs of an aging population and their increasing demand for services. As a result, employment for occupational therapists and occupational therapy assistants is expected to grow 29% between 2012 and 2022.[14,15]

Challenges

A challenge facing occupational therapists in hospitals or skilled nursing facilities is the stress that comes from trying to meet productivity demands. Most facilities measure productivity by factoring the therapists' minutes of time worked over the number of minutes billed. For example, if a therapist is required to be 80% productive, he or she should bill for 385 minutes of treatment in an 8-hour (or 480-minute) day. The failure to meet a productivity standard can result in loss of merit increases, promotion, and, in severe cases, loss of job. Those who have difficulty meeting an employer's productivity standard often suffer from job-related stress. The frustration of not having ample time to complete treatments, meet client goals, and complete documentation creates a cycle the occupational therapist might feel powerless to change. Occupational therapists should reflect on the proper fit for a work environment where they can be productive and adequately challenged.[16]

Another common challenge in occupational therapy is the risk of back injury. Occupational therapists who work with large, deconditioned clients must have strength, agility, and stamina to help clients move in and out of beds and wheelchairs and on and off toilets and bath benches; they must be able to physically support these clients while assisting them in daily life activities.[16]

Opportunities

The occupational therapy profession continues to evolve. Areas of emerging practice include driver rehabilitation and

Reflections on a Daily Life Activity

To understand the "occupational nature" of a person today, one must understand the importance of daily life activities in one's own life. Occupational stories are told in many ways in our culture (e.g., obituaries, introducing oneself to people, casual conversations, and autobiographies). Write about one daily life activity and how important and meaningful that activity is to you as an occupational being.

training and universal design consulting. Additionally, the AOTA has a "Centennial Vision" focus on children and youth and mental health, in addition to other fields of occupational therapy.

Role of the Occupational Therapist

Occupational therapy's role in health care and within public health teams is to return an individual to daily life activities or occupations that are meaningful, purposeful, and goal directed. When one is faced with limited capacity to engage in these activities, it becomes the role of the occupational therapist to (1) improve the individual's capacity or skills, (2) use proficient and well-designed tasks and activities to develop skills, and/or (3) modify the environment for improved engagement in supporting life tasks and to recover

Aptitude Profile

The typical profile and aptitude of an occupational therapist is one who is creative and a problem solver—specifically one who is able to elicit information from the client and his or her family to design an individualized solution that addresses the primary concerns of the client. The occupational therapist establishes a therapeutic relationship with clients and their families and effectively explains to them that such adaptions are created for meeting the client's needs, values, and goals. Therefore, it is integral for an occupational therapist to cultivate effective listening skills, and then be able to clearly communicate options for the client. Following are key skills for success in occupational therapy:[17]

Advocate	Excellent communicator
Comfortable with ambiguity	Excellent listener
Compassionate	Logical
Creative	Motivating
Diverse interests and background	Sees more than one solution to a problem
Empathic	Self-aware and aware of others

the maximum level of independence. When the individual's skills are aligned with the individual's desires, there is greater quality of life, function, and independence. Occupational therapists work with infants, children, and adults of all ages who are experiencing physical, cognitive, developmental, and/or emotional impairment(s). Occupational therapists work in hospitals, private practice clinics, skilled nursing facilities, community mental health centers, and schools (Fig. 20-5). Their intended outcome is always to help the individual accomplish daily tasks with more self-confidence and independence.

Occupational therapists are skilled at interpreting the impact disease, developmental disabilities, injuries, mental illness, aging, and social and physical environmental barriers have on daily life activities. This occurs through skilled observations, interviewing techniques, and the use of standardized and nonstandardized assessments. With this knowledge, the occupational therapist designs individualized treatment plans to align with the individual's interests, capabilities, and environment (Fig. 20-6). The occupational therapist may recommend adaptation for the home, work, or community environment and may introduce adaptations and tools to make engagement in daily life activities easier. Occupational

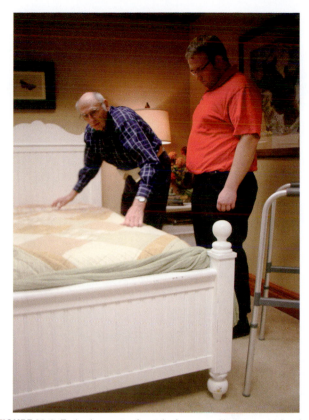

FIGURE 20-6 Tasks that most of us take for granted become a major challenge for those using a walker. The occupational therapy student is observing this patient make his bed. Many patients value their independence, so teaching them how to safely live independently is an important aspect of the therapist's role.

therapists review the treatment plans and treatment strategies, evaluate the individual's progress, and adjust the treatment plan accordingly. Role responsibilities of an occupational therapist and an occupational therapy assistant are similar; however, it is the occupational therapist who assumes the responsibility of directing the evaluation, designing the plan of care, and implementing the occupational therapy process. [18]

Role of the Occupational Therapy Assistant

The associate degree is the minimum standard degree required to practice as an **occupational therapy assistant.** Occupational therapy assistants work alongside occupational therapists in hospitals, community health centers, nursing facilities, mental health centers, and substance abuse agencies; they must, however, receive supervision from an occupational therapist to provide occupational therapy services (Fig. 20-7). The occupational therapist may direct the occupational therapy assistant to administer selected assessment tools and then interpret the information provided by the occupational

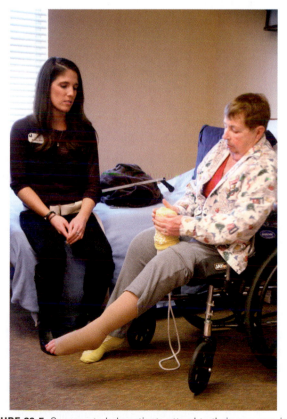

FIGURE 20-5 One way to help patients attend to their own care is for them to practice. In this photo, the occupational therapist is showing a patient how to put a sock onto a sock-aid. This practice will enhance the learning application for the patient's own needs.

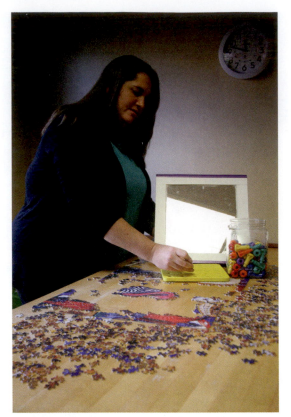

FIGURE 20-7 Learning ways to use fine motor skills improves application and enhances overall improvement. In this photo, the occupational therapy assistant is demonstrating the fine motor pegboard to a patient.

therapy assistant. Often, the occupational therapist and occupational therapy assistant collaborate with a client to develop a treatment plan. The occupational therapist determines when to delegate responsibilities to an occupational therapy assistant within the parameters of state law. [18]

Working Together

Occupational therapists collaborate with those in medicine, pharmacy, nursing, nutrition, physical therapy, health services and information management, rehabilitative counseling, and contractors. The collaboration with the other disciplines helps provide a holistic plan of care for the client. Formal collaborative meetings enable the primary-care team to understand each other's roles and provide strategies to support the client. In a structured program, particularly one that addresses a chronic and complex disease, care providers can develop common client goals and discuss a shared vision of service delivery. The occupational therapist might identify available programs that would benefit the client or discuss a gap in the client's options and suggest the development of a new program. This interprofessional care team works to ensure appropriate treatment and quality care.

CASE STUDY

Carol, a 55-year-old woman, was involved in a single-car motor vehicle accident and sustained multiple traumas, including traumatic brain injury, left upper-arm fracture, nerve injuries, and a crush injury of the left leg. The crush injury and infections of the left-lower leg led to three progressive amputations, resulting in an above-knee amputation. She is single with no children and currently living independently in a single-story house with a basement. Before her car accident, she was a faculty member at a local community college. After 2 years of rehabilitation, she has recently returned to her teaching role at the community college.

The rehabilitation team and I plan to reassess Carol's cognitive functions because her traumatic brain injury is causing damage to the exterior layer of the brain. The exterior brain tissue is responsible for executive function, or complex high-level processes such as thinking, remembering, and reasoning. Carol is given a battery of assessments by the psychologist, speech therapist, and me, the occupational therapist, to assess her cognitive abilities. The results indicate that Carol is performing strongly in the verbal domain, but is having difficulty in the areas of reasoning, perceptual speed, and memory. These cognitive deficits have a large impact on her work. Her difficulties in memorizing multiple work-related details make it hard for her to remember all of her meetings and appointments and arrive on time. She also has problems prioritizing work tasks due to the decreased ability to reason and process information quickly.

Carol's joint range of motion and strength in her arms and hands are decreased due to the peripheral nerve damage she sustained in the automobile accident. She continues to have limited-hand function due to flexion contractures of the left and right finger joints of the middle, ring, and little finger joints. Carol had been seen by a local occupational therapist who specializes in hand therapy for passive range of motion and functional activities. Carol is right-hand dominant, so these losses to her range of motion and strength, especially in her right hand, make it difficult to word process efficiently. She needs more time to prepare her course syllabus and lecture topics. These losses also decrease her e-mail communications with colleagues and students.

The amputation of her left lower leg affects Carol's ability to walk and impairs her balance; her walking speed is decreased, as is her endurance for walking, due to the increased energy demands that an amputation and prosthetic limb require. Carol requires extra time to get from her office to meetings or classes and greater endurance to negotiate the long hallways.

Carol has returned to a half-time faculty position. The Americans with Disabilities Act (ADA) requires employers to make reasonable accommodations to the workspace and/or job description to allow individuals with disabilities to return to work. Initially, Carol felt that she was being discriminated against in the workplace because of her disabilities. Her supervisor, a human resources representative, a physical therapist, a speech therapist, her physician, a vocational rehabilitation representative, and the occupational therapist meet to establish her needs and accommodations. Together the team agrees on a revised job description for Carol. It is noteworthy that Carol's decrease in cognitive functioning is a major reason why she is having trouble completing tasks necessary to maintain her classes. Carol contends that she was minimally involved in the team meeting and believes the college's needs have been put before her own needs. How can the interprofessional team work in collaboration with Carol and her college and keep her central to the care plan and outcome?

Questions

1. What disciplines must be involved in meeting Carol's goals and outcomes?
2. What are the goals for Carol's care?
3. How can the interprofessional team address Carol's concerns?
4. Why is interprofessional collaboration important in this case?
5. Why do you think Carol is disenfranchised from her plan of care?
6. What recommendations would enhance interprofessional collaboration and enhance Carol's involvement with her plan of care?

Review Questions

1. What historical event and philosophy has had the largest impact on the development of the occupational therapy profession?
   A. Revolutionary War
   B. Civil War
   C. Moral Treatment
   D. Affordable Care Act

2. What is one of the most common challenges in the occupational therapy profession?
   A. Back injuries
   B. Fatigue
   C. Meeting production standards
   D. Attending meetings

3. What health and human services setting is the largest employer of occupational therapy?
   A. Hospitals
   B. Home health agencies
   C. Behavioral health centers
   D. Community health programs

4. The scope of practice for an occupational therapist is based on evaluation and intervention focusing on which of the following considerations?
   A. Improve human capacity
   B. Engage in all daily life activities
   C. Modify and adapting the environment
   D. All the above

5. The largest employer of occupational therapists and assistants is:
   A. School systems
   B. Home health agencies
   C. Hospitals
   D. Nursing homes

6. What service requires the occupational therapist to interpret the information provided by the occupational therapy assistant after establishing service competencies?
   A. Treatment planning
   B. Evaluation
   C. Home adaptation
   D. Driver's rehabilitation

7. What are the key beliefs of occupational therapy?
   A. Recognize human capacity for growth and self-understanding
   B. Understand the power of occupation
   C. Understand the influence of the social and physical environment
   D. All of the above

8. After completing academic courses in occupational therapy, an occupational therapy student must complete how many weeks of fieldwork?
   A. 10 weeks
   B. 20 weeks
   C. 24 weeks
   D. 30 weeks

9. What level of degree must a student attain currently to practice as an occupational therapist?

   A. Bachelor's of occupational therapy

   B. Master's of occupational therapy

   C. Doctor of occupational therapy

   D. B and C

10. When occupational therapists and occupational therapy assistants work collaboratively, which tasks require supervision by the occupational therapist?

    A. Evaluations

    B. Implementation of treatment

    C. Treatment planning

    D. All of the above

Glossary of Key Terms

Occupational therapist—a health-care professional charged with improving a client's function and skills through meaningful activities, adapting a client's environment, and educating the client and the client's family to facilitate enhanced performance of daily activities

Individuals with Disabilities Education Improvement Act (IDEA) of 2004—a law requiring public schools to create and implement an individual educational plan (IEP) for every child between the ages of 3 to 20 who qualifies and receives special education services.

Individual educational plan—a planning document indicating the learning needs of the child, the services the school will provide, and indicators of success for learning and participation.

Affordable Care Act of 2010—a law to improve access, quality, and affordability of health-care services in the United States

Occupations—the everyday life activities that have meaning, purpose, and goal directedness for the individual to participate in roles and situations in home, school, workplace, community, and other settings

Activities of daily living (ADLs)—essential everyday activities a person does to care for oneself and protect one's health

Moral Treatment—a belief of treating mental illness with human kindness, respect, and a daily structure originating both from psychiatry and religious or moral concerns between the 18th and 19th centuries

Occupational performance—the capacity to perform daily life activities that fulfill one's roles according to one's life stage, cultural norms, and environments

American Disabilities Act of 1990 (ADA)—a law guaranteeing people with disabilities to have the same opportunities as all people to participate in employment, purchase goods and services, and participate in all government programs and services

Occupational therapy assistant—a health-care professional who collaborates with the occupational therapist to improve a client's function and skills through meaningful activities, adapting a client's environment, and educating the client and the client's family to facilitate enhanced performance of daily activities. The occupational therapy assistant is supervised and works under the license of the occupational therapist.

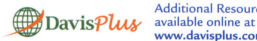 Additional Resources are available online at www.davisplus.com

Additional Resources

Accrediting Body

Accreditation Council for Occupational Therapy Education—www.aota.org/Educate/Accredit.aspx

The Accreditation Council for Occupational Therapy Education (ACOTE) is the accrediting agency for occupational therapy education; it ensures and enhances the quality of occupational therapy education.

Educational and Professional Resources

American Journal of Occupational Therapy—www.aota.org/Pubs/AJOT_1.aspx

The *American Journal of Occupational Therapy* (AJOT) is a refereed professional journal with a focus on research, practice, and health-care issues in the field of occupational therapy.

The Occupational Therapy Practice Framework: Domain and Process, 3rd Edition—http://myaota.aota.org/shop_aota/prodview.aspx?TYPE=D&PID=786&SKU=1227A

The *Occupational Therapy Practice Framework* is a document to communicate interrelated ideas that define and guide the practice of occupational therapy and promoting health through engagement in occupation.

American Occupational Therapy Association (AOTA)—www.aota.org

The American Occupational Therapy Association (AOTA) is the largest membership organization of professional occupational therapists in the world. The association supports professional development, ensures professional standards, and supports health policy.

Considering an Occupational Therapy Career?—www.aota.org/Education-Careers/Considering-OT-Career.aspx

This link provides stories about how students discovered a career in occupational therapy, describes how occupational practitioners work with clients, and discusses future job prospects.

World Federation of Occupational Therapists (WFOT)—www.wfot.org

The World Federation of Occupational Therapists (WFOT) is an international association of occupational therapists that began in 1951 to promote occupational therapy internationally.

Regulatory Body

National Board of Certification in Occupational Therapy (NBCOT)—www.nbcot.org

The National Board of Certification in Occupational Therapy (NBCOT) is a credentialing agency that provides certification for the occupational therapy profession.

Research

American Occupational Therapy Foundation (AOTF)—www.aotf.org

The American Occupational Therapy Foundation (AOTF) is a nonprofit organization supporting occupational therapy research and understanding of the relationship between daily life activities and health.

References

1. American Occupational Therapy Association. Occupational therapy practice framework: Domain and process.

   http://ajot.aota.org/.
   Accessed October 11, 2013.

2. Vallance JT. *The Lost Theory of Asclepiades of Bithynia*. Oxford, UK: Clarendon Press; 1990.

3. Peloquin SM. Moral treatment: Contexts considered. *Am J Occup Ther.* 1989;43(8):537–544.

4. Bockoven JS. *Moral Treatment in American Psychiatry*. New York, NY: Springer Publishing; 1963.

5. Bing RK. Occupational therapy revisited: A periphrastic journey. *Am J Occup Ther.* 1981;35:499–518.

6. Levine RE. The influence of the Arts and Crafts movement on the professional status of occupational therapy. *Am J Occup Ther.* 1987;41(4):248–254.

7. Quiroga VAM. *Occupational Therapy History: The First 30 Years, 1900 to 1930*. Bethesda, MD: American Occupational Therapy Association; 1995.

8. Law M, Polatajko H, Baptiste W, Townsend E. Core concepts of occupational therapy. In: Townsend E, ed. *Enabling Occupation: An Occupational Therapy Perspective*. Ottawa, ON: Canadian Association of Occupational Therapists; 1997.

9. Vanier J. *Community and Growth*. New York, NY: Paulist Press; 1979.

10. Downey M. *A Blessed Weakness: The Spirit of Jean Vanier and l'Arche*. San Francisco, CA: Harper & Row; 1986.

11. Coppard BM, Dickerson A. A descriptive review of occupational therapy education. *Am J Occup Ther.* 2007; 61:672–677.

12. American Occupational Therapy Association, Accreditation Council for Occupational Therapy. *Education Standards for Occupational Therapy, 2011 Edition*.

    http://www.aota.org/Education-Careers/Accreditation/Overview.aspx.
    Accessed October 23, 2013.

13. American Occupational Therapy Association, Accreditation Council for Occupational Therapy. *Education Standards for Occupational Therapy, 2011 Edition*.

    http://www.aota.org/Educate/Accredit/Standards Review.aspx.
    Accessed October 11, 2013.

14. American Occupational Therapy Association. *AOTA 2010 Occupational Therapy Compensation and Workforce Report*. Bethesda, MD: AOTA Press; 2010.

15. Bureau of Labor Statistics, U.S. Department of Labor. Occupational outlook handbook, 2012–2013 edition, occupational therapy assistants and aides.

    http://www.bls.gov/ooh/. . ./occupational-therapy-assistants-and-aides.htm.
    Accessed December 16, 2013.

16. National Career Services. Job profile: Occupational therapist.

    https://nationalcareersservice.direct.gov.uk/advice/planning/jobprofiles/Pages/occupationaltherapist.aspx.
    Accessed October 24, 2014.

17. American Occupational Therapy Association. Guidelines for supervision, roles, and responsibilities during the delivery of occupational therapy services. *Am J Occup Ther.* 2009;63: 797–803.

18. Ohio Occupational Therapy, Physical Therapy, and Athletic Trainers Board. Comparison of responsibilities of occupational therapy practitioners in school-based practice.

http://otptat.ohio.gov/Portals/0/Pdfs/Comparison%20of%20Responsibilities%20of%20Occupational%20Therapy%20Practitioners%20in%20School%20March%202011.pdf.

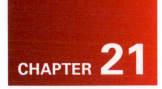
Physical Therapy

Deanna Dye, PT, PhD

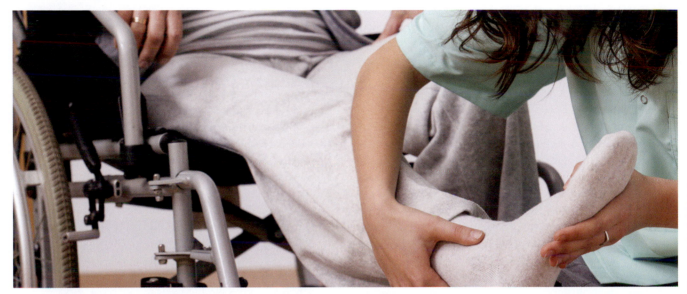

Photo credit: istock/Thinkstock

Learning Objectives

After reading this chapter, students should be able to:

- Articulate the history, development, and current role of the physical therapy professional
- Describe the different educational and licensing requirements of the physical therapist and the physical therapist assistant
- Identify the various practice settings for physical therapy professionals
- Recognize the patient management process of the physical therapist
- Discuss the relationships of the physical therapy professional with other health-care professionals
- Articulate the various opportunities and challenges facing the physical therapy profession

Key Terms

- Evaluate
- Range of motion
- Strength
- Vital signs
- Exertion tolerance
- Movement
- Life span
- Interventions
- Therapeutic exercise
- Manual therapy
- Functional activities
- Therapy
- Autonomous practice
- Specialization
- Practice setting
- Rehabilitation
- Anatomy
- Physiology
- Kinesiology
- Diagnosis
- Body systems
- Examination
- Plan of care
- Lymphedema

"A Day in the Life"

Hello, my name is Jason and I am a physical therapist (PT) working in an acute-care hospital. I work with the patients who are currently in the hospital for a variety of reasons. This is the fifth day of my 7-day shift. I work 7 days straight and then have 7 days off. I am off to our daily planning meeting to identify the patients I will be treating today. There are four PTs and three physical therapist assistants (PTAs) working today in our facility. At our daily planning meeting I learned that in addition to the seven patients I worked with yesterday, I have three new patients to see. Their diagnoses vary. We will be seeing Mrs. Brown, who had a stroke, on the neurological floor; Mr. Vasquez, who had open heart surgery, on the cardiac floor; and Jamie Jones, who broke her ankle and just had surgery this morning. Before heading to the patient rooms, I checked their past medical histories. I checked Mrs. Brown's laboratory reports, Jamie's surgical report, and Mr. Vasquez's daily reports. I recently read a research article that used a sit-to-stand test to predict a patient's likelihood of being discharged to home. I plan to apply this test with my care of Mrs. Brown.

I've asked Gail, the PTA, to come with me while I **evaluate** Mrs. Brown, who had a stroke. First, I'm stopping at the nurses' station to speak with Mrs. Brown's nurse, Nick, to discuss any concerns before working with the patient. I need to know if she has complained of any dizziness when she gets out of bed or if she has reported any other medical concerns today.

After introductions and a check of Mrs. Brown's blood pressure and heart rate, we were able to evaluate her performance of **range of motion** and **strength** of her arms and legs. We helped her work on her balance by having her sit on the edge of the bed and reach in multiple directions while we constantly watched and monitored her **vital signs.** Gail had to physically guard Mrs. Brown as she performed the reaching to prevent her from falling. Due to her lack of strength and balance, we decided not to perform any standing or walking at this time.

Next we went to see Jamie, who had surgery on her ankle. She needed instruction on how to walk with crutches while keeping all the weight off her injured ankle. We also had to show her how to move from sitting to standing and how to go up and down stairs. First, we checked her strength and general mobility to make sure she would be safe to get out of bed. She then demonstrated the ability to perform all the activities with minimal instruction and guarding. I will go speak with the social worker and let her know that from a physical therapy standpoint, Jamie is able to be discharged from the hospital. Next, we went to see Mr. Vasquez, who was just completing a breathing treatment with a respiratory therapist when we arrived at his room. We discussed his condition with the respiratory therapist and determined we should use 4 liters of oxygen when walking today. Before we worked with Mr. Vasquez, we again checked with his nurse to make sure she knew we were going to be having him exercise and walk and to be sure she had no concerns. While carefully monitoring Mr. Vasquez's vital signs, we had him perform some easy range-of-motion exercises while sitting and standing. Then we had him walk in the hallway while we kept track of his vital signs, distance, and time spent walking. We were able to determine his **exertion tolerance** with the data collected and will compare his progress day to day. All in all, it's been a pretty exciting day. Now I'll go back to the office to finish documenting all our care.

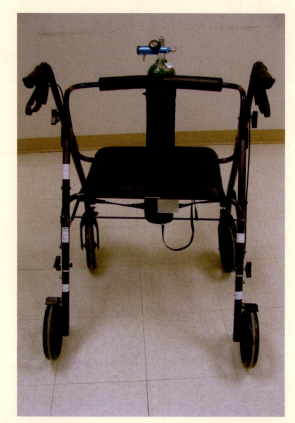

This type of walker can be used to assist patients with walking. The walker provides mobility and independence for patients.

Introduction to Physical Therapy

What Is Physical Therapy?

According to the *Guide to Physical Therapy Practice*,[1] "physical therapy is defined as the care and services provided by or under the direction and supervision of a physical therapist." Well, that is perfectly clear. So, who is a physical therapist (PT), and what does a PT do? A PT has a degree in physical therapy from an accredited graduate-level program. The World Confederation for Physical Therapy (WCPT)[2] provides this definition of physical therapy: "Physical therapy provides services to individuals and populations to develop, maintain and restore maximum **movement** and functional ability throughout the **life span.** This includes providing services in circumstances where movement and function are threatened by ageing, injury, pain, diseases, disorders, conditions or environmental factors. Functional movement is central to what it means to be healthy."

Physical therapists are often helped by physical therapist assistants (PTAs), who usually have an associate degree from an accredited physical therapist assisting program. Physical therapist assistant is another career choice in physical therapy. PTAs help carry out physical therapy interventions directed by the PT and are a valuable part of the profession.

Physical therapists primarily apply physical **interventions** to restore a person's ability to engage in life with the fewest physical restrictions possible. Some of the interventions a PT uses include **therapeutic exercise; manual therapy,** including massage, soft tissue, or joint mobilization; **functional activities;** and application of heat or cold. The PT examines the patient to determine what he or she is able and unable to do and then decides if the cause of the inability is something the PT can address, such as weakness, inflexibility, muscle spasm, discoordination, or pain. If the PT determines that physical **therapy** can help, a plan of care is developed with the patient. We look at that process in more detail later in the chapter.

History and Professional Organization

Physical therapy began, as did many allied health professions, from a societal need. Contrary to the conventions of the time, soldiers injured during World War I received recovery assistance from restoration aides who were exclusively women (Fig. 21-1). In fact, the first national association was called the American Women's Physical Therapeutic Association founded in 1921. Men were included into the profession in the 1930s and the association's name was changed to the

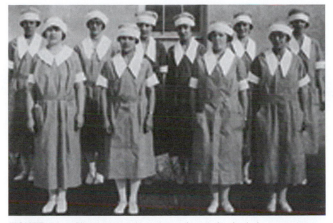

FIGURE 21-1 First graduating class. Army physical therapy course, 1923. (From U.S. Army Medical Department, Office of Medical History. Accessed March 31, 2015. Photo from U.S. Army Medical Department Office of Medical History website. http://history.amedd.army.mil/corps/medical_spec/chapterIII.html.)

American Physiotherapy Association. Physical therapy merged into the medical community largely during the polio epidemic and after World War II in the 1940s and 1950s.[3-5] Physical therapy's foundation is a combination of physical education and medical knowledge. The first PTs used exercise, braces, electrical therapy, aquatic therapy, and heat and cold application. Children afflicted with polio lost the use of their muscles because of nerve damage. Physical therapists frequently worked with these children in pool settings to help strengthen their muscles. In addition to strengthening, braces were fitted to support the legs so the child could learn to walk again. With soldiers, group classes for strengthening and flexibility were conducted in addition to individual care (Fig. 21-2). The goal was to get the person, child, or soldier back to living fully with the least amount of mobility restriction.

Since its beginnings, physical therapy has been represented by a national organization currently named the American Physical Therapy Association (APTA). It has over 77,000 members, mainly licensed physical therapists and PTAs, and serves to promote the profession by sharing information with the public, insurance companies, Congress, and of course its own members.[3] Members of the APTA may be seen on Capitol Hill speaking with congressional representatives about issues important to the profession. APTA-created advertisements promoting and highlighting the benefits of physical therapy appear in magazines and on television. Members may meet directly with insurance company representatives to share and educate them on the practice of physical therapy. The APTA is driven by the membership and has chapters in every state. These chapters promote and support the profession at the state level. Being a member

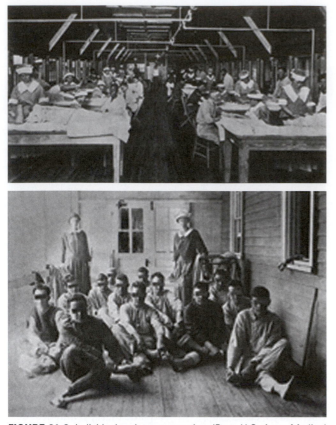

FIGURE 21-2 Individual and group exercise. (From U.S. Army Medical Department, Office of Medical History. Accessed March 31, 2015. Photo from U.S. Army Medical Department Office of Medical History website. http://history.amedd.army.mil/corps/medical_spec/chapterIII.html.)

of the APTA is a great way for a physical therapy professional to stay up to date with current practice and network with colleagues.

The APTA helps unify the profession through a common vision and set of values. It also helps define best practices. The APTA's vision statement expresses the long-term goal that physical therapists be recognized as the first-line health-care provider of choice for people with movement disorders. In addition to its vision, the APTA has an established Code of Ethics and Core Values identifying and defining exemplary professional conduct. A major accomplishment helping to explain the practice of physical therapy is the APTA's *Guide to Physical Therapist Practice.*[1] This book helps identify the types of disorders addressed, the method of examination, and the common tests, measures, and interventions used by physical therapists. A wealth of information is available at APTA's website (www.apta.org).

Today there are over 200,000 PTs and over 66,000 PTAs in the United States.[6] Women still outnumber men, 68% to 32%.[3,5] The median salary for a PT in 2013 was $81,000 with an average salary range from $56,000 to $113,000.[7] The median salary for a PTA in 2013 was $53,000 with an average

salary range from $32,000 to $73,000.[8] Physical therapists and their assistants work in a variety of settings and with all types of injuries and dysfunctions. The goal, as always, is to return people to their highest level of physical function.

Work Settings

Acute-Care Hospital

Although PTs first began by working in hospitals and the military, only about 11% of PTs practice in acute-care

Food for Thought

"By definition then, physical therapy is a health profession that emphasizes the sciences of pathokinesiology and the application of therapeutic exercise for the prevention, evaluation, and treatment of disorders of human motion."

—Helen Hislop[9]

hospitals today.[3,10,11] Working in acute care requires special knowledge to monitor exercise tolerance and manage complex problems. Patients often have many medical issues requiring a highly organized team approach to care. A PT's role may be to help someone walk who is currently using a ventilator to breathe. A patient may have multiple fractures and need to be taught certain restrictions to movement. The skill of an acute-care PT consists of sound judgment and keen observation. The acute-care PT's primary role is to keep patients mobile to avoid the detrimental effects of bedrest while balancing proper rest for optimal healing.

Outpatient Clinic

As the profession has expanded in scope and autonomy. The majority of PTs and PTAs (55%) work in outpatient clinics, either privately or group owned, or as part of a hospital system.[2,10] Patients who come to an outpatient clinic can have a variety of issues. The clinic may specialize in a particular area. Some clinics treat patients with spinal dysfunctions such as low back pain or whiplash. Other clinics primarily treat athletes who have sustained a sports-related injury. Still other clinics may see patients with neurological problems such as a spinal cord injury or balance dysfunction. Patients live at home and come to the clinic for continued care. They

may need care 5 days a week or only require 1 day a week. The amount of care depends on the patient's needs.

Skilled Nursing Facility or Long-Term Care

Only about 5% of PTs and 18% of PTAs work in long-term care. This area of practice is growing along with the aging population (over 65).[3,10,11] Physical therapists working in long-term care may have **specialization** in geriatrics to provide optimal care to the elderly. Knowing the anatomical and physiological changes that occur with aging is essential when prescribing appropriate exercises and activities. In addition to natural changes with age, many older adults have chronic medical problems such as heart disease, chronic lung problems, or degenerative arthritis that must be addressed. Individualized attention is the key to working in this **practice setting.**

Home Health

Home health is a unique practice setting. Nearly 7% of PTs choose to treat patients in the patients' own home.[10,11] Patients can be any age but must have significant difficulty leaving their home. Special regulations and criteria must be met for a patient to be eligible to receive home health. The home health therapist has to be very resourceful because there is often limited equipment and space. Creative use of the patient's own home items makes for effective care. For strengthening, the PT might have the patient carry a load of laundry; for balance, the PT could have the patient reach into cupboards or walk around obstacles in the room. The home health therapist also has to be medically astute. Often the therapist may be the one to alert the medical team of a decline in the patient's medical condition that may warrant

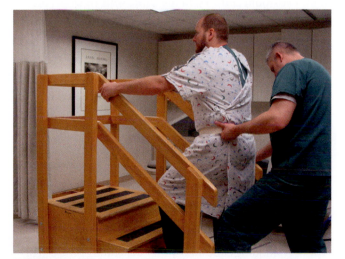

FIGURE 21-3 Physical therapist teaching a patient to climb stairs.

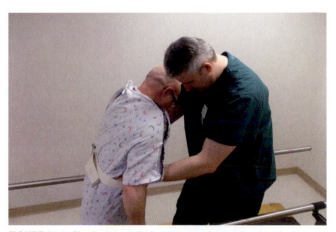

FIGURE 21-4 Physical therapist helping a patient walk using the balance bars.

either a visit to the physician or a trip to the hospital. There is never a dull moment when working in home health.

Teaching

About 10% of PTs and 5% of PTAs engage in teaching within the profession as faculty members of a physical therapy program.[10,11] Those who teach primarily work at universities and need to have a doctorate degree. Many programs prefer that the faculty member also has a specialist certification as well. Those teaching at the PTA level usually have a minimum of a bachelor's degree, but most have a master's degree.

Other Practice Settings

About 3% to 5% of PTs and PTAs work in inpatient **rehabilitation** centers. These centers have patients staying in the facility and learning skills to be able to return home. Usually the patient has suffered a catastrophic injury such as a spinal cord injury, stroke, or traumatic brain injury. Patients stay at the facility between 1 and 12 weeks depending on their needs.

About 7% of PTs and 1.5% of PTAs work in the school system addressing the needs of children with disabilities. This setting is unique, and service is mandated by law. All care must be targeted toward improving the child's ability to learn and engage with peers.

A few PTs work with industry, helping companies with wellness programs or workplace ergonomics.[10,11]

Education

Physical therapy education has changed dramatically over the years as the professional knowledge and skill base has expanded. The first education program was through the military and in the 1920s consisted of 4 months of training; this was expanded to 12 months in the late 1930s (Fig. 21-5). Today, students training to be PTs need to have at least a bachelor's degree before applying for acceptance into a graduate program in physical therapy. The bachelor's degree can be in any field as long as it fulfills the prerequisites of the physical therapy program. Currently, all physical therapy programs are at the doctorate degree level. Most programs last 3 years with combined classroom and clinical course work. Programs range from 90 to 120 credit hours. The curriculum consists of courses in **anatomy, physiology, kinesiology,** neuroscience, pathology, biomechanics, physical therapy–specific **diagnosis,** and in-depth study of four **body systems**—musculoskeletal, neuromuscular, cardiovascular and pulmonary, and integumentary. About 80% of time is spent in the classroom and 20% in the clinical setting with an average of 27.5 weeks of clinical experience/internships.[12]

Subject	Hours
Anatomy:	
Theory	38
Laboratory	61
Physiology:	
Theory	16
Laboratory	16
Massage:	
Theory	38
Laboratory	74
Hydrotherapy	4
Electrotherapy	6
Remedial exercise:	
Theory	33
Laboratory	33
Pathology	26
Kinesiology	6
Psychology	10
Hospital management	2
Emergency treatment and bandaging	23
Personal hygiene	3
Ethics of nurses	2
Surgical clinic	15
Reconstruction clinic[1]	163
Development group exercise	28
Recreational exercise	23
Total hours	620

[1] Practical experience in the actual treatment of patients.

FIGURE 21-5 Original curriculum—1918. (From U.S. Army Medical Department, Office of Medical History. Accessed March 31, 2015. Photo from U.S. Army Medical Department Office of Medical History website. http://history.amedd.army.mil/corps/medical_spec/chapterIII.html.)

Students interested in becoming a PT can choose from over 200 accredited programs in the United States.[3,13]

Students training to be PTAs will need to obtain an associate degree. Most programs are within community colleges, though some are within universities and private colleges as well. Many programs have a competitive enrollment, and often students with current bachelor's or even master's degrees apply. Programs last 2 years, and many students take 1 additional year to complete general education requirements. The programs have both classroom and clinical coursework. Courses cover content in the areas of anatomy, physiology, biomechanics, kinesiology, clinical pathology, behavioral sciences, communication, ethics, and specific physical therapy interventions, as well as some tests and measures. On average, PTA students spend 75% of time in the classroom and 25% in the clinic with 16 weeks of full-time clinical experience/internship. Students interested in becoming a PTA can choose from over 300 accredited programs in the United States.[13,14] Prospective students can find a wealth of information at the APTA website (see www.apta.org/ProspectiveStudents).

Continuing Education

All PTs and PTAs must be committed to learning throughout their careers. Most states require that therapists engage in continuing education every year. Most physical therapy licensing boards require an average of 20 hours of continuing education per year for the licensee to maintain licensure.[3] The type of continuing education varies depending on the area of expertise for the therapist. Therapists can attend conferences and weekend workshops, do home study or online courses, or engage in scholarly writing. The main requirement is to be up to date with the best practice for the profession. Science in rehabilitation and health is constantly changing, and professional PTs must stay current to provide the best care for their patients.

Physical Therapists' Specialization Areas (Year Established)

- Cardiovascular and pulmonary physical therapy (1981)
- Clinical electrophysiological physical therapy (1982)
- Geriatric physical therapy (1989)
- Neurological physical therapy (1982)
- Orthopedic physical therapy (1981)
- Pediatric physical therapy (1981)
- Sports physical therapy (1981)
- Women's health (2006)

Note: Wound care has a residency but is not a specialty of the APTA.

Author Spotlight

Deanna Dye, PT, PhD

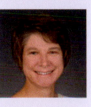

I have been practicing physical therapy for over 25 years. I graduated with a bachelor's degree and practiced in many different settings. My first job was at a hospital that had a satellite clinic 1 hour away in a rural county. I drove to the clinic each day seeing home health patients in route and also provided care for two nursing homes. I spent time working at a rehabilitation hospital with people who had sustained injury to their spinal cord resulting in various amounts of paralysis. This position led me to the area of adaptive recreation, which has been very rewarding. I have taught people with paralysis how to ski, paddle a canoe, and rock climb.

I discovered that I loved to teach, so I pursued my advanced degrees in education and taught for 17 years at both PTA and PT programs. While teaching I pursued specialized clinical training in vestibular dysfunction and wound care. I co-directed a dizziness and balance clinic during my time teaching at the PT program. Now, I work in a hospital clinic specifically in wound care. My career, so far, demonstrates how flexible and variable the profession can be. It allows you to keep your balance in life while constantly learning new skills and meeting new challenges. It is truly a profession that provides you a lifelong career.

After graduation, therapists may choose to specialize in a particular area of care. They can begin this process by performing a residency in one of nine areas of specialty, eight of which are recognized by the American Board of Physical Therapy Specialties.[3]

Scope of Practice of Physical Therapy

Patient Management Process

Physical therapy practice is directly guided by the patient-therapist relationship. There are three foundations of care: the scientific evidence, the therapist's experience, and the patient's goals. Applying these three foundations, the therapist uses an evaluative patient management process to design a plan of care for the patient (Fig. 21-6). The patient management process begins with an **examination.** The examination is a thorough process during which the PT gathers data about the patient. The data consist of several things related to the patient's reason for seeking physical therapy care. The patient's medical, social, and mental history is gathered primarily through an interview with the patient and with family members if indicated, or through the patient's medical record. A screen of the patient's general health requires assessing the condition of several body systems which include the function of the heart, lungs, muscles, nerves, and even digestion, hormones, and skin. A good portion of the screen occurs through the interview. It is this process that informs the PT if other medical professionals should be involved with the patient's care.

The physical examination is more specific to the patient's issue. Based on a hypothesis of the likely cause of the patient's symptoms, the therapist will choose certain tests and measures to confirm or refute this hypothesis. The PT may conduct muscle strength and endurance tests, special ligamentous and joint tests, or joint range of motion and muscle flexibility tests (Table 21-1). Based on the data, the PT decides on the course of action and treatment needed. An individualized **plan of care** is devised and various interventions implemented. That is where the fun begins. Depending on the condition, PTs spend much of their time actively moving. Whether it is teaching strengthening exercises, playing balancing games, setting up aerobic exercise programs, or physically stretching a patient's muscles, PTs are physically engaged in caring for their patients. In less complex patient cases, the plan may be carried out by a PTA instead.

Body Systems

Physical therapists work with disorders of four major body systems: the musculoskeletal system, the neuromuscular

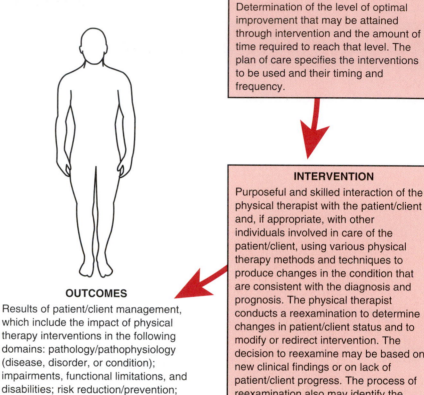

FIGURE 21-6 Elements of patient management leading to optimal outcomes. Reprinted with permission from American Physical Therapy Association.

system, the cardiovascular and pulmonary system, and the lymphatic and integumentary system.[1] Each system has unique issues and dysfunctions that can develop or occur at birth. The PT has a wealth of knowledge of each system and can choose appropriate tests and measures and design a plan of care with specific interventions to address that system.

Musculoskeletal

Within the musculoskeletal system, PTs address muscle, joint, and bone injuries or dysfunctions. This area of practice is often considered orthopedics. Patients may have a muscle strain or ligamentous sprain such as a hamstring tear or an ankle sprain. Patients may be recovering from surgery to replace a joint such as a total knee replacement or to repair a

fracture. Patients could be recovering from surgery to repair soft tissue damage such as a rotator cuff repair or a bicep tendon repair. All these conditions would fall under the musculoskeletal system. Physical therapists who work primarily in this system may specialize in orthopedic or perhaps sports physical therapy.

Neuromuscular

Within the neuromuscular system, PTs address issues of muscle control and coordination, balance, and overall functional mobility. This area of practice is often considered neurology. Physical therapists working with disorders of the neuromuscular system may work with children who have disorders from birth, such as cerebral palsy or muscular

TABLE 21-1 Common Tests and Measures and Interventions Used in Physical Therapy

Tests and Measures	Interventions
Aerobic capacity testing	Aerobic exercise
Breath sounds	Aquatic therapy
Breathing capacity	Balance activities
Balance	Electrical stimulation
Coordination	Gait training
Ergonomic analysis	Heat and cold application
Flexibility	Manual therapy
Gait analysis	Prosthetic and orthotic training
Joint integrity and mobility	Resistant exercise
Ligamentous integrity	Soft tissue mobilization
Muscle strength	Stretching
Posture assessment	Transfer training
Proprioception	Work retraining
Skin integrity and sensation	Wound care

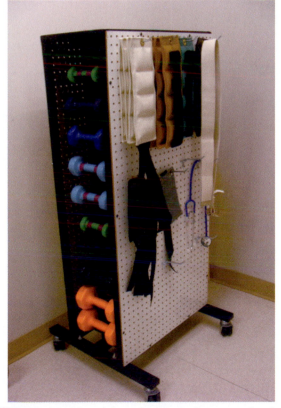

FIGURE 21-7 A weight rack is used to store various types of equipment used for patient care.

dystrophy. They can also work with adults who have sustained a traumatic brain injury, stroke, or spinal cord injury. Therapists can also work with patients who have multiple sclerosis or Parkinson's disease. Therapists who work primarily in this system may specialize in neurological physical therapy. If therapists are working primarily with children, they may have a pediatric specialty.

Cardiovascular and Pulmonary

Within the cardiovascular and pulmonary system, therapists address issues of exercise tolerance, endurance, and overall aerobic conditioning. Patients with primary dysfunction in the cardiovascular system may have had a heart attack or have a heart valve disorder. They may be recovering from open heart surgery to repair damage. Patients may have issues with circulation in their legs and have the condition of peripheral arterial disease. Patients with primary dysfunction in the pulmonary system may have chronic obstructive pulmonary disease (COPD) or may have exercise-induced asthma. Therapists who work primarily in this system may specialize in cardiovascular pulmonary physical therapy.

Lymphatic and Integumentary

Within the lymphatic and integumentary system, therapists address issues of swelling from poor lymphatic flow and skin damage from various wounds. This area of practice is often considered lymphatic therapy and wound and/or burn care. Patients may need lymphatic therapy if they have **lymphedema** acquired or as a result of surgery such as a mastectomy due to breast cancer. Patients needing wound care can present with a variety of wounds. Wounds can develop from lack of sensation such as ulcers on the feet of a patient with diabetes or from pressure on the sacrum of a patient with a spinal cord injury. Burns often require a very delicate and painful recovery. Many require a skin graft. Special knowledge of skin healing, bandaging, topical agents, and specialized dressings is required. Therapists working primarily with this system often have additional training in lymphatic therapy and wound care and hold additional certifications. (See Table 21-2 for common pathologies.)

Licensure

Physical therapists are licensed in all 50 states. Each state has specific licensing requirements along with a physical therapy practice act that identifies scope of practice and rules and regulations. To be licensed to practice as either a PT or a PTA, all states require candidates to pass the national physical therapy examination (NPTE), either the PT or PTA version, and graduate from an accredited or equivalent PT or PTA program. The NPTE is offered four times a year and is taken at specified testing centers within each state. In addition, most states require candidates to pass

TABLE 21-2 **Pathologies and Injuries Treated in Physical Therapy (Almost A–Z)**

Amputations	Ligament sprain/repair
Back pain	Meniscus tear
Burns	Myocardial infarction (heart attack)
Carpal tunnel syndrome	
Cerebral palsy	Multiple sclerosis
Chronic obstructive pulmonary disease	Osteoarthitis
	Parkinson's disease
Degenerative joint disease	Peripheral arterial disease (PAD)
Fractures	
Guillain-Barré syndrome	Rotator cuff tear/repair
Hamstring strain	Spinal cord injury
Herniated disc	Stroke
Incontinence	Traumatic brain injury
Knee replacement surgery	Vestibular neuritis
Labrum tear	Wounds
Lateral epicondylitis (tennis elbow)	

an examination that covers the state's specific rules and regulations, which is called a *jurisprudence* examination. Licenses can be transferred from state to state but are only valid in the state where they were issued. More information can be found at the Federation of State Boards of Physical Therapy's website (see www.fsbpt.org).

Trends, Challenges, and Aptitude

The future for physical therapy is bright. The aging population and improvements in medicine lead to a high demand for physical therapy professionals in the future. In fact, it is predicted that demand will likely exceed the supply of professionals.[3, 15] According to *U.S. News and World Report*, the Bureau of Labor Statistics believes the employment of physical therapists will increase by 36% by 2022.[16] In 2011, physical therapy was one of the "Ten Happiest Jobs" according to *Forbes*,[15] and it has consistently ranked high in the best 100 jobs in *U.S. News and World Report* (ranked eighth in 2013[15] and seventh in 2014[16]). Among health-care professions, physical therapy is ranked fifth.[16]

The profession continues to grow, with continued research honing the effectiveness of physical therapy interventions. This ongoing research will provide more and more evidence-based guidelines and best practices. The challenge will be for the profession to stay current and cost effective in a challenging health-care environment. Physical therapy professionals must be able to show that physical therapy improves a person's quality of life and is worth the cost of care. Physical therapy professionals must stay up to date with the latest changes in health care and scientific evidence. They must be efficient with their time and effective with their care. Physical therapy is a wonderful profession, whether as a PT or a PTA. It is always challenging, never boring, and extremely rewarding.

Aptitude Profile

Characteristics needed to succeed as a physical therapy professional can be summed up by the "five *C's*":

Natural Talent		Professional Characteristic
Cares for others	→	Compassionate
Likes to solve problems or puzzles	→	Critical thinker
Enjoys learning new things	→	Continued learner
Friendly, talkative, people person	→	Communicator
Makes decision after looking at all options	→	Clinical judgment

Working Together

Physical therapists work with many other health professionals. The amount of collaboration largely depends on the work setting and the health needs of the patient. Physical therapists working in a private practice outpatient clinic have the least direct collaboration. They interact primarily with the patient's medical physician and perhaps a social worker. In the hospital or inpatient rehabilitation setting, PTs interact with nurses, medical physicians and their assistants, social workers, respiratory therapists, occupational therapists, speech therapists, pharmacists, and dietitians on a regular basis. Each profession gives its unique insight and expertise regarding a patient's care. For instance, if a PT is working with a patient who has a pressure ulcer, the medical physician will be monitoring and coordinating the overall comprehensive plan of care for the patient. The PT needs to know the patient's nutritional status and consult with the dietitian regarding the recommended diet to encourage the patient to eat the proper foods needed for healing. Nursing will ensure proper bed mobility and hygiene care. The pharmacist assesses the patient's medications and checks for any medications that may impair healing, such as steroids. The social worker might investigate living arrangements needed once the patient leaves the hospital. All members of the interprofessional team must collaborate to ensure quality patient care.

CASE STUDY

Mrs. Maple is working with physical therapy after her 2-week stay in the hospital because of issues with congestive heart failure. Her past medical history includes a heart attack 15 years ago, type 2 diabetes, obesity, and high cholesterol. She quit smoking 5 years ago but still has difficulty with sustaining a healthy eating plan. She has returned to Good Sam's Nursing Home for some rehabilitation in the hope that she can then go back to her own home where she lives with her husband of 55 years. On examination, the physical therapist finds that Mrs. Maple has difficulty walking and low aerobic endurance with shortness of breath that limits her walking distance to 50 feet before needing a rest. She has been able to go up 2 steps with moderate assistance. She also has difficulty getting in and out of bed, showering, and getting dressed, primarily because of general decreased strength. Her difficulty walking requires her to use a walker for short distances. For longer distances she needs a wheelchair. She uses 3 liters of supplemental oxygen at rest and up to 6 liters when walking. To get in and out of bed, she has been using a hospital bed so that she can elevate the head of the bed to help her sit up and then needs moderate physical assistance to stand. She needs additional adaptive equipment for dressing and showering. Her husband is 75 years old and in good health. For her to successfully return home, she will need to walk 150 feet, get in and out of bed independently, shower with minimal assistance, and ascend and descend 5 steps. Their two children live within an hour's drive. Both work full-time jobs and have children of their own.

Questions

1. What are the barriers facing Mrs. Maple's personal goal to return home?
2. What are the primary physical therapy goals for Mrs. Maple's care?
3. What disciplines should be involved with Mrs. Maple's care?
4. Why is interprofessional collaboration important in this case?
5. Develop an interprofessional plan of care based on your knowledge from other chapters.
6. What are some barriers facing interprofessional collaboration?

Review Questions

1. Physical therapy was first used during which war?
   A. World War I
   B. World War II
   C. Vietnam War
   D. Korean War

2. Physical therapists were originally called:
   A. Physiotherapists
   B. Restoration aids
   C. Restorative nurses
   D. Physical education aids

3. Today, the national association that represents the profession of physical therapy is called the:
   A. National Physical Therapy Association
   B. Association of Physical Therapists and Assistants
   C. American Physical Therapy Association
   D. American Physiotherapy Women's' Association

4. Accredited academic programs for physical therapists award which entry-level degree?
   A. Associate
   B. Bachelor's
   C. Master's
   D. Doctorate

5. Approximately how many PTs are working in the United States?
   A. 50,000
   B. 200,000
   C. 500,000
   D. 1 million

6. During the physical examination of a patient, the PT will likely:
   A. Ask the patient to rate his or her pain
   B. Ask the patient his or her past medical history
   C. Perform specific tests and measures
   D. Develop the plan of care

7. A patient with an ankle sprain would be classified into which body system?
   A. Musculoskeletal
   B. Neuromuscular
   C. Cardiovascular
   D. Integumentary

8. PTs are licensed in every state.

   A. True

   B. False

9. Which of the following reasons were given for physical therapy to be in demand in the future?

   A. Schools are decreasing in number.

   B. Extreme sports are gaining popularity.

   C. The population is aging.

   D. All of the above are correct.

10. Characteristics to succeed as a physical therapy professional include compassion, critical thinking, communicating, creativity, and:

    A. Continued learning

    B. Cautiousness

    C. Capability

    D. Clarifying

Glossary of Key Terms

Evaluate—the interpretation of the results of the patient's examination, including all internal and external factors and determining whether treatment will help a patient and to what degree

Range of motion—the degree of movement of a joint that a person can obtain

Strength—the amount of tension a muscle can produce

Vital signs—measurements of the body's basic functions (heart rate, blood pressure, temperature, and respiratory rate)

Exertion tolerance—the amount of activity or work a person can do without exhaustion or injury

Movement—the complex interaction of the joints, muscles, and nervous system that results in motion

Life span—the entire life of an individual from birth to death

Interventions—any activity, device, or action used for treating an individual

Therapeutic exercise—movements or activities performed to address a specific need

Manual therapy—an intervention that uses the therapist's hands directly on the patient to mobilize muscles, soft tissues, or joints.

Functional activities—movements or activities that allow people to perform daily needs such as walking, moving from one position to another, climbing stairs, cooking, and bathing

Therapy—treatment of a disorder or condition

Autonomous practice—the ability to work with patients without the direction of another health professional, such as needing a prescription from a medical physician

Specialization—obtaining in-depth knowledge and skills in a particular area of practice

Practice setting—locations or organizations where therapists work

Rehabilitation—applying interventions to assist a person in recovery from an injury or illness

Anatomy—the structure of a body such as the bones, muscles, and organs

Physiology—the study of how the body works and functions

Kinesiology—the study of how a body moves

Diagnosis—assigning a label to a cluster of signs and symptoms that result in a dysfunction

Body systems—a group of the body's organs that work together to perform a function

Examination—the close inspection of a person through observation and conduction of tests and measures

Plan of care—an agreement between the patient and healthcare professional that details the service to be provided including frequency, length of time, and interventions

Lymphedema—swelling caused by a dysfunction of the lymphatic system

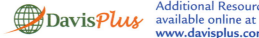

Additional Resources are available online at www.davisplus.com

References

1. American Physical Therapy Association. *Guide to Physical Therapist Practice,* rev 2nd ed. Alexandria, VA: American Physical Therapy Association; 2003.

2. World Confederation for Physical Therapy. Policy statement: Description of physical therapy. 2013. London, UK.

   http://www.wcpt.org/policy/ps-descriptionPT.
   Accessed December 20, 2014.

3. American Physical Therapy Association. *Today's Physical Therapist: A Comprehensive Review of a 21st-Century Health Care Profession.* Alexandria, VA: American Physical Therapy Association; 2011.

4. Murphy WB. *Healing the Generations: A History of Physical Therapy and the American Physical Therapy Association.* Alexandria, VA: American Physical Therapy Association; 1995.

5. American Physical Therapy Association. *APTA History*. Alexandria, VA: American Physical Therapy Association; 2013.

    http://www.apta.org/History/.

    Accessed January 24, 2014.

6. Federation of State Boards of Physical Therapy, Jurisdiction licensure reference guide topic: Number of PTs and PTAs by state. 2006.

    http://www.fsbpt.org/download/JLRG_Number OfPTsAndPTAs_200806.pdf.

    Accessed January 22, 2014.

7. Bureau of Labor Statistics. Occupational employment statistics May 2013. Physical therapist.

    http://www.bls.gov/oes/current/oes291123.htm.

    Accessed December 20, 2014.

8. Bureau of Labor Statistics. Occupational employment statistics May 2013. Physical therapist assistants.

    http://www.bls.gov/oes/current/oes312021.htm.

    Accessed December 20, 2014.

9. Hislop HJ. Tenth Mary McMillan Lecture: The not-so-impossible dream. *Phys Ther.* 1975;55:1069–1080.

10. American Physical Therapy Association. *Physical Therapist Member Demographic Profile 2010*. Alexandria, VA: American Physical Therapy Association; 2011.

    http://www.apta.org/WorkforceData/Demograph-icProfile/PTMember/.

    Accessed January 24, 2014.

11. American Physical Therapy Association. *Physical Therapist Assistant Member Demographic Profile 2010*. Alexandria, VA: American Physical Therapy Association; 2011.

    http://www.apta.org/WorkforceData/ DemographicProfile/PTAMember/.

    Accessed January 24, 2014.

12. American Physical Therapy Association. *Physical Therapist (PT) Education Overview*. Alexandria, VA: American Physical Therapy Association; 2013.

    http://www.apta.org/PTEducation/Overview/.

    Accessed January 24, 2014.

13. Commission on Accreditation in Physical Therapy Education. *Home Page: Quick Facts*. Alexandria, VA: American Physical Therapy Association; 2014.

    http://www.capteonline.org/home.aspx).

    Accessed February 2, 2014.

14. American Physical Therapy Association. *Physical Therapist Assistant (PTA) Education Overview*. Alexandria, VA: American Physical Therapy Association; 2013.

    http://www.apta.org/PTAEducation/Overview/.

    Accessed January 24, 2014.

15. American Physical Therapy Association. *Physical Therapist (PT) Careers Overview*. Alexandria, VA: American Physical Therapy Association; 2013.

    http://www.apta.org/PTCareers/Overview/.

    Accessed February 2, 2014.

16. *U.S. News & World Report*. Best healthcare jobs. 2014. http://money.usnews.com/careers/ best-jobs/physical-therapist and

    http://money.usnews.com/careers/best-jobs/ rankings/the-100-best-jobs?int=d97792.

    Accessed December 20, 2014.

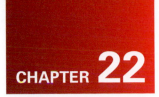

CHAPTER 22

Physician Assisting

Amanda Moloney-Johns, MPAS, PA-C

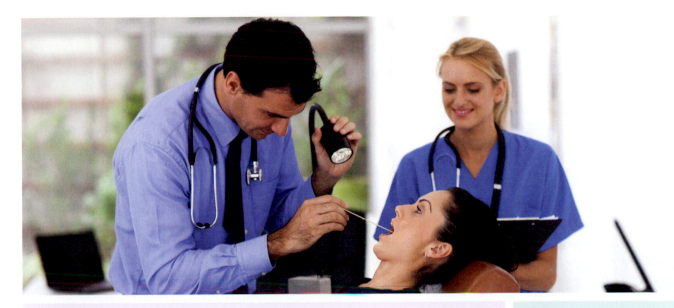

Photo credit: istock/Thinkstock

Learning Objectives

After reading this chapter, students should be able to:

- Describe the physician assistant profession
- Explain the role of the physician assistant on the medical team and in our current health-care system
- Discuss the scope of practice of a physician assistant
- Outline the required education and licensure requirements for physician assistants
- Describe the current opportunities and challenges for the physician assistant profession

Key Terms

- Physician assistants
- Collaboration
- Workforce
- Supervising physician
- Delegation of Services Agreement
- Physician Assistant National Certifying Exam (PANCE)
- Continuing medical education

 ## "A Day in the Life"

Hello! My name is Amanda and I am a physician assistant (PA). I work in an outpatient primary-care clinic and typically see about 25 patients per day. My day usually starts around 8:00 a.m. and ends around 6:00 p.m., and I usually work 45 to 50 hours per week. In primary care, I manage patients of all ages with a wide range of both acute and chronic health-care issues. Some patients require only a few minutes while others require much more time, but I typically spend an average of 15 minutes with each patient. This requires me to manage my time effectively, sometimes working with more than one patient at a time. My job continually interests and challenges me because no two days are ever the same. Here are some examples of patients that I treated recently in clinic:

- A 2-year-old well-child check. I examined the patient and discussed his immunizations, development, behavior, and overall health with his parents.
- A 24-year-old woman with a sore throat. After some tests it was found that she had strep throat, so I prescribed

(continued)

antibiotics and gave her some additional instructions on how best to improve her condition.

- A 46-year-old man who cut himself on the job and needed stitches. I cleaned his wound, provided local anesthesia, and placed six stitches. I also gave him instructions on how to watch for infection and how to care for his wound until his follow-up appointment with me.

- A 56-year-old man with diabetes and hypertension. We discussed his medications and other details like diet and exercise. I referred him to a nutritionist so that he can improve his diet. I also ordered blood tests to monitor his disease.

- A 42-year-old man with a back injury who needed a referral to an orthopedic surgeon. I consulted with

my supervising physician and then talked to the orthopedic surgery PA on the phone and arranged a consultation. This will be the same PA who will perform a preoperative and postoperative assessment, assist the surgeon during the surgery, and see the patient during his hospital stay. We will touch base to arrange follow-up care once the patient leaves the hospital after his operation.

When I am not seeing patients, I document details of each patient's visit in his or her chart, review phone and e-mail messages from patients, complete paperwork required by insurance companies and pharmacies, call patients about lab and other test results, and consult with other health-care professionals about care for my patients. The days are very busy, but I love my job!

Introduction to Physician Assisting

Description

Physician assistants (PAs) are licensed health-care providers who are trained to provide health care to people of all ages in a wide variety of specialties and settings. PAs are partnered with and trained to practice medicine under the supervision of a physician, and are able to evaluate and assess patients of all ages with both acute and chronic conditions. They can take medical histories, perform physical examinations, order and interpret laboratory and imaging studies, perform procedures, diagnose injuries and illnesses, prescribe medications, and provide education, counsel, and treatment for patients with illness or injury. They must also document their findings in the patient's medical record and work with other health-care professionals regularly to help coordinate the best care for their patients.[1]

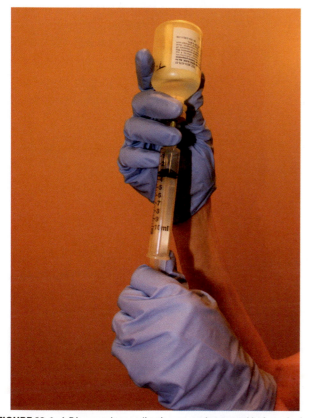

FIGURE 22-1 A PA preparing medication to numb a wound before placing stitches.

History

The PA profession was created to provide a solution to the shortage of primary-care physicians in the 1960s. However, the origins of the idea of the profession date back to the 1940s when a general practice physician from North Carolina, Dr. Amos Johnson, hired and trained Henry "Buddy" Treadwell as a "doctor's assistant" to care for patients in his rural practice so that he could attend medical meetings. As Dr. Johnson and Buddy Treadwell's relationship became known and accepted in North Carolina, Dr. Eugene Stead used it as a model to develop the first physician assistant program at Duke University in 1965, enrolling former military corpsmen as students.[2] The first PA class graduated from Duke University on October 6, 1967.[1] With an increase in specialization of physicians and the introduction of Medicare and Medicaid, the shortage of primary-care physicians, especially in rural areas, became evident and PAs were seen as a possible solution to the need for increased access to health care. By the end of the decade, the American Medical Association formally recognized the idea of the PA. The profession quickly became more established in the 1970s, with the development of a national certification examination and accreditation standards. By the 1980s, the PA profession had gained nationwide acceptance and continued rapid growth. All states and territories of the United States had accepted the practice of PAs by the end of the 1990s. The globalization of the profession expanded in the 2000s with increased international interest in the PA concept to improve health-care delivery and offer an effective response to physician shortages.[2]

According to the National Commission on Certification of Physician Assistants (NCCPA), there are currently more than 95,000 certified PAs in the United States.[3] There are also PAs who currently practice in Canada, India, and The Netherlands, among other countries.[1]

Scope of Practice

PAs are formally trained in general medicine, and for this reason they have flexibility to meet different health-care needs and can adapt to meet these needs as they change and evolve in our society. PAs can practice in settings including rural and urban, outpatient and inpatient, hospitals, clinics, and nursing homes. PAs can also practice in all areas of medicine, ranging from primary care to surgery, and subspecialties such as cardiology or oncology. The American Academy of Physician Assistants 2010 Census reported that approximately one-third of PAs work in primary care and two-thirds work in specialties. The U.S. government also employs PAs, and they can work for the armed services, including Army, Navy, and Air Force, or federal government entities such as the Indian Health Services or the Department of Veterans Affairs.

A wide range of services can be performed by PAs, including the diagnosis and treatment of preventive, emergent, urgent, acute, and chronic illnesses and injuries across the life span. Although most PAs practice medicine with a great deal of autonomy, they always work under the supervision of a physician. However, this does not mean that the **supervising physician** must be physically present at all times or directly participate in each individual case. Instead, physicians delegate an appropriate level of autonomy to the PA to fit their practice setting and type. The scope of practice of PAs is determined by several factors, including state laws and the delegation of duties by the individual physician, which are detailed in a document called a **Delegation of Services Agreement.**[4]

Each state has its own laws and regulations, which determine what tasks a PA is allowed to perform in that state. Outlined examples in the Delegation of Services Agreement include the amount and type of supervision a PA will receive, what services the PA can perform, and the percentage

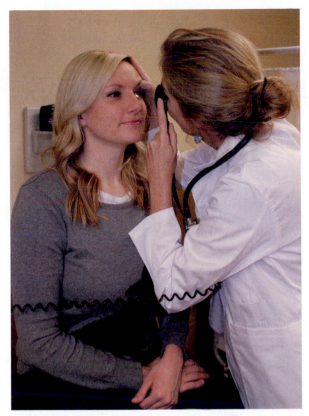

FIGURE 22-2 A PA using an ophthalmoscope to examine a patient's eye.

of charts that require review and cosignature by the physician. These details often depend on the PA's experience and education in a particular area of medicine.[5] For instance, a PA who has been practicing in an area of medicine for 20 years may be granted more autonomy than a new graduate, who may require more direct supervision initially and acquire more autonomy as abilities increase with time and experience. Practice setting also contributes to the PA's scope of practice. A PA in a rural practice may be the only provider consistently present in the clinic, whereas the physician is physically present in that clinic only a few days per month. The PA can manage the care of patients, consulting the physician on cases for which additional advice is required, thus allowing the physician to dedicate time to more complicated cases. In contrast, a PA in cardiothoracic surgery may work side by side with the supervising physician on a daily basis, and the physician may delegate duties such as assisting in surgery, performing hospital rounds, and managing preoperative and postoperative care. The flexibility of physician-delegated autonomy allows the physician to customize the relationship with the PA to best fit in the practice. PAs always represent their supervising physician, working collaboratively and practicing medicine as directed by their supervising physician. A PA may not perform any

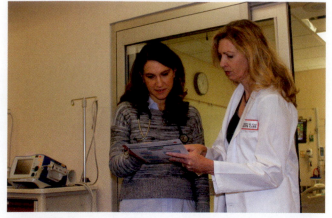

FIGURE 22-3 Two PAs discussing a care plan for a patient in the intensive care unit.

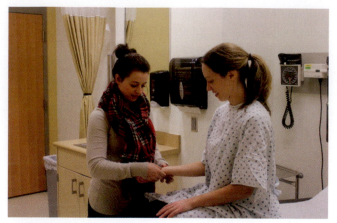

FIGURE 22-4 Two PA students practicing physical examination skills.

duties that are outside the supervising physician's scope of practice. Individual institutions may also affect the scope of practice of a PA. Hospitals, health maintenance organizations, and other facilities require PAs to be credentialed and allow certain privileges based on their own organizational requirements.[5]

The American Medical Association House of Delegates adopted the *Guidelines for Physician/Physician Assistant Practice.* These guidelines state the following[5]:

- The physician is responsible for managing the health care of patients in all settings.

- Health-care services delivered by physicians and physician assistants must be within the scope of each practitioner's authorized practice, as defined by state law.

- The physician is ultimately responsible for coordinating and managing the care of patients and, with the appropriate input of the physician assistant, ensuring the quality of health care provided to patients.

- The physician is responsible for the supervision of the physician assistant in all settings.

- The role of the physician assistant in the delivery of care should be defined through mutually agreed on guidelines that are developed by the physician and the physician assistant and based on the physician's delegatory style.

- The physician must be available for consultation with the physician assistant at all times either in person or through telecommunication systems or other means.

- The extent of the involvement by the physician assistant in the assessment and implementation of treatment will depend on the complexity and acuity of the patient's condition and the training, experience, and preparation of the physician assistant, as adjudged by the physician.

- Patients should be made clearly aware at all times whether they are being cared for by a physician or a physician assistant.

- The physician and physician assistant together should review all delegated patient services on a regular basis, as well as the mutually agreed on guidelines for practice.

- The physician is responsible for clarifying and familiarizing the physician assistant with his or her supervising methods and style of delegating patient care.

Required Education

PAs are trained in the medical model, meaning that the curriculum of PA education is similar to that of medical school and complements physician training.[6] A PA must have graduated from an accredited PA training program to obtain licensure. Currently, there are 190 accredited programs in the United States. PA programs are accredited by the Accreditation Review Commission on Education for the Physician Assistant, Inc. (ARC-PA). Each program must comply with Standards of Accreditation determined by ARC-PA.[7]

Most PA programs offer a master's degree as an entry-level and terminal degree for the profession. At minimum, an applicant typically must complete at least 2 years of course work in science courses to obtain the necessary prerequisites for admission to a PA program. Most programs require coursework in anatomy, physiology, chemistry, and microbiology. Generally, most applicants have a bachelor's degree before admission to a PA program, though this can be in any field of study as long as the necessary prerequisites are completed before matriculation. Requirements differ between PA programs, but many applicants also have several years of health-care experience before they are accepted into a PA program. Examples of health-care experience can include, but are not limited to, emergency medical technicians, paramedics,

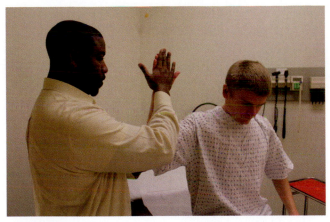

FIGURE 22-5 PA students practicing a shoulder examination.

radiology technicians, medical assistants, nurses, athletic trainers, respiratory therapists, and patient-care technicians.

The curriculum of a PA program is intense. The average length of a PA program is 27 months, designed to train competent health-care providers quickly and cost-effectively.[1] PA programs typically have a didactic phase and a clinical phase. The didactic phase consists of classroom education in the following core courses: anatomy, physiology, pharmacology, physical diagnosis, clinical medicine, and behavioral science.[1,8] Students also experience more than 2,000 hours of clinical education in the clinical phase of the program.[1] Clinical rotations include managing patients across the life span in family medicine, internal medicine, emergency medicine, general surgery, pediatrics, obstetrics/gynecology, and behavioral health in outpatient, inpatient, emergency, and operating room settings.[8]

License

To practice as a PA after completion of an accredited PA program, graduates must pass the **Physician Assistant National Certifying Exam (PANCE),** which is administered by the NCCPA. If graduates successfully pass the examination, they can apply for state licensure or registration, which is required to practice as a PA in any state. To maintain certification, PAs must pass the Physician Assistant National Recertifying Examination (PANRE) every 10 years and obtain 100 hours of **continuing medical education** (CME) every 2 years. Some required CME hours must focus on self-assessment and performance improvement. Each state also has specific CME requirements necessary for maintenance of licensure.

Salary

The salary of PAs varies depending on geographical location, level of experience, type of organization, and area of practice.

According to the U.S. Bureau of Labor Statistics, the median annual salary for all PAs in 2012 was $90,930, and the mean annual salary was $92,460. The highest-paying states were reported to be Rhode Island, Connecticut, Washington, Oregon, and Nevada. The National Physician Assistant Salary Report in 2010 reported that the median salary for PAs with 20 years or more of experience was $101,000.[9] The median salary range for PAs working in primary-care specialties (family medicine, general internal medicine, and general pediatrics) was $80,000 to $89,000. Internal medicine subspecialty median salaries ranged from $83,000 to $100,000, and surgical subspecialties ranged from $87,750 to $115,500, though years of experience also influence salary amount.[9]

Trends

The outlook for PAs in the next decade is very good. The Patient Protection and Affordable Care Act will potentially insure up to 30 million more Americans in the next few years, increasing the demand for health-care providers. Additionally, the Association of American Medical Colleges reports that by 2020 there will be a shortage of more than 90,000 physicians, with at least half of those in primary care. There will also be significant growth in the percentage of patients over 65 years of age, resulting in increased health needs by this population. These shortages will most significantly affect rural and underserved populations.[10]

Physician assistants are in a perfect position to help fill in the gaps of the physician shortage and provide increased access to health care in a cost-effective way. It can take up to a decade to train a physician, whereas PA training is considerably shorter and less expensive, allowing PAs to enter the **workforce** more quickly and provide health care to those with a critical need.[12] The U.S. Bureau of Labor Statistics projects that the PA profession will be the second fastest growing profession in the next 10 years and that the need for PAs will increase by 30% between 2010 and 2020. The American Academy of Physician Assistants predicts that the number of PAs will increase from approximately 74,000 in 2008 to between 137,000 and 173,000 by 2020. The job outlook is very good in both primary care and specialty areas, and also those working with rural and underserved populations.[1,11]

Challenges

All professions have challenges. One of the challenges the PA profession faces is the wide discrepancy of legislation between states. National and state organizations work diligently to break down barriers to care provided by PAs, which varies from state to state. Because the PA profession is relatively young, many people are unfamiliar with PAs and what they

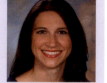

Author Spotlight

Amanda Moloney-Johns, MPAS, PA-C

I graduated from the University of Utah Physician Assistant Program in 2006. I have practiced as a PA in the fields of pain management and urgent care, and currently work as an assistant professor and the Director of Clinical Education at the University of Utah Physician Assistant Program. I became a PA because it combined my interests of practicing medicine, making a difference in the lives of others, working as part of a team, and having a career that provides the opportunity for lifelong learning. I enjoy being able to form meaningful relationships with my patients while providing them education about how to improve their health. I also love working with PA students and working in PA education.

can do. This unfamiliarity often requires PAs to educate patients about the profession and their qualifications to provide health care, though this can be seen as an opportunity rather than a challenge.

Another challenge of the PA profession is that PAs can work very long hours, including nights, weekends, and holidays. PAs can also be "on call," which may require them to come to work unexpectedly or on very short notice. PAs are often required to see many patients per day, and there may be time pressures associated with a busy schedule. As with any profession involving long hours and time pressures, this type of work can lead to high stress levels and burnout. Caring for patients is a privilege, but also a tremendous responsibility. Some of the greatest satisfaction PAs get from their work is the relationships they

Aptitude Profile

The following list offers a general overview of some of the characteristics and skills needed when working as a physician assistant:

Aware of limitations	Integrity
Collaborative	Intelligent
Compassionate	Problem solver
Critical thinker	Professional
Emotional stability	Respect
Empathetic	Responsible
Ethical	Sound judgment
Good interpersonal skills	Team player

develop with their patients. However, dealing with difficult situations, such as the death of a patient, can be emotionally taxing.

Last, PAs act as advocates for their patients, especially for vulnerable populations such as those in rural and underserved communities. PAs can act tirelessly to obtain proper resources to provide the best care for their patients, but these resources may not be available to every patient because of their insurance status or lack of ability to afford certain aspects of their care, such as medications or procedures. Social injustices can be challenging for PAs, though being a PA means being part of the solution to improved health-care access and better patient outcomes.

Working Together

By definition, the PA profession is one of **collaboration.** Not only will PAs work directly with physicians, they often work with multiple other professions, including pharmacists, nurses, medical assistants, nutritionists, social workers, physical therapists, occupational therapists, speech therapists, audiologists, dentists, and medical laboratory scientists. Often it is the PA who coordinates the care for the patient and the team works together to provide the best possible care. Having a PA as part of an interprofessional medical team results in high-quality care, improved coordination of care, decreased costs, decreased waiting time for patient appointments, increased patient satisfaction, and improved patient outcomes.[7]

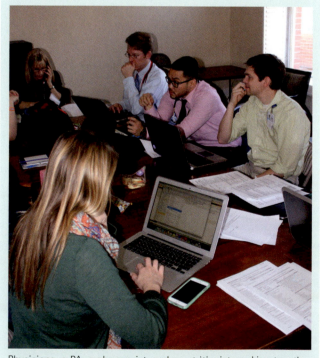

Physicians, a PA, a pharmacist, and a nutritionist working together on the care of an elderly patient at an assisted-living facility.

CASE STUDY

Jack is a 52-year-old white man who arrives in clinic today with a chief complaint of low back pain. He is a construction worker and does not have insurance. He states that he was working in his yard a few weeks ago, and suddenly felt pain in his low back as he was gardening. His pain has not resolved and he is having difficulty walking. These symptoms are interfering with his ability to work his construction job, as he is in constant pain throughout the day. He also has type 2 diabetes, high blood pressure, and high cholesterol. Jack has been prescribed medications for these issues in the past but has not taken them "for months." He states that because he lives in a rural area, it is difficult for him to seek care on a regular basis and obtain his medications. He is also unsure of how to take the medications, and because he "doesn't feel sick," he does not feel that he needs them. He is married and has three children, and states that he must work to support his family. He has taken a few days off work because of the pain, but he cannot afford to take much time off and is coming in for help to diagnose and improve his condition.

Questions

1. In what ways can a PA be involved in Jack's care?

2. What are the social issues facing Jack?

3. What other health professionals should be involved in this case?

4. Why is a team approach important in this case?

Review Questions

1. The PA profession was started in what decade?

    A. 1920s

    B. 1960s

    C. 1980s

    D. 2000s

2. Physician assistants can work in which area of medicine?

    A. Primary care

    B. Cardiology

    C. Orthopedic surgery

    D. All of the above

3. Which of the following factors determines scope of practice?

    A. Supervising physician

    B. State laws and regulations

    C. Individual organizations who employ the physician assistant

    D. All of the above

4. Physician assistants must work under the supervision of a physician to be able to practice medicine.

    A. True

    B. False

5. Currently, most PA programs award which degree on completion of the program?

    A. Associate degree

    B. Bachelor's degree

    C. Master's degree

    D. Doctoral degree

6. To practice as a PA, which of the following is/are required?

    A. Graduation from an accredited PA school

    B. Passing the Physician Assistant National Certifying Exam (PANCE)

    C. Obtaining state licensure

    D. All of the above

7. In addition to individual state requirements, PAs are required to obtain how many hours of continuing medical education every 2 years?

    A. 25

    B. 50

    C. 100

    D. 200

8. Growth is projected for the PA profession in the next 10 years because of:

    A. Projected physician shortage

    B. Potentially more Americans becoming insured through the Patient Protection and Affordable Care Act

    C. The increasing age of the U.S. population

    D. All of the above

9. Which of the following characteristics are valuable in the PA profession?

   A. Need for independence

   B. Compassion

   C. Unidisciplinary

   D. Judgmental

10. Physician assistants often work with which of the following professions?

   A. Physical therapists

   B. Nurses

   C. Pharmacists

   D. All of the above

Glossary of Key Terms

Physician assistant—a medical professional who is nationally certified and state licensed to practice medicine; always works with a supervising physician

Collaboration—working with another person or group to achieve or accomplish something

Workforce—the number of people in a nation or region who are employed or available for work

Supervising physician—a licensed physician partner under whom a physician assistant practices medicine; a supervising physician determines the scope of practice of a physician assistant

Delegation of Services Agreement—a document formulated by a physician assistant and his or her supervising physician; it outlines what types of medical services a physician assistant can perform and how these services are performed, on behalf of the supervising physician

Physician Assistant National Certifying Exam (PANCE)—a computer-based test consisting of questions that assess basic medical and surgical knowledge

Continuing medical education—required education by physician assistants to maintain competency and licensure and to keep current on new medical information

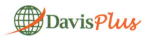 **Additional Resources are available online at www.davisplus.com**

Additional Resources

The American Academy of Physician Assistants (AAPA)—www.aapa.org

Information on state chapters of the AAPA—www.aapa.org/about_aapa/constituent_organizations/chapters

National Commission on Certification of Physician Assistants—www.nccpa.net

Physician Assistant History Society—www.pahx.org

Physician Assistant Education Association—www.paeaonline.org

Accreditation Review Commission on Education for the Physician Assistant, Inc.—www.arc-pa.org

References

1. American Academy of Physician Assistants. http://www.aapa.org.

   Accessed December 8, 2013.

2. Physician Assistant History Society. http://www.pahx.org/period02.html.

   Accessed December 9, 2013.

3. National Commission on Certification of Physician Assistants. http://www.nccpa.net.

   Accessed December 10, 2013.

4. American Academy of Physician Assistants. *State Law Issues: Supervision of PAs: Access and Excellence in Patient Care.* October 2011.

   http://www.aapa.org/uploadedFiles/content/The_PA_Profession/Federal_and_State_Affairs/Resource_Items/SLI_PASupervision_110811_Final.pdf.

   Accessed December 10, 2013.

5. American Academy of Physician Assistants. *Professional Issues: PA Scope of Practice.*

   http://www.aapa.org/uploadedFiles/content/The_PA_Profession/Federal_and_State_Affairs/Resource_Items/PI_PAScopePractice_110811_Final.pdf.

   Accessed December 10, 2013.

6. American Academy of Physician Assistants. *Professional Issues: PA Education—Preparation for Excellence.*

    http://www.aapa.org/uploadedFiles/content/ The_PA_Profession/Federal_and_State_Affairs/ Resource_Items/PI_PAEducation_v3.pdf.
    Accessed December 11, 2013.

7. Accreditation Review Commission on Education for the Physician Assistant, Inc.

    http://www.arc-pa.org/about/about_pa.html.
    Accessed December 10, 2013.

8. Accreditation Review Commission on Education for the Physician Assistant, Inc. *Accreditation Standards for Physician Assistant Education, Fourth Edition.* March 2010.

    http://www.arc-pa.org/documents/Standards 4theditionwithclarifyingchanges9.2013%20FNL.pdf.
    Accessed December 11, 2013.

9. American Academy of Physician Assistants. *National Physician Assistant Salary Report, Research and Statistics, Results from AAPA's 2010 Census.*

    http://www.pasconnect.org/aapa-10-29-2013-46170/ 2010_Salary_Report.pdf.
    Accessed December 11, 2013.

10. Association of American Medical Colleges. *Physician Shortages to Worsen Without Increases in Residency Training.*

    https://www.aamc.org/download/286592/data/.
    Accessed December 11, 2013.

11. Bureau of Labor Statistics, U.S. Department of Labor. Occupational outlook handbook, 2012–2013 edition, physician assistants.

    http://www.bls.gov/ooh/healthcare/physician-assistants.htm.
    Accessed December 9, 2013.

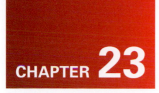

CHAPTER 23

Radiography

Amy Freshley-Lebkuecher, MS, and Rex Ameigh, MSLM

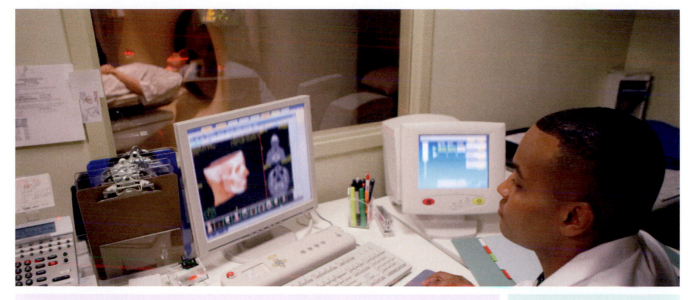

Photo credit: Fuse/Thinkstock

Learning Objectives

After reading this chapter, students should be able to:

- Identify the professional organizations related to radiography
- Identify the accrediting agency for radiography
- Identify the registry/certification agency for radiography
- Identify equipment used by radiographers
- Demonstrate understanding of paths to certification/registration eligibility in radiography
- Explain the difference between licensure and certification/registry

Key Terms

- Computed tomography (CT)
- Radiologic technologist
- Primary-care provider
- Radiologists
- Medical doctor (MD)
- Doctor of osteopathy (DO)
- Physician assistant
- Nurse practitioner (NP)
- Accreditation
- Magnetic resonance imaging (MRI)
- Cardiovascular interventional technologist (CVIT)
- Mammography
- Bone densitometry

"A Day in the Life"

Good morning. My name is Jay and I am a radiographer. When I arrived at the hospital at 6:55 a.m., I proceeded to the radiography core to check my day's assignment. The duty board shows I'm assigned to the emergency department (ED). So I'm off to the ED x-ray room to relieve the night crew. Then I'll check with the ED nurses and physicians to see if they need any exams. I'll let you know what I learn a bit later.

Things were quiet when I checked in at the ED triage desk so I went back to the x-ray room to clean up in preparation for the beginning of the morning exams. It looked like the night shift radiographer had been busy! The x-ray table and upright chest stand needed disinfecting. Some of the imaging receptors looked soiled, so I cleaned them too. After that, I logged onto the computer in preparation for the day's exams. It wasn't long until the ED let me know a patient needed a chest x-ray. I checked the computer to ensure the exam was ordered. It was, so I headed to the patient's cubicle. When I arrived, I introduced myself as a technologist who would be performing the chest exam. Before leaving the ED, I verified the patient's identity by asking for name and date of birth. I also checked the patient's armband ID. Once I was sure I had the correct patient, I headed to the x-ray room for the procedure. While I transported the patient, I explained the exam. The ED nurses had the patient dressed for the images, so I proceeded to get a history of the patient's current complaint. The patient was able to stand unassisted, so I positioned him against the chest stand for a posteroanterior (PA) chest film. I asked the patient to take in a deep breath, blow it out, and then take in another deep breath. The exposure was made at the point of the second inspiration. That procedure was repeated for the lateral projection. Once the images were completed, they were checked for technical accuracy and sent electronically to the doctor. After that task was completed, I returned the patient to the cubicle. When I got back to the x-ray room, I checked the emergency "crash" cart. Several medications were past the expiration date, so I called the pharmacy for a new med tray. About that time, I heard a page for lifting help in **computed tomography** (CT). They need my assistance, so I'll check back with you when I return.

When I got back from CT, the new medication tray was delivered. The pharmacy tech and I verified that a security tag was attached to the cart. The ED called to notify me that a trauma patient was due momentarily. The trauma protocol requires portable cervical spine, chest, and abdomen images. I took the mobile x-ray machine and image receptors to the ED trauma room. After the patient was stabilized, the ED nurse helped me lift the fracture board for placement of the image receptors and monitored the patient as I obtained the images. The images were processed in the x-ray suite, checked for technical accuracy, and forwarded to the doctor. About that time, my lunch relief arrived, so I grabbed a quick bite. When I got back, I helped the radiographer complete an exam in progress. As I was returning the patient to the ED, a nurse told me the patient in room 2 needed a portable chest x-ray. After retrieving the portable unit, I checked the chart to verify the exam, room, and patient identity. A respiratory therapist was administering a treatment so I waited until she finished. When the treatment was complete, I took the machine into the room and introduced myself. After explaining the exam, the nurse and I pulled the patient up in the bed and placed the image receptor behind the patient's back. The patient was given breathing instructions and I made the exposure. The cassette was removed from behind the patient's back and placed in the mobile unit. After removing the unit from the room, I ensured everything was back in its proper place. The image was processed and sent to the physician. After imaging several patients, the ED x-ray room was a mess! The housekeeper came by to change the laundry basket, restock the linen, and clean the room. My shift was about over, so I cleaned the image receptors and table again. I made sure I logged off the computer and closed out all the exams. When the evening radiographer arrived, I briefed him on the day's activities and pending exams. After that, all I had left to do was clock out and head home. It was another interesting day working in the ED. It was gratifying to know I helped patients get appropriate medical treatment by providing the practitioners with quality images.

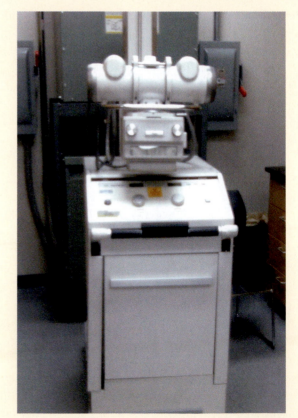

Introduction to Radiography

Description

Radiologic technologists (or **radiographers**) are specialized health-care professionals working in hospitals, clinics, education, and, in some instances, medical sales. Radiographers primarily produce radiographic images of patients as ordered by physicians or physician extenders. When patients see their **primary-care provider** (PCP) because of an injury or other pathological condition, the provider often orders x-rays or other diagnostic examinations such as a computed tomography (CT) scan. These images are produced with ionizing radiation that is produced when high-speed electrons bombard a tungsten target in an x-ray tube. This radiation is selectively absorbed by body tissue, providing the practitioner with images of structures invisible to the naked eye. These x-ray "pictures" play a vital role in the diagnosis and treatment of a variety of diseases and injuries. They are interpreted by specially trained physicians called **radiologists.** The radiologist's findings are reported to the PCP, who creates a treatment plan based on those findings. The PCP can be a **medical doctor** (MD), **doctor of osteopathic medicine** (DO), **physician assistant** (PA), or **nurse practitioner** (NP).

Origins of Radiography

The profession of radiography began when "x-rays" were discovered by Wilhelm Conrad Roentgen on November 8, 1895. It was immediately evident that these rays had medical applications. What was less clear was who would use these rays to image patients. Initially, individuals performing examinations had no medical training. Professional photographers purchased equipment and performed "Roentgen photography." In the early 1900s, anyone could purchase x-ray equipment. Chemists, engineers, and electricians were commonly the owners of these medical devices.[1] However, around 1910, the novelty waned and physicians began to purchase x-ray units for diagnosis. In the beginning, the physicians were owner/operators, obtaining and interpreting the images.[2] This practice was abandoned fairly quickly. The equipment was rudimentary and did not have much penetrating power. It could take up to 20 minutes of exposure for a hip image, and development of the glass plates took as long as 4 hours.[2] It did not take long for physicians to relegate the technical work of obtaining images to their office staff, training them to perform examinations. Many of these "technicians," typically women, were clerical workers with no medical knowledge.[1]

Reports of biological damage caused by x-radiation appeared as early as 1896. Thomas Alva Edison is credited with the invention of the fluoroscope. A fluoroscope is an x-ray machine that allows the operator to see internal structures in real time. For example, the operator can watch the heart as it is beating. Edison displayed the fluoroscope at the Electrical Exhibition in New York City that year. However, Edison's experimentation with the device resulted in significant radiation exposure to his friend and assistant, Clarence Madison Dally. Dally subsequently died of radiation-induced cancer in 1904, and he is regarded as the first radiation fatality. Edison abandoned his work with x-radiation after Dally's death.[3]

As the field expanded, it became apparent that the new technology was not harmless as initially believed. The technicians felt a need to discuss experiences with their peers to share what they learned and to minimize the potential hazards associated with the profession. There were essentially no instruction manuals, so equipment settings and positioning were devised using methods of trial and error.[1] It was clear that education of the technicians needed to be formalized and standardized.

In October 1920, Eddy C. Jerman, a Civil War veteran, collaborated with 13 other technicians to form the first professional society. About half of the attendees were female, which was consistent with the number of women working in the field. Dr. Jerman and his colleagues called the society the American Association of Radiologic Technicians (AART). The newly formed society, which later became the American Society of X-Ray Technicians (ASXT), published its first journal, *The X-Ray Technician,* in 1929.[4] This society was the precursor to the current society for imaging professionals.

Technology expanded rapidly, and personnel had trouble keeping pace. Physicians continued to train x-ray technicians. The doctors and technicians worked together to form formalized training programs in hospitals. In 1944, x-ray technology joined with other allied health professions in championing the establishment of standards of education and **accreditation.** The ASXT joined with the American Medical Association (AMA) to publish the first "Essentials of an Acceptable School for X-Ray Technicians." By the 1950s, ASXT membership had grown to 4,000 and about 125 schools offered training in x-ray technology.[2,4] In 1964, the ASXT changed its name to the American Society of Radiologic Technologists (ASRT).[4]

As x-ray technologists continued to grow professionally, the field of radiography also evolved. Initially, images were captured on a glass plate that was coated with emulsion. Glass continued to be used until the First World War. Glass was in short supply, so alternative materials were needed. The first alternative material used was cellulose nitrate; however, this substance proved to be flammable, and it was replaced by cellulose triacetate in the 1920s. By 1960, a polyester base was introduced and it is still in use today.[5] In the early days of radiography, development of the latent (undeveloped) images produced by the x-rays required open tanks of chemicals. Glass plates were slid into metal tracks for submersion in the chemical tanks. When film replaced glass plates, the film was clipped to racks and "hand tanked." The technician taking the exposure would literally submerge the film hanger in the developer tanks and move them up and down. They would agitate the film in this method for a few minutes and hold the film up to a light. If the image was too light, they would repeat the process. If the image was dark enough, they would rinse the film and put it in the fixer. In emergency cases, the wet film would be taken to the radiologist for interpretation. This practice was the origin of the term "wet reading," because the films were actually wet when interpreted. In the 1940s, automatic processors were introduced. Manual processing generally took about an hour to get a dry image. Some modern automatic processors take only about 45 seconds.

Image intensifying screens were the next breakthrough. These screens fluoresced, so light actually exposed the film, not the x-rays. This led to reduced radiation doses to the patient and operator by requiring less exposure to obtain a diagnostic image. By the 1970s, nearly all hospital imaging departments used intensifying screens. The efficiency of the screens continued to improve by using new materials, such as rare earth minerals. All of these improvements required technologists to change their radiographic technical factors. Innovations meant the personnel constantly honed their skills to keep pace.

The computer age that began in the 1970s had a major impact on imaging. Computed tomography was invented early in that decade and made it possible to visualize anatomy in three dimensions.[5] As computers became more powerful, their application in radiography expanded.

Currently, virtually all modalities are able to store images in a digital format. That format has many advantages. Images may be enhanced after exposure, viewed remotely, and stored in a computer. Potentially, patients may receive lower doses by eliminating repeat exposures due to technical factor errors. Images can be sent to multiple physicians simultaneously, facilitating easier access and earlier reporting. Finally, there is no need for a film room or archive space. One drawback to digital imaging is the initial capital expense. Currently, some facilities continue to produce images as a hard-copy radiograph, which requires chemical processing (Fig. 23-1). However, most hospitals now have the capability to produce computer-generated digital images (Fig. 23-2).

The radiography modality has several subspecialties. Radiographers can work in computed tomography, **magnetic resonance imaging**, **cardiovascular intervention technology, mammography, bone densitometry,** and quality management.

Tips and Tools

When radiography began, the term *x-ray technician* (or just *technician*) was used to describe workers making images. The literature of the day reflected that term, which is why it is used at the beginning of this chapter. As the educational standards grew and the workers became professionals, the title was changed to *radiologic technologist*. Today, radiology professionals are radiologic technologists. However, the types of images they make also describe them. Technologists working in general imaging areas may be referred to as *radiographers*. Technologists working in women's services are often referred to as *mammographers*.

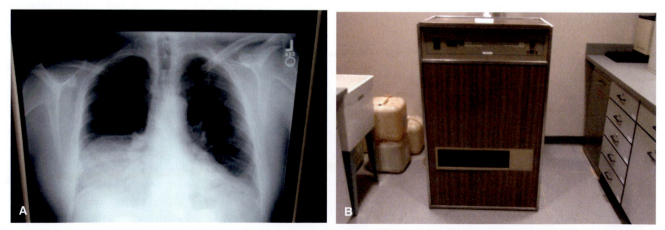

FIGURE 23-1 (A) Analog chest x-ray. Before the advent of digital x-rays in the 1980s, analog x-rays were used. **(B)** Chemical radiographic processor. This equipment is essential for x-ray departments because this machine processes images taken by x-ray equipment.

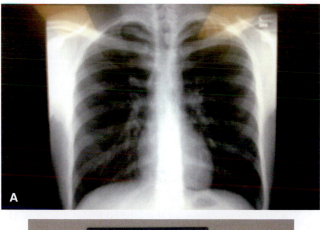

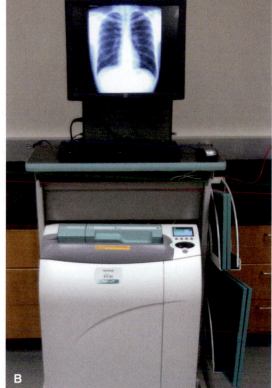

FIGURE 23-2 (A) Digital chest x-ray. Due to the multiple advantages of digital imaging, most radiology facilities now offer digital imaging. **(B)** Digital chest x-ray with processor. Digital processors work with digital x-rays and use computer algorithms to perform image processing.

Scope of Practice

The American Society of Radiologic Technologists (ASRT) defines the scope of practice of medical imaging. All registered radiologic technologists—credentialed as RT(R)—are qualified to image patients using a variety of equipment. The scope of practice of the radiographer also includes performing diagnostic radiographic and noninterpretive fluoroscopic procedures as prescribed by a licensed independent practitioner.[2]

To maintain certification through the American Registry of Radiologic Technologists (ARRT), radiographers must complete appropriate continuing education to meet requirements to sustain a level of expertise and awareness of changes and advances in practice. The general scopes of practice are as follows[2]:

- Receive, relay, and document verbal, written, and electronic orders in medical record
- Assess patient's clinical history for appropriateness of ordered procedure
- Ensure documentation is available for use by licensed independent practitioner
- Verify informed consent
- Assume responsibility for patient needs during procedures
- Prepare patients for procedures
- Determine appropriate technical exposure factors
- Keep dose as low as reasonably achievable (ALARA) to patient, self, and others by applying strict radiation safety principles
- Perform venipuncture as prescribed by a licensed independent practitioner
- Start and maintain intravenous access as prescribed by a licensed independent practitioner
- Identify, prepare, and/or administer medications as prescribed by a licensed independent practitioner
- Evaluate images for technical quality, ensuring proper identification is recorded
- Identify and manage emergency situations
- Provide patient education
- Educate and monitor students and other health-care providers
- Perform ongoing quality assurance activities

Required Education

Currently, individuals can be trained as a radiographer through three educational methods, a certificate program, an associate degree program, or a bachelor's of science degree program. Each method has different general education requirements before the professional portion of the program. For example, students pursuing an associate degree are usually required to complete approximately 1 year of general education courses before admission into the program. Students pursuing a bachelor's of science degree must typically complete at least 2 years of core/required courses before starting the program. Each program sets requirement criteria, which include minimum grade point average (GPA) requirements. Acceptance is competitive, so students are not guaranteed a seat in the program. In 2015, the ARRT national registry examination requirements include completion of an associate degree. Examples of an associate of applied science or bachelor's of science radiography courses include the following:

- Medical terminology
- Introduction to radiologic technology
- Patient care and interaction
- Radiographic procedures
- Radiographic image analysis
- Clinical education
- Radiobiology and radiation protection
- Radiation physics
- Radiographic pathology

Licensure

Not all states require licensure at this time. In June 2012, an ASRT introduced a bill before Congress which would require minimum levels of education for anyone administering radiation for diagnostic or therapeutic purposes. The goal of the bill is to ensure patient safety and diagnostic quality images. The bill is known as Consistency, Accuracy, Responsibility and Excellence in Medical Imaging and Radiation Therapy (CARE).[2] Passage of this bill would set federal education and certification standards. Until federal standards are set or licensure is mandated, it is advisable to check with local departments of health services to determine if licensure is required in your state.

Salary

According to the Bureau of Labor Statistics, the median pay for radiographers was $55,910 ($26.88 per hour) in 2012.[6] Salaries vary widely by geographical area, but entry-level radiographers typically start at about $15.00 per hour ($31,200 per year). Compensation also depends on where a radiographer works. Hospitals, imaging centers, physician practices, and urgent-care clinics are all potential employers. Hospitals typically pay more than physician offices. This is due in part to hospitals' need to be open 24 hours a day, 7 days a week. Weekend, afternoon, and night shifts usually offer a salary differential for individuals working shifts other than the standard 5-day workweek.

Trends

According to the Bureau of Labor Statistics, the employment opportunities for the field will increase by about 28% through 2020.[6]

Challenges

As is the case with most health professions, radiographers are challenged by the "graying" of the population. As people age, their health typically deteriorates and they need more health-care services. Meanwhile, many radiographers are nearing retirement age, so there may be a shortage of qualified professionals to perform the required examinations. At the same time, uncertainty about health-care reimbursements may lead hospital executives to not fill vacated positions. The end result of these factors may be doing more examinations with fewer radiographers.

The obesity epidemic in the United States presents another challenge for imaging professionals. When positioning a patient for an examination, radiographers depend on palpation of (manually feeling for) bony landmarks. It is difficult to locate these landmarks on obese patients. The examination tables have weight limits, which some patients may exceed. In computed tomography (CT) and magnetic resonance imaging (MRI), these patients may literally not fit into the aperture (opening) of the scanner. These circumstances put radiologic technologists in the awkward position of asking patients for their weight. Obese patients also cause additional physical stress for the technologists, especially if they are not ambulatory or are in need of assistance getting on the examination table.

The technology used to produce images has changed dramatically in the last decade. Many radiographers in practice

Aptitude Profile

A career in radiography is not a good fit for everyone. Someone investigating medical imaging opportunities should be outgoing and helpful. When considering the field, it is important to determine if you have the personality traits to be a successful radiographer. Following are some characteristics required to be a good imaging professional:

Able to interact with diverse populations	Computer literate
Able to meet deadlines	Dependable
Ability to manipulate x-ray equipment	Empathetic
Able to work independently	Good communication skills
Ability to work in dimly lit area	Like to help others
Adaptable to changing work environment	Good manual dexterity
Attentive to detail	Task oriented
	Team player
	Willingness to walk/ stand about 80% of a workday

today began their careers taking x-rays using film and chemical darkroom processing. The vast majority of facilities have transitioned to computed or digital radiography, which produce electronic images on a receptor plate. Technologists who are not computer literate may feel intimidated by these new technologies.

Role of the Radiologic Technologist (Radiographer)

On successful completion of an educational program, a prospective radiologic technologist is determined to be registry eligible by the program director. If the student's scaled score is 75 or above on the American Registry of Radiologic Technologists (ARRT) examination, the graduate may use the credentials RT(R) and is a certified radiographer. Radiography is a primary certification. The radiographer is now qualified to perform a variety of different diagnostic examinations, including fluoroscopy (Fig. 23-3). Most radiographers work in hospitals where they use ionizing radiation to make diagnostic images. Physicians interpret these images to identify fractures and diseases. Some radiographers may work in private medical practices where they may also perform medical assisting duties such as monitoring vital signs, drawing blood, and giving injections. All radiologic technologists work with sophisticated equipment (Fig. 23-4) and computers. Radiographers are valued members of the health-care team.

In addition to general radiography, there are also several secondary certifications. These certifications require documentation of performance of proctored examinations, as well as passage of an additional examination. The roles of these radiologic technologists are discussed next.

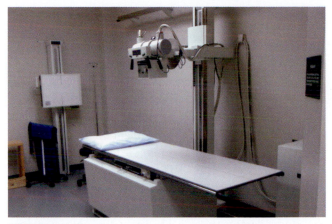

FIGURE 23-4 Diagnostic radiography room. Radiographers work with various types of equipment that aids in diagnosing health conditions.

Computed Tomography (CT) Technologist

A CT technologist uses sophisticated equipment (Fig. 23-5) that employs a rotating x-ray tube to produce cross-sectional images of patients. These images may be used to find kidney stones, tumors, fractured vertebral bodies, arterial stenosis, or ruptured vertebral discs. These technologists must be knowledgeable about viewing anatomy in three dimensions. Many of the examinations require use of contrast media (x-ray dye), so CT specialists must be proficient in administration of intravenous contrast. Trauma victims, whether involved in motor vehicle accidents or invasive trauma such as a gunshot wound, routinely have CT examinations. These technologists often work with critically ill patients. They must be efficient and ready to deal with emergency situations.

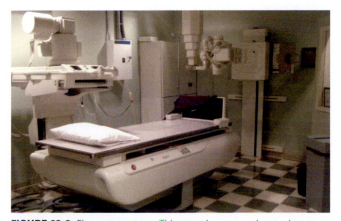

FIGURE 23-3 Fluoroscopy room. This room houses equipment known as a fluoroscope that uses imaging techniques to perform real-time moving images. Images such as a pumping heart can be seen in real time to aid in diagnosing.

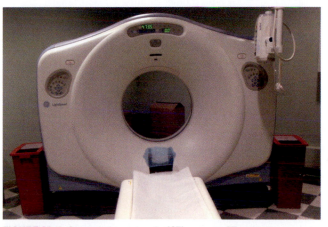

FIGURE 23-5 Computed tomography (CT) scanner. CT scanners use computer-processed x-rays to view images of a specific area. These images allow for inside views without cutting through the object.

Cardiovascular Interventional Technologist

A cardiovascular interventional technologist (CVIT) images the heart and/or peripheral vessels. To visualize the vasculature, contrast agents are instilled in the vessels with a power injector. These procedures are highly invasive. To examine the arterial system, an interventional radiologist or cardiologist inserts a catheter into the femoral artery under sterile conditions. The CVIT may scrub in to assist the physician. The technologist sets the injection and filming rates as directed by the physician. If the diagnostic phase of the study demonstrates a blockage, the physician may choose to perform an interventional procedure called an *angioplasty.* The blocked vessel may be expanded using a special balloon catheter and a stent may or may not be deployed to help keep the vessel open. CVITs may work in

the cardiac catheterization laboratory or interventional radiography. Regardless of where they work, they must know how to prepare and maintain a sterile field and be highly familiar with vascular anatomy.

Magnetic Resonance (MR) Technologist

An MR technologist uses a scanner (Fig. 23-6) that uses strong magnetic fields and radiofrequencies to obtain cross-sectional images of patients. MR images do not show bones very well, but they are excellent for demonstration of soft tissue. These images are extremely useful for soft tissue injuries such as ligament damage. MR is also used to image the central nervous system to diagnose ruptured discs in the spine and nerve diseases such as multiple sclerosis. To create the images, a very strong magnet is needed. The MR technologist must carefully

Author Spotlight

Amy Freshley-Lebkuecher, MS

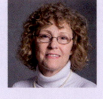

My name is Amy Freshley-Lebkuecher, and I've been a radiography professional for almost 30 years. As a radiographer and a radiation therapist, I've worked in many capacities in diagnostic imaging and radiation oncology. Like many high school juniors, I was unsure of what I wanted to do with my life. Although I knew I wanted to work in health care, I wasn't sure about what field. I was anxious to start my career, and I felt 4 years of college was not an option. At that time, respiratory therapy was a hospital-based, 1-year certificate program. One evening I was speaking with one of my babysitting clients. She asked about my future plans and I told her about respiratory therapy. She said, "Well, do you know what I am?" Since I knew her only as a full-time mother of three, I was clueless. She revealed that she was a radiologist, a specialized physician who interpreted medical images. She took a break from her practice while her children were young, but was about to resume her career. She advised me to consider radiology, explaining that there were several career paths within the profession. I did some research, found a program nearby, and was on my way. While working full time, I pursued bachelor's and master's degrees. After 25 years of clinical practice, I accepted a faculty appointment at Austin Peay State University. As the clinical coordinator in the bachelor's degree radiologic technology program, I taught radiography courses and provided clinical oversight. In June 2012, Austin Peay added a radiation therapy concentration to the radiography program. I am the director of that concentration. Radiation therapy is my true passion, so I am thrilled to play a role in the training of the next generation of therapists.

Rex Ameigh, MSLM

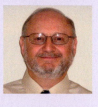

My name is Rex Ameigh, and I served my country for 20 years in the U.S. Army. After retirement, I was unsure about the path I wanted to pursue. Initially, I interviewed with a few companies that were similar to my active duty experience. Those experiences left me with the feeling I wanted to do something different. I reflected back to occupations I considered after high school graduation. At that time, I thought about going to medical school, nursing, or radiography school. The educational requirements for medical school required so many classes; I would need to complete a bachelor's degree to meet the application requirements. The educational requirements for nursing were within reason, but I didn't think long-term patient care was a good fit for me. That realization led me back to radiography. My research reinforced my suspicions—radiography was the right occupation for me. After graduation, I was hired as a weekend technologist at a level one trauma center. I enjoyed this position because I like helping people. Providing a public service is very rewarding. After working as a technologist for a few years, I was given the opportunity to teach. In the ensuing years I've held several teaching positions. I also enjoy this aspect of the profession. Although now I mostly help students, I still feel I'm helping patients by training competent, caring professionals. As I've gotten older, I've decided that it's not work if you enjoy what you're doing. I do really enjoy what I'm doing, and I plan to continue teaching as long as that is the case. If you like helping people in a patient care setting, you will enjoy this occupation. It is very rewarding both professionally and financially.

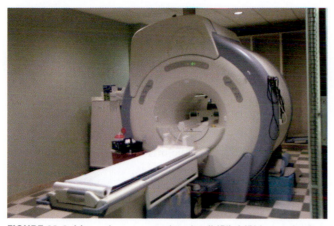

FIGURE 23-6 Magnetic resonance imaging (MRI). MRI is a technology that uses magnetic fields and radio waves to create images of the body without exposing the patient to ionizing radiation.

screen each patient before a scan is performed. Patients with cardiac pacemakers or implanted ferromagnetic devices could be seriously injured if subjected to the strong magnetic fields. MR technologists may also inject contrast material.

Mammographer

Mammography is a radiographic examination that uses a dedicated x-ray unit (Fig. 23-7) to image breast tissue. A mammogram, a radiographic examination of the breast, can determine whether a breast lump is a cyst or a solid tumor. Mammography can detect very small breast cancers, often before a lump is felt. Mammographers play a vital role in early detection of breast cancer. Early detection saves lives, so mammographers provide a valuable service. Many mammographers cross-train in bone densitometry. Bone density scans are performed on a dual-energy x-ray machine (Fig. 23-8) and are used to evaluate women for osteopenia or osteoporosis. These conditions are most prevalent in postmenopausal women. Women over age 40 should have routine screening mammograms, and women 50 or older should have a baseline bone density scan. The demographics of these groups are similar, so it makes sense to offer both services in one location. Cross-training the mammography staff is a good use of human resources.

Quality Management (QM) Technologist

A QM technologist reviews radiographic images for technical accuracy. The radiographer taking the images does an initial review. However, the QM technologist is responsible for ensuring the images meet the radiologist's criteria for diagnostic purposes. QM technologists may also perform quality control tests on the radiographic equipment.

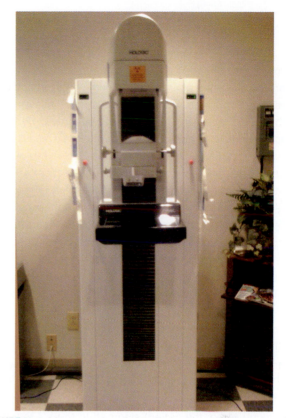

FIGURE 23-7 Mammography unit. Mammography machines use low-dose radiation to produce breast tissue images for purposes of diagnosing and screening.

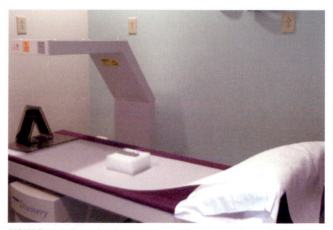

FIGURE 23-8 Bone density scanners produce images for evaluation of osteopenia or osteoporosis, which is a condition resulting in an increased risk of bone fractures.

Working Together

Radiographers work with a variety of clinical and support staff. The radiographer interacts with clinicians, nurses, and allied health professionals, as well as support staff including housekeeping, central supply, pharmacy, admitting, and dietary services. Additionally, they work with patients, their families, and the general public.

CASE STUDY

At 6:30 p.m., a 37-year-old man was admitted to the emergency department (ED) complaining of severe back pain. The patient, a construction worker, stated he may have "pulled something" in his back while on the job. The ED physician reviewed the electronic medical record (EMR) and noted that the patient had a past history of kidney stones. The physician decided to order some tests to determine the cause of the patient's pain. Initially, an x-ray examination of the lower (lumbar) spine was requested. The radiographer was contacted, and the patient was transported to the imaging department. The images were obtained, and the patient returned to the ED to await the results. The lumbar images were interpreted as normal.

The patient's pain was still severe, and the physician suspected a kidney stone. Laboratory findings were inconclusive. A computed tomography (CT) examination without contrast media is a highly reliable method of diagnosing renal calculi. The physician decided to request a CT scan. The imaging staff was contacted and the CT technologist performed the scan using a kidney stone protocol. Again, the patient returned to the ED to wait for results. The CT was reported as negative for kidney stones.

The patient's pain continued to intensify. As time passed, the patient noticed some tingling and intermittent numbness in the lower extremities. This finding prompted the ED physician to consider magnetic resonance imaging (MRI). The decision was made to admit the patient for pain management and a 24-hour observation. In most hospitals, the MRI department does not operate around the clock. The MRI was requested for 8:00 a.m. the next day.

The MRI of the lumbar spine revealed a ruptured disc. A neurologist was consulted and the decision was made to prescribe bedrest in the short term. The patient was discharged with a referral to an orthopedic surgeon who would determine a long-term plan. The plan would probably include physical therapy featuring back-strengthening exercises and instruction on proper lifting techniques.

Questions

1. What medical professionals and ancillary staff were involved in the patient's care?

2. Why were radiographs of the lumbar spine requested?

3. Why was a CT scan performed?

4. When the patient complained of numbness and tingling, what procedure was requested and why?

Review Questions

1. Wilhelm Conrad Roentgen discovered x-rays in:
   A. 1589
   B. 1859
   C. 1895
   D. 1995

2. The radiologic technologist most likely to image a patient with a possible ankle fracture is:
   A. A radiographer
   B. A CT technologist
   C. An MRI technologist
   D. A cardiovascular technologist

3. The radiologic technologist most likely to image a patient with a possible ruptured disc is:
   A. A radiographer
   B. A CT technologist
   C. An MRI technologist
   D. A cardiovascular technologist

4. The radiologic technologist most likely to image a patient with a possible kidney stone is:
   A. A radiographer
   B. A CT technologist
   C. An MRI technologist
   D. A cardiovascular technologist

5. The radiologic technologist most likely to work in interventional radiography is:
   A. A radiographer
   B. A CT technologist
   C. An MRI technologist
   D. A cardiovascular technologist

6. Which of the following is not a challenge facing radiographers?
   A. The obesity epidemic
   B. Lack of computer skills
   C. Too many young radiography professionals
   D. Influx of patients due to the aging population

7. The radiologic technologist most likely to image a patient with a breast mass is:
   A. A radiographer
   B. A mammographer
   C. A CT technologist
   D. A quality management technologist

8. The radiologic technologist most likely to perform quality control tests on radiographic equipment is:

    A. A radiographer

    B. A mammographer

    C. A CT technologist

    D. A quality management technologist

9. The earliest x-ray images were recorded:

    A. Digitally

    B. On glass plates

    C. Electronically

    D. On polyester bases

10. Which of the following is the national professional society for imaging professionals?

    A. ARRT

    B. JRCERT

    C. ASRT

    D. ISRRT

Glossary of Key Terms

Computed tomography (CT)—a computerized radiographic procedure that produces cross-sectional images of the anatomy

Radiologic technologist—a person who operates diagnostic radiologic equipment to perform radiographic examinations of patients with the supervision of a physician

Primary-care provider (PCP)—a health-care provider who manages the health care provided to a patient

Radiologist—a medical specialist who is trained in imaging for purposes of diagnosing and treating diseases

Medical doctor (MD)—a physician who has completed medical school and residency in a specific area of medicine

Doctor of osteopathy (DO)—a physician with additional training in the manipulation of muscles and bones to promote healing

Physician assistant (PA)—a specially trained and licensed individual who performs tasks usually done by a physician and works under the direct supervision of a physician

Nurse practitioner (NP)—a registered nurse with advanced training who can practice medicine with the supervision of a licensed physician

Accreditation—the voluntary process of recognizing that a facility or institution has met established standards

Magnetic resonance imaging (MRI)—a radiologic technology modality that uses magnetic fields to image parts of the body using a computer system

Cardiovascular interventional technologist (CVIT)—a technologist with special training in both invasive and non-invasive cardiovascular techniques

Mammography—radiographic examination of the breast

Bone densitometry—a method to determine the mineral density of bones using a specialized radiographic procedure

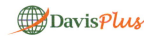 Additional Resources are available online at www.davisplus.com

Additional Resources

American Society of Radiologic Technologists (ASRT)—www.asrt.org

ASRT is the professional society of radiologic technologists and radiation therapists.

American Registry of Radiologic Technologists (ARRT)—www.arrt.org

ARRT is the credentialing agency for radiologic technologists and radiation therapists.

International Society of Radiographers and Radiologic Technologists (ISRRT)—www.isrrt.org

ISRRT is an international organization that fosters communication with radiologic technologists worldwide to advance education and the practice of radiologic technology.

Joint Review Committee on Education in Radiologic Technology (JRCERT)—www.jrcert.org

JRCERT promotes excellence in education and elevates quality and safety of patient care by offering external accreditation of radiologic technology programs.

References

1. Harris EL. The birth of science. In: Young PT, McElveny C, Pongracz-Bartha B, eds. *The Shadowmakers: A History of Radiologic Technology,* 1st ed. Albuquerque, NM: American Society of Radiologic Technologists; 1995.

2. Joint Review Committee on Education in Radiologic Technology. History.

    http://www.jrcert.org/history.

              Accessed November 13, 2013.

3. Sherer MAS, Visconti PJ, Ritenour ER. Radiation quantities and units. In: Wilke J, Hutchinson M, eds. *Radiation Protection in Medical Radiography,* 5th ed. St. Louis, MO: Mosby Elsevier; 2006.

4. American Society of Radiologic Technologists. About ASRT.

    http://www.asrt.org.

    Accessed November 13, 2013.

5. Carlton RR, Adler AM. *Principles of Radiographic Imaging: An Art and a Science,* 4th ed. Clifton Park, NY: Thomson Delmar Learning; 2006.

6. Bureau of Labor Statistics, U.S. Department of Labor. Occupational outlook handbook, 2012–2013 edition, radiologic technologists.

    http://www.bls.gov/ooh/healthcare/radiologic-technologists.htm.

    Accessed November 11, 2013.

CHAPTER 24

Radiation Therapy

Jennifer L. Harper, MD

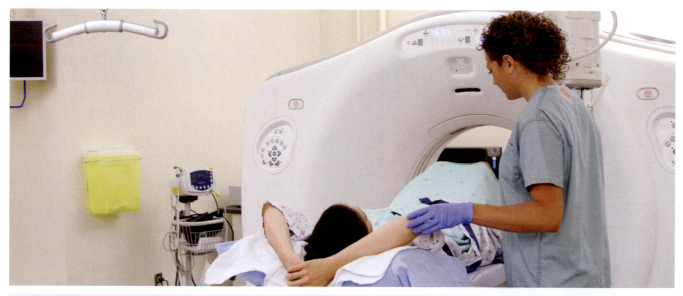

Photo credit: istock/Thinkstock

Learning Objectives

After reading this chapter, students should be able to:

- Explain the role of a radiation therapist in patient care and safety
- Describe the education and credentialing process
- Identify the members of an interprofessional team within a radiation oncology department and describe their respective roles
- Describe the opportunities and challenges of a career in radiation therapy

Key Terms

- Linear accelerator
- Simulation
- Oncology
- Radiation oncologist
- Medical physicist
- Medical dosimetrist
- Radiation therapist

"A Day in the Life"

Hi, my name is Ashley and I am a radiation therapist. I am a member of a tightly coordinated interprofessional team, composed of doctors, nurses, medical physicists, medical dosimetrists, and radiation therapists, involved in the treatment of cancer with radiotherapy. As I review my schedule this morning, it reflects many of the skills and responsibilities of a radiation therapist. The first half of the day, I will be working with my partner treating patients on a **linear accelerator,** a technologically advanced machine that generates the high-energy x-rays used in the treatment of cancer. The radiation therapists begin each day by measuring the x-ray beam's energy output to ensure it is accurate. These measurements must be performed and must meet protocol standards before

treating any patients. Undetected errors in energy output could result in undertreating the patient, resulting in cancer recurrence, or overtreating the patient, resulting in patient injury. If the measurements do not meet our quality standards, I will contact our medical physicist, who will perform further diagnostic tests on the equipment to identify the problem. In this way, radiation therapists are essential to ensuring patients are safely and accurately treated.

My first patient of the day is undergoing a series of daily radiation treatments over a course of several weeks, which is commonly prescribed. He has a diagnosis of oral cavity cancer. As a result of both the cancer and sores in the mouth, a common side effect of radiation therapy to this region, he is not

(continued)

able to eat very well. I notice he looks like he has recently lost weight. I review the recorded weights in the medical record and confirm that he has lost 8 pounds in under a week. I alert the doctor and the nursing staff to his state of malnutrition. The patient will be referred to a dietitian for consultation. As a radiation therapist, I am the primary liaison between our patients and the medical staff. I am actively involved in assessing the needs, both medical and social, of our patients during the course of treatment and reporting those to the physicians and nurses as illustrated by this patient encounter.

My second patient of the day is undergoing radiation therapy for the diagnosis of lung cancer. Before delivering a treatment, a series of radiographic images is obtained by the radiation therapist to ensure the lung tumor is encompassed by the radiation beam. These images can be either two-dimensional x-rays or three-dimensional computed tomography (CT) images. Our linear accelerator has the capability of capturing CT images, so I obtain and review the CT images of the patient on the treatment table. During this process, I confirm the position of the lung tumor relative to the planned radiation dose distribution and confirm that all treatment parameters match those prescribed. Radiation therapists make minor adjustments to the patient position parameters to ensure the tumor is localized accurately, if necessary. This process of daily imaging and real-time modification of patient position on the treatment machine is called *image-guided radiation therapy.* Finally, I contact the physician for final review and will administer the patient's treatment. Radiation therapists use their knowledge of radiographic anatomy, skills in medical imaging, and understanding of equipment capabilities to ensure the prescribed course of radiation is accurately administered.

During today's lunch hour we are having a staff meeting to review updated hospital procedures, such as appropriate measures for reducing risk of infections, emergency evacuation preparedness, and radiation safety protocols. In our department, it is extremely important to remind the radiation therapy team of our responsibilities in minimizing the occupational exposure to radioactivity.

This afternoon I will be working as the simulation therapist in our simulation procedures. The process of developing a radiation therapy treatment plan is personalized for every patient and requires extensive initial planning. The first step is called a **simulation.** During this collaborative procedure the physician, an expert on dose calculations, the medical dosimetrist, and the simulation therapist determine how best to position a patient for the daily course of treatment, what devices can be used to aid in replicating that position daily, and what barriers to reproducibility may exist.

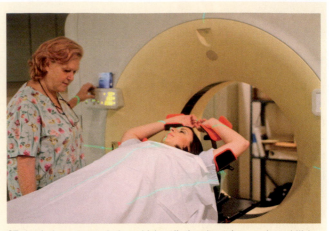

CT simulation process during which radiation therapists use immobilizing devices and help determine optimal patient positioning. CT images of the patient in the treatment position are then obtained.

Once these issues are addressed, the simulation therapist will perform a CT scan of the patient in the treatment position. These three-dimensional CT images will be a "virtual model" of the patient that is used for defining the tumor volume and modeling the radiation dose distribution in the treatment planning software program. After a radiation treatment plan is developed, it is critical that the patient's positioning at the time of the simulation be replicated by the radiation therapist with each treatment to ensure the prescribed dose to the tumor and adjacent healthy tissue is accurately delivered. Radiation therapists administering daily treatments regularly face equipment-related and patient-related challenges to reproducing patient positioning. Thus, their input is invaluable at the time of simulation.

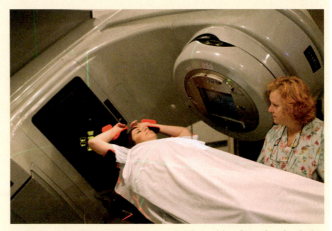

Radiation therapists replicate the patient's position from the simulation on the treatment couch of a linear accelerator as they prepare to deliver the treatment.

Introduction to Radiation Therapy

Radiation Therapy in Cancer Treatment

Radiation therapy is a cancer treatment modality which uses high-energy x-rays, called photons, or radioactive materials to kill cancer cells by damaging their DNA. Radiation therapy can be used in patients with both curable and incurable stages of cancer. Depending on the type and location of the tumor, radiation therapy may be used as a standalone treatment or may be combined with surgery and chemotherapy. For those patients with incurable or metastatic stages of cancer, radiation therapy can be used to relieve cancer-related symptoms such as acute neurological injury or bone pain.

History of Radiation Therapy

Shortly after the development of the x-ray tube and the discovery of x-rays, cancer-fighting applications were postulated. Many of the pioneers in x-ray technology suffered burns and soft tissue necrosis of their hands because the harmful effects of overexposure to x-rays were not yet fully understood. This led to the hypothesis that if radiation exposure from x-rays could produce injury to healthy tissue, it may curb the uncontrolled growth of cancerous tissue. Emil Grubbe, a Chicago medical student, was the first American to test this hypothesis when he employed x-rays to treat a patient with recurrent breast cancer along the chest wall in 1896.[1] Grubbe was able to demonstrate a treatment response, although his patient ultimately died of disease progression to other organs.[2] The early x-rays used by Grubbe and others were very low energy and thus only superficially penetrating. This limited the application for therapeutic x-rays to only superficial tumors. A tremendous breakthrough in the field of radiation oncology occurred with the development of the linear accelerator in the 1960s. The linear accelerator was capable of producing much higher energy x-rays and thereby afforded the opportunity to treat tumors deeply seated within the body without causing excessive injury to normal tissue.

In 1902, Marie and Pierre Curie discovered radium, a radioactive element that emits a naturally occurring form of x-ray called a gamma ray. Radium and other radioactive materials began to be implemented in the treatment of tumors arising in anatomical sites where the radioactive sources could be temporarily or permanently implanted. Radioactive materials are still being used to treat common cancers such as prostate and cervical cancer. The application of radioactive sources to treat tumors is termed *brachytherapy*.

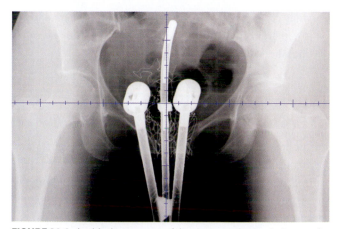

FIGURE 24-1 A critical component of the treatment for cervical cancer involves placing radioactive sources, harbored within a brachytherapy applicator, into the uterus and vaginal vault. This is a radiograph of the female pelvis with a brachytherapy applicator in place.

Modern Radiation Therapy

Modern **oncology,** the medical field of cancer care, involves multiple treatment modalities, including surgery, chemotherapy, and radiation therapy. Physicians representing the surgical, medical, and radiation oncology fields collaborate in a multidisciplinary team to determine which modalities should be used, and in what sequence, to optimize patient outcomes. Within a radiation oncology department, there is also an interprofessional team who design, implement, and ensure the quality of a radiation therapy treatment plan. These teams include radiation oncologists, medical physicists, medical dosimetrists, and radiation therapists:

- The **radiation oncologist** is the physician who determines the indications for radiation therapy and prescribes the dose and duration of an individual patient's treatment.

- The **medical physicist** has a background in physics that is applied to the field of radiation oncology. The medical physicist's role is to assist in the development of treatment plans and monitor the safety and functionality of all imaging and therapy equipment with the radiation oncology department.

- The **medical dosimetrist** has expertise in radiation dose calculation and distribution. Using advanced computer software modeling, radiation dosimetrists work with medical physicists and radiation oncologists to develop a radiation therapy plan.

- The **radiation therapist** has expertise in the operation of radiation therapy delivery machines, such as linear accelerators. Radiation therapists participate in radiation treatment planning and treatment delivery. They have daily contact with patients undergoing treatment and are the primary liaison between the patient and the other members of the interprofessional team.

Types and Conditions of Employment

Employment opportunities can be found in hospitals and freestanding cancer centers. Radiation therapists generally work 8-hour days Monday through Friday. Current regulations require that two therapists at a time must be assigned to a treatment machine. This process helps ensure patient safety. Although emergent patient treatments are uncommon, radiation therapists may be required to be on call over nights, weekends, or holidays to cover emergent cases. These on-call times are shared among all the therapists working within a radiation oncology center.

Required Education

Accredited educational programs in radiation therapy provide students with a background in human anatomy, cancer pathophysiology and staging, physics of radiation therapy, radiation safety, and radiobiology. Students learn the clinical applications of these topics for radiation treatment planning and delivery. Programs provide supervised clinical experiences where students demonstrate proficiency in patient care, simulation, and treatment administration.

As of 2013 in the United States, there were 1- and 2-year certificate programs, associate-degree programs, and baccalaureate-degree programs in radiation therapy. The Joint Review Committee on Education in Radiologic Technology (JRCERT) is the accrediting agency for all radiation therapy programs recognized by the U.S. Department of Education. Only those students who have completed training in a JRCERT-accredited program are eligible to take the national certificate examination. The American Registry of Radiologic Technologists (ARRT) is the recognized certifying agency for radiation therapists. The ARRT has asserted that as of January 1, 2015, candidates for certification in radiation therapy must earn an associate degree, baccalaureate degree, or graduate degree from an accredited program to be eligible for certification examination. There are also ethics requirements for ARRT certification. The ARRT requires candidates to undergo an ethics review. The questions in this review process address any prior convictions, court-martials, disciplinary action by regulatory or other certification boards, and education honor code violations. Candidates who complete the certification process may use the credential RT(T) after their name. The RT designates registered technologist and the (T) denotes

radiation therapist. To maintain certification, a radiation therapist must obtain 24 hours of appropriate continuing education credits every 2 years.

Trends

In 2013, the Institute of Medicine issued a report on U.S. cancer care. The report asserts that the U.S. cancer care delivery system is in crisis due to factors that include an aging population and workforce shortages.[3] These issues have direct implications for the field of radiation therapy. The U.S. Bureau

---

Aptitude Profile

When considering a career in radiation therapy, one of the primary considerations should be an honest assessment of one's desire to participate in patient care. Radiation therapy, like most health-related professions, is a service industry and thus it is imperative that a radiation therapist enjoy the daily interaction with patients and their caregivers. Prospective radiation therapist should also be aware that the clinical work environment of a radiation oncology department exposes radiation therapists to communicable diseases, blood and other body fluids, and noxious odors. Radiation therapists should be compassionate and empathetic because the cancer patient population they are serving is facing life-threatening medical events or may be at the end of life. Further, radiation therapists should be able to maintain poise in stressful or changing work conditions.

There are physical demands that are essential to performing the duties of a radiation therapist. Radiation therapists generally work 8-hour shifts and are on their feet more than 80% of that time. Radiation therapists also frequently transfer patients with limited ambulation on and off of a treatment table. Therefore, many training programs require applicants to be able to lift 20 to 50 pounds occasionally and 10 to 25 pounds regularly.

Radiation therapists must also have attention to detail because they are a critical component in ensuring patient safety and accurate treatment administration. They should also be proficient in basic computer skills because the operation of the linear accelerators and imaging equipment such as CT scanners requires computer interface. Characteristics and skill sets are summarized in the following list:

Able to maintain calm and poise in stressful situations	Compassionate
	Desire to participate in patient care
Able to meet physical demands such as standing for long periods	Empathetic
	Proficient in basic computer skills
Attention to detail	

of Labor Statistics forecasts a faster than average growth rate of employment in the field of 20% from 2010 to 2020.[4] The median annual wage of a radiation therapist in May 2010 was $74,980 according to U.S. government reports.[4]

Challenges

Although the direct patient interaction and interprofessional care model make a radiation therapy career gratifying, there are challenges as well. The technology in the field of radiation therapy is rapidly evolving. The incorporation of new imaging technologies and new types of treatment delivery equipment are decreasing treatment-related side effects and improving cancer outcomes following radiation therapy. These advances in technology are also requiring radiation therapists to frequently acquire new skill sets to incorporate these emerging technologies into the clinical practice. Radiation therapists who quickly become proficient in new skills

will be an asset to their department, but those who do not can become obsolete.

An additional challenge facing radiation therapists can be the pressure of maintaining a tight daily schedule while ensuring accurate and safe treatment delivery. Generally, patients undergoing a course of radiation therapy will be given an appointment time for treatment. However, delays to a daily treatment schedule invariably occur. Delays may include such impediments as treatment machine malfunction, emergent add-on treatments, and patients presenting late for treatment. As the primary liaison with the patients in a radiation oncology department, radiation therapists bear the brunt of disgruntled patients required to wait for their treatment due to circumstances outside the therapists' control.

Author Spotlight

Jennifer L. Harper, MD

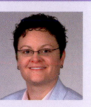

My first exposure to the field of radiation oncology was through the multidisciplinary tumor conferences I attended as a medical student. Faculty members representing the disciplines of surgical, medical, and radiation oncology participated in these conferences. I so enjoyed the case presentations, the discourse about treatment strategies, and the weighing of risk and benefit with each treatment modality. The concept of doctors working as a team to develop a personalized treatment recommendation for an individual patient was very appealing to me.

During my residency training in radiation oncology, I came to appreciate that a similar interprofessional team exists within a radiation oncology department. Radiation therapists are an essential component of that team. In my current position as a faculty radiation oncologist, I recognize and appreciate the radiation therapists' contribution to patient care. My patients frequently comment on the kindness and hospitality of the radiation therapist and how they have made their course of treatment a positive experience. I also rely on the radiation therapists to communicate with me about medical and social issues that arise with the patients during their course of treatment. On multiple occasions, radiation therapists have alerted me to acute patient changes in mentation, ease of breathing, or neurological status. These findings represented medical emergencies and the patients were managed appropriately. Working in this type of interprofessional teams is a very gratifying part of my profession.

Working Together

Radiation therapists are members of an interprofessional team within a radiation oncology department. The primary responsibilities of a radiation therapist include the administration of radiation to patients for cancer treatment, participating in development of radiation therapy treatment plans, and ensuring patient safety. Each of these duties requires collaboration with physicians, medical physicists, medical dosimetrists, and other radiation therapists.

CASE STUDY

Mr. Drayton is a 68-year-old African American man who was recently diagnosed with small-cell lung cancer. This type of smoking-related lung cancer often presents at advanced stages. In Mr. Drayton's case, he was found to have a primary tumor in the right lung and metastasis in the liver and bone. He was admitted to the hospital for worsening shortness of breath as a result of his progressing lung cancer. During the hospitalization, he had acute onset of weakness in bilateral lower extremities. Magnetic resonance imaging (MRI) of the spine revealed multiple soft tissue masses within the thoracic spine that were compressing the spinal cord. Tumor deposits that compress the spinal cord can impede nerve signal transduction, resulting in loss of motor strength and sensation below the level of the compression. Radiation therapy is the primary treatment of malignant spinal cord compression from small-cell lung cancer, a highly radiosensitive tumor. However, it is imperative that treatment begin as quickly as possible after the onset of neurological deficits. Delays in treatment can dramatically reduce the opportunity for neurological recovery. Thus, spinal cord compressions represent oncologic emergencies.

(continued)

The radiation oncologist saw Mr. Drayton in consultation after reviewing his MRI. She obtained a history; performed a physical examination, which confirmed bilateral lower extremity weakness; and recommended a palliative course of radiation therapy. The physician then discussed the plan with the radiation therapist staffing the simulation procedures. She communicated that the area of treatment was within the thoracic spine. This information instructs the radiation therapist as to what region of the spine should be encompassed by the CT scan images during the simulation. Recognizing the emergent nature of this case, the radiation therapist quickly coordinates a time to treat the patient on the linear accelerator following treatment planning. When Mr. Drayton is transported to the radiation oncology department, the radiation therapist greets him and explains the simulation process. He will be positioned on the CT scanner table in a supine position.

Mr. Drayton has back pain from the bone metastasis that is exacerbated by lying on the very firm CT scanner table. The simulation therapist noted his discomfort and thought his pain might be relieved by the placement of padding onto the CT table. However, the simulation therapist also was aware that the patient positioning, including the padding, would have to be replicated at the time of treatment. To treat the spine, the radiation beam would have to pass through any padding placed underneath the patient. She conferred with the medical physicist before placing the padding, to be certain that the padding had no properties that would attenuate or alter the radiation dose distribution at the time of actual treatment. After the medical physicist confirmed that it would be safe to place the padding, the simulation therapist obtained a CT scan of the thoracic spine. The medical dosimetrist imported the CT images into a treatment-planning software program. The radiation oncologist identified the levels of the cord compression on the CT images and defined the target volume. The medical dosimetrist developed a radiation treatment plan that delivered the prescribed dose to the target volume.

After the physician approved the plan, the dose calculations were confirmed by the medical physicist to ensure accuracy. Then Mr. Drayton was transferred to the radiation therapy treatment area and placed on the treatment couch of the linear accelerator. Using the treatment parameters that were communicated to the radiation therapist by medical dosimetry, the radiation therapist will position the patient and capture two-dimensional x-rays to ensure that the tumor will be accurately targeted by the radiation beam. After physician approval of the imaging and setup parameters, the radiation therapist will administer the first dose of radiation therapy.

Questions

1. How is interprofessional communication important in the simulation process?

2. In what way is the radiation therapist involved in ensuring the accuracy of the treatment administration?

3. In what way is the radiation therapist involved in ensuring the safety of the patient?

4. In what ways do the radiation therapists use their skills in image acquisition and knowledge of human anatomy to successfully design and implement a radiation therapy plan?

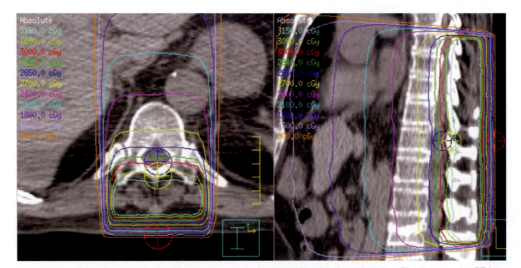

FIGURE 24-2 CT-based three-dimensional radiation therapy treatment plan targeting the thoracic spine. The lines on the CT image represent lines of equal radiation dose, called *isodose lines.*

Review Questions

1. Which of the following is not a member of the inter-professional care team within a radiation oncology department?

    A. Radiation oncologist

    B. Medical physicist

    C. Radiation therapist

    D. Phlebotomist

2. The role of a radiation therapist is to:

    A. Diagnose cancers and prescribe treatments

    B. Use computer modeling of radiation dose distribution on a virtual patient to develop a treatment plan

    C. Participate in radiation therapy treatment planning and administration of radiation to patients

    D. Manage human resources within a radiation oncology department

3. To be eligible for the radiation therapy certification examination in 2015, which of the following criteria must be met?

    A. Completion of a graduate program in radiation physics

    B. Completion of an associate degree, baccalaureate degree, or graduate degree from an accredited program

    C. Completion of an associate degree, baccalaureate degree, or graduate degree from an accredited program and completion of an ethics review by ARRT

    D. Completion of a 1- or 2-year certificate program in radiation therapy

4. During the initial planning phase of developing a radiation therapy treatment plan, called a simulation, the radiation therapist may perform a/an:

    A. MRI

    B. CT scan

    C. Radiation therapy treatment using high-energy x-rays

    D. Radiation exposure measurement

5. The agency responsible for credentialing radiation therapists is:

    A. The American Registry of Radiologic Technologists (ARRT)

    B. The American Society of Therapeutic Radiology (ASTRO)

    C. The American Radium Society (ARS)

    D. The American Joint Commission on Cancer (AJCC)

6. The challenges of a radiation therapy career include the:

    A. Relatively few positions anticipated in the future

    B. Requirements for credentialing by multiple agencies

    C. Need to quickly master emerging technologies

    D. Need to frequently relocate

7. The machine that generates the high-energy x-rays most commonly used in treating cancer is a:

    A. Linear accelerator

    B. CT scanner

    C. Thermography unit

    D. Hygrometer

8. Radiation therapists help ensure patient safety by:

    A. Accurately administering radiation therapy treatment

    B. Performing daily measurements of radiation beam output

    C. Assisting in evacuation procedures during emergencies

    D. All of the above

9. Educational programs in radiation therapy provide students with a background in which of the following?

    A. Human anatomy

    B. Biochemistry

    C. Medical billing and coding

    D. Human resource management

10. The credentialing process for radiation therapists involves an ethics review and would require reporting of which of the following?

    A. Military court-martials

    B. Divorce

    C. Parking violations

    D. Traffic citations

Glossary of Key Terms

Linear accelerator—a technologically advanced machine that generates the high-energy x-rays used in the treatment of cancer.

Simulation—a collaborative procedure in which the physician, the medical dosimetrist, and the simulation therapist determine how best to position a patient for the daily course of treatment, what treatment devices can be used to aid in replicating that position daily, and what barriers to reproducibility may exist. A CT scan is then obtained with the patient immobilized with appropriate treatment devices, in the treatment position. This CT scan will be used for three-dimensional radiation treatment planning.

Oncology—the medical field of cancer care which involves multiple treatment modalities, including surgery, chemotherapy, and radiation therapy.

Radiation oncologist—A physician who determines the indications for radiation therapy and prescribes the dose and duration of an individual patient's treatment

Medical physicist—Members of the interprofessional team within a radiation oncology department with a background in physics that is applied to the field of radiation oncology. The medical physicist's role is to assist in the development of treatment plans and monitor the safety and functionality of all imaging and therapy equipment with the radiation oncology department.

Medical dosimetrist—Members of the interprofessional team within a radiation oncology department with expertise in radiation dose calculation and distribution. Using advanced computer software modeling, medical dosimetrists work with medical physicists and radiation oncologists to develop a radiation therapy plan

Radiation therapist—members of the interprofessional team within a radiation oncology department expertise in the operation of radiation therapy delivery machines, such as linear accelerators. Radiation therapists participate in radiation treatment planning and treatment delivery.

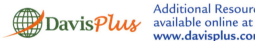

Additional Resources are available online at www.davisplus.com

Additional Resources

Radiation Therapy Accrediting Body
Joint Review Committee on Education in Radiologic Technology (JRCERT)—www.jrcert.org

Educational and Professional Resources
American Registry of Radiologic Technologists (ARRT)—https://www.arrt.org
ARRT is the agency that credentials radiation therapists after completing their training. Candidates for certification must pass the ARRT examination, as well as an ethics review.

American Society of Radiologic Technologists (ASRT)—www.asrt.org
ASRT is the leading professional society of radiologic science professionals. This includes radiation therapists.

References

1. Grubbe, Emil H. M.D. F.A.C.P. (obituary). *Br Med J.* August 20, 1960;2(5198):609.

2. Grubbe EH. *X-Ray Treatment: Its Origins, Birth, and Early History.* St. Paul and Minneapolis, MN: Bruce Publishing Company; 1949.

3. National Research Council. *Delivering High-Quality Cancer Care: Charting a New Course for a System in Crisis.* Washington, DC: National Academics Press; 2013.

4. Bureau of Labor Statistics, U.S. Department of Labor. Occupational outlook handbook, 2012–2013 edition, radiation therapist.

   http://www.bls.gov/ooh/Healthcare/Radiation-therapists.htm.

   Accessed January 18, 2014.

CHAPTER 25

Recreational Therapy

Mary Ann Keogh Hoss, PhD, and Missy Armstrong, MS

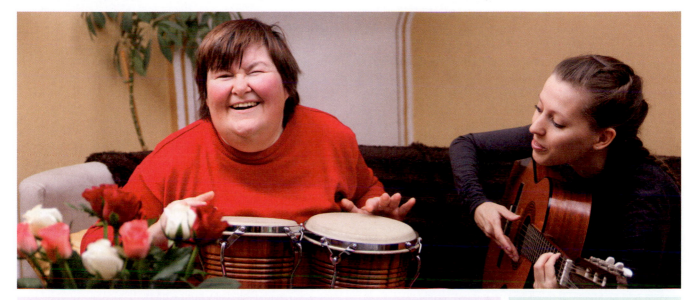

Photo credit: istock/Thinkstock

Learning Objectives

After reading this chapter, students should be able to:

- Define recreational therapy
- Define the role of a recreational therapist
- Describe the education and credentialing process for a recreational therapist
- Discuss the continuum of services provided in recreational therapy
- Explain the relationship between recreational therapists and other members of the health-care team
- Identify the opportunities and challenges for those working in the field of recreational therapy

Key Terms

- Certified therapeutic recreation specialist (CTRS)®
- Recreational therapist
- Quality of life
- Community integration
- Leisure
- Play
- Outcomes
- Function
- Wellness
- Chronic disease management
- Assessment, planning, implementation, and evaluation (APIE) process
- Addiction
- Community Skills
- Therapeutic recreation
- Nonpharmacological interventions

"A Day in the Life"

I am a **certified therapeutic recreation specialist** (CTRS)® presently working in an inpatient rehabilitation hospital-based unit. Rehabilitation units are only one of the many sites where a certified recreational therapist may work, but the hospital will probably be the first to introduce patients and families to the role of the **recreational therapist,** whose purpose is to improve **quality of life** through activity and **community integration** to improve physical, cognitive, emotional, social, and **leisure** and **play** needs.[1] This rehabilitation unit specializes in working with patients who have had spinal cord injuries, traumatic brain injuries, or strokes. The population of this hospital-based unit tends to be younger, individuals who engage in high-risk sports or personal behavior, and who value returning to their previous leisure experiences.

I'll decide on who to see based on the goals or **outcomes** that the patients have set for themselves. Each patient has had an assessment that includes standardized tests designed to identify attitudes and behaviors toward leisure and play and interests that could be used during treatment, or explored for modifications.[1] The goals for treatment will be in the area of physical and cognitive **function,** emotional attitudes toward their injury and change in lifestyle, and social skills and abilities. I'll need to know what family support is available, what kind of work the patient did, and, most important, with whom and what they did in their nonwork or leisure time. I'll want to know what community setting they are returning to and what the community has to offer in terms of activity and resources. My goal in all cases will be how I can get the individual back to his or her previous leisure interests with the fewest adaptations, with the people he or she enjoyed being with, with the fewest changes. If I can't, then, based on what I know about their function, I'll introduce new options for leisure. The treatment plan will consider the immediate needs of the patient, a long-term health and **wellness** plan, and the management of the patient's condition or **chronic disease management.** This is often referred to as the *four phases of the therapeutic recreation process,* or the **assessment, planning, implementation, and evaluation (APIE) process.**[1] This process leads to outcomes that promote those values unique to the individual.

My first patient is a current senior in high school. His injury occurred after a fall while water-skiing when another person ran over him with a motorized water ski. He suffered a traumatic brain injury, his left leg was severed above the knee, and he has multiple contusions. His transfer to inpatient rehabilitation was delayed when he developed pneumonia after he aspirated water. His brain injury has required that he relearn the basic skills for dressing and bathing; he has difficulty with his memory and attention and is unaware of any limitations he might have in those areas. His family reports that he doesn't seem to understand what has happened to him, is very quick to get angry, and has been combative. I will provide resources of reading materials, community services, and support organizations. I have been asked to spend time with the patient's younger sister, educating her to the changes that she will see, and to help her understand that her brother's condition will improve. We draw a picture together for his wall.

During our assessment, the patient reports that he isn't interested in being fitted with his new prosthetic leg and talks mostly about what he can't do because of the limb loss. He demonstrates limited insight into his brain injury as he verbalizes the unrealistic plan to drive home from the hospital and return to school the next day. He has a large group of friends who will require education and resources to help him cope with the increase in activity and stimulus that high school will bring. He states that he had a very active athletic lifestyle before his injury playing water polo, swimming competitively, and skiing both on water and on snow. He assumes that part of his life is over. He states that what he most wants to get back to is hanging with friends. He also reports that during the off season for swimming he drank and used marijuana daily, but he doesn't consider himself to have an **addiction.**

The recreational therapy goal will be to focus on how he will return to his social structure of friends and his active leisure lifestyle. His plan will include aquatic therapy, reengagement and education with his friends, and adapted equipment and experience for his prosthetic limb. He will be at risk for seizures and will be counseled to not drink alcohol or use marijuana for 1 year. He isn't agreeable to all of the goals but is very interested in the idea of getting back into the water, although he expresses some fear that it won't be like before.

During his inpatient stay he will be scheduled for regular aquatic therapy time. The first session will include desensitization to the water and, depending on how he is feeling, some initial adaptation to his limb. He admits that his fear of the water he loves is more dramatic than he thought and we introduce relaxation techniques. These appear to help, and we then address how he will get in and out of the water without his prosthetic leg, how he will dress, and any lower limb adaptations he might benefit from. I am aware that an above-the-knee amputation will change his kicking pattern and I may suggest a temporary flipper to even out his kick. His upper body stroke will probably remain the same. As skiing is a passion, we will guide him to research adapted ski programs, both water and snow, and discuss other adaptations he might use. To help him better acclimate to his previous social life, I will contact his friends and offer education about individuals with brain injuries and how, as friends, they can best help him. The patient denies that he has a brain injury, so the more information I can provide to his friends, the more equipped they will be to handle the personality changes that brain injuries can sometimes have. Research suggests that social structure and support will be critical to his recovery.

His outpatient recreational therapist will continue the goals but will integrate additional **community skills** necessary for independence. He has agreed to meet with other individuals with amputations. He and a friend have agreed to go skiing together and since I volunteer for the winter skiing program, I've promised that I will be his guide using the adapted ski sled during his first downhill snow run.

Introduction to Recreational Therapy

Description

The American Therapeutic Recreation Association (ATRA) serves as the professional membership organization for recreational therapists. As such, it provides information to individuals about the profession. The following is information regarding the profession based on frequently asked questions from the ATRA website.[2]

Recreational therapists use a wide range of activity- and community-based interventions and techniques to improve the physical, cognitive, emotional, social, and leisure needs of their clients. Recreational therapists assist clients to develop skills, knowledge, and behaviors for daily living and community involvement. The therapist works with the client and his or her family to incorporate specific interests and community resources into therapy to achieve optimal outcomes that transfer to the client's real-life situation.

Research supports the concept that people with active, satisfying lifestyles will be happier and healthier. Recreational therapy/**therapeutic recreation** (RT/TR) provides services based on individuals' interests and lifestyle and allows them to better engage in therapy and apply these functional improvements to all areas of their life. Ultimately, it allows them to generalize their therapeutic outcomes to their life after the health-care team is no longer involved, resulting in greater health maintenance over time. RT/TR aims to improve individuals' functioning and keep them as active, healthy, and independent as possible in their chosen life pursuits.

Recreational therapists may work with a wide range of individuals requiring health services, including geriatric, mental health, addictions, general medicine, physical medicine and rehabilitation, developmental disabilities, and pediatric clients.

Most recreational therapists are employed by health-care agencies and work in traditional inpatient hospitals or health facilities, but an increasing number are being hired in residential facilities, community mental health centers, adult day-care programs, substance abuse centers, hospice care, community centers, and school systems. There is a growing trend for recreational therapists to work in private practice providing services in the home and community as well.

RT/TR embraces a definition of "health" that includes not only the absence of "illness," but extends to enhancement of physical, cognitive, emotional, social, and leisure development so individuals may participate fully and independently in chosen life pursuits. The unique feature of RT/TR that makes it different from other therapies is the use of recreational modalities in the designed intervention strategies. RT/TR is extremely individualized to each person by his or her past, present, and future interests and lifestyle. The recreational therapist has a unique perspective regarding the social, cognitive, physical, and leisure needs of the patient. Incorporating the client's interests and the client's family and/or community makes the therapy process meaningful and relevant. Recreational therapists weave the concept of healthy living into treatment not only to ensure improved functioning, but also to enhance independence and successful involvement in all aspects of life.

Recreational therapy means a treatment service designed to restore, remediate, and rehabilitate a person's level of functioning and independence in life activities, to promote health and wellness, and to reduce or eliminate the activity limitations and restrictions to participation in life situations caused by an illness or disabling condition.[3] Recreational therapists are standard treatment team members in rehabilitation services. Recreational therapy is listed as a rehabilitation therapy service in The Joint Commission (TJC) standards. In addition, recreational therapists are designated as treatment team members (based on need) in the acute brain injury, postacute brain injury, and inpatient rehabilitation standards of the Commission on Accreditation of Rehabilitation Facilities (CARF). The Centers for Medicare and Medicaid Services (CMS) includes recreational therapy in the mix of treatment and rehabilitation services used to determine federal compliance in skilled nursing, rehabilitation (physical and psychiatric), and long-term care facilities. Therapeutic recreation is specifically indicated as a related service under the Individuals with Disabilities Education Act. A few states regulate this profession through licensure, certification, registration, or regulation of titles.

Recreational therapists plan, direct, and coordinate treatment programs for people with or at risk for disabilities, addictions, chronic disease, illness, or injury. Health promotion and wellness programs may be used to maintain or improve function and/or quality of life. Recreational therapists use a variety of techniques, including arts and crafts, drama, music, dance, sports, games, and community trips. These programs help maintain or improve a client's physical and emotional well-being. Recreational therapists are different from and should not be confused with recreation workers, who organize recreational activities primarily for enjoyment.[4] Recreational therapists may be referred to by many names, such as RT, CTRS®, recreation therapist, recreational therapist, activity therapist, inclusion specialist,[1] and therapeutic recreation specialist.

History

"Recreation is one of those special aspects of civilization which has the potential to contribute to the sustaining of life, the prevention of dysfunction and the treatment of pathology."[5] *Recreation* is defined by Webster as "refreshment of one's mind or body after work."[6] Because recreation is a common element of everyday life, recreational therapy is often not considered a serious profession. After all, how hard

can it be? The use of recreation and retreats to aid and cure illness has been traced back to ancient civilizations.

Recreation has served as a tool in rehabilitation since the early 1900s in the United States.[5] During World War I, "the American Red Cross initiated the provision of recreation services to military personnel in hospitals and convalescent centers overseas and stateside ... these services were considered diversional as well as therapeutic, were introduced into public health hospitals by the Red Cross."[7] The Veteran's Bureau gradually took over the care, treatment, and rehabilitation of servicemen with the replacement of Red Cross workers. Before World War II, several national movements took place that had an impact on the development of therapeutic recreation services. These included services for the blind or mentally retarded and the park and recreation movement.[7] The development of the profession has its roots in both hospital and clinical areas, with special populations such as the blind (now known as the visually impaired) and mentally retarded (now known as the developmentally delayed), as well as in the community with the park and recreation movement. Those multiple directions are where recreational therapists can still be found today.

Author Spotlight

Mary Ann Keogh Hoss, PhD

When I was in grade school, there was for a short time a person in my class who could not speak very well and had hearing aids. She was not able to keep up with the rest of the class and had to leave. I always thought, Why couldn't she have stayed and we help her to keep up? Later, when I was in high school, I did a lot of work in leading groups both at school and at work. I worked part time in a hospital in the kitchen. In the kitchen we had a 3-hour time block to serve, deliver, and clean up 600 meals for patients daily. While I learned my job as a soup person, I quickly got to know every job on the tray line. I became the *caller,* the person who starts the tray line. I had to be aware of the job and pace of eight other workers who were putting food on the tray. This taught me to be aware of who was doing what at what pace. Finally, I became the *checker.* This is the last person on the tray line who checks to make sure everything is on the tray correctly and places the tray for delivery. Knowing all aspects of a job and being responsible to monitor others' progress let me know that I could lead a group and pay attention to how each person was doing in the group. I liked learning about the variety of types of disabilities and impairments. It was an adventure and challenge to see how a person's recreation and leisure pursuits could improve his or her functioning and quality of life. In

college I was taught about the assessment process that needed to be put in place to look at each person's needs and functioning level. After assessing the person, a plan needed to be developed and implemented to reach goals the person had set. If the goals were or were not being met, an evaluation needed to be done. These experiences have helped me in all of the work I have done in my career.

Missy Armstrong, MS

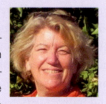

During my senior year of college my fiancée fell while skiing and became a tetraplegic. During our 6-month rehabilitation at one of the top three centers in the nation, we left the building once. No one seemed invested in teaching skills that would enhance our quality of life and leisure. Through trial and error, personal investment, research, and the support of our friends we were able to reengage with modifications to our previous interests. The teaching of basic community skills and the adaptations necessary for us to return to our previous interests became an ongoing passion and a lifelong professional commitment. I validated my interests with an MS in recreational therapy at University of Oregon, then on to Seattle where I have worked in pediatrics, geriatrics, physical rehabilitation, and psychiatry at Harborview Medical Center. Now a manager for an interdisciplinary team on rehabilitation and psychiatry, I am impressed at the functionality of play as a tool to reengage in life.

The first university educational programs in recreational therapy were started in 1950 with master's degree programs at Springfield College in Springfield, MA, the University of Minnesota, and Columbia University. In 1953, Sacramento State College offered a bachelor's degree in recreational therapy. San Francisco State College developed a hospital recreation program. Further development of the profession was seen with the creation of the Council for the Advancement of Hospital Recreation (CAHR) in 1953. This brought together four associations: the American Recreation Society, Hospital Section, established in 1948; the American Association of Health, Physical Education, and Recreation, established in 1952; the National Association of Recreational Therapists, established in 1953; and the National Recreation Association's Hospital Consultant, established in 1953.[8]

In 1955, CAHR published the first hospital recreation personnel standard suggesting national registration. This registration plan was in place as a national program until 1966, when the National Recreation and Park Association accepted the National Therapeutic Recreation Society (NTRS). At that time NTRS took over the national credentialing program. In 1981, the National Council for Therapeutic Recreation Certification (NCTRC), formerly the NTRS Board of Registration, became a completely autonomous national credentialing body for recreational therapists.[8]

In 1984, another professional membership organization was created, the American Therapeutic Recreation Association (ATRA), where professional services in health-care organizations were viewed by their effectiveness in improving functional capacity, health status, and/or quality of life of the client.[6] The 1980s saw the development of a body of knowledge and standards of practice. NTRS and ATRA worked jointly in the 1990s on areas of common interest to promote the profession. Throughout the 1990s and early 2000s, NCTRC revised and updated certification criteria and examinations, conducted job analyses, and reported on the growth of the field.[8] The NTRS branch of the National Recreation and Park Association was dissolved in 2010, leaving ATRA as the sole professional membership organization with NCTRC remaining as the national credentialing body.

Scope of Practice

The following description of practice scopes is taken from the National Council for Therapeutic Recreation Certification (NCTRC)[12]:

The primary purpose of recreation therapy practice is to improve health and quality of life by reducing impairments of body function and structure, reducing activity limitations, participation restrictions, and

environmental barriers of the clients served. The ultimate goal of recreation therapy is to facilitate full and optimal involvement in community life.

The scope of recreational therapy practice includes the following areas[9]:

- Patient/client assessments
- Planning an individualized approach
- Designing interventions specific to individuals
- Implementation of the plan for the person
- Documentation of the response to specific therapeutic interventions
- Evaluation of progress toward meeting rehabilitation goals
- Management of overall therapeutic recreation services
- Consultation to programs and individuals regarding therapeutic recreation services
- Research of therapeutic recreational interventions and outcomes
- Education, for either individuals or groups that require specific therapeutic recreation or recreational therapy intervention

Outcomes of service interventions may include the following[10]:

- Improvement in physical health status
- Improvement in long-term health status
- Reduction in health risk factors
- Improvement in cognitive functioning
- Improvement in psychosocial health and well-being
- Reduction in reliance on the health-care system
- Reduction in complications related to secondary disability
- Reduction in symptom levels of chronic or degenerative disorders
- Improvement in social interaction skills and social network
- Decrease in manifestations of stress and depression
- Reduction in medical complications and increase in rate of healing

Recreational therapists work with all of the therapies, including physical, occupational, and speech, as well as physicians, case managers, nursing, social workers, and other health-care professionals, especially in inpatient clinical settings. Recreational therapy differs from other therapies in its use of leisure and involves physical, cognitive, social, or emotional activity that is freely chosen and intrinsically motivated.[11] In clinical settings recreational therapists work with patients when the service has been ordered by a physician. In outpatient and community settings they may work alone or with a wide

Overcoming Obstacles

Although people who have had accidents or debilitating diseases may be temporarily challenged or barred from performing their previous activities, they do not necessarily give up on their dreams of returning to their previous functional capacity. They have to overcome many obstacles to achieve their goals, but it is immensely rewarding for them when they do.

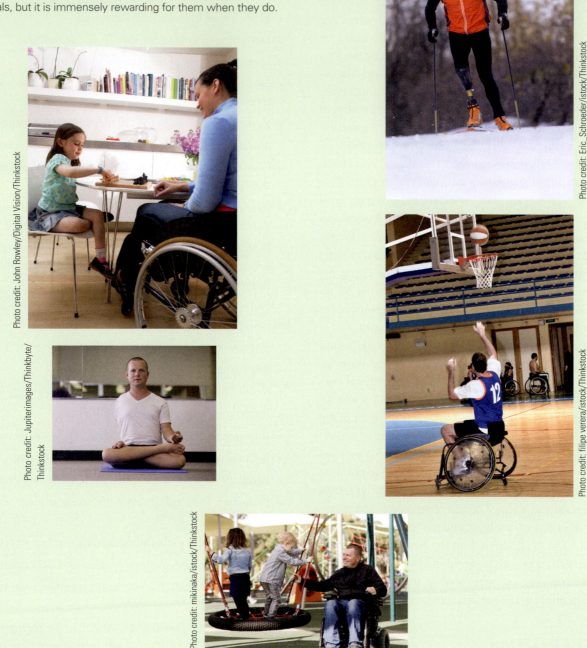

Photo credit: John Rowley/Digital Vision/Thinkstock

Photo credit: Eric_Schroeder/istock/Thinkstock

Photo credit: Jupiterimages/Thinkbyte/Thinkstock

Photo credit: filipe verera/istock/Thinkstock

Photo credit: mikinaka/istock/Thinkstock

variety of specialists with or without a physician order. When services are offered through a park and recreation department, these are open to the public for individuals and their families wanting the service. Recreational therapists may work in the home with individuals regardless of age who have need of the service. In states with Medicaid waivers, recreational therapists often work with individuals and their families to meet various needs. In some states using the patient-centered medical home approach, recreational therapists may be available. Recreational therapists are available by a variety of methods.

Required Education

As the governing body that credentials all recreational therapists in the United States and Canada, NCTRC suggests a bachelor's degree in therapeutic recreation or a related field. Master's and doctoral degrees are encouraged for educators and researchers.

Therapeutic recreation programs include courses in assessment of physical, cognitive, social, emotional, and behavioral function as it relates to leisure knowledge, skills and abilities, and functional independence in life activities, human anatomy and kinesiology, medical and psychiatric conditions, characteristics of illnesses and disabilities, and the use of assistive devices and technology. Bachelor's degree programs include an internship.[12]

Certification and License

Most employers prefer to hire certified recreational therapists. Hospitals and other clinical settings often require certification by the NCTRC. The council offers the certified therapeutic recreation specialist (CTRS)® credential to candidates who pass a written certification examination and complete a supervised internship of at least 480 hours. The CTRS® is the credential therapists use after their signature when documenting the therapeutic process as the setting requirements demand.

NCTRC also offers specialty certification in five areas of practice: geriatrics, behavioral health, physical medicine and rehabilitation, developmental disabilities, or community inclusion services. Therapists need a minimum of a bachelor's degree in recreational therapy to qualify for certification. Once certification is obtained, an annual maintenance process is in place. Every 5 years therapists must demonstrate work experience in therapeutic recreation and 50 hours of continuing education credit or pass the national examination to maintain their credential.[12]

Some states require recreational therapists to be licensed; requirements vary by state. As of 2010, only Oklahoma, North Carolina, Utah, and New Hampshire required recreational therapists to hold a license. For specific requirements, contact the state's medical/health board.

Salary

According to the Bureau of Labor Statistics (BLS)[13] in 2014 the mean hourly wage for recreational therapists was $22.14 and the mean annual wage was $46,060. Continuing-care retirement communities and assistive-living facilities for the elderly tend to have the lowest wages with the hourly mean wage at $18.54. General medical and surgical hospitals tend to have the highest hourly mean wage at $23.81. Salaries differ based on the type of setting in which a recreational therapist chooses to work.[13]

Trends

According to the BLS, the growth projections for the demand in the field is at 13%. The growth rate for all occupations is at 11%. The growth rate for recreational therapists is slightly higher than the national average, which indicates a good probability for the availability of jobs. Reasons for the positive employment trend include the following:

- As the large baby-boom generation ages, they will need recreational therapists to help treat age-related injuries and illnesses, such as strokes. Additionally, age-related declines in general physical ability, and sometimes mental ability, may also be treated with recreational therapy.

- Legislation requiring federally funded services for disabled students will continue to shape the need for recreational therapists in education settings.

- Third-party payers will continue to use therapists' services as a way to reduce the costs of inpatients' recoveries from injuries or illnesses, moving treatment to outpatient settings rather than more costly hospital settings.[4]

Challenges

All health-care professionals face challenges in the competitive health-care market. In recreational therapy, ongoing dilemmas include a lack of acknowledgment of the discipline as a health profession because of the value judgment placed on the term *recreation*. This term confuses both the public and other clinical professionals. Within the profession's context, recreation is play with a purpose. Recreational therapy is used as an intervention to achieve a specific outcome for an individual. In clinical settings, use of recreational therapy interventions is based on medical necessity. This means that recreational therapy services are reasonable and necessary for the treatment of illness or injury or to improve function. In community settings the promotion is health and wellness for special populations. The selection of a treatment or activity is based on the recognition of the different demographics and settings. This activity may be used to reinforce a skill or ability, to introduce a new skill for function, or to maintain and reinforce skills. All of these interventions are with intent to improve function and quality of life.

For example, in a long-term care facility where the population is primarily geriatric, the activity might be supported dancing to old swing tunes; in a hospital, the recreational therapist would work toward the community skills necessary to return to previous leisure interests at discharge; and in a facility managing patients with psychiatric illness, the recreational therapist might educate the depressed patient on skills that would provide structure, such as daily exercise, to promote wellness and recovery. To reinforce healthy behaviors, a community-based recreational therapist would need to recognize the unique needs of the chronic condition and to know the limits of the people they serve.

Health and wellness promotion is a rapidly growing area within recreational therapy, providing programs to meet community needs. Although acknowledged as valuable by the World Health Organization, the fulfillment of these concepts poses another challenge. Despite the benefits of community integration, leisure, and play to the rehabilitation process, the insurance companies want to cap costs through reduced lengths of patient hospital stays. A patient need only demonstrate 50 feet of ambulation with a walker to be considered ready for discharge; however, without supporting activity once home, the patient may not succeed. The national health picture recognizes the value of socialization, exercise, and reinforcing activity as critical to a positive attitude.

The national emphasis on health and wellness will place further demands on recreational therapists. Recreational therapists have long practiced in the community with both individuals and families. The demand to institute and expand programs and offerings to meet the needs of populations regarding obesity, mental health, and an aging population will tax existing resources.

Another demand on the profession is the growth of prison populations. Prison populations encounter issues such as untreated mental health, chronic disease management, and multiple disabilities. Program demands will continue to challenge practitioners. Youth detention facilities are another setting needing health and wellness promotion programs as well as therapeutic interventions.

There is some speculation within the broader rehabilitation community that the recreational therapist is only interested in introducing sports activity. To the contrary, most therapists are trained in many hands-on techniques for relaxation, symptom reduction, and socialization. A skilled recreational therapist will know the limitations of a given disease process. For example, the patient interested in art can be connected with an artist through the recreational therapist, but it will be the recreational therapist who manages the patient positioning, the manipulation of the brush (if there are hand limitations), and the management and placement of supplies for greatest independence.

Finally, it is a challenge for recreational therapists to be accepted as members of teams with many different health professionals. Again, because of misconceptions about the word "recreation," misunderstandings about recreational therapy can occur. In some clinical settings recreational therapy may be referred to as a **nonpharmacological intervention** because of the outcomes achieved with the interventions. Inclusion in interprofessional educational offerings is necessary for all disciplines to effectively understand that their role is achieving positive patient outcomes.

Role of the Recreational Therapist

The role of the recreational therapist supports the "playing to learn" approach to rehabilitation in all settings and with all ages. Children with disabilities may require a "learn to play" concept; developing social skills, situational learning opportunities, and life skills. Teens and young adults often have a "risk" (possibility of suffering harm) component to play that can be used as a treatment

Aptitude Profile

The BLS[4] identifies the following as attributes a person should possess if researching recreational therapy as a profession:

Compassion. Recreational therapists should be kind, gentle, and sympathetic when providing support to clients and their families. They may deal with clients who are in a great deal of pain or under severe emotional stress.

Critical-thinking skills. Recreational therapists should be able to quickly think of adaptations to activities when a client's therapy plan requires adjustment.

Leadership skills. Recreational therapists must be organized and able to plan, develop, and implement intervention programs in an effective manner.

Listening skills. Recreational therapists must listen to a client's problems and concerns. The therapist can then determine the course of intervention in the work treatment or therapy program appropriate for that client.

Patience. Recreational therapists may work with clients who need more time and special attention than other clients.

Speaking skills. Recreational therapists need to communicate well with their clients. They need to be able to give directions during activities or instruct a client on healthy coping techniques.[4]

intervention for positive behaviors and alternative approaches for alcohol/drug use. Adults have a similar opportunity using recreation, leisure, and play activities to integrate into the community, build tolerance/endurance, and organize and self-manage nonwork time. The therapist should be skilled in the ability to identify patient attitudes about leisure, the development of positive and safe leisure behaviors, and link to the age, ability, and access of the community. What is acknowledged is that all individuals learn through leisure and play.

As a member of an interdisciplinary team, the recreational therapist also supports and complements other team members' goals. The skills learned in one therapy provide the building blocks for other learning. The physical therapist may teach a patient to walk, but the recreational therapist will provide skilled oversight for the same person to walk in many different environments, such as with heavy traffic or in wet weather. This skill may be linked to independent transportation, advocacy for self,

and greater independence, including recreation and leisure. This educational process helps the patient integrate into the community.

For recreational therapists working in the community through a nonprofit organization or parks and recreation department, their role is to improve health by focusing on healthy behaviors and maintaining or improving one's quality of life. A recreational therapist should have knowledge of client behaviors and functional modification interventions, including techniques to adapt attitudes, knowledge, skills, and abilities. For example, the recreational therapist is trained to recognize the potential risks of ongoing alcohol abuse and to help identify the triggers to negative behavior and support alternatives.

Working Together

The team aspect of rehabilitation care depends on all disciplines having a unique role but sharing expertise and knowledge. It does not matter whether the setting is an acute-care hospital, a rehabilitation center, long-term care, a community center, or a camp for special populations or schools; it only matters that the unique and routine information built with the individual consumer in mind supports the long-term plan. The team links each skill set for the patient to greater independence. For example, the recreational therapist might seek out the nurse to determine how long the patient can sit in a chair comfortably; the physical therapist would provide valuable information regarding the patient's quality and distance of gait; the occupational therapist might suggest modifications that could be made to the patient's clothes that would promote independence; and the speech therapist would provide necessary information on memory and attention. Additionally, the social worker would have information about the possible discharge location, as well as the patient's family structure and dynamics. This combined information, and the assessment by the recreational therapist of the patient's knowledge, skills, and abilities as they relate to leisure and community independence, ensures a return to a positive, reinforcing, and as close to previous leisure lifestyle as possible. Although the patient has a limited inpatient stay, all therapies should progress the patient to greater independence and teach the necessary skills to be successful. The skill building continues in the community.

CASE STUDY

Ms. S is a 55-year-old woman admitted to the emergency department who was found to have had a rupture of a left posterior inferior cerebellar aneurysm and left cerebellar stroke that resulted in cognitive and mobility impairments. She was transferred to the inpatient rehabilitation unit, completed her course of treatment, and left the facility to home with supervision. At discharge she was able to ambulate 50 feet with a front-wheeled walker; was able to complete all activities of daily living (ADLs) independently; and, with the support of a memory book, was 90% for basic memory. Her swallow has improved to include thin liquids.

As an outpatient she is being referred to physical therapy, speech therapy, recreational therapy, and vocational rehabilitation. She was referred specifically to aquatics to improve ambulation, strength, and activity endurance. Additionally, her physician has expressed concern about the lack of community access and decreased socialization.

Medical history: Patient is post aneurysm with craniectomy, bypass, clipping, and external ventricular drain (EVD) placement, which is used to drain fluid from the brain. The patient also experienced left cerebellar stroke and ventriculoperitoneal (VP) shunt placement, which is used to relieve brain pressure. History of hypertension, breast cancer, osteopenia. No allergies to food/medications.

Functional abilities, strengths and limitations, and adaptations necessary: She is motivated to ambulate with a single-point cane from a front-wheeled walker, improve her memory, and return to work. She reports a fear of falling and reports being very tired by the afternoon. She is motivated and willing to learn to use public transportation to promote her independence. Her limitations

(continued)

include decreased activity endurance, strength, and safety. She is a fall risk.

Assessment of skills, abilities, interests, attitudes, and knowledge of resources: Physical: Patient ambulates independently with four-wheeled walker, walks up to 1 hour a day for exercise. She reports fatigue in the evening. She is continent and has no open wounds. Social: Lives alone in the city but was supported immediately after discharge from inpatient by a brother and sister. She has strong support from family and friends, but they all work during the day. She reports feeling lonely, and misses her group of friends.

Transportation: She has transitioned the training she received from recreational therapy, using a shuttle to get back and forth to the hospital. She is anxious to feel more confident and use the city bus to gain access to more shopping, bank, friends, and recreation resources.

Cognitive: She denies impairments. Speech reports a significant improvement in her memory except when in a stressful situation.

Patient reports that she continues to adjust and process the changes she has had to make. She reports that she feels as if she is coping with her new disability but wants to move on and return to the activities and people that she enjoyed.

Leisure/recreation: Patient enjoys reading, walking, hiking, going to the gym, and spending time with friends. She reports daily exercise of walking and would like to add swimming. She is using a supported shuttle system but would like to use the city bus for greater options.

Individual recreational therapy treatment plan, including goals and objectives: Goals include safe entrance and exit of pool using the stairs; ambulation up to 2 laps in the pool without rest or support; independent use of the community bus to pool; energy conservation techniques with planned rest periods during activity; map route adjustment to promote safe walking; and use of ramps, elevators, and handrails.

Outcomes of implementing the treatment plan as documented in progress notes: Patient demonstrated progress in the following swimming techniques: elementary backstroke pull with pull buoy, elementary backstroke with verbal cues when at wall, breaststroke with limited kick coordination. Patient obtained goggles and demonstrated improved head position and independent

buoyancy with use, after initial adjusting to use. Patient is agreeable to transition to lap pool and deep water, tolerating 6 laps with fins, long rest between laps. Patient making progress toward transition between breaststroke rolling to supine for elementary backstroke when fatigued due to decrease stroke mechanics and anxiety related to catching breath. Patient agreeable to continuing work in lap pool so she can be independent without floatation equipment.

Education: Primary learner: patient.

Patient challenges to learning: Coordination anxiety, fatigue.

Topics taught: Aquatic safety, adaptive swim techniques, aquatic exercise, community integration, transportation options, value of socialization.

Posteducation response: Demonstrated understanding.

Six-session review: Patient continues to make steady progress in water ambulation. Team feels as if this has improved her stamina dramatically and she will be able to transition to single-point cane. She remains motivated and has increased her community lap swims, demonstrating improved technique, improved endurance, and safe techniques. She has had two supervised trips using public transport and reports less fear of falling. She has met several women in her gentle aerobics class and was thrilled when they invited her for tea after the pool, and even more thrilled when they suggested lunch the next day. She personally attributes these outcomes to the skills she learned in the pool and the experiences in the community.

Questions

1. Why is this therapist so concerned about what the patient's goals are?

2. Why is it so important to incorporate them into the treatment plan?

3. What is the most significant clinical risk to the success of this woman's treatment plan?

4. She had other leisure interests; how will her three individualized treatment goals help her to return to these activities? What else could be built into her treatment plan, for example, to return to hiking?

5. What do you think are the key therapy treatments that the recreational therapist provided for this patient that she could not do for herself?

Review Questions

1. The profession of recreational therapy in the United States is traced back to the:

   A. Veterans Bureau

   B. Red Cross

   C. Park and recreation department

   D. City government

2. Recreational therapy can be practiced by:

   A. An art therapist

   B. Park and recreation personnel

   C. A hospital technician

   D. A certified therapeutic recreation specialist

3. To become a recreational therapist, the education one needs is:

   A. An associate degree

   B. A bachelor's degree

   C. A master's degree

   D. A doctoral degree

4. To become a certified therapeutic recreation specialist, one must:

   A. Complete an internship and pass a national test

   B. Graduate from college

   C. Register at the state

   D. Sign up online

5. Recreational therapists use a range of activity- and community-based interventions to improve:

   A. Physical needs

   B. Cognitive skills

   C. Leisure needs

   D. All of the above

6. A quality one should possess if considering recreational therapy as a profession is:

   A. Compassion

   B. Critical thinking

   C. Listening skills

   D. All of the above

7. The projected job growth for recreational therapists is:

   A. Lower than the projected average

   B. Very close to the national average

   C. Significantly higher than the national average

   D. None of the above

8. Challenges for recreational therapists include:

   A. Confusion about the profession

   B. Having enough play time

   C. Being physically active

   D. All of the above

9. The scope of practice for recreational therapists includes:

   A. Listening to the person needing services

   B. Assessment

   C. Pleasing the family

   D. Moving the person receiving services to a new home

10. A rapidly growing area within recreational therapy is:

    A. Health and wellness

    B. Hospital work

    C. Rehabilitation units

    D. None of the above

Glossary of Key Terms

Certified therapeutic recreation specialist (CTRS)®—a person who has been granted the credential of a recreational therapist by the National Council for Therapeutic Recreation Certification

Recreational therapist—person practicing the profession of recreational therapy with a credential

Quality of life—subjective assessment of psychological and spiritual well-being characterized by feelings of satisfaction and contentment

Community integration—process of reintroducing a person to activities offered in the community

Leisure—experiences that support the development of capacities and resources leading to positive well-being

Play—activity related to development of the individual

Outcomes—expected changes in functional capacity, health status, and quality of life based on interventions

Function—potential ability to perform specific activities in daily life management

Wellness—the active process of becoming aware and making choices towards a healthy and fulfilling life

Chronic disease management—process of managing ongoing disease; heart disease, diabetes, failure, spinal cord injury, head injury, stroke

Assessment, planning, implementation, and evaluation (APIE) process—four phases of the therapeutic recreation process—Assessment, Planning, Implementation and Evaluation

Addiction—dependent on or abuse of substances such as alcohol or cocaine

Community skills—identified skills necessary to successfully maneuver in the community; curb cuts, open doors, elevators, carrying items, and using adapted devices

Therapeutic recreation—holistic process that purposefully uses recreation and experiential interventions to bring about a change

Nonpharmacological interventions—behavioral and social interventions, such as good hygiene or use of face masks, used to prevent communicable diseases

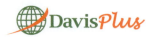

Additional Resources are available online at www.davisplus.com

Additional Resources

American Therapeutic Recreation Association—www. atra-online.com
National Council on Therapeutic Recreation Certification—www.nctrc.org
The Joint Commission—www.jointcommission.org
Commission on Accreditation of Rehabilitation Facilities (CARF)—www.carf.org

References

1. Carter MJ, Van Andel GE. *Therapeutic Recreation: A Practical Approach.* Long Grove: Waveland Press, Inc., 2011.

2. American Therapeutic Recreation Association. Frequently asked questions.

    https://www.atra-online.com/.
    Accessed April 17, 2014.

3. American Therapeutic Recreation Association. Definition of therapeutic recreation.

    http://www.atra-online.com/displaycommon.cfm?an=12.
    Accessed April 17, 2014.

4. Bureau of Labor Statistics. U.S. Department of Labor. Occupational outlook handbook, 2012–2013 edition, recreational therapists.

    http://www.bls.gov/ooh/healthcare/recreational-therapists.htm.
    Accessed December 19, 2013.

5. Avedon EM. *Therapeutic Recreation Services: An Applied Behavioral Science.* Englewood Cliffs: Prentice-Hall Inc., 1974.

6. *Webster's II New College Dictionary.* Boston: Houghton Mifflin Company, 2001.

7. Reynolds RP, O'Morrow GS. *Problems, Issues and Concepts in Therapeutic Recreation.* Englewood Cliffs: Prentice-Hall Inc., 1985.

8. Therapeutic Recreation Directory. Dixon C. Recreational Therapy—1940–2006.

    https://www.recreationtherapy.com/history/rthistory3.htm.
    Accessed April 18, 2014.

9. National Council for Therapeutic Recreation Certification. NCTRC scope of practice.

    http://nctrc.org/wp-content/uploads/2015/02/RP3-nctrc-scope-of-practice.pdf.
    Accessed December 10, 2013.

10. Coyne C, Kinney W, Riley B, Shanks J, eds. *Benefits of Therapeutic Recreation: A Consensus View.* Marysville: Adyll Arbor, 1998.

11. Robertson T, Long T. *Foundations in Therapeutic Recreation.* Champaign: Human Kinetics, 2008.

12. National Council for Therapeutic Recreation. Become a CTRS.

    http://nctrc.org/new-applicants/become-a-ctrs/.
    Accessed December 10, 2013.

13. Bureau of Labor Statistics. U.S. Department of Labor. Occupational employment and wages May 2014, recreational therapists 29-1125.

    http://www.bls.gov/oes/current/oes291125.htm#nat.
    Accessed September 3, 2015.

CHAPTER 26

Rehabilitation Counseling

Linda Holloway, PhD, CRC

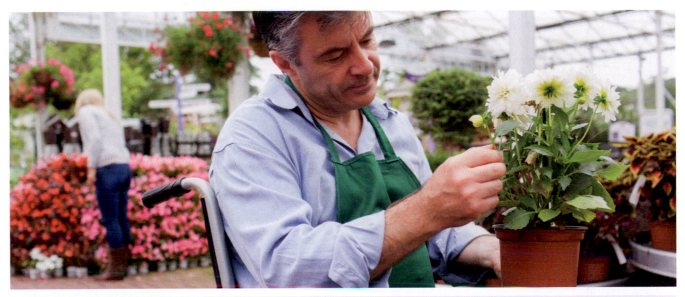

Photo credit: Wavebreak Media LTD/Thinkstock

Learning Objectives

After reading this chapter, students should be able to:

- Understand the role of the rehabilitation counselor
- Identify the various practice settings in which rehabilitation counselors are employed
- Describe the education, licensing, and certification process
- Understand the relationship between rehabilitation counselors and other stakeholders
- Discuss opportunities and challenges for working in the field of rehabilitation counseling

Key Terms

- Transition vocational rehabilitation counselor (TVRC)
- Vocational rehabilitation (VR)
- Transition
- Assistive Technology (AT)
- Holistic approach
- Empowerment

- Advocacy
- Autonomy
- Integration
- Inclusion
- Consumers
- Case management
- Disability management

- Certified rehabilitation counselor (CRC)
- Vocational Rehabilitation and Employment Services (VR&E)
- Disability accommodations
- Forensic rehabilitation

"A Day in the Life"

Hello, my name is Kelly and I am a **transition vocational rehabilitation counselor (TVRC).** I work in a state vocational rehabilitation agency and I am off to an admission, review, and dismissal (ARD) meeting. I am also meeting with some new school counselors later today. I love my job—I'm always on the run!

It's now later that morning. I'm just leaving the school and have only a few minutes to catch you up on my day. The ARD meeting went very well. The ARD committee is designated with making educational plans for students with disabilities. It consists of the student, one or both parents (or guardian), the child's teacher, the TVRC, representatives from the school (the teacher, a special education assessment team member, and an administrator who can commit resources), and other individuals at the discretion of the agency or the parents. The student is 19 years old and has a diagnosis of autism. He is graduating next year and does not plan to attend college, so we developed a vocational plan that matches his interests and abilities. I explained the services the state **vocational rehabilitation (VR)** agency can provide and how we can assist the student in making the **transition** from school to work. He was very excited about getting part-time work so that he could not only develop skills but have money to purchase videogames.

It's now afternoon and I'm on my way to a local pharmacy to discuss a part-time job opening that I think will be a great fit for one of my students. This is a company that has hired individuals with disabilities before, and they have a great reputation for being a good employer. The student that I am working with has a spinal cord injury and hopes to attend pharmacy school. I worked with a physical therapist to help him get the right wheelchair. I discussed his strengths and why I thought he would be a good match for the opening, especially since we sponsored him at a summer internship at Walgreen's Pharmacy where he really excelled. I also discussed some of the job accommodations that would be needed, such as installing a ramp with a platform so that he can reach the counter. I told them that the state agency would pay for these accommodations and also gave them information about targeted job tax credits available for hiring a person with a disability. They were very interested so I scheduled an interview for him the following week. I can't wait to call him and give him the news.

After dinner, I read a new journal article about various behavioral supports that might assist a person with autism in the workplace. Tomorrow I am attending training on autism and employment hosted by an expert in the state and I want to be prepared. Even though I've been at my job for several years, the agency provides a lot of continuing education and training to keep me abreast of new developments and techniques. I really look forward to these trainings as I strive to be a very good rehabilitation counselor. Besides, I can share this information with my students. As a certified rehabilitation counselor, I am required to have continuing education to ensure that I am current, and I can use this training toward that requirement.

Introduction to Rehabilitation Counseling

Description

According to the 2010 U.S. Census, nearly 20% of Americans have some type of disability. This trend is expected to continue as the U.S. population ages. With age comes the likelihood of experiencing some type of disability. Additionally, thanks to medical advances and technology, individuals with disabilities are living longer and fuller lives. With this growing population comes an increased demand for rehabilitation counselors.

Rehabilitation counselors assist people with all types of disabilities—physical, mental, sensory, cognitive, and emotional—to meet their life goals, such as living more independently or finding a meaningful job. They are counselors who have additional knowledge of medical and psychosocial aspects of disabilities. Rehabilitation counselors integrate this knowledge with their understanding of disability and employment law, **assistive technology,** and community resources. It is a very challenging job that requires a lot of creative thinking, similar to putting the pieces of a puzzle together.

History

Rehabilitation counseling began after World War I and first served veterans with disabilities.[1] Many rehabilitation counselors still work with veterans, but services were expanded to civilians in 1920. It is still a relatively new occupation compared with other health-care professions. Rehabilitation counselors were originally trained to assist veterans and those with occupational disabilities to return to work. In the 1950s this was expanded to include individuals with mental illness and intellectual disabilities. During the 1960s, services were expanded to those with substance use disorders and socially "handicapping" issues such as low education and criminal histories. Those with substance use disorders are still eligible for services, but criminal offenders and those with limited education no longer qualify for state/federal services. However, many rehabilitation counselors still work with this population in other settings.

Today, the skills of rehabilitation counselors are used in a variety of work settings, such as rehabilitation facilities, addiction treatment and mental health agencies, residential programs, specific disability organizations, higher education, businesses, state and federal agencies, and private practice. They provide counseling and guidance, case management and referral services, consultation to businesses and employers, and recommendations for accommodations and assistive technology in the workplace, school, and home. They work with consumers of any age, gender, ethnicity, or religion, but they work primarily with those age 14 and older. Some focus on working with a specific population, such as veterans; others focus on working with a specific disability group, such as individuals with traumatic brain injury.

Rehabilitation counselors use a **holistic approach** to ensure that all aspects of a person's life are taken into consideration. They also use a strengths-based approach that focuses on capacity rather than disability. **Empowerment** and **advocacy** are key components of their work. They work "with" rather than "doing for" the person they serve. The "dignity of risk" is an expression that means rehabilitation counselors help support a person's goals, and the person's right to **autonomy** outweighs the potential risks associated with living a full life. This does not mean intentionally putting a person in harm's way, but understanding that all of us take risks every day. **Integration** and **inclusion** are also important to rehabilitation counselors—everyone has the right to live, work, and play in their communities.

Tips and Tools

Typically, the term **consumer** is used to describe the person that you are serving. However, in some settings the term *client, job seeker, student, resident,* or *patient* may be used. One key principle is to use "people first" language whenever possible. For instance, a person *has a disability* rather than *is disabled.* The term *handicapped* should never be used to refer to an individual; rather, the person's environment may be "handicapping" because, for example, there are no curb cuts for easier access. There are some exceptions to the rule of using "people first" language. For instance, most people who are congenitally deaf say "I am deaf" because they do not view deafness as a disability.

Scope of Practice

The scope of practice varies greatly depending on the work setting. In general, rehabilitation counselors help people manage the personal, social, physical, and vocational effects of their disabilities. They assess the strengths and limitations of their **consumers** to help them find new ways of accomplishing their goals. Rehabilitation counselors may do the following:

- Provide individual or group counseling
- Evaluate abilities, interests, skills, health, and experience
- Conduct vocational assessments
- Arrange for psychological or medical services
- Provide **case management** and referral to other services
- Deliver psychiatric rehabilitation services
- Conduct addiction assessments
- Recommend accommodations and modification for school, work, and home
- Develop, implement, and monitor treatment plans and goals
- Arrange for additional training or services that facilitate independence or employment
- Work collaboratively with medical and other providers

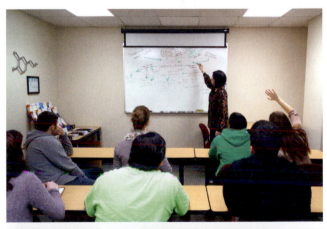

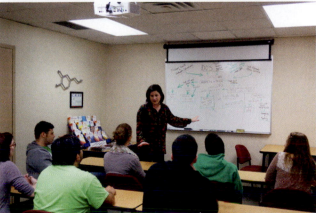

FIGURE 26-1 The rehabilitative counselor leads a recovery group.

- Provide consultation to businesses and employers on return-to-work and **disability management** programs
- Advocate for the rights of individuals with disabilities
- Give court testimony
- Engage in job development and placement
- Develop life care plans
- Facilitate school-to-work transition services

Required Education

A master's degree in rehabilitation counseling is typically required, although some individuals with related degrees and experience can also be employed as rehabilitation counselors. Most rehabilitation counseling programs are accredited by the Council on Rehabilitation Education (CORE).[2]

An individual with the appropriate credentials can become a **certified rehabilitation counselor (CRC)** by passing a national examination offered through the Commission on Rehabilitation Counselor Certification (CRCC).[3] Many rehabilitation counselors are eligible to become licensed as professional counselors, although many state and federal agencies are exempt from licensure requirements.

Salary

According to the National Occupational Information Network (O*NET),[4] the median pay for rehabilitation counselors in 2012 was $33,880. This pay can vary greatly depending on work setting. However, the salary survey conducted by the CRCC in 2007 showed that the average salary of those responding was $57,176. Those working in forensic/expert witness settings earned the highest salaries, with an average of $93,000; those working in a state agency (other than state rehabilitation) had the lowest salaries at $45,000. The difference between the CRCC data and O*NET may be that those who are CRCs usually have at least a master's degree (as well as some with a PhD) whereas O*NET data includes bachelor's degree personnel who have the title of rehabilitation counselor. A 2014 salary survey by the American Counseling Association[5] found that rehabilitation counselors had better benefits and were the highest paid counseling specialty, earning over $13,000 more than clinical mental health counselors and community counselors.

Trends

The job outlook for rehabilitation counselors is expected to grow faster than average—28% according to the *Occupational Outlook Handbook*.[5] Because there has been a shortage of rehabilitation counselors for several decades (particularly in rural areas), the Rehabilitation Services Administration, the federal agency that oversees the state VR programs, has been providing scholarships to fund graduate-level education for rehabilitation counselors. Additionally, the average CRC is over 50, so many will be retiring in the next decade.

As previously mentioned, the aging baby boomers will be likely to acquire disabilities that may affect their ability to live or work independently. Another current trend is an increase in the number of veterans returning from war with new disabilities. These veterans need rehabilitation counseling to adjust to their disabilities and develop new independent living or employment skills. Yet another trend is the tremendous increase in the incidence of autism spectrum–related disorders and learning disabilities. Some rehabilitation counselors are specifically trained to assist individuals on the spectrum in living independently or finding and keeping a job.

Assistive technology is another area that is changing rapidly within the field of rehabilitation. Rehabilitation counselors not only use technology to manage their case loads, but they also make recommendations to consumers on types of assistive technology, such as speech output software or the latest advances in hearing aids. Some rehabilitation counselors obtain certification in assistive technology, but all need to be aware of resources and stay current on the newest devices on the market.

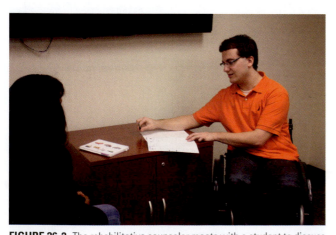

FIGURE 26-2 The rehabilitative counselor meets with a student to discuss testing and accommodations.

Challenges

One of the biggest challenges faced by rehabilitation counselors is time management. There is always more to do than the day allows. Rehabilitation counselors face multiple demands from many different directions—the need to respond to consumers, the need to contact referral sources, the need to keep current on disability issues and technology, and the need to understand employers and employment trends. Most work within complex systems and need to understand legislation and policies that affect disability. It is imperative that rehabilitation counselors develop an effective system to manage their workload and respond to requests in a timely manner. Good supervision and training can facilitate the workload a great deal.

Resource management is another major challenge for rehabilitation counselors. Some rehabilitation counselors manage a budget of over $200,000 to purchase goods and services for their consumers (such as wheelchairs, vocational training, etc.), yet there are always more needs than the budget can accommodate. It is the ethical obligation of a rehabilitation counselor to distribute resources in a fair and equitable manner. That often means making some hard choices, such as choosing to spend $50,000 on home modifications for an individual with a high-level spinal cord injury when it might mean that others may not get needed services. Finding resources in the community, leveraging the available funds, and always considering the implications of decisions made for others requires a high level of integrity and thoughtfulness.

Stress is common in human services and allied health careers. Individuals in these fields have a huge impact on the lives of the individuals they serve, and this should never be taken lightly. Most rehabilitation counselor education programs help students learn ways to cope with stress and develop strategies to prevent burnout so they can remain effective counselors.

Role of the Vocational Rehabilitation Counselor

Vocational rehabilitation counselors often work in state vocational rehabilitation agencies or the Veterans Administration within the **Vocational Rehabilitation and Employment Services (VR&E)** unit, although some work for nonprofit and for-profit agencies. They provide counseling and guidance and develop a comprehensive, individualized plan to allow the individual to achieve his or her employment goals. Their effectiveness is measured by their ability to help a person become employed in a job that matches his or her strengths, interests, and abilities. Those in state vocational rehabilitation and the VR&E manage a fairly large budget that allows them to purchase services that help reduce or eliminate the barriers so that the individual can be more independent. They work with many community agencies and employers.

Aptitude Profile

Choosing a career involves finding a good match between a person's skills, abilities, and interests and the requirements of the job. Many health-care occupations require some of the same characteristics—empathy, compassion, resourcefulness, and emotional maturity, to name a few. However, some require much more hands-on patient care, such as nursing, physical therapy, and occupational therapy. Social workers tend to focus more on advocating within the community and changing policies and systems to better serve their clients, although some do quite a bit of one-on-one work with their clients. Rehabilitation counselors also advocate for systems change, but most spend a significant amount of their time working with the consumer and other service providers. Unlike other allied health providers, rehabilitation counselors who work for the state and federal government have a significant budget from which to purchase services for their consumers, so they must be diligent in allocating resources. In addition to interfacing with other social services providers, many rehabilitation counselors interface with employers, human resources managers, and insurance companies.

According to Leierer and his colleagues,[6] rehabilitation counselors possess a "Holland's code" of social, artistic, and investigative (SAI). *Social* means they are highly social beings who like working with others. *Artistic* refers to those who are creative and curious. *Investigative* means they like to solve problems, perform experiments, or conduct research. So, if you like a challenge, like putting the "pieces of a puzzle together," and are creative and social, rehabilitation counseling might be a good fit for you.

The following list includes some of the necessary skills and abilities to consider when entertaining the idea of becoming a rehabilitation counselor. Although this list is not exhaustive, all of these characteristics are required to be effective in the rehabilitation field.

Able to handle stress	Excellent communicator
Active listener	Good at complex problem-solving
Advocator	Independent worker
Collaborative	Nonjudgmental
Critical thinker	Objective
Detail oriented	Perceptive
Empathic	Responsible

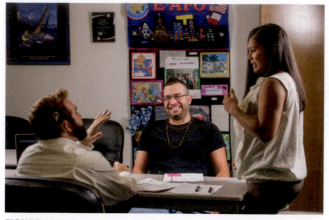

FIGURE 26-3 A vocational rehabilitation counselor meets with a student to discuss employment opportunities.

Author Spotlight

Linda Holloway, PhD, CRC

I knew as a small child that I wanted to help people, but I didn't find the field of rehabilitation counseling until I was a junior in college. What attracted me to the field was that it was very person-centered and action-oriented—helping people accomplish their life goals. It combined my love of people, my interest in medical and psychological issues, and my commitment to social justice. The most rewarding aspect is seeing people really blossom and overcome their disability by accomplishing things they did not think were possible, such as moving into their own apartment or getting their dream job.

Role of Transition Counselors

Transition counselors work closely with the school, the student, and the student's family to provide vocational support to students who are leaving school. Services provided include training programs, job tryouts, interest evaluations, counseling, and referral to other agencies. They work with schools, providers, students, parents, employers, and other stakeholders to assist the student in transitioning from school to work or higher education.

Role of Rehabilitation Counselors in Mental Health and Addiction

An increasing number of rehabilitation counselors work in mental health and addiction treatment programs. They provide counseling and develop treatment plans to help individuals with their mental health or substance use issues. The goal is to help individuals manage their disability and achieve greater independence and a better quality of life. Some provide psychiatric rehabilitation services such as supported employment and independent living skills.

Role of Rehabilitation Counselors in Business and Industry

Some rehabilitation counselors work in business or industry. They may help individuals return to work after an injury or illness or provide disability management to reduce or mitigate the effects of disability in the workplace. They may work in the insurance industry to help injured workers find another

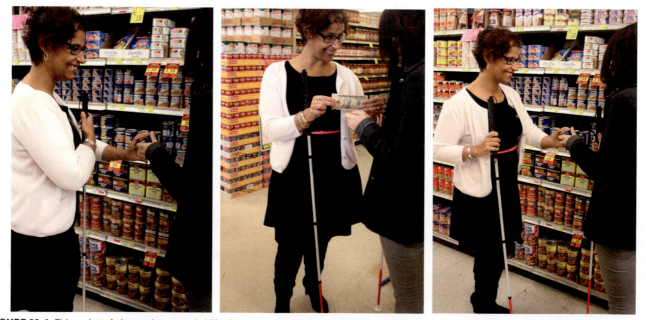

FIGURE 26-4 This series of photos shows a rehabilitation counselor helping a visually impaired student learn how to live independently.

job that they can perform. Others work in employee assistance programs (EAPs) providing counseling and/or substance abuse treatment. They perform job analysis, analyze transferable skills, and recommend accommodations and modifications to reduce the impact of the disability. Some provide disability awareness training, and others serve as equity and diversity officers to help businesses hire and retain individuals with disabilities.

Role of Rehabilitation Counselors in Higher Education

Rehabilitation counselors may work in higher education in roles such as **disability accommodation** specialists, academic counselors, or career counselors. Their goal is to remove accessibility and environmental barriers in school environments to promote student success. Knowledge of assistive technology and disability legislation is often used. They may administer occupational assessments, provide career counseling, or offer academic advising to help students select a major and ultimately a career.

Rehabilitation counselors may also teach in rehabilitation counseling and related fields. Although most tenure-track positions require a doctoral degree, there are opportunities for those with master's degrees and strong experience to teach at the undergraduate level and to provide clinical and internship supervision at the graduate level. Those with a master's degree are typically hired as lecturers or as clinical faculty.

Role of the Forensic Rehabilitation Counselor

Forensic rehabilitation counselors are consulted when there is either a significant injury or disability and the stakes are high. It may be a case involving medical malpractice in which they are asked to assess the person's injury, quality of life, or ability to return to work in any capacity. They provide expert testimony in cases where injury or disability is in question.

Role of Rehabilitation Counselors in Rehabilitation Facilities

Some rehabilitation counselors provide a range of services that support individuals living as independently as possible within their community. These services may allow individuals to remain living in their home and/or transitioning them from an institutional setting or care facility into the community. Services may provide assistance in benefit planning, arrangement for housing or transportation, assistance in

managing finances, or helping to get services from other agencies. Some work with individuals with specific disabilities such as intellectual disabilities, cerebral palsy, or brain injury. These rehabilitation counselors provide cognitive remediation to help individuals develop coping strategies to aid in memory or decision-making skills. They also provide personal and adjustment services to help clients improve their interpersonal skills. The type of settings and services they provide is almost unlimited.

Role of Baccalaureate-Prepared Rehabilitation Specialists

The title *rehabilitation counselor* is typically reserved for those with a master's degree who are trained to do counseling. However, a number of programs prepare individuals to work with individuals with disabilities in a variety of community settings. These professionals typically work in nonprofit programs and provide case management, skills training, discharge planning, advocacy, or employment services. The roles of bachelor's-level rehabilitation professionals vary greatly depending on the work environment. They may be managing programs, developing treatment plans, or working one on one with consumers to assist in living more independently. Currently, about 50 universities offer bachelor's degrees in rehabilitation studies, but many individuals from other human service degree programs provide these same types of services. However, these programs typically lack the focus on disability.

Working Together

Rehabilitation counselors work with a variety of medical and allied health professionals, as well as schools, businesses, and community agencies. When working in an inpatient or residential facility, rehabilitation counselors typically interact with physicians, nurses, and occupational, speech, and physical therapists, as well as technicians. In mental health and addiction treatment facilities, they interact regularly with psychiatrists, social workers, and case managers.

If they are providing vocational rehabilitation services, rehabilitation counselors will interact with many allied health professionals, such as physicians, physical and occupational therapists, and psychologists, as well as employers, human resources personnel, rehabilitation engineers, and other community agencies.

Those working in forensic rehabilitation and workers' compensation will also interact with attorneys and judges. They provide testimony in court cases to determine whether or not a settlement should be given based on the level of disability and who was at fault.

SUMMARY

Rehabilitation counseling is a rewarding career that allows individuals to practice in a wide variety of settings. Rehabilitation counselors work with individuals with any type of disability to help them achieve their life goals. They use an individualized, person-centered, and strengths-based approach to help individuals overcome the challenges and barriers they face in their daily lives. There is a high demand for rehabilitation counselors, and this is expected to increase due to the large number of rehabilitation counselors who will be retiring in the next decade, as well as the growing number of individuals who are affected by disability and chronic health conditions. If you are interested in a challenging job that truly affects the lives of others, consider the profession of rehabilitation counseling.

CASE STUDY

DJ is a 21-year-old veteran who acquired a mild traumatic brain injury (TBI) when the vehicle he was driving hit an improvised explosive device. He is also experiencing posttraumatic stress disorder (PTSD). Before the accident, he was the kind of guy who lived for the moment and had no long-range plans. He joined the military because he didn't know what he wanted to do and he just wanted to get his parents off his back. Now, he is severely depressed and just wants to be left alone.

After his release from the hospital, he was referred to VR&E, where he was assigned a vocational rehabilitation counselor (VRC). His VRC first reviewed all his medical and psychological information from the Veterans Administration (VA) hospital to determine the extent of his injuries and his psychological reaction to them. She listened to his story and recommended that he attend a support group for veterans with disabilities. She also arranged to meet with him weekly to provide counseling and develop an individualized employment plan. She referred him for an extensive vocational assessment to determine his skills, interests, and abilities and to the VA psychiatrist for a psychiatric evaluation to determine if antidepressants were needed. She also contacted the pharmacist to discuss the side effects related to his medication so that these could be taken into account when considering a good job match.

After reviewing all the assessment information, DJ and his VRC determined that he was a good fit for a career in forestry. He loved the outdoors, had an aptitude for science, and preferred to be alone. In addition

to the counseling and medication that he was receiving, his VRC recommended some new apps for his iPhone that were developed for veterans with PTSD. When he is feeling anxious and stressed out, he can use the relaxation app on his phone. His VRC showed him how to use his VA benefits to pay for his college expenses and helped him locate a university that has a good forestry program. She helped him to get the documentation that he needed to apply for disability support services at the university. She also referred him to a cognitive remediation program with an occupational therapist at a local brain injury clinic that will help him explore assistive devices and develop compensatory strategies for living with his brain injury. She will continue to see him regularly throughout his academic program and will assist him with job placement when he graduates. At that time, she will do a job analysis to determine if any accommodations are needed and also help him to discuss his functional limitations and needs.

DJ is feeling very optimistic. He is anxious about returning to school, but feels that he has the skills to manage his PTSD and his TBI. He also knows that he can contact his VRC whenever he feels the need. He is learning to manage the symptoms of his PTSD and has knowledge of environmental issues that he can control to minimize his disability.

Questions

1. What are the pressing issues facing DJ?
2. What disciplines should be involved with DJ's care?
3. Why is collaboration important in this case?
4. What are ultimately the goals for DJ's care?
5. What are some barriers to collaboration?

Review Questions

1. The rehabilitation counseling profession arose from which of the following major social issues?
   A. Injured workers
   B. Veterans returning from World War I
   C. Prohibition
   D. Veterans returning from Iraq

2. One of the most common challenges in the rehabilitation counseling profession is:

    A. Time pressures

    B. Low pay

    C. Abundant resources

    D. Patient diversity

3. The area of rehabilitation counseling that requires court testimony in high-stakes cases is called:

    A. State VR

    B. VA VR&E

    C. Mental health

    D. Forensic rehabilitation

4. The agency that certifies that rehabilitation counselors are competent to practice in the field is:

    A. The Commission on Rehabilitation Counselor Certification

    B. State Vocational Rehabilitation

    C. Counselor Educator programs

    D. State LPC boards

5. When considering rehabilitation counseling as a profession, it would be wise for the individual to have the following as a characteristic:

    A. Good communication skills

    B. Strong math aptitude

    C. Pity toward persons with disabilities

    D. Excellent IT skills

6. The scope of practice for a rehabilitation counselor in a state VR agency includes:

    A. Court testimony

    B. Psychotherapy treatment

    C. Housing modifications

    D. Counseling

7. Assistive technology is:

    A. A component of case management

    B. Used to increase, maintain, or improve functional capabilities

    C. The same as IT

    D. A cool game

8. Individuals who want to demonstrate their expertise in rehabilitation counseling usually hold this credential:

    A. BSW

    B. CRC

    C. LPC

    D. PhD

9. The Holland's code that is most like rehabilitation counselors is:

    A. SEC

    B. SRI

    C. SAI

    D. SCI

10. Which of the following uses "people first" language?

    A. Wheelchair bound

    B. Wheelchair user

    C. A person who uses a wheelchair

    D. A person who is handicapped

Glossary of Key Terms

Transition vocation rehabilitation counselor (TVRC)— term used to describe a professional working with individuals in transition positions

Vocational rehabilitation (VR)— a program that assists people with disabilities in getting or keeping a job

Transition— moving from school to work or to postsecondary education

Assistive Technology (AT)— a term used to describe devices that are used by people with disabilities to assist them in doing everyday activities (computers, wheelchairs, a screen reader, and hearing aids are examples of AT)

Holistic approach— treating the whole person, including social and environmental factors

Empowerment— to promote self-actualization; to enable individuals to speak up for themselves

Advocacy— actions taken to support the rights of people with disabilities; to ensure social justice and participation in the community for individuals with disabilities

Autonomy— allowing a person to make their own choices

Integration— living and working in the community, not in a segregated setting

Inclusion— being a part of one's community or group; typically used in reference to schools

Consumers— the person receiving rehabilitation services; a client; a student with a disability

Case management— a collaborative process that includes assessing, planning, implementing, monitoring, and evaluating the services required by individuals with disabilities; coordination of services for individuals with disabilities

Disability management—a program that assists employers in maximizing productivity by reducing the impact of absenteeism and disability

Certified rehabilitation counselor (CRC)—term used to describe a professional working in the field of rehabilitation who has passed the national certification exam

Vocational Rehabilitation and Employment Services (VR&E)—the term used for vocational rehabilitation services provided by the Veterans Administration

Disability accommodations—a reasonable adjustment to a job or work environment that makes it possible for an individual with a disability to perform the job duties

Forensic rehabilitation—the provision of scientific, unbiased assessment and consulting services within litigated settings, particularly in relation to economic damages

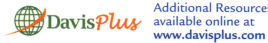 Additional Resources are available online at www.davisplus.com

Additional Resources

Accrediting Body
Council on Rehabilitation Education (CORE)—www.core-rehab.org
CORE is a national organization that accredits graduate programs that provide academic preparation for a variety of professional rehabilitation counseling positions. CORE also accredits undergraduate programs in rehabilitation and disability studies.

Certification
Commission on Rehabilitation Counselor Certification (CRCC)—www.crccertification.com
CRCC is an independent, not-for-profit organization dedicated to improving the lives of individuals with disabilities by promoting quality rehabilitation counseling services to individuals with disabilities through the certification of rehabilitation counselors and providing leadership in advocating for the rehabilitation counseling profession.

CRCC Career Center—www.crccertification.com/crccareers
The CRCC Career Center provides a wealth of information on the many facets of a career in rehabilitation counseling.

Education and Professional Resources
National Council on Rehabilitation Education (NCRE)—www.ncre.org
NCRE is a professional organization of educators dedicated to quality services for persons with disabilities through education and research. NCRE advocates up-to-date education and training and the maintenance of professional standards in the field of rehabilitation.

American Rehabilitation Counseling Association (ARCA)—www.arcaweb.org
ARCA is an organization of rehabilitation counseling practitioners, educators, and students who are concerned with improving the lives of people with disabilities. Rehabilitation counselors are counselors with specialized training and expertise in providing counseling and other services to persons with a disability. It is a subdivision of the American Counseling Association.

International Association of Rehabilitation Professionals (IARP)—www.rehabpro.org
IARP is a global association for professionals involved in private rehabilitation.

National Rehabilitation Counseling Association (NRCA)—http://nrca-net.org
NRCA is a national organization representing rehabilitation counselors practicing in a variety of work settings: private nonprofit agencies, hospital medical settings, educational programs, private for-profit businesses, state/federal agencies, private practice, unions, and others.

Rehabilitation Counselors and Educators Association (RCEA)—http://rehabcea.org/
RCEA comprises educators and counselors employed in both public and private rehabilitation settings. Recognizing the broad base of persons with disabilities, RCEA promotes training opportunities and continuing activities to ensure that those in the field of rehabilitation stay up to date about their profession

References

1. Sporner M. Service members and veterans with disabilities: Addressing unique needs through professional rehabilitation counseling. *J Rehabil Res Dev.* 2012;49(8):xiii–xvii.

2. Council on Rehabilitation Education. (n.d.). http://www.core-rehab.org.
   Accessed September 7, 2015.

3. Commission on Rehabilitation Counselor Certification. http://www.crccertification.com.
   Accessed September 7, 2015.

4. O*NET Center. Summary report for:_21-1015.00-Rehabilitation Counselors.

http://www.onetonline.org/link/summary/21-1015.00.

Accessed September 7, 2015.

5. Bureau of Labor Statistics. U.S. Department of Labor. Occupational outlook handbook, 2012–2013 edition: rehabilitation counselors.

http://www.bls.gov/ooh/community-and-social-service/rehabilitation-counselors.htm.

Accessed September 7, 2015.

6. Leierer S, Blackwell T, Strohmer D, Thompson R, Donnay D. The newly revised Strong Interest Inventory: A profile interpretation for rehabilitation counselors. *Rehabil Counseling Bull.* 2008; 51(2):76–84.

CHAPTER 27

Respiratory Care/ Cardiopulmonary

Jennifer Keely, MEd, RRT-AACS; and Kathryn Rollins, MEd, RRT-NPS

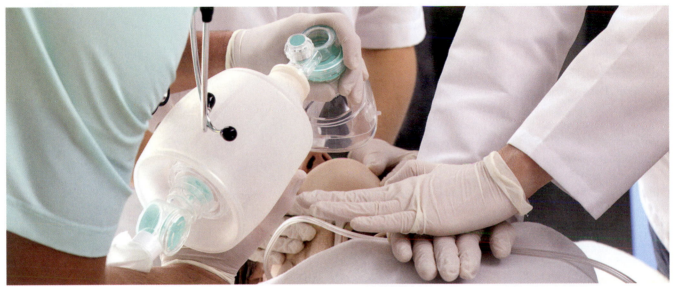

Photo credit: istock/Thinkstock

Learning Objectives

After reading this chapter, students should be able to:

- Understand the role of a respiratory therapist
- Identify the various respiratory care specialties
- Describe the education and licensing process
- Understand the relationship between respiratory therapists and other members of the health-care team
- Discuss opportunities and challenges for working in the field of respiratory care

Key Terms

- Mechanical ventilator
- Nebulizer treatments
- Endotracheal tube
- Arterial blood gas (ABG)
- Cardiopulmonary
- Resuscitation team
- Respiration
- National Board for Respiratory Care (NBRC)
- American Association for Respiratory Care (AARC)
- Board examinations
- Physician extender
- Organ procurement coordinators
- Wheeze

"A Day in the Life"

Hello! My name is Ann and I am a respiratory therapist. I work in all areas of the hospital but today I'm staffing in the intensive care unit (ICU). I begin each day by hearing a report about patients from the previous shift. Then I develop a schedule for the day and gather any equipment I may need. My days are often unpredictable; therefore I need to be prepared for anything.

After shift report, I began my assessments on each of the patients who are on a **mechanical ventilator,** which helps them breathe when they are too sick or sedated to breathe effectively on their own. Assessments include a physical evaluation as well as reviewing recent laboratory results and x-rays. It's important to communicate any findings with other members of the health-care team, such as the patient's nurse or physician. I also assess each patient's response to the mechanical ventilator and discuss any recommended changes with the physician. After I assess the more critical patients, I can begin my treatment rounds. Treatment rounds often consist of giving patients **nebulizer treatments,** evaluating their need for supplemental oxygen, and performing various therapies to improve lung function. This process usually repeats every 4 hours.

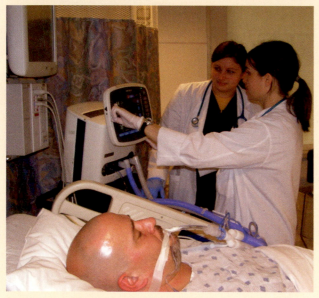

A patient on mechanical ventilation.

The first patient we'll see today has been admitted for pneumonia. A respiratory therapist gives her a nebulizer treatment every 4 hours. The medication in the nebulizer helps open the patient's airways, making it easier for her to breathe. Before we start any treatment, the patient's lung sounds and vital signs will be assessed. These values are compared with a posttreatment assessment to see if any changes occurred.

I just heard a page for "respiratory stat" to room 12. The patient arrived after heart surgery a few hours ago; we need to check on his status right away. This patient has a low oxygen level and appears to have secretions stuck in his breathing tube, called an **endotracheal tube.** I need to increase his oxygen and suction the blockage immediately before his condition deteriorates.

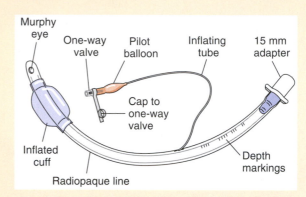
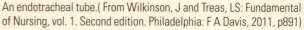

An endotracheal tube.(From Wilkinson, J and Treas, LS: Fundamental of Nursing, vol. 1. Second edition. Philadelphia: F A Davis, 2011, p891)

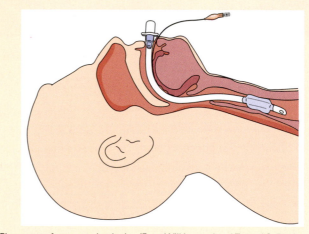

Placement of an orotracheal tube. (From Wilkinson, J and Treas, LS: Fundamental of Nursing, vol. 1. Second edition. Philadelphia: F A Davis, 2011, p891)

The patient is breathing normally again and his oxygen level is returning to normal. The physician has ordered a routine blood test called an **arterial blood gas (ABG)** to further evaluate the patient's condition. You can watch as I draw blood for the ABG and then we'll discuss how the test results affect our choice in ventilator setting.

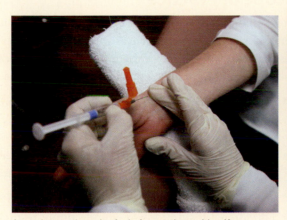

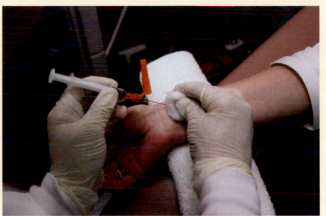

A respiratory therapist feels for a pulse to identify an artery. (From Stasinger, SK and Di Lorenzo, MS: The Phlebotomy Textbook. Third edition. Philadelphia: FA Davis, 2011, p356)

A blood sample is collected from an artery for ABG analysis. (From Stasinger, SK and Di Lorenzo, MS: The Phlebotomy Textbook. Third edition. Philadelphia: FA Davis, 2011, p356)

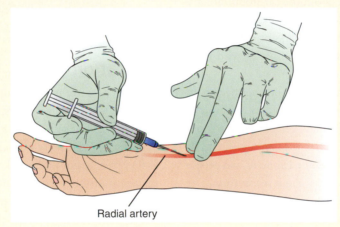

Radial artery

A view of the artery under the skin.

The patient's ABG results were in the normal range, but he continues to need the help of a mechanical ventilator to breathe. He will be closely monitored over the next few hours to check for any other signs of respiratory distress. He will also be started on additional nebulizer treatments and breathing exercises to prevent any lung infections.

A physician just requested a smoking cessation consultation for a patient before discharge. Patient and family education is another important element of a respiratory therapist's job.

Providing education about home medications and healthy lung tips decreases the number of hospital visits and can significantly improve the quality of a patient's life.

The next shift will be arriving soon. The new staff will cover the ICU for the next 12 hours, until I'm back tomorrow. It may seem like a long day, but working 12-hour shifts 3 days a week is normal for my job. Today, I hope you have seen how important communication, organization, and quick thinking are in the world of respiratory care.

Introduction to Respiratory Therapy

Description

Respiratory therapy is a profession that focuses on one primary body system: the **cardiopulmonary** system. The cardiopulmonary system consists of the heart and lungs, which work together to provide oxygen to the body and eliminate carbon dioxide. When one or both sets of organs are not functioning properly, the body's ability to function is affected. Respiratory therapists, also called respiratory care practitioners (RCPs), focus primarily on dysfunction of the lungs, which can be caused by conditions present since childhood, such as cystic fibrosis or asthma; traumatic events, such as car accidents, that require life-supporting mechanical ventilation; or conditions that develop over time, such as bronchitis, pneumonia, or emphysema.

One of the more unique aspects to being a respiratory therapist is the opportunity to work with patients of all ages, in all areas of the hospital, sometimes during the course of one 12-hour shift. A respiratory therapist might start the day as part of the **resuscitation team** at the birth of a premature infant and finish the shift by caring for mechanically ventilated patients at the end of their life span. Therapists in smaller hospitals or in supervisory positions at larger facilities are more likely to work with varied patient populations in one day, whereas staff therapists at larger hospitals often have the opportunity to specialize in one area of respiratory therapy. You will learn more about these different areas later in the chapter.

History

Compared with professions such as nursing and physical therapy, which came about during the mid-1800s and 1920s, respectively, respiratory therapy is a relatively young profession. The first professional respiratory therapy organization, the Inhalational Therapy Association, was organized in 1947. Though today's respiratory therapists must have extensive knowledge about the cardiopulmonary system and understand how to select and use complicated equipment, in the early years of the profession a respiratory therapists' duties were fairly limited compared with what they are today.

Interest in the function of the human body has been documented as early as 350 BC when a Greek philosopher, Aristotle, discovered that animals that had been placed in airtight boxes did not live for very long.[1] Over the centuries that followed, philosophers and scientists studied animals and people to develop increasingly precise theories about **respiration.** The use of oxygen to treat people with asthma and heart problems began in the late 1700s.[1] This treatment continued into the early 20th century when those who transported oxygen tanks around the hospital were known as oxygen orderlies. When the polio epidemic in the United States struck in the early 1900s, negative pressure ventilators, commonly called "iron lungs," were a revolutionary means of providing ventilation to patients whose muscles were paralyzed by disease.

It could be argued that the development of the respiratory therapy profession was partially due to medical practices used during World War II. When flying at high altitudes, U.S. pilots were at risk of becoming disoriented and losing consciousness in the cockpit due to the lower level of oxygen at high altitudes. The solution to this dangerous dilemma came in the form of a special oxygen mask that delivered oxygen under pressure. As often happens with medical equipment and practices used in wartime, their use spread to civilian hospitals during and after the war. As oxygen delivery equipment became more sophisticated and understanding about the pulmonary system advanced, it became clear that more training was required for people giving oxygen therapy and inhaled medication. This need for trained personnel provided the momentum for the start of the respiratory therapy profession as we know it today.

Scope of Practice

Today's respiratory therapists are equipped with a diverse array of skills that allow them to assess and treat patients with respiratory ailments in a variety of settings. Respiratory therapists can be found working in the following areas:

- Hospitals—working as staff therapists, staff educators, researchers, infection control specialists, computer administrators, or management
- Home health agencies—providing respiratory care services to patients in the private home or nursing home setting
- Sales representatives for drug and equipment companies
- Educational institutions to educate future respiratory therapists
- Organ procurement agencies—serving as organ procurement coordinators to facilitate the process of organ donation

Education

Respiratory therapists' training has evolved considerably over the past several decades. Initially called "inhalational therapy," early education came in the form of on-the-job training. People simply learned by observing experienced practitioners as they went about their workday. Under the watchful eyes of their mentors, they gained hands-on experience with patients in the clinical setting until it was determined they were ready to work independently. The phrase, "see one, do one, teach one," probably provides an accurate picture of what training looked like in those days. At that time, therapists' primarily responsibilities included delivery of supplemental oxygen, aerosolized medication, and various types of therapy to help expand the lungs and maintain clear airways. However, with the rapid evolution of life-supporting mechanical ventilators and the development of blood gas analysis, it became clear that formal education programs needed to be developed to provide more thorough, consistent training.[1] Respiratory therapy certification programs flourished during the 1960s. Graduates of these programs, which were typically completed in 1 year, received only a certificate of completion, rather than an actual degree. These certification education programs continued until 2002, when the **National Board for Respiratory Care (NBRC)** mandated that the entry-level degree required to practice respiratory therapy be an associate or 2-year degree. An entry-level degree is the minimum degree a practitioner must earn to be able to enter the professional field. There are currently 449 respiratory therapy education programs in the United States, with only 12% of those programs offering baccalaureate, or 4-year, degrees in respiratory therapy.[2] Recently, the **American Association for Respiratory Care (AARC),** a professional organization for respiratory therapists, made a series of recommendations for the profession, including a recommendation that all therapists should have a minimum of a baccalaureate degree to practice respiratory therapy. Whether or not this recommendation comes to fruition remains to be seen. In recent years, some universities have begun offering master's-level programs in respiratory therapy. Currently, less than 1% of the programs in the country offer these graduate degrees. Students in these graduate degree programs usually focus on one of several career paths, such as management, research, or respiratory therapy education.

Licensure and Salary

Successful completion of an academic program is only the first step toward being able to practice respiratory therapy in a professional capacity. Regardless of the type of degree earned, the student must pass examinations designed by the NBRC after graduating. The NBRC is a voluntary group of respiratory therapists who, as a group, evaluate the competency of respiratory therapists through the process of board examinations.[3] **Board examinations** are computer-based tests given to ensure that new practitioners have the necessary skills and knowledge to be safe and effective. New graduates must take the Therapist Multiple Choice (TMC) examination, a 160-question examination that has two established cut scores. This examination is designed to measure essential knowledge, skills, and abilities required of entry-level respiratory therapists and determine eligibility for the Clinical Simulation Examination (CSE). The CRT and RRT credentials are used as the basis for the licensure in all of the 49 states that regulate the practice of respiratory care.[4] Candidates who earn only the lower cut score obtain the credential of certified respiratory therapist (CRT) and are not eligible to take the CSE. Some people choose not to pursue further credentials beyond the certification level and are, from a human resources perspective, considered entry-level respiratory therapists. Others may decide to retake the examination in an attempt to earn the higher credential of registered respiratory therapist (RRT). It is common for hospitals to require that certified respiratory therapists only work in the general care areas of the hospital rather than in ICUs, but this requirement is not universally true. Candidates who earn the higher cut score on the TMC are then eligible to take the CSE. This computer-based examination consists of 22 problems with various clinical settings and patient scenarios designed to simulate realistic situations in patient care. Candidates who successfully pass this examination earn the RRT credential. RRTs are generally understood to possess a more advanced set of clinical skills than certified respiratory therapists and are more likely to work in areas of the hospital with critically ill patients, such as the ICU. It has also become increasingly common for hospitals to hire only registered therapists.

After successful completion of the board examinations, the therapist must apply for a license to practice respiratory therapy in his or her state of residence. Drug screens and background checks are part of the licensure application process, and licensure fees vary considerably from state to state. Traveling therapists who work for temporary employment agencies must often hold multiple state licenses. According to the U.S. Bureau of Labor Statistics, a newly credentialed therapist entering the workforce can expect to earn between $42,000 and $47,000, and the median salary for therapists nationwide is just over $54,000 per year.[5]

Continuing Education

As with any health profession, it is essential that respiratory therapists ensure that their professional knowledge and practices are up to date and supported by strong medical research. In an effort to ensure the competency of all practicing therapists, state licensure generally requires that each person complete a minimum of 24 hours of continuing respiratory care education (CRCE) over a 2-year period. All therapists must maintain a record of the CRCE they have received so that they can provide proof to the licensing agency in their state. If a therapist fails to provide proof of the minimum number of CRCE to the licensing agency, his or her license to practice respiratory therapy in that state might be suspended. Most therapists find that obtaining the minimum amount of CRCE is not difficult because CRCE opportunities are widely available at professional conferences, hospital educational programs, and online learning opportunities.

Trends and Challenges

As of 2010, over 112,000 people listed respiratory therapy as their profession in the United States. As with other health professions, the demand for respiratory therapy is expected to grow as the baby boomer population (those born between 1946 and 1964) continues to age and develop conditions such as pneumonia and chronic obstructive pulmonary disease (COPD), a disease most often developed as a result of cigarette smoking. According to the U.S. Bureau of Labor Statistics, while other professions are expected to grow by 14% in the years between 2010 and 2020, the respiratory therapy profession is expected to grow by 28%.[5]

Greater numbers of respiratory therapists are returning to graduate school to earn master's and doctoral degrees. These therapists often have jobs in management, education, or research that require more education than a 4-year degree can provide. There is a move toward therapists with advanced degrees serving as physician extenders. A **physician extender** is someone who performs some of the duties of a physician under the supervision of a physician. Nurse practitioners and physician assistants have traditionally served as physician extenders, but there is growing interest in respiratory therapists working in this capacity as well.

Perhaps the biggest controversy in the profession at this time is the minimum required education level of respiratory therapists. As mentioned, there are practitioners, such as physicians and nurses, who believe that for the good of the profession, all respiratory therapists should have at least a baccalaureate degree. They reason that baccalaureate graduates are better prepared for critical thinking and problem-solving than are associate-degree therapists. Additionally, students in 4-year programs have more time in school to learn about management and research. Currently, there is legislation underway that will allow physicians to be reimbursed for services provided by baccalaureate-degreed respiratory therapists who work in their offices. If this legislation passes, the demand for baccalaureate programs will likely increase.

Opponents of this move toward a requisite baccalaureate degree have expressed serious concerns about the effects the change would have on students' accessibility to respiratory therapy programs.

It is unlikely that all 390-plus associate degree programs would be able to transition to baccalaureate programs. This move would result in the closure of many programs, reducing the number of programs available. There are many students for whom a 4-year college is not accessible for a variety of reasons. Working adults who want to enter the respiratory therapy field as a second career are often not able to devote the time required for a 4-year academic program. Last, a 4-year school is financially out of reach for many people. Proponents of the baccalaureate requirement point out that practitioners in the rehabilitative professions, such as physical therapy and occupational therapy, which have higher degree requirements, earn higher salaries and generally have more autonomy in the practice of their professions. Having more autonomy means they have more freedom to make decisions that guide the care of their patients. Meanwhile, those who oppose the requirement feel that respiratory therapy education requirements should match those of the nursing profession, which still requires only an associate degree to practice. People on both sides of the debate feel very strongly about their position. Although many are not comfortable with disagreement, we can take comfort in the fact that these passionate arguments reflect industry practitioners' care and

concern about the profession, as well as a desire to see it flourish.

Role of General Acute-Care Therapists

The majority of respiratory therapists work in an acute-care setting. This setting is often identified as a general-care floor within a hospital or similar facility. As an acute-care therapist, therapists actively treat patients on a short-term basis for injury, illness, acute and chronic medical conditions, or postoperative recovery. As part of their role in the acute-care setting, respiratory therapists apply principles to prevent, identify, and treat conditions of the cardiopulmonary system. Therapists working in an acute setting can expect to manage the care of several patients during their shift and travel throughout the hospital. At a minimum, facilities require therapists to hold the CRT credential, and many expect therapists to have the advanced-level RRT credential as well.

Role of Critical-Care Therapists

Critical-care respiratory therapists work in the intensive care settings within a hospital. They may work with patients of all ages with a variety of medical conditions. Critical-care settings include adult, pediatric, and neonatal intensive care units. There may be some overlapping in the roles between general acute-care therapists and critical-care therapists; however, there are distinct differences between the two. The critical-care therapist has often obtained advanced education and/or experience in the critical-care setting. The NBRC offers additional testing beyond the initial CRT and RRT credentials. The Adult Critical-Care Specialist (RRT-ACCS) and

Aptitude Profile

A good respiratory therapist possesses the following characteristics:

Ability to function in a high-stress environment

Adequate physical strength and mobility for moving patients and equipment

Excellent communicator and collaborator

Friendly and strong patient advocate

Interested in human anatomy and physiology

Lifelong learner

Sensitivity and compassion

Strong critical thinker

Strong troubleshooting skills

Tolerant of working with bodily fluids, sights, and smells

Author Spotlight

Jennifer Keely, MEd, RRT-ACCS

The field of respiratory therapy has a significant number of therapists who entered the profession as a second career. This was true for me as I discovered respiratory therapy toward the end of my enlistment as an Air Force musician. Having been diagnosed with asthma while in the Air Force, I started to learn firsthand about inhaled medication, pulmonary function testing, and the debilitating effects of decreased lung function. As I sought out career opportunities to pursue after the military, it became clear to me that a profession specializing in disorders of the lungs was a perfect fit.

What I love most about respiratory therapy is the wide variety of patient care environments in which I can work. I can provide asthma education to kids in a rural clinic one day, and the next day care for the most critically ill patients in the intensive care unit. I can assist with the resuscitation of a premature infant immediately after birth and also provide breathing treatments to elderly patients on the general-care floors. There is always variety and rarely time to be bored!

For those of you considering a career in respiratory therapy, understand that as a relatively young profession, current and new members have the opportunity to shape and define it in a way that ensures that respiratory therapists are viewed by all as essential members of the health-care team. We have an essential role in helping people in every stage of their lives, from beginning to end.

Kathryn Rollins, MEd, RRT-NPS
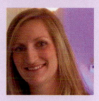

Why respiratory therapy, you might ask? My interest in the health-care field began in high school. I decided to start with a job as a certified nursing assistant (CNA) while I continued to research health-care careers. When I was introduced to various careers areas, such as radiology, respiratory therapy, and nursing, I recall having a strong interest in the tasks and education related to the respiratory system. I wanted to understand the how and why of the respiratory system, as well as its connection to the rest of our body.

I applied to a respiratory therapy program during my sophomore year of college. After completing 2 challenging but worthwhile years, I obtained my bachelor's of science in respiratory therapy. After graduation I was presented with numerous career opportunities. I decided to move over 600 miles from home to pursue a specialty career in neonatal respiratory care. Over the years I've increased my scope of practice to adult care, pulmonary rehabilitation, and education. The variety of opportunities for respiratory therapists is one of the things I love most about the profession.

I feel very fortunate to have worked with several respiratory therapists who always provide passionate care to their patients and am thankful for the opportunity to have worked in various health-care settings. My tips for success for those of you considering respiratory care is to always ask questions, never be afraid to speak up for your patients, and strive for a strong relationship with other health professionals.

Neonatal/Pediatric Respiratory Care Specialist (CRT-NPS or RRT-NPS) examinations ensure individuals have essential knowledge, skills, and abilities required of respiratory therapists in their particular specialty area[4] (Fig. 27-1).

Respiratory therapists working in the critical-care setting have a passion for fast-paced and intricate care environments. As part of their role in the critical-care setting, respiratory therapists treat critically ill patients with the most advanced medical equipment.[6] The role of the respiratory therapist includes assessment and treatment of patients. Respiratory therapists employ a range of cardiopulmonary therapies, including airway management, administering therapeutic medications and treatments, obtaining and analyzing blood gas samples, and managing mechanical ventilators.

Role of Transport Therapists

Respiratory therapists with advanced critical-care skills are well suited for careers in ground and air transport. As part of the transport team, therapists work closely with nurses, physicians, and emergency medical technicians (EMTs) to transport patients to the appropriate facility. Therapists should enjoy traveling by ambulance, helicopter, or fixed-wing airplane. When they are not actively participating in a transport, therapists may work in other areas of the hospital, including the emergency department and ICU.[6]

Role of Pulmonary Function Therapists

Therapists who enjoy the diagnostic aspects of respiratory care may specialize in pulmonary function testing. These therapists work in hospital- or physician-based pulmonary function laboratories, where they perform the testing required to determine whether a person has a lung disease and, if so, which type.[6] Therapists in this area generally specialize in pulmonary diagnostics, earning credentials as a certified pulmonary function technologist (CPFT) or registered pulmonary function technologist (RPFT).

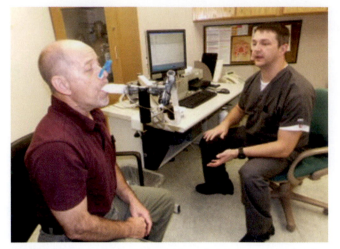

FIGURE 27-1 A respiratory therapist is performing pulmonary function tests on a patient.

Working Together

Respiratory therapists are health-care professionals who prevent, evaluate, and treat dysfunctions of the cardiopulmonary system. To care for patients in the most effective manner, respiratory therapists focus heavily on communication, collaboration, and problem-solving with an interprofessional health-care team. In every type of work environment, respiratory therapists interact with several disciplines, including medicine, nursing, radiology, pharmacy, and many other fields. For example, a respiratory therapist working in a hospital ICU will work with a radiographer to obtain a chest x-ray for a patient, followed by collaboration with physicians and nurses to develop a care plan for the critically ill patient based on the x-ray results.

Role of Polysomnography Therapists

Respiratory therapists are increasingly being called on to specialize in the area of sleep care. Respiratory therapists who work in sleep care are generally employed by sleep laboratories and often work the night shift, when polysomnography or sleep studies are conducted. Sleep studies assist therapists evaluating individuals with suspected sleep disorders. Additionally, therapists learn the function and use of polysomnographic equipment to provide safe and effective treatment to patients. In 2007, the NBRC developed the sleep disorders specialist (SDS) credential for respiratory therapists. Therapists who specialize in sleep care hold the CRT-SDS and/or RRT-SDS credentials, but may also want to earn the registered polysomnographic technologist (RPSGT) credential.[4]

Role of Home Care Therapists

Therapists who enjoy independent thinking outside of the hospital setting may seek a career in home care. Respiratory patients with long-term illnesses receive health-care services in their homes from respiratory therapists. Respiratory therapists who like to visit with patients and work outside office or hospital walls do well in home care. These therapists often have previous experience and have earned the CRT and/or RRT credential.

Role of Nonclinical Respiratory Therapists

The career outlook in respiratory care continues to expand. Many respiratory therapists work outside of the clinical setting as managers, educators, and sales representatives.

Each respiratory care department has managerial personnel responsible for everything from budget preparations to implementing hospital policies. Typically, individuals become managers after several years of respiratory care experience. Most managers have the RRT credential, and many have earned a higher level of education.[6]

Respiratory therapy educators serve both current and future practitioners. Educators serve as professors and instructors in school programs, including those at the community college and university levels, as well as continuing education coordinators for hospital respiratory therapy departments.[6] Most educators hold advanced degrees in education, in addition to experience in the clinical setting.

Those who enjoy marketing and education find careers in respiratory drug or equipment sales to be a great fit. Sales representatives establish and maintain relationships with physicians, hospitals, local professionals, and other resources in the medical community. Job responsibilities include marketing services, educating clients, and meeting monthly sales quotas. Respiratory therapists who seek a career in sales are often motivated, self-driven, and strong team players. Respiratory therapists have also been known to work as hyperbaric technicians, case managers, **organ procurement coordinators,** infection control officers, and researchers.

SUMMARY

The role of a respiratory therapist can span several areas of health care. Individuals who become respiratory therapists have the flexibility to find the area of respiratory care that most ideally fits their personality and goals. Whether you prefer working with infants to adults or acute to critical care, you can find your place in respiratory care.

CASE STUDY

Ben, a 5-year-old boy, and his parents arrive in the emergency department (ED). The physician is helping with a critical case and has asked you to help evaluate Ben's condition. You begin by introducing yourself to Ben and his parents, and continue by asking questions related to his medical history. Ben's parents noticed a runny nose and frequent dry cough over the past 2 days and also report Ben has been reluctant to join in gym class at school. They had an appointment with Ben's pediatrician scheduled for Monday, but Ben started having trouble breathing, so they rushed him to the ED.

On physical examination, Ben appears to be in moderate respiratory distress. He has to breathe very hard and deep to get a full breath of air. You use your stethoscope to listen to Ben's lungs while the nurse measures his body temperature and blood pressure. You hear a **wheeze** as he takes each breath and notice that his blood oxygen level is low. A radiographer comes to take an x-ray of Ben's chest to allow detection of problems in his lungs, such as pneumonia. As you await the results from Ben's chest x-ray, you gather the necessary treatment equipment and start him on supplemental oxygen. You've decided that a medicated nebulizer treatment will help Ben's breathing. He is very apprehensive and scared of the therapy you have for him and begins to cry. As an experienced therapist, you know Ben desperately needs his breathing treatment and gently hold the mask over his nose and mouth to deliver the aerosolized medication. You continue to comfort Ben during his breathing treatment while continually monitoring his physical condition for any changes (Fig. 27-2). The physician arrives to evaluate Ben along with the nurse to administer medications. You relay your assessment of Ben's condition, including his vital signs and physical assessment before and after the treatment. After the physician carries out an assessment you will work as a team to discuss Ben's next step of care.

Questions

1. The respiratory therapist's primary goal in this case study was to improve Ben's breathing. Why do you think this was an appropriate goal for the respiratory therapist?

2. Which specialty in respiratory care would be most helpful in this situation?

3. Respiratory distress can be a frightening and life-threatening situation for any patient. Do you feel the additional training toward advanced credentials would help therapists in this situation?

4. What other health-care disciplines do you think the therapist would interact with while treating Ben in the ED?

Review Questions

1. The respiratory therapy profession was first recognized in:
   A. 350 BC
   B. The 1940s
   C. The 1800s
   D. 2002

2. The minimum education level required of respiratory therapists is:
   A. A certificate of completion
   B. An associate degree
   C. A baccalaureate degree
   D. A master's degree

3. The primary patient population cared for by respiratory therapists is:
   A. Premature babies
   B. Adults
   C. The elderly
   D. All of the above

4. The organization responsible for creating the examinations new graduates must take to earn their respiratory therapy credentials is the:
   A. Inhalation Therapists' Association
   B. American Association for Respiratory Care
   C. National Board for Respiratory Care
   D. American Lung Association

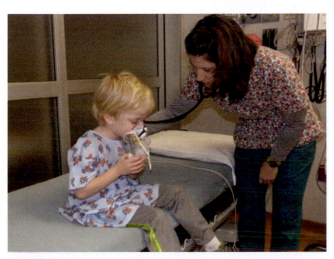

FIGURE 27-2 A pediatric patient is receiving nebulized medication.

5. Chronic obstructive pulmonary disease (COPD) is a disease that is usually caused by:

    A. Bad genetics

    B. Cigarette smoking

    C. Air pollution

    D. Inhaling noxious fumes

6. One of the biggest issues being discussed in the respiratory profession is:

    A. Determining the minimum education requirement

    B. Job burnout

    C. Patient diversity

    D. Autonomy

7. Respiratory therapists can work in several areas of health care, including:

    A. Marketing and sales

    B. Case management

    C. Research

    D. All of the above

8. When considering respiratory therapy as a profession, it would be wise for the individual to have the following as a characteristic:

    A. Prefers a slow-paced work environment

    B. Prefers to work alone

    C. Shy when interacting with others

    D. Strong interpersonal skills

9. Individuals who want to work in a critical-care setting usually hold this certification in respiratory care:

    A. Certified respiratory therapist (CRT)

    B. Registered respiratory therapist (RRT)

    C. Certified pulmonary function technologist (CPFT)

    D. Registered sleep disorders specialist (RRT-SDS)

10. A respiratory therapist must successfully pass ____ examination(s) before obtaining the registered respiratory therapist (RRT) credential.

    A. 1

    B. 2

    C. 3

    D. 4

Glossary of Key Terms

Mechanical ventilator—a machine that makes it easier for patients to breathe until they are able to breathe completely on their own

Nebulizer treatments—a drug delivery device used to administer medication in the form of a mist inhaled into the lungs

Endotracheal tube—a plastic tube used as a pathway for air and oxygen during mechanical ventilation; the tube is placed into the trachea (windpipe) through the mouth or nose until the patient can breathe unassisted

Arterial blood gas (ABG)—a diagnostic test that measures the amount of oxygen (O_2) and carbon dioxide (CO_2) in arterial blood

Cardiopulmonary—of or relating to the heart and lungs

Resuscitation team—trained medical staff that provide clinical expertise during a life-threatening medical emergency

Respiration—the act of breathing

National Board for Respiratory Care (NBRC)—certifying board created to evaluate the professional competence of respiratory therapists

American Association for Respiratory Care (AARC)—professional membership association for respiratory care professionals and allied health specialists interested in cardiopulmonary care

Board examinations—licensing examinations administered by the NBRC to individuals seeking a certification in respiratory therapy

Physician extender—Medical professional who is not a physician but who performs the duties typically done by a physician; usually nurse practitioners or physician assistants

Organ procurement coordinators—are responsible for all aspects of organ procurement from the initial hospital referral through the organ recovery procedure

Wheeze—a continuous, coarse, whistling sound produced in the respiratory airways during breathing

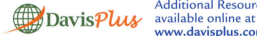 Additional Resources are available online at www.davisplus.com

Additional Resources

Accrediting Body

National Board for Respiratory Care—www.nbrc.org
The NBRC is the national certifying board that evaluates the professional competence of respiratory therapists.

Educational and Professional Resources

American Association for Respiratory Care—www.aarc.org
AARC is a professional membership association for respiratory therapists and other medical professionals interested in cardiopulmonary care.

Respiratory Care—http://rc.rcjournal.com
Respiratory Care is a refereed, professional journal that focuses on research in respiratory care.

References

1. Kacmarek RM, Stoller JK, Heuer AJ. *Egan's Fundamentals of Respiratory Care.* St. Louis, MO: Elsevier; 2013.

2. Ward JJ. History of the respiratory care profession. In: Hess DR, MacIntyre NR, Mishoe SC, Galvin WF, Adams AB. *Respiratory Care Principles and Practice,* 2nd ed. Sudbury, MA: Jones & Bartlett Learning; 2012.

3. Commission on Accreditation for Respiratory Care. 2012 report on accreditation in respiratory care education.

   http://www.coarc.com/.

   Accessed September 7, 2013.

4. National Board for Respiratory Care. About NBRC. http://www.nbrc.org.

   Accessed September 4, 2013.

5. Bureau of Labor Statistics, U.S. Department of Labor. Occupational outlook handbook, 2012–2013 edition, respiratory therapists.

   http://www.bls.gov/ooh/healthcare/respiratory-therapists.htm.

   Accessed October 1, 2013.

6. American Association for Respiratory Care Careers. http://aarc.org/careers/.

   Accessed September 4, 2013.

Social Work

Patricia Royal, EdD, MSW

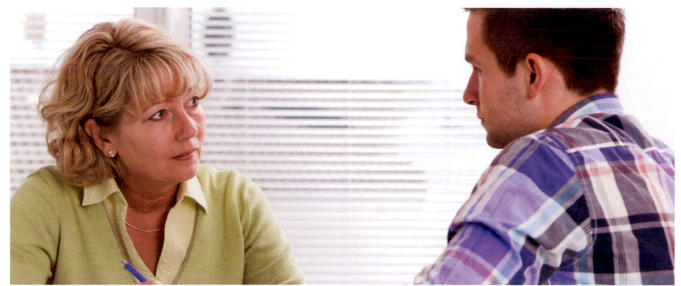

Learning Objectives

After reading this chapter, students should be able to:

- Describe the role of a social worker
- Differentiate the various types of social workers
- Describe the education and licensing process
- Explain the relationship between social workers and other members of the health-care team
- Discuss opportunities and challenges in the field of social work

Key Terms

- Psychosocial assessment
- Advocacy
- Case management
- Health-care social worker
- Child and family social worker
- Mental health social worker
- Substance abuse social worker

 ## "A Day in the Life"

Hello, my name is Becky and I am a medical social worker. I work in a dialysis unit and I am off to a patient care plan meeting. I have a busy agenda today but will try to provide you with details of the events as they happen. I also have a new admission today, which will happen after the care plan meeting. A care plan meeting is where the interprofessional team discusses the patient's progress. Today, we discussed a patient who has now been placed on the kidney transplant list. She is a 39-year-old mother of three who suffered with uncontrolled high blood pressure and diabetes for a number of years and as a result developed end-stage renal disease. She's been on dialysis for 3 years and has been compliant with her regimen. She completed the necessary physical and **psychosocial assessments,** reviewed all the required documents explaining the process, and is a good candidate for the transplant. At this time, she is just waiting for the kidney.

Now, I have a new admission to complete. This process includes talking with the patient and family members. I need to

(continued)

explain the financial requirements of treatments, which include her insurance benefits and co-pays, HIPAA forms, authorization forms, advance directives, living wills, transplant options, and resources available for her. I also need to discuss transportation options for the patient and let her know about transient treatment. Although most dialysis patients receive treatments three times per week, they are also allowed to travel and receive treatments at other locations during the travel. This type of service is called transient and is not used too often, but the service is available if needed. I am responsible for setting up the dialysis treatments at the closest facility where the patient plans to visit. The transient treatment does take some time to arrange so I ask patients to notify me at least a month in advance of the travel dates.

Whew, what a day. It's finally over. It is almost 6:30 p.m. and I have been at work since 8:30 this morning. It's been a long day but that is normal for my job. After the new admission, I had to deal with a couple of emergency situations. One matter was related to transportation issues. One patient who usually rides the county van to dialysis missed her ride. On the way to the patient's home the van was involved in an accident. The patient was becoming anxious because she was afraid of

missing her dialysis treatment and since today is Friday, she knew she would not be back until Monday. She was concerned she would have to wait too long until her next treatment. I had to figure out some means of transportation for this patient while keeping in mind her payer source might only pay for specific transportation. The patient is in a wheelchair, so finding an accessible mode of transportation took some time, but fortunately the patient was able to get here and receive her treatment before the weekend. Another patient came into my office and was upset about a letter he received from his insurance company regarding co-pays for treatments and medications. I spent about an hour talking with him and the insurance carrier before reaching an agreement. Just when I thought things were calm, I received a call from another dialysis unit regarding a transient patient. A patient from another state had an unexpected death in family living in this area. The patient needs to come to this facility for treatment while she stays with her family here. I spent the rest of the afternoon working on the paperwork for the transient patient to be treated at our facility.

So, there you have it—just a typical day in the life of a dialysis social worker.

Introduction to Social Work

Description

The number of baby boomers reaching retirement age is growing, and so is the need for social workers, particularly medical social workers. Social workers are vital to the healthcare team and provide patients and family members with resources and tools needed for quality care. The roles of social workers and the environment in which they work are varied, allowing many choices for individuals seeking this profession.

Social work can be defined as seeking to improve quality of life for individuals or groups of people and promoting social change to society. This improvement may occur through policy development, teaching, **advocacy,** or direct practice, which includes psychosocial therapies. Although the social work profession was not truly recognized until around the 19th century, its underlying premises can be dated back over a thousand years.[1]

Historical Perspective

The origin of social work dates back before the 11th century, when almshouses for the poor and handicapped were established in England. It was during this time that people, usually women, began to provide charity to less fortunate individuals. This type of charity continued until the bubonic plague hit Europe in the 1300s, causing the death of over one third of the working population. With the loss of needed workers, all able-bodied men were expected to work, and charity to them was forbidden; however, within the next decade, with

the rise of Christianity, charitable acts were no longer prohibited, and in fact were expected. The church provided for the poor who were unable to work, disabled, widows, and children until the state intervened in the 1500s. During the 1600s to 1800s, workhouses were established as a means to prevent assistance to individuals deemed able to work, which included the handicapped, the elderly, and young children. Between 1800 and 1900, many of the workhouses were closed and the new movement focused on women's rights for education, work opportunities, and equality. The government no longer emphasized helping the poor, but rather the idea of self-sufficiency was dominant. Some religious leaders and volunteers continued to provide for those less fortunate. In 1889, Jane Addams and Ellen Gates Starr, social reformers and activists, opened one of the first settlement houses, which were established to provide educational and social opportunities to working-class citizens. The first settlement house was known as the Hull House and was started in Chicago, Illinois. In 1898, the first school for social work was established and centered on training volunteers and friendly visitors to become advocates for the less fortunate.[2]

Much like the nursing field, social workers were seen as a group of individuals who provided charity to those less fortunate. Obviously, the social work terminology was not used during this time; however, the underpinning philosophy was present and the evolution of the social worker was started. The theoretical frameworks that advanced social work to a profession included philosophies from medicine, education,

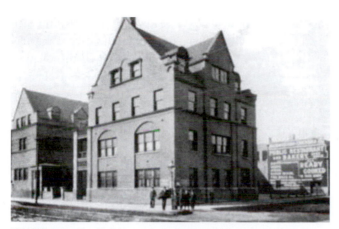

FIGURE 28-1 The Hull House in Chicago, Illinois, around 1920. (Photo credit: The Grainger Collection, New York)

anthropology, politics, education, and psychology. By combining bits and pieces of the aforementioned disciplines, social work was recognized as an interdisciplinary field and has maintained that status through the years.[2]

Individuals with a strong desire to help others and create social change often consider social work. There are many fields in the realm of social work, and altruistic individuals are presented with numerous opportunities in selecting an area of interest. Some individuals prefer to engage in counseling services to patients and families. Some of these services are in the areas of bereavement, adoption issues, marriage counseling, financial difficulties, unemployment, and job performance. Some social workers prefer to work in school environments and help children and families with the various transitions within the educational realm. Other social workers prefer to work with abused children and train for child protective services roles. Social workers are renowned as resource specialists, and some social workers focus on working in environments that require resource allocation and referrals. Referrals are a vital part of the social worker's job. Individuals who need assistance in paying for medications or other medical expenses often seek advice from social workers. Referrals for other reasons, such as alcohol and drug abuse, are common. Some social workers work in **advocacy** or patient education; others hold advanced degrees and have careers in research or teaching in an academic environment.

These are just a few of the many opportunities for individuals who desire to become a social worker.

Scope of Practice

The scope of practice for social workers relates directly to the education and licensure of the individual and the requirements of the state. Additionally, state and federal regulations may place restrictions and limitations on scope of practice. This issue is further addressed later in this chapter. Here we focus on the general scope of practice either by baccalaureate- or master's-prepared social workers.

- Assessments, including psychosocial (includes patients in medical settings, children in school environments, and families in community arenas)
- Advocacy for individuals and communities
- Crisis intervention, planning, and evaluation
- **Case management** (including child welfare)
- Child custody assessments
- Community organization
- Coordination and evaluation of service delivery
- Consulting
- Counseling skills
- Diagnosis of mental, emotional, or substance abuse disorders
- Interviewing patients/clients
- Life skills training
- Policy development
- Private practice skills (macro and clinical)
- Psychotherapy with adults and children
- Referral assistance
- Supervision
- Teaching/education to patients/clients
- Treatment planning and evaluation

Tips and Tools

Depending on the type of service, the term *patient* is used whereas in other areas the term *client* is used. Using the term *patient* usually indicates that the social worker is in a medical setting and using the term *client* usually means the person is in a community setting, such as social services or child protective services. Sometimes the combined term *patient/client* is used.

Tips and Tools

Psychosocial assessments are completed on new patients and updated regularly on existing patients within many health-care facilities. These assessments help the treatment team determine the patient's mental and psychosocial status to enhance the benefits of the treatments. The psychosocial assessments may also provide family updates that might affect the patient's outcomes. In addition to mental and social status, other items of note might include data such as exercise, diet, and sports and leisure activities.

Required Education

The majority of the states recognize three degrees of education for social workers: the baccalaureate degree (BSW) and the advanced degrees of master's of social work (MSW) and doctorate of social work (DSW). Although some states allow individuals with an undergraduate degree to work as social workers, often it is only in entry-level positions. With the increases in demand in health-care fields, many organizations and agencies require an advanced degree and license. Accrediting bodies and health-care payers are putting demands on the health-care environments to provide at least one on-site MSW to supervise or sign off on patient records. As these restrictions continue, the number of advanced-degree social workers will increase. To obtain a license as a social worker, one must have an MSW and a set number of supervised hours. These supervised hours must be managed by another MSW or a DSW. The number of required hours varies by state but the average is approximately 3,000 to 4,000.[4] Core courses one might expect to take in either the BSW or MSW include the following:

- Introduction to social work practice
- Research methods
- Group and individual counseling
- Psychopathology
- Ethics in social work
- Individual differences
- Policy and development
- Internship

Salary

The average salary range for social workers varies according to their specific area of practice. According to the Bureau of Labor Statistics, the median salary ranges are divided among **health-care social workers; child, family, and school social workers; mental health and substance abuse social workers;** and all other social workers. Health-care social workers encompass those working in hospitals, home health-care services, local government, nursing and residential care settings, and individual and family services. Under the umbrella of child, family, and school social workers are jobs in elementary and secondary schools, local and state governments, and individual and family services. The third category, mental health and substance abuse, includes those working in hospitals, including psychiatric and substance abuse hospitals, local government, outpatient mental health and substance abuse centers, and individual and family services.[3] The last category, all others, comprises

social workers in fields not already described. Within each of these subcategories, the median annual salary range may differentiate as much as $20,000 depending on the job market and specific degrees or training needed. The chart in Figure 28-2 shows the four overall broad categories with the annual median salaries and the distribution of salaries by category.[4]

Trends

As stated, the number of baby boomers reaching retirement age continues to increase, which in turns increases the need for medical social workers. Seniors in the age bracket of 85 and older are the fastest-growing group in the U.S. population. As the number of older seniors climbs, the more likely they are to need hospitalizations, medical procedures, and/or nursing home placements. Therefore, the employment projections for medical social workers will be slightly higher than those in other areas. Overall social work employment is expected to increase by 25%; however, when broken down by occupational areas, the percentages are as follows: health care (34%); mental health and substance abuse (31%); and child, family, and school (20%). An increase of 16% is expected for all other social work categories.[1] Employment projections are also high for social workers in mental health and substance abuse due to the increase of court-ordered treatment programs. For individuals who are interested in pursuing careers in social work, opportunities should continue in an upward trend because the field is expected to grow faster than average for all occupations (Fig. 28-3).

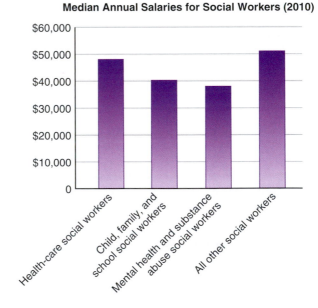

FIGURE 28-2 Median annual salaries for social workers in 2010.

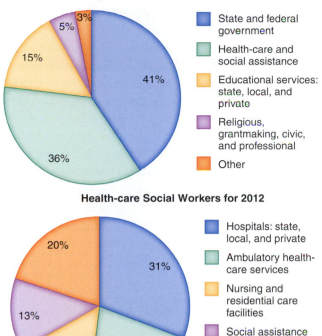

Child, Family, and School Social Workers for 2012

- State and federal government
- Health-care and social assistance
- Educational services: state, local, and private
- Religious, grantmaking, civic, and professional
- Other

3%, 5%, 15%, 41%, 36%

Health-care Social Workers for 2012

- Hospitals: state, local, and private
- Ambulatory health-care services
- Nursing and residential care facilities
- Social assistance
- Other

20%, 31%, 13%, 15%, 21%

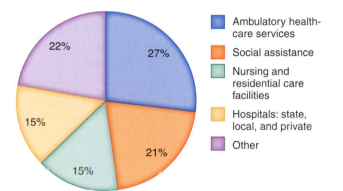
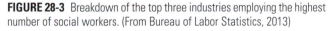

Mental Health and Substance Abuse Social Workers for 2012

- Ambulatory health-care services
- Social assistance
- Nursing and residential care facilities
- Hospitals: state, local, and private
- Other

22%, 27%, 15%, 15%, 21%

FIGURE 28-3 Breakdown of the top three industries employing the highest number of social workers. (From Bureau of Labor Statistics, 2013)

Challenges

As with most careers, social work can have many challenges. One of the more common challenges is job burnout due to stress. Social workers often get so involved in the lives of their patients/clients that it becomes difficult to separate work and home time. This involvement is more specific in the areas of health care and counseling. Social workers who work in facilities such as home health, nursing homes, and hospice facilities often become attached to the patients and families. The patients and families often become a part of the social worker's family, and when it is time for discharge, or if the

patient dies, the social worker has to grieve for the loss as well. The relationship that has been formed has to be severed, and this constant process of building bonds and then severing them begins to take a toll on the social worker.

Another social work area that sees more job burnout is in child protective services. Individuals who have difficulty separating their emotions from the job will endure more job-related stress leading to burnout. The frustration of seeing child abuse on a regular basis portrays a hopeless cycle in which the social worker may feel that nothing can be done and his or her involvement is meaningless. In these circumstances, it is much better for the social worker to step back and examine other alternatives.

Another challenge for social workers is the lack of resources available for patients/clients in need. Part of the role of the social worker is to bridge the gap between the patient/client and resources. When resources are scarce, the social worker may feel frustrated because she or he is not able to provide assistance as needed. Depending on the political climate, some programs or funds may be altered or totally cut, even when the need for that resource is still substantial. The social worker may feel helpless and question a career change.

Often there is a lack of collaboration within the social work arena. Although some social work jobs promote interprofessional collaboration, others do not. This lack of a team approach often creates barriers between social work and other disciplines. To be effective, social workers need

Aptitude Profile

When deciding on a career, the individual should take into consideration the skills and abilities needed to be successful in that particular job. Many jobs in the health-care fields require some of the same characteristics; however, some skills are more specific to social work. The following list includes some of the necessary skills and abilities to consider when entertaining the idea of becoming a social worker. Although this list is not exhaustive, all of these characteristics are required to be effective in the social work field.

Able to handle stress	Independent worker
Advocator	Nonjudgmental
Altruistic	Objective
Compassionate	Resourceful
Emotionally mature	Responsible
Empathic	Self-aware
Ethical	Sensitive
Good communicator	Skillful in interviewing

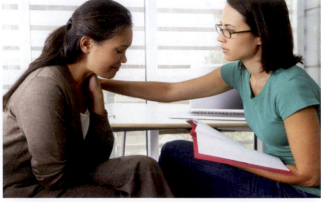

FIGURE 28-4 Some social workers provide bereavement counseling such as shown in this photo. Providing emotional support while allowing grieving individuals to freely express their thoughts without judgment enhances the grieving process and closure.

to understand other issues that may be going on in clients'/patients' lives, and not being privy to this information may create a wedge between social workers and other disciplines. This team-based approach is especially useful in the health-care field.

Role of the Master's-Prepared Social Worker

There are some similarities between the baccalaureate-prepared social worker (BSW) and the master's-prepared social worker (MSW); however, the BSW is usually supervised by the MSW. In organizations or facilities that can suffice with a BSW, supervision is often done by a nursing supervisor or director of nursing (DON).

Master's-prepared social workers usually have an area of concentration that helps determine some of the roles the social worker will eventually play. The typical choices include mental health, health care, gerontology, and family and children concentrations. Some universities are beginning to offer another option called *leadership and management*. This newer concentration represents individuals who desire to be supervisors and managers or provide evaluations of social work programs. The roles of social workers are determined by their areas of concentration, and some are discussed next.

Role of Medical Social Workers

Medical social workers are one of the fastest-growing concentrations in social work. Individuals working as medical social workers hold jobs in both inpatient and ambulatory settings. As part of their roles for the inpatient settings, medical social workers complete discharge evaluations, which includes coordinating home health service, hospice service,

durable medical equipment, and referrals for long-term care facilities or rehabilitative centers. Medical social workers also provide assistance and/or direction in the application process for Social Security, Medicare, and Medicaid. They provide both supportive counseling and financial counseling depending on the need. Medical social workers often provide crisis intervention for both patients and families. Some medical social workers are employed by managed-care organizations and are responsible for collecting and analyzing medical information as needed for other health professions. They are always the patient's advocate and are helpful in the organization of support groups applicable to the patient's or family's own health issues. As part of an interprofessional team, medical social workers provide evaluations and recommendations regarding a patient's support, finances, resources, and mental status.

Role of Clinical Social Workers

There is some overlapping in roles and places of employment between medical social work and clinical social work; however, there are some distinct differences between the two types. The clinical social worker has obtained a clinical license in the state of practice, in addition to holding a master's degree from an accredited program and at least 3,000 hours of postmaster's experience in a supervised clinical setting.[2] The role of the clinical social worker includes diagnosis, assessment, and treatment of patients/clients in a variety of settings. They employ a range of psychotherapy treatments when dealing with emotional, mental, and behavioral disorders. These patients/clients are often found in settings such as hospitals, community and primary health centers, child welfare agencies, mental health centers, and substance abuse

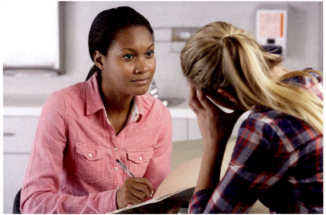

FIGURE 28-5 Medical social workers complete psychosocial assessments on patients, which are evaluations of mental, physical, and emotional health. These assessments help the interprofessional team create an individualized plan of care.

agencies.[2] In most states, clinical social workers' services are billable to insurance companies, Medicare, and Medicaid. Additionally, clinical social workers may have their own private practice.

Role of Child, Family, and School Social Workers

The role of social workers in this category provides some of the same interventions as those already discussed. The main difference between this category and the ones already discussed is that the focus is not health care-related. These social workers still provide counseling, assessments, and referrals; however, the overall center of attention revolves around personal, family, home, community, and school functions. Roles in this arena may include the removal of children from their homes due to abusive situations, evaluation of home environments for both adoption and child removal, assisting with employment, seeking shelter for the homeless and victims of domestic violence, and making referrals as needed. School social workers provide some of the same interventions; however, they generally are confined to school-related issues such as helping students with behavioral and emotional issues that interfere with the child's ability to learn. Some school social workers provide crisis intervention inside and outside of the school environment, particularly in the areas of violence and drug- or alcohol-related matters. These social workers often depend on teachers to recognize problems, so they need to work closely with teachers and administrators at the school.

Role of Mental Health and Substance Abuse Social Workers

Some of the roles for social workers in mental health and substance abuse may also occur in other categories; however, the overall focus for this type of social worker is prevention and treatment of mental health disorders and substance abuse. The work setting may be in a psychiatric hospital, mental health center, or substance abuse facility. Completing admission screenings and performing psychosocial assessments are routine for these social workers. Both supportive and psychological counseling are provided for individuals dealing with mental health and/or substance abuse issues. As in other categories, patient/client advocacy and referrals are a vital component for these social workers. Clients with substance abuse problems may be court-ordered to a substance abuse facility for treatments. These clients may be angry about their situation, creating a hostile environment for the social worker.

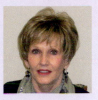
Role of Baccalaureate-Prepared Social Workers

To be recognized as a social worker, the minimum standard degree required is usually the baccalaureate degree in social work (BSW). These social workers may work in a variety of settings and include varied roles and responsibilities. Many provide case management in areas such as social services or child protective services. Other BSWs work as discharge planners in hospitals and other health-care facilities. Resource allocation and referrals are a common but important role for many BSWs. Providing patients/clients with appropriate resources or assistance in acquiring the resources occurs in most work environments. Other roles for BSWs include career counseling, mediating, consulting, advocating, and developing policies. The roles for BSWs are much like those for MSWs, meaning the working environment will generally dictate some of the responsibilities along with the supervision required. As noted, these social workers are usually supervised by an MSW.

Required Continuing Education

Licensed social workers must take continuing education credits either yearly or every 2 years, depending on the state where the license was obtained. The number of credit hours also depends on the state, but all states require continuing education. The number of hours ranges from 20 to

Working Together

Due to the many roles social workers play, a number of disciplines are directly involved in the social worker's day. Social workers must be cognizant of the various needs to be met by other professionals. Depending on the environment, some of the disciplines with which social workers regularly collaborate are medicine, pharmacy, nursing, nutrition, physician assisting, occupational therapy, physical therapy, health services and information management, and rehabilitative counseling. The collaboration among these disciplines ensures adequate resources are met. Having the collaboration of the other disciplines helps provide a holistic plan of care for the patient. All of these disciplines, along with some others, are usually part of the interprofessional care team of which the social worker is a member. This interprofessional team works to ensure appropriate treatment and resources to provide quality care.

50 credit hours every 2 years, with the initial renewal somewhat different from subsequent renewals for many states. Some states require specific topics for continuing education, such as substance abuse, cross-cultural education, aging and long-term care, and domestic violence. Most states require some form of continuing education in the area of professional ethics or law. The manner in which the education may be obtained varies as well. Options include courses, workshops, practice-oriented seminars, and training by accredited programs. Home study and online courses are allowed in many states, which makes it somewhat easier to obtain the required hours without the interruption of daily work schedules.[4]

CASE STUDY

Maria is a 61-year-old Hispanic woman. She has been in the United States for only 5 years and speaks very little English. She had been living in Naucalpan, Mexico, until her husband died 6 years ago. She then moved to the United States to join her only son and his family. Her son and his family moved to the United States about 15 years ago and are acclimated to U.S. culture; however, it is much harder for Maria because of her age and limited time spent here. Maria's son gets frustrated with her because she is having a very difficult time adjusting and he is constantly telling her she needs to work harder on becoming an American citizen. Maria tries to hold on to her heritage and had begun to distance herself from her son due to her feelings of inadequacy. Recently Maria was diagnosed with prehypertension and insulin-dependent diabetes mellitus. Her physician started her on daily injections, but Maria has difficulty understanding the injection process and the amount of insulin needed. Because of her poor comprehension, as well as limited funds to buy her medications, she often skips taking her insulin. Additionally, Maria planned to purchase a glucose monitoring kit at her local pharmacy as directed by her physician but became so frustrated with her inability to communicate with the pharmacist that she just gave up and left. Although Maria's doctor has not started her on hypertensive medication yet, he plans to check her blood pressure at the next appointment and make a determination at that time; however, in the meantime he has provided Maria with a low-sodium diet written in English. Her physician is not aware that she does not comprehend the information because she nods her head in the affirmative when asked if she understands. Maria can only read bits and pieces of information on the diet plan and refuses to ask her son for help. There is a neighborhood senior center that Maria has visited a couple of times, but the walk is a little far for her and she does not have regular transportation. Maria has thought of trying to get a job but is aware of her limited skills. She also has a back injury from 20 years earlier that caused her to quit work and become a housewife. Her husband had been providing all the financial support until his death. Maria's husband had a small life insurance policy, which sustained her for a few months before she sold her house and moved in with her niece until her decision to move to the United States; however, that money is almost completely depleted. Maria feels lost and confused. She is tempted to move back to Mexico but knows she is better off staying close to her only immediate family. Who can help Maria?

Questions

1. What are the pressing issues facing Maria?
2. What disciplines should be involved with Maria's care?
3. Why is interprofessional collaboration important in this case?
4. Develop an interprofessional plan of care based on your knowledge from other chapters.
5. What are ultimately the goals for Maria's care?
6. What are some barriers facing interprofessional collaboration?

Review Questions

1. The social work profession was recognized in the:

   A. 18th century

   B. 20th century

   C. 19th century

   D. 21st century

2. One of the most common challenges in the social work profession is:

   A. Time pressures

   B. Job burnout

   C. Abundant resources

   D. Patient diversity

3. The area of social work with the highest projection of increase in employment is:

   A. Child, family, and school

   B. Medical or health care

   C. Mental health

   D. Substance abuse

4. Although each state varies on licensing requirements, the average number of required supervised hours is:

   A. 1,000–1,500 hours

   B. 1,500–2,000 hours

   C. 2,000–2,500 hours

   D. 3,000–4,000 hours

5. When considering social work as a profession, it would be wise for the individual to have the following as a characteristic:

   A. Subjective attitude

   B. Judgmental attitude

   C. Altruistic nature

   D. Sympathetic nature

6. The scope of practice for a social worker in the school environment includes:

   A. Advocacy

   B. Psychotherapy treatment

   C. Evaluation

   D. Counseling

7. The theoretical frameworks that advanced social work include:

   A. Education and anthropology

   B. Geography and anthropology

   C. Mathematics and education

   D. Medicine and journalism

8. In many health-care settings, the state and/or federal government may require a/an _____ to sign off on a BSW in a patient chart.

   A. Nurse

   B. MSW

   C. Physician

   D. Administrator

9. Individuals who want to do research or teach in academic settings usually hold this degree in social work:

   A. BSW

   B. MSW

   C. DSW

   D. ASW

10. When various disciplines work collaboratively to create a patient plan of care, this is called:

    A. Interprofessional

    B. Unidisciplinary

    C. Independent

    D. Broad scope of practice

Glossary of Key Terms

Psychosocial assessment—evaluation of a patient's psychological and social issues

Advocacy—the appeal for support by an individual or group for resources or political influence

Case management—coordination of services on behalf of an individual, particularly in health-care environments

Health-care social worker—individual working in a health-care environment who provides services to patients in a hospital or clinical environment

Child and family social worker—individual working as a social worker who deals with child and family issues such as family dynamics

Mental health social worker—individual working in a mental health facility who provides services to patients who have mental health issues such as depression

Substance abuse social worker—individual who works with patients with substance abuse problems

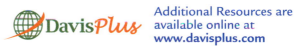

Additional Resources are available online at www.davisplus.com

Additional Resources

Accrediting Body

Council on Social Work Education—www.cswe.org
CSWE is a national association of social work education programs and individuals that ensures and enhances the quality of social work education.

Educational and Professional Resources

Journal of Social Work Education—www.cswe.org/Publications/JSWE/PurchasingJSWE.aspx
The *Journal of Social Work Education* (JSWE) is a refereed professional journal concerned with education in social work and social welfare.

The Social Work Dictionary, 5th Edition, by Robert L. Barker—www.naswpress.org/publications/reference/dictionary.html
The Social Work Dictionary captures more than 9,000 terms, cataloging and cross-referencing the nomenclature, concepts, organizations, historical figures, and values that define the profession.

National Association of Social Workers (NASW)—www.naswdc.org
The NASW is the largest membership organization of professional social workers in the world. The association enhances the professional growth and development of its members, creates and maintains professional standards, and advances sound social policies.

Society for Social Work and Research (SSWR)—www.sswr.org
The SSWR encourages the design, implementation, and dissemination of rigorous research that enhances knowledge about critical social work practice and social policy problems.

Society for Social Work Leadership in Health Care (SSWLHC)—www.sswlhc.org
The SSWLHC supports emerging leaders in all roles, by providing leadership knowledge and skills in health-care arenas.

International Association for Social Work with Groups, Inc. (IASWG)—http://iaswg.org
IASWG is a not-for-profit organization of group workers, group work educators, and friends of group work who support its program of advocacy.

Clinical Social Work Association (CSWA)—www.clinicalsocialworkassociation.org
The CSWA is the leading organization ensuring the efficacy, stability, and viability of clinical social work.

Substance Abuse and Mental Health Services Administration (SAMHSA)—www.samhsa.gov
SAMHSA enhances the professional growth of social workers in the fields of substance abuse and mental health.

Regulatory Body

Association of Social Work Boards (ASWB)—www.aswb.org
The ASWB provides support and services to the social work regulatory community for advancing competent and ethical practices.

References

1. Reamer FG. The evolution of social work ethics. *Social Work.* 1998;43(6):488–500.

2. National Association of Social Workers.
   http://www.socialworkers.org/pressroom/features/general/history.asp.
   Accessed March 14, 2013.

3. Bureau of Labor Statistics, U.S. Department of Labor. Occupational outlook handbook, 2012–2013 edition, social Workers.
   http://www.bls.gov/ooh/Community-and-Social-Service/Social-workers.htm.
   Accessed January 23, 2013.

4. National Association of Social Workers. *NASW Standards for Clinical Social Work, 2005 Edition.*
   http://www.socialworkers.org/practice/standards/NASWClinicalSWStandards.pdf.
   Accessed March 4, 2013.

CHAPTER 29

Speech-Language Pathology

Elaine Shuey, PhD

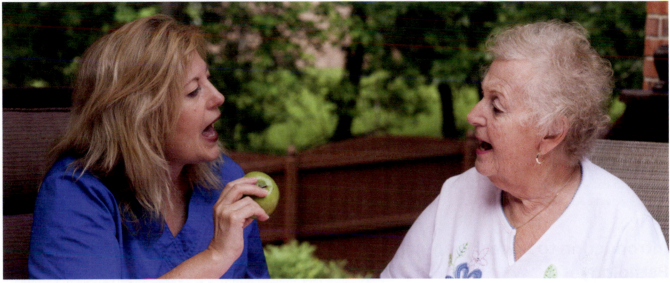

Photo credit: i stock/Thinkstock

Learning Objectives

After reading this chapter, students should be able to:

- Discuss the disorders that are targeted by a speech-language pathologist
- Name the primary work environments in which speech-language pathologists are employed
- Describe the education, certification, and licensing process for this field
- Explain how a speech-language pathologist interacts with members of other professions in a variety of work settings
- Discuss the outlook for employment in this field

Key Terms

- Communication disorder
- Developmental communication disorder
- Acquired communication disorder
- Speech
- Language
- Dysphagia
- Certificate of Clinical Competence

"A Day in the Life"

I'm Louise, a speech-language pathologist (SLP) who works in the schools. Thank goodness for tablets. I mean the computer type. Because of them, I can now fit groceries in the trunk of my car. Like many school-based SLPs, I serve more than one school. In fact, I serve four. However, in only one school do I have space assigned to me where I can store materials and tests. In the other schools, I share space with other therapists, and none of us has storage. In the past, that meant the trunk of my car was filled with toys, therapy work sheets, tests I needed to evaluate, tools to assess communication skills, and copies of students' individualized education plans (IEPs). Of course, my spare tire was there too, but I could never reach it. As tablets have improved and the number of applications has blossomed, I have been able to leave a lot of my materials behind. I can now even give some tests via the tablet.

(continued)

Today I'm working at the middle school all day. My population here is very diverse, which is not unusual. School-based SLPs probably treat a greater variety of disorders than any other SLP. My first student is a sixth-grader who has a serious fluency disorder. We are working hard to find a technique that he can use to reduce his stuttering. Then I'll see two boys who have Down syndrome. They are both hard to understand and I'm working to make their speech clearer, and to improve their abilities to follow directions in the classroom. Then I have a meeting with a parent, and two more group sessions. My last group of the morning is four children who have a language delay. They are starting a new section in science class, and I will work to help them learn the vocabulary they need for the new section. The science teacher gave me a list of terms and some photos to use for this task. One of the girls in the group uses an augmentative and alternative communication (AAC), device and I'll keep her a bit longer so we can program the new vocabulary into the device. Later, I'll check on her at lunch because she has dysphagia. The dietary staff alters her food to make it safer and easier to eat, and I trained a classroom aide to help her eat safely. About once a month I like to check to see that things are going well. The resource room teacher and I will be seeing a group of students who have autism spectrum disorder. This group has good articulation and basic language skills, but they have a lot of difficulty with pragmatics. For example, the one student stares at the person he is talking to. He never looks away. It makes the listener uncomfortable. Another student doesn't understand when the topic has changed and keeps talking about the previous topic. Things like this not only make communication difficult, but also lead to the students being picked on, ignored, or made fun of. To work on these things, I create scenarios to target the students' problem areas and the resource room teacher and I work through them with the students. We also create videos to evaluate behaviors. I'll end the day with an IEP meeting. Every student who receives special services has to have an IEP, which has the goals or objectives from all the specialists who will work with the child. Most of them will be at the meeting, along with the parents. We'll discuss our goals and lay out a plan for the upcoming year. This can be overwhelming for the parents, but we all try to make them comfortable. After work, I'm going to stop by the grocery store and fill that empty trunk with food.

Introduction to Speech-Language Pathology

Description

Many people are familiar with the term *speech therapist,* but the correct name for this professional is *speech-language pathologist.* Since that is a mouthful (no pun intended), it is usually shortened to SLP. SLPs work with individuals who have communication or swallowing disorders, with clients ranging from newborns to older adults. Depending on work environment, the people with whom an SLP works might be called *students, patients, residents,* or *clients.* The term *client* will be used here.

History

The field of SLP grew out of a variety of other areas. Teachers of rhetoric, speech, or debate tried to help those with communication problems and pushed for a professional organization and skills to deal with these. Theater, music, education, psychology, and other areas have contributed to the development of the field. In 1925, the first professional group devoted to communication disorders was started. The scope of disorders then was much narrower than it is now.

Scope of Practice

A **communication disorder** is difficulty creating, sending, receiving, or understanding a message. For example, a person who had a stroke might have difficulty putting the words together, or formulating a message, to ask for something. A person with multiple sclerosis might be able to formulate the message in his thoughts, but be unable to produce the speech, writing, or sign language needed to get the message across. An individual with a hearing loss may not be able to hear or receive the message someone is saying. A person who had a brain injury may hear the message but be unable to understand it.

A **developmental communication disorder** exists from birth or from the person's first attempts to communicate, or it may be acquired, as with someone who has a stroke or neuromuscular disease. An **acquired communication disorder** usually occurs after the individual has already developed communication skills, which are now impaired by the stroke or other incident. Following is an overview of the specific areas where there may be communication problems and which an SLP might evaluate/diagnose and then target in therapy. This is a very brief summary of a variety of complex concepts. The American Speech-Language-Hearing Association (ASHA) has more in-depth information about these areas on its website.[1] These areas constitute the SLP's scope of practice.

Aspects of Communication

Speech

Speech includes three areas: articulation, voice, and fluency. Articulation is the act of producing speech sounds such as consonants or vowels. A child who has not developed sounds at an expected age would have a developmental articulation delay. This could be an isolated delay or part of another disorder such as Down syndrome or cerebral palsy. An articulation disorder can be acquired as well, as in the case of some neuromuscular disorders such as Parkinson's disease or multiple sclerosis. SLPs are trained to write speech sounds by using the International Phonetic Alphabet (IPA).[2] The IPA has symbols for sounds in all languages, and these symbols make it easier to explain what sound a person is producing (Figs. 29-1 and 29-2). For example, in English the letter "c" might be pronounced as several different sounds. The IPA allows the SLP to write exactly what it is, such as /k/ in cough or /s/ in cent.

Voice is the tone produced in your voice box, or, more correctly, your larynx (Fig. 29-3). If you whisper, you are not using voice, even though you are articulating. If you hum, you are producing voice, but not articulating. Voice disorders can be the result of excess use of the voice or of a disease process. The voice might be characterized as harsh, hoarse, breathy, or strained. Pitch might be too low or too high. It is not unusual for someone who uses the voice extensively for a job or hobby to develop a voice problem. Teachers, coaches, and cheerleaders are prone to this type of disorder. The SLP can help that person learn to use the voice more efficiently and to conserve it when possible. A voice disorder that results from a bacterial or viral infection or cancer will first require treatment by a physician, followed by work with an SLP to recover the best voice possible. Occasionally, because of the presence

of cancer, the larynx is removed and the SLP will help the person learn a method of *alaryngeal* (without a larynx) speech.

Fluency refers to how speech flows. Everyone has likely had a fluency problem at one time or another, such as when nervous about giving a speech or when trying to explain the dent in the car to a parent. One may hesitate between words or add fillers such as "um," "uh," or "like." When a lack of fluency occurs consistently and interferes with communication, it is a fluency disorder. Stuttering is often used to describe this type of disorder and is characterized by hesitations and repetitions of sounds, syllables, or even whole words.

Language

Speech is only one method of getting a message across to someone else. Other ways are signing, gestures, writing, and other symbol systems. The content of the message, however, is called **language.** A language is a shared set of rules and vocabulary that allows people within a culture to communicate with each other. As with speech, a language disorder can be developmental or acquired. It can be primarily receptive (understanding language) or expressive (producing language).

There are several aspects of language, including syntax, semantics, and pragmatics. *Syntax* means grammar, those rules English teachers, and sometimes moms, drill into us. Dialectic differences, such as "y'all" or "come with," are not disorders, just variations of the standard American dialect based on region and/or culture. An example of a developmental syntactic delay might be if a child overuses the rule on plurals. For most words, adding an "s" indicates the plural as in *cars, cats,* or *houses,* but

The International Phonetic Alphabet (revised to 2005)

Consonants (pulmonic)

	Bilabial	Labiodental	Dental	Alveolar	Postalveolar	Retroflex	Palatal	Velar	Uvular	Pharyngeal	Glottal
Plosive	p b			t d		ʈ ɖ	c ɟ	k ɡ	q ɢ		ʔ
Nasal	m	ɱ		n		ɳ	ɲ	ŋ	N		
Trill	ʙ			r					R		
Tap or Flap		ⱱ				ɽ					
Fricative	ɸ β	f v	θ ð	s z	ʃ ʒ	ʂ ʐ	ç ʝ	x ɣ	χ ʁ	ħ ʕ	h ɦ
Lateral fricative				ɬ ɮ							
Approximant		ʋ		ɹ		ɻ	j	ɰ			
Lateral approximant				l		ɭ	ʎ	ʟ			

Where symbols appear in pairs, the one to the right represents a voiced consonant.
Shaded areas denote articulations judged impossible.

FIGURE 29-1 IPA symbols for consonants. (IPA chart. https://internationalphoneticassociation.org/content/ipa-chart. Available under a Creative Commons Attribution-Sharealike 3.0 Unported License. Copyright © 2005 International Phonetic Association.)

VOWELS

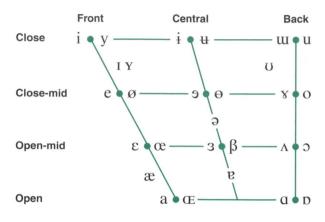

Where symbols appear in pairs, the one to the right represents a rounded vowel.

FIGURE 29-2 IPA symbols for vowels. (IPA chart. https://www.international phoneticassociation.org/content/ipa-vowels. Available under a Creative Commons Attribution-Sharealike 3.0 Unported License. Copyright © 2005 International Phonetic Association.)

that rule does not work for irregular plurals such as *geese, mice,* or *deer.* A child who says "gooses," "mouses," or "deers" is displaying overgeneralization of the rule. Some generalization is normal at early ages but is evidence of a delay at later ages.

Semantics is an interesting area of language that deals with the meanings of words. As language has evolved, we have "assigned" words to objects or concepts. Some are rather concrete and easy to define. A car is a four-wheeled object we get in and drive around. Other terms are more abstract or subjective. Try explaining *delicious, creepy,* or *valuable* to someone. Some words have multiple meanings. *Fly* means to soar through the air, although it is also an obnoxious bug. Meanings are often added or changed over time. To describe something as "fly" has nothing to do with soaring or bugs, but instead means something is great or admirable. Advances in technology regularly add new words

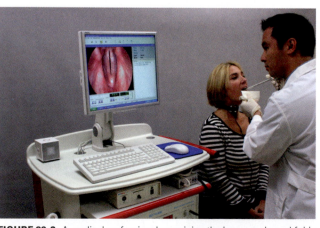

(Photo courtesy of Pentax Medical.)

FIGURE 29-3 A medical professional examining the larynx and vocal folds of a client.

and meanings such as *texting, selfie,* or *to google something.* Meanings may vary by dialect or region as well. A pie might have a crust and fruit, but in some areas it could also be a pizza. Semantics is indeed a fascinating area of study.

Semantic disorders or delays can make communication difficult because the words needed to communicate the message may be missing or wrong. This can happen developmentally, after a stroke or head injury, or as a result of certain disorders. To say that someone is saving money to attain a car is a semantic error. Instead, the person would *obtain* a car, but the error is minor and the message will probably still be understood. More serious errors, or the use of terms that are not actually words, will cause a much greater problem in communication. If a client asks you to get the "smither," you may have no idea what she means and communication will fail, because the word has no meaning in standard or regional dialects.

Pragmatics refers to the rules of how to use language in a social context. Pragmatic rules are much harder to define than syntactic or semantic rules. Pragmatics include issues such as how close you should stand to someone when talking, how long you should maintain eye contact, or whether you can call someone by his or her first name or should instead use some other means of address. Pragmatics vary by culture, region, and even age.

In certain environments, the SLP works extensively with individuals who have autism or pervasive developmental disorders. People who have these disorders often have difficulty with language, particularly pragmatics, although they may have a problem in any area of communication. The SLP would work with teachers and other therapists to help the person with autism be as good a communicator as possible.

The phrase *English as a second language* (ESL) refers to the act of learning English after having learned another language first. Individuals learning English may have difficulty with both speech sounds and with many aspects of language. This is not considered to be a disorder, but it is not unusual for an SLP to work with such clients to improve their English skills, coordinating efforts with the ESL teacher.

Additional Areas of Practice

Reading

SLPs often work collaboratively with reading specialists and classroom teachers to improve children's literacy or reading skills. Remember that the definition of a communication disorder includes the inability to understand or decode a message. This includes both a spoken and a written message. The SLP works on many of the underlying skills needed for literacy. Children must be able to match letters with the sounds they represent. They need to be able to decode what happens when letters are combined to form syllables or words. Rhyming; identification of syllable breaks; and understanding that sounds occur at the beginning, middle, and ends of words are all aspects of literacy that an SLP might target.[3]

Augmentative and Alternative Communication

An interesting tool that SLPs use is called *augmentative and alternative communication* (AAC).[4] This term is used to indicate any means of expressing a message other than verbal. Signs, gestures, writing, and facial expressions are all aspects of AAC. However, many people think of AAC as being the use of pictures for communication when the client's speech is too difficult to understand without assistance. Before the advent of personal computers, this meant a sheet of paper or a board covered with photos or drawings that helped the individual to communicate. The photos might include family or pet pictures, drawings of food and drink, or drawings to indicate pain or the need to go to the bathroom (Figs. 29-4 and 29-5). This type of AAC may still be used for specific situations. If a patient is temporarily unable to speak because he is on a ventilator or just had his larynx removed, the SLP would provide the nursing staff with this type of AAC to help the client meet his basic needs. When thirsty, the client

would point to a representative picture. However, technological advances have created computer-based devices that can allow the individual to express simple to complex language. A very young child might have a device programmed only with words such as *mommy, cookie,* or *truck,* because that is his appropriate language level. When he wants his truck, he touches that picture on his device and it says "truck" for him. As he matures and develops more language, his device will become more complex, eventually allowing him to produce the same syntactically complex, situationally relevant statements that any teenager or adult might produce. He will go from a simple "truck" to "my dad traded the minivan for a Ford F-250 with the extended cab and Mom is really mad." Even if the client has severely impaired motor skills and cannot point, adaptations can still be made to allow him to use an AAC device.

Hearing

It is the responsibility of the audiologist to perform complete hearing testing and to make a diagnosis of hearing loss. However, it is within the SLP's scope of practice to perform basic screenings of hearing to determine if referrals for further testing should be made. SLPs frequently provide therapy to clients who have hearing loss. The SLP might work to improve the

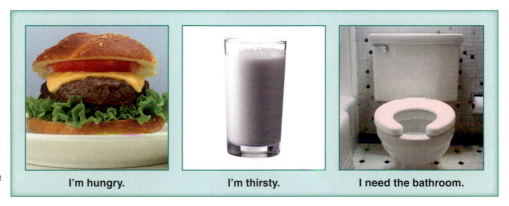

FIGURE 29-4 Clip art used for a simple AAC device.

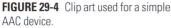

I'm hungry.   I'm thirsty.   I need the bathroom.

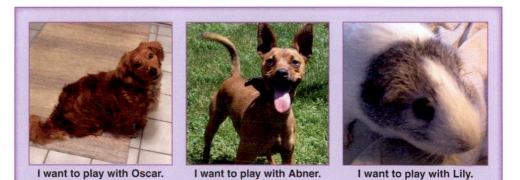

FIGURE 29-5 Personal photos for a simple AAC device.

I want to play with Oscar.   I want to play with Abner.   I want to play with Lily.

client's hearing skills, a process called *aural rehabilitation*. The client might be taught to turn down the television or other noise sources, to improve lighting, and to watch a speaker's lips, face, and hands for improved communication. The hearing loss might also be accompanied by speech or language problems that the SLP would target in therapy. As cochlear implants are becoming more common, SLPs are learning how to help the recipients achieve the best hearing and speech possible. A cochlear implant is a device that is surgically implanted to provide sound to a person who is deaf or severely hard of hearing.

An audiologist might determine that a client has a (central) auditory processing disorder. This client may have normal hearing, but be unable to accurately process the spoken message. This is not the result of a stroke or head injury, but was probably present at birth. The SLP will work to strengthen the client's listening skills. Targeted areas might be improving the ability to listen in noisy environments, learning to follow increasingly longer directions, or establishing compensations such as note taking to retain auditory information. If the client is a child, both the SLP and the audiologist would work with the classroom teacher to be sure classroom accommodations are made to compensate for the child's auditory problems.

Dysphagia

Dysphagia means difficulty swallowing and it is often a major part of the SLP's caseload in health-care settings. Dysphagia can occur at any age, but it is a common problem following stroke, head injury, or various neuromuscular diseases such as multiple sclerosis, amyotrophic lateral sclerosis (ALS, also known as Lou Gehrig's disease), or Parkinson's disease. The process of swallowing actually starts when the person sees, smells, or thinks about food. There are several steps involved in getting food from the plate to the stomach. The person must first get the food into the mouth by either using a utensil or by biting off a piece to be chewed. The tongue and teeth must work together to chew the food enough to be swallowed. Several stages are involved in the actual swallow, starting in the mouth and eventually leading to the stomach. If this process breaks down, there is a danger of malnutrition, dehydration, choking to death, or developing pneumonia because fluids leaked into the lungs. Dysphagia therapy involves techniques to improve the actual swallow. The SLP may also work with the family or other caregivers to change the consistency of food. Food that is of a consistency like that of applesauce or pudding is easiest to control. Therefore, harder foods such as meat might be pureed, and thinner liquids may be thickened to make them safer to swallow. If the swallowing problems create an extreme danger for the client, tube feeding might be used on either a temporary or permanent basis.

Therapy Setting

Traditional speech therapy consisted of an SLP and a client in a room, working on some aspect of the client's communication. This still occurs frequently and is appropriate for many clients. However, therapy is administered in a variety of other ways as well. Clients may be seen in small groups because they are working on the same skills. Groups are also used to improve pragmatic skills or to provide mutual support. The client's family or other professionals may be involved in the session. Therapy might be conducted in a "therapy room," a hospital room, a resident's room at a residential facility, a classroom, the dining room, or a client's home (Fig. 29-6). Therapy might not even be conducted indoors. Work with a coach or cheerleader might be done on the athletic field. The advent of telepractice has led to therapy where the client and therapist are communicating via a secure computer program and are not even in the same building, or possibly even the same state.

Required Education

Most SLPs complete an undergraduate/bachelor's degree in speech-language pathology, communication disorders, speech pathology/audiology, or a similarly named program. In general, this program is considered to be a preprofessional degree, because it prepares you to go on for a graduate degree, rather than for an immediate job in the field. The entry-level degree is the master's degree. Master's programs are accredited by the Council on Academic Accreditation in Audiology and Speech-Language Pathology[5] and take a full 2 years to complete. A list of programs

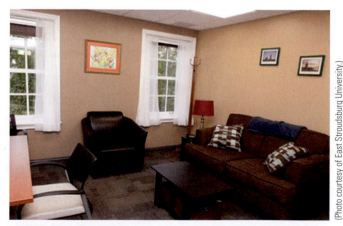

FIGURE 29-6 Naturalistic speech-language therapy room at the East Stroudsburg University Speech and Hearing Clinic.

is available on the ASHA website.[6] Some programs are called 5-year programs because students complete the undergraduate portion in 3 years followed by the 2-year graduate program. Competition for graduate school is intense, and students must maintain good undergraduate grades to increase their chances of being accepted into a graduate program.

Speech-language pathology's sister field, audiology, has shifted to an undergraduate degree followed by a 4-year clinical doctorate instead of a master's degree. It may be that speech-language pathology will do the same sometime in the future.

License/Credentials

The **Certificate of Clinical Competence** (CCC) is the nationally recognized credential for SLPs. It is awarded by ASHA. To earn this, the SLP must complete a master's degree from an accredited institution, pass a PRAXIS test specific to the field, and complete a Clinical Fellowship experience. The Clinical Fellowship is a 9-month, full-time job experience supervised by an SLP who already has his or her CCC. This is an actual job, not an internship or volunteer experience. Obtaining the CCC implies that the individual practices ethically, uses therapy techniques that are supported by research, and keeps the client's well-being and success as the primary focus.

Most states require that the SLP obtain a professional license from the state. Just as a driver's license makes it legal for a person to drive, the professional license makes it legal

for the SLP to practice *in that state.* In addition, if the SLP will be practicing in the schools, he or she may be required to obtain a teaching certificate from the department of education in that state. Rules for both licensure and teaching certificates vary from state to state.

Most professionals must demonstrate that they are staying current with changes in their fields through continuing education. There are many ways to obtain continuing education credits, including journal reading; attendance at conferences, workshops, or in-services; or using online sources such as webinars or courses. ASHA requires an average of 10 continuing education hours or units per year over a 3-year period. Continuing education may also be required to maintain state licensure or teaching certificates, but again, this varies by state.

Salary

As with most professions, SLP salaries vary somewhat by geographical region and by work environment. A school-based SLP usually earns the same as a teacher in that district who has the same level of education and number of years of experience. Historically, SLPs employed in a health-care environment have earned more than their school-based counterparts. This salary gap has been narrowed somewhat over the years as schools shifted from the bachelor's to the master's degree as the required level of education. Further, the shortage of SLPs has served to drive up SLP salaries regardless of work environment. According to ASHA,[7] in 2014 the median academic year salary of school-based SLPs was $60,000. The median annual salary for SLPs working in a health-care setting was $75,000 in 2013.[8]

Trends

In recent years, more and more children have been identified as having special needs, including the need for speech therapy. At the other end of the spectrum, the population of individuals over age 65 has been rapidly increasing. That population also has increasing health-care needs, including the need for speech therapy. Further, almost 25% of SLPs currently in the field are age 55 or older, meaning that they will be looking toward retirement in the near future.[9] The math is clear: (more children needing therapy) + (a growing older adult population) + (an SLP workforce facing retirement) = a national shortage of SLPs. An SLP who has the proper credentials, prepares an accurate and appropriate resume, learns good interviewing techniques, and is willing to seek a job should have no difficulty finding one.

Author Spotlight

Elaine Shuey, PhD

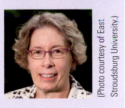

(Photo courtesy of East Stroudsburg University.)

Like most high school students, I seriously considered what I wanted to do with my life. Did I want to go into music? I played three instruments and sang in various groups. Or did I want to go into a health-care field? I joined the high school's health career club to explore that option. On a field trip to a state hospital, I got to see the audiologist in action. I was amazed. I applied to colleges where I could become an audiologist. Part way through my undergraduate program, I realized I was better suited to be a speech-language pathologist. Communication is essential for success, for safety, and for a rich life. I knew that a career in which I might help people to communicate better would be both professionally and personally fulfilling. So that's the path I chose, and I never looked back.

Challenges

SLPs have a very broad scope of practice. That scope can make it difficult and time consuming for professionals to keep up to date on research and trends in the field. The shortage of SLPs has created a situation where there are fewer professionals to treat more clients. Caseloads have grown, making it difficult to keep up with both therapy and the paperwork/reporting requirements of most jobs. The shortage has also led some employers, schools in particular, to hire unqualified individuals to serve the communicatively impaired population. This unethical practice is a threat to both the client and the field of speech-language pathology. Finally, cuts in health care and insurance coverage impede an SLP's ability to adequately serve his or her clients.

Role of the School-Based SLP

According to ASHA,[9] the majority of SLPs, 57%, work in an educational setting. An elementary school is the most common of these settings, but others include preschools, secondary schools, a combination of levels, special schools, or colleges and universities. School-based SLPs see clients from infancy through 21 years of age. An infant may have a disorder known to affect communication or feeding, such as Down syndrome or cleft palate. The SLP works with the family, often in their own home, to encourage speech and language development and sufficient feeding. School-based SLPs may see clients with any of the communication disorders listed previously.

Role of the Health-Care Facility–Based SLP

Employment in a health-care facility makes up 38.1% of SLP work settings. Within this category, the largest single employer is acute-care hospitals. Some SLPs work in residential health-care facilities such as skilled nursing homes or rehabilitation centers. *Residential* means that the client lives at that facility, at least while receiving treatment. Other SLPs work in nonresidential health-care facilities. As the name implies, the client probably lives at home but receives therapy from the agency that employs the SLP. This could be a home health agency where the SLP goes to the client's home to provide services. It could also be a private physician's office, a speech and hearing center, or an SLP's private practice. The SLP in this setting might see clients who have a variety of different communication problems. On the other hand, the facility might be focused on just one type of rehabilitation, such as the speech, language, and swallowing difficulties associated with stroke.

Aptitude Profile

Speech therapy has been described as requiring a combination of art and science. An SLP has to understand the anatomy, physiology, neural control, and physics that underlie speech, language, hearing, and swallowing. He or she must develop therapy skills and learn how to apply them with a population that may vary greatly in terms of age, type of disorder, severity of communication impairment, ability to cooperate in therapy, and many other factors. Following is a list of basic skills that an SLP needs to succeed both educationally and professionally.

A desire to work collaboratively	Objectivity
A sense of responsibility	Patience
Compassion	Respect for ethnic, cultural, religious, age, and other human differences
Ethics	
Good speech and language abilities	
Good writing skills	Strong math and science skills
Hearing adequate to evaluate the communication skills of clients	Strong organizational abilities

Working Together

SLPs interact closely with a variety of other professionals. These professionals vary somewhat by work environment. The school-based SLP is likely to work closely with the classroom teacher, special education or resource room teachers, the educational audiologist, the school psychologist, and other therapists who are providing services to the client. An example of coordination might occur at the preschool level between the occupational therapist (OT) and the SLP. The OT may be working to get the client to hold a pencil properly. The SLP might be working on concepts such as "under," "over," and "around." The two would share these goals. When the SLP is using a writing or coloring task with the client, she reinforces the OT's goals for holding the pencil or crayon. Likewise, when the OT is working with the pencil or crayon, she will have the child put lines "under," "over," or "around" a picture. Both goals are reinforced collaboratively.

The SLP is also likely to work with other therapists in a health-care setting. These include occupational, physical, recreational, and respiratory therapists. The SLP would get input from and give suggestions to the nursing staff regarding communication and feeding. Social workers, physicians, dietary workers, and nutritionists would also all work closely with the SLP. In all work environments, the client's family is an essential part of the therapy team.

CASE STUDY

Marie is an SLP at a university clinic. She supervises graduate students as they provide therapy at the on-campus clinic where they see a variety of clients from the campus and community. Mike, a student majoring in vocal music, has been referred by his voice instructor because he has become hoarse. Mike plans to become a professional voice instructor and singer, so this change in voice is worrisome. Mike's vocal folds were examined by an otolaryngologist, who is a specialist in disorders of the ear, nose, and throat and is often referred to as an ENT. The ENT diagnosed vocal nodules and recommended speech/voice therapy. Vocal nodules are growths on the vocal folds or vocal cords caused by phonotrauma or vocal abuse. This means Mike is doing something, probably not consciously, that is damaging his vocal folds and his voice.

Marie and her students conducted a thorough evaluation of Mike's voice, which included objective data, a review of the ENT's report and video, and perceptual data. He was given a hearing screening, which he failed, something that is not uncommon in musicians. The majority of the evaluation was a careful history to try to determine what vocal behaviors lead to the vocal nodules. Mike has been taking vocal lessons and performing in concerts and plays since junior high, so he knows how to sing in a healthy manner. What has changed? Does he have a new hobby or job that requires voice? Has he been ill lately or had surgery that affected voice? Is he on any new medications? Two issues became clear. First, Mike reports symptoms of gastric reflux. This is when stomach acid backs up into the esophagus. Reflux does not cause vocal nodules but can hinder their healing. Second, about 6 months ago, Mike took a job as an assistant coach for a junior high soccer team. Like any coach, he has to yell to be heard across an open field. He enjoys coaching and needs the money so quitting is probably not an option. Instead a voice therapy program was devised that included the following: learning how to yell more efficiently; using amplification during practice; increasing hydration, that is, drinking more water during practice to increase overall and vocal fold hydration; and practicing vocal function exercises to improve voice. If therapy is not successful, Mike will have to make a decision about coaching versus his career as a performer.

Questions

1. What professional should Marie refer Mike to for a complete hearing evaluation?

2. What professional should Marie refer Mike to regarding the reflux symptoms?

3. Which other professionals should Marie work with to ensure Mike's success in therapy?

4. Why is it better to do speech/voice therapy to eliminate vocal nodules rather than surgery?

5. Can you think of something else Mike can do as a coach that would conserve his voice?

Review Questions

1. An SLP working in Ohio has her CCC, state professional license, and Ohio teaching certificate. She is moving to Alabama. Which of these credentials will move with her?

   A. CCC

   B. State professional license

   C. Teaching certificate

2. What is currently the entry-level degree for an SLP?

   A. Associate degree

   B. Bachelor's degree

   C. Master's degree

   D. Doctorate

3. A person who cannot pronounce sounds correctly has what kind of disorder?

   A. Voice

   B. Fluency

   C. Articulation/speech

   D. Language

4. The term *dysphagia* refers to difficulty with:

   A. Hearing

   B. Swallowing

   C. Speech

   D. All of these

5. The majority of SLPs work in what type of setting?

   A. Hospitals

   B. Nursing homes

   C. Rehabilitation centers

   D. Schools

6. An SLP can _____ a client's hearing.

   A. Comprehensively test

   B. Screen

   C. Observe

7. A communication disorder might be:

   A. Developmental

   B. Acquired

   C. Either of the above

   D. Neither of the above

8. Professionals must stay current in their fields by engaging in:

   A. Clinical practice

   B. Continuing education

   C. Reading the newspaper

   D. Using the IPA

9. AAC is often adopted when the client's speech is too difficult to understand. It can be used:

   A. Only if the client has good motor skills and can point with his finger

   B. Only if the client has adult language skills

   C. By clients of any age, language level, or motor abilities

10. Communication involves:

    A. Speaking

    B. Listening

    C. Reading

    D. Writing

    E. Signing

    F. All of the above and more

Glossary of Key Terms

Communication disorder—difficulty creating, sending, receiving, or understanding a message

Developmental communication disorder—difficulty with communication that exists from birth or from the person's first attempts to communicate

Acquired communication disorder—difficulty with communication that develops after a person has already developed communication skills, as might happen after a stroke or head injury

Speech—the act of producing a message that can be heard by others; includes *articulation,* the production of speech sounds such as consonants or vowels; *voice,* the production of the tone with which one speaks; and *fluency,* how well speech flows

Language—a shared set of rules and vocabulary that allows people within a culture to communicate with each other

Dysphagia—difficulty swallowing; can be a problem anywhere in the act of swallowing from getting food into the mouth, to chewing it well enough to be swallowed, to actually swallowing it

Certificate of Clinical Competence—the nationally recognized credential for speech-language pathologists, awarded by the American Speech-Language-Hearing Association following completion of a master's degree and other requirements

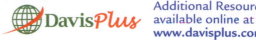

Additional Resources are available online at
www.davisplus.com

Additional Resources

American Speech-Language-Hearing Association (ASHA)—www.asha.org

- Provides the Certificate of Clinical Competence for qualified SLPs
- Produces professional journals
- Supplies information for the public about communication disorders
- Has resources for students interested in the field
- Provides and certifies continuing education

National Student Speech-Language-Hearing Association (NSSLHA)—www.asha.org/students

- Student branch of ASHA
- Chapters on most campuses where speech-language pathology programs exist
- Provides educational information and experiences
- Allows access to ASHA materials

State Speech-Language-Hearing Associations

- All states and the District of Columbia have an association that is affiliated with ASHA
- Provide continuing education and professional advocacy in that state
- Named [*state name*] Speech-Language-Hearing Association

State Licensing Agency

- Most states require that SLPs be licensed
- Search "speech-language pathology" or "professional licenses" on the state government website to locate the administering agency

State Education Agency

- Most states require that school-based SLPs have teacher certification from that state
- Search "department of education" or "teacher certification" on the state government website to locate appropriate information

References

1. American Speech-Language-Hearing Association. Communication for a Lifetime.
   http://www.asha.org/public.
   Accessed September 4, 2015.

2. The International Phonetic Association. Full IPA Chart.

   https://www.internationalphoneticassociation.org/content/full-ipa-chart.

   Accessed September 4, 2015.

3. American Speech-Language-Hearing Association. Welcome to ASHA's literacy gateway.

   http://www.asha.org/publications/literacy.

   Accessed September 4, 2015.

4. American Speech-Language-Hearing Association. Augmentative and alternative communication.

   http://www.asha.org/slp/clinical/aac.

   Accessed September 4, 2015.

5. American Speech-Language-Hearing Association. Academic program accreditation.

   http://www.asha.org/academic/accreditation.

   Accessed September 4, 2015.

6. American Speech-Language-Hearing Association. CAA accredited program listing.

   http://www.asha.org/uploadedFiles/CAAAccredited Programs.pdf.

   Accessed September 4, 2015.

7. American Speech-Language-Hearing Association. Schools survey report: SLP annual salary and hourly wage trends 2004–2014.

   http://www.asha.org/uploadedFiles/2014-Schools-Survey-SLP-Salary-Trends.pdf.

   Accessed September 4, 2015.

8. American Speech-Language-Hearing Association. SLP healthcare survey, 2013.

   http://www.asha.org/uploadedFiles/2013-SLP-Health-Care-Survey-Annual-Salaries.pdf.

   Accessed September 4, 2015.

9. American Speech-Language-Hearing Association. Highlights and trends: Member and affiliate counts, year-end 2012.

   http://www.asha.org/uploadedFiles/2012-Member-Counts-Final.pdf.

   Accessed September 4, 2015.

The Professional Work Environment

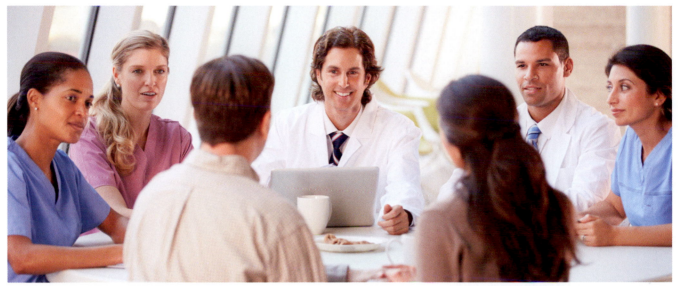

Photo credit: monkeybusinessimages/istock images/Thinkstock

Chapter 30
Professionalism and Ethics in Health Care

Chapter 31
Professionals Working Together

Professionalism and Ethics in Health Care

Patricia Royal, EdD

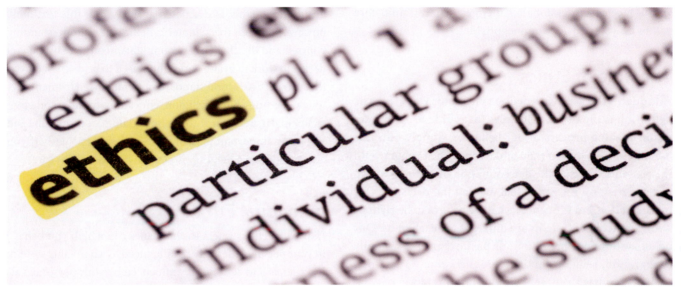

Photo credit: istock/Thinkstock

Learning Objectives

After reading this chapter, students should be able to:

- Discuss the professional and ethical issues related to a profession in health care
- Discuss personal and professional values that might affect their potential career in health care
- List ethical issues that might be encountered in health care
- Identify legal ramifications regarding professional choices while working in health care

Key Terms

- Ethical
- Values
- Ethics
- Discretion
- Reputation
- Morals
- Emotional stability
- Empathy
- Values conflict

Introduction to Professionalism and Ethics in Health Care

This chapter introduces some of the **ethical,** legal, and **values**-related issues that arise in the health-care professions. If you are seriously interested in becoming a health-care professional, you need to be aware of some of the challenges that you may face both personally and professionally. Health-care professionals, like anyone else, are people with their own personalities, values, and ethics.

However, unlike many other professions, health care has a specific set or code of ethics that may directly influence the health, safety, well-being, and care of patients. These codes specify ethical and moral behaviors and can be traced back to the beginning of medicine as a science. The Hippocratic Oath specifically identifies a professional code to which all physicians must adhere: do no harm. Although this professional code may seem simplistic and easy to abide by, one has to determine what "harm" means, and determine what is in the best interest of the patient. These codes are based on professional ethics, but personal ethics occasionally clash with professional codes because of one's differences in values and ethics. It is important not only to recognize when and why these clashes occur but also to understand how to resolve these challenges. Knowing yourself, your habits, your core values, and your personality traits is an important part of evaluating your preference when determining a career in the health professions. If it is in the best interest of the patient, can you put your personal preferences aside to provide nonjudgmental care? In the face of professional challenges, what, if any, core values do you consider nonnegotiable?

The Role of Ethics

Although **ethics** can be defined in many ways, a basic definition is the moral principles that guide us in our decision-making process or our behavior. Simply put, it is the difference between right and wrong. The problem with this statement is that the determination of right or wrong is dependent on the individual making the decision. Our own belief system influences what we believe to be right or wrong, and belief systems are different for each of us. Our belief systems are based on our past experiences, family background, religious affiliations, and values. Therefore, each person has a different view or interpretation of what is right or wrong, and these views often clash, especially within teams.[1,2]

Ethics in health care is not based on an individual view but rather on the core principles involved in health care. Health-care professionals can no longer view ethics from personal values or morals but instead must consider what is in the best interest of the patient. There are four central principles of ethics in health care: autonomy, beneficence, nonmaleficence, and justice.[3]

- *Autonomy* represents the patient's right to make his or her own decisions. An example of autonomy would be allowing the patient to make a decision on beginning dialysis treatments.
- *Beneficence* means to do good. An example of beneficence would be providing medicines or other treatment to someone who is in obvious pain.
- *Nonmaleficence* means to do no harm. An example of nonmaleficence would be withholding treatment or medicines that have not been deemed safe.
- *Justice* indicates fair treatment for all. An example of justice would be allowing all patients the same opportunity for resources (e.g., the flu vaccine).

Other guiding principles in delivering ethical health care consist of four standards of treatment: veracity, privacy, confidentiality, and fidelity.[3]

- *Veracity* means to always be honest and tell the patient the truth.
- *Privacy* refers to the patient's right to remain private.
- *Confidentiality* refers to only sharing patient information on a need-to-know basis with others.
- *Fidelity* indicates loyalty and duty to care for the patient.

Ethics, as an important element in interprofessional health-care teams, is discussed at the end of this textbook; however, because this chapter is dedicated to understanding yourself and the challenges you might encounter should you decide to work in health care, ethics need to be discussed from that perspective. Moral standards are influenced by many factors, including family, religion, education, friends, and environmental issues. Ethics are an important part of your life and will be an important part of your career, particularly if you are considering a helping profession such as health care.

Individual Ethics

Individual ethics refers to the manner in which you behave in your personal life and are influenced by your value system. Your goals and actions are influenced by your personal values and moral reasoning and your belief about obligations.[1] Lawrence Kohlberg identified six stages of moral development, which he associates with personal obligations and the moral perspectives of the individual. These stages change throughout life as we mature and grow as individuals. Our focus becomes less on self and more about others and societal concerns. The stages of moral development are the preconventional, conventional, and postconventional levels.[1]

- *Preconventional level*—at this level, behavior is guided by self-interest and individual perspectives. Decisions are made on what is best for the individual regardless of the effect on others or society. There are two stages within the preconventional level: (1) obedience and punishment and (2) instrumental purpose and exchange. Both of these stages reflect an individualistic nature without regard for others. An example of the preconventional level is a child who eats all of his vegetables so he can have dessert. The child is operating in the best interest of self because of his desire for ice cream, not because of the benefits of the vegetables.
- *Conventional level*—at this level, behavior is based on the need to conform to other individuals or society. Decisions are made on the expectations of meeting

obligations imposed by societal laws rather than personal self-interest. There are two stages within the conventional level: (1) conformity to group norms and (2) societal accord. An example of the conventional level is an individual who always obeys the traffic rules. In this case, the individual is following the rules because they are there, rather than the punishment that might be associated with disobeying the traffic rules—a traffic ticket. Additionally, this individual views the rules being in accordance with societal interest.

- *Postconventional level*—at this level, behavior is based on personal values and ideology. The internal belief system guides the behavior; fundamentally, the belief is based on the "it is the right thing to do" philosophy. There are two stages within the postconventional level: (1) social contract and consensus and (2) the greater good for all. An example of the postconventional level is an individual who recycles based on the philosophy of protecting resources for the next generation. This individual views societal needs above self-interest. Individuals who reach this stage of development seek out ways to solve problems and focus on others while reasoning that the benefits will be reaped by all. Unfortunately, less than one fourth of individuals function at this level; the majority of people are in the conventional level.

Professional Ethics

Professional ethics refer to the way individuals behave in the work environment. Although it is important to be ethical in all jobs, it is critically important in health-care settings because your behavior may affect someone's life.[4,5] Patients may be frightened, very ill, confused about treatments, or unsure about their diagnosis. They need health-care professionals who represent the facility in a positive light and have strong work ethics. They need individuals who take their work seriously and follow through with patient needs. Additionally, patients need health-care professionals who are professional and ethical. Many factors represent professional ethics, including attendance, reliability, attitude, competence, appropriate attire and language, and discretion.

Attendance

Attendance refers to the commitment made by the employee to be present for work unless extenuating circumstances dictate otherwise. If you are constantly absent for work, others have to fill in for you, and sooner or later your reputation will suffer. Health-care organizations often work with a lean staff, so absenteeism greatly inhibits the work schedule. It is expected that individuals will be absent from work occasionally, for sick days, vacation days, and other legitimate reasons, but those who are regularly absent or tardy may be viewed as people who do not value their job or the patients. Attendance refers to not only being physically present at the work setting, but also being engaged in the work. Therefore, one should always strive for attendance and punctuality and always be engaged as a health-care professional.

Reliability

Reliability refers to consistency of following through with tasks.[4,5] Others may depend on you to complete a task before they can move to the next phrase. Reliable individuals always complete their assigned tasks or job duties in a timely manner. Reliability also implies that the individual is confident and can be trusted to do a job well. If jobs are left undone or not completed in a timely manner, it is possible that patient care is compromised. A patient may be waiting on a referral to a specialist and if the referral is not completed or is late, the patient's health could be jeopardized. Because health care is dependent on so many timely processes, individuals who choose a career in health care should be aware of the importance of reliability and accountability in delivering quality care.

Attitude

Attitude refers to the manner in which an individual approaches work or life. Attitudes can be positive or negative, but more important, they can be infectious. People with negative attitudes can sometimes influence others to share in their negativity, thus lowering the morale of a group. On the other hand, a positive attitude can reinforce morale, teamwork, and enthusiasm. You can decide whether you want to be a pessimist or an optimist.

Being an optimist does not mean that you never feel bad or have bad days, but rather that your overall attitude toward life is positive and the influence you have on others is generally a positive encounter. Optimistic people usually smile more and are more pleasant to work with, which enhances the work environment. Patients, who may already feel bad, would probably rather deal with an optimistic health-care professional than a pessimistic one. People working in health-care environments need to be positive, especially when engaging with patients.

Competence

Competence refers to the skills, knowledge, education, and experience one needs to work in a specific field or discipline.[4] These assets are needed for individuals to be effective health-care professionals. If individuals are not competent in those areas, the task at hand or the job itself may suffer, possibly affecting patient care. Health-care professionals recognize the importance of maintaining the required education, license, certification, or other types of competency-based education or skills. Individuals adequately trained in the required areas will be confident in their decision-making skills, thereby increasing quality patient care.

Appropriate Attire

Dressing appropriately in the work environment is often determined by your role in health care. Your attire will be tied to your role, but all employees need to be cognizant of the image they may be projecting. To portray a professional status, professional dress attire should be worn at all times when in the work environment. Professional dress also includes areas other than clothing, such as hair and nails. Hair and nails, especially in health-care environments, should be clean and groomed. When people enter a health-care facility, often the first person seen is a receptionist or administrative assistant. This first image may create a lasting image, and may either reflect positively or negatively when considering return appointments or referrals to others. Professional attire typically includes slacks, shirts, and ties for men, and slacks, skirts, and dresses for women. For those working in surgery or laboratories, clean, neat scrubs, laboratory coats, or uniforms are appropriate. Many organizations have a dress code informing the employee of acceptable attire; however, a true professional is prepared to dress appropriately regardless of the policy.

Appropriate Language

When talking with your friends, you may find yourself using slang or jargon that seems appropriate for your age or group of friends; however, this type of language is not acceptable in the work environment. Professionals should never use demeaning, disrespectable, or offensive language regardless of the situation. When you decide to work in health care, you must take into account the patient populations, the work environment, and the work atmosphere and be aware that patients and their families deserve to be treated with respect and may be offended by "after hours" language. Even something as innocent as using someone's first name without permission might be disrespectful to some individuals. Therefore, it is best to err on the side of caution and always practice respectful language. It is also good to practice appropriate language away from work because practice becomes routine and you are less likely to say something inappropriate.

Discretion

Discretion refers to diplomacy, privacy, and the use of good judgment when working in all settings, but particularly in health-care environments.[4] Not only is discretion mandated under the Health Information Portability and Accountability Act (HIPAA) rules, but it is also expected for all professionals working in health care. HIPAA was established to protect patient information while transferring data to and from databases. Additionally, this law also requires written consent before a health-care provider delivers any type of examination or treatment on patients, except in emergency situations. Violation of HIPAA laws may result in civil and criminal penalties. Aside from the legalities of HIPAA, all professionals are expected to be discrete in discussing patient issues and are not allowed to discuss any patient with others without signed consent forms. Additionally, the discussion of patients outside of the office environment is prohibited due to the possibility of someone overhearing the comments.

Social Media

An area of concern in today's society is that of social media. Due to technology, we are able to connect with individuals around the world, which has created a smaller world for us. Usually technology brings us closer together and we are able to learn from this advanced equipment; however, there is another side that may be problematic. We are able to see what others are doing, and they can see what we are doing. Therefore, although it might seem like a good idea to post your photos of the weekend for all your friends to see, you must realize that other people will see them as well. Being a professional means you must be aware of your social devices and where your pictures might show up. Employers may use social media such as Facebook when hiring for a professional position. They want to know as much about the potential employee as possible, and social media is one way for them to find out. What may seem like an innocent post could possibly cost you a job. Therefore, always think about anything that can be misconstrued and who will actually end up seeing the information. If there is ever a doubt about something you might post, do *not* post it.

Ethical Issues

All work environments deal with ethical issues, but no work environment is more diverse or morally divided than health care. Therefore, before engaging on a career as a health-care professional, you may want to think about the ethical issues you might encounter and self-assess to determine which, if any, may cause you turmoil or uneasiness. Many ethical issues arise in health care. Possible questions/concerns follow. As you read each one, reflect on your feelings and ethics.

- Is it possible for me to remain neutral in this situation?
- Would I have trouble working with this population or condition?
- Is my value system creating internal chaos in this issue?
- Could I treat/counsel the patient without judging him or her?
- Would I be able to refer this individual without feeling like I failed?
- Would I be able to handle this situation without seeking consultation?

Potential ethical issues/concerns in health care include the following:

- Abortion—refers to the termination of pregnancy for either medical or personal reasons. Many U.S. states allow abortions but impose restrictions such as waiting periods, required counseling, required ultrasound, physician or hospital only performed, or parental signatures. Other states do not allow abortions except for certain exemptions such as rape or incest, or danger to the woman's health.[6]

- End-of-life decisions—refers to living wills and how individuals decide to live their last days, weeks, or months. Individuals may request that all heroic measures be administered, such as breathing tubes, cardiopulmonary resuscitation (CPR), and tube-feeding, to prolong life; or individuals may elect to receive no treatments regardless of the situation. An alternative is to choose a single option, such as CPR but nothing else. End-of-life decisions are preferably made by the patient while still possessing full awareness. Individuals also have the option of allowing someone else to make the decision for them based on the conditions at that time. Individuals can appoint a family member as health-care power of attorney that will allow future decisions to be made as needed.

- Euthanasia—refers to the administration of a lethal dose of medicine to a terminally ill patient. This medication, used to ease pain, is administered by a physician or another third party and is illegal in all U.S. states. However, there are continued debates in this area and the legal status may change before long, largely because Americans seeking euthanasia travel to other countries where it is permissible, such as The Netherlands. Should U.S. laws be changed to accommodate those individuals who choose to die?

- Physician-assisted suicide (PAS)—refers to the administration of a lethal dose of medicine by the patient under the advice or direction of a physician. The qualifications for the use of the medicines require the patient to be terminally ill. Only a few U.S. states allow PAS, but a number of states have considered making it legal.

- Human immunodeficiency virus/acquired immunodeficiency syndrome (HIV/AIDS)—refers to individuals who are HIV positive or are AIDS symptomatic. The ethical issue for some individuals is not the disease itself but the contraction method, which may be through sexual activity or drug use. Once considered a stigma, the perception of an HIV/AIDS infection has changed over time, but for many, the disease represents a way of life that is inconsistent with some individuals' values.

- In vitro fertilization—refers to a method of fertilization in which sperm fertilizes eggs outside of the woman's body (in vitro), generally in a test tube. Although the first test-tube baby was born in 1978, some schools of thought have continued to view this event as unnatural. Those among that population believe that all women are not meant to be mothers and when medicine intervenes to "right this inequality," it is not a natural choice.[6]

- Surrogate pregnancies—refers to pregnancies that occur outside of the natural mother's body. The surrogate may be a family member, a friend, or a paid individual who allows the egg and sperm from the parents to be implanted in her body. This other woman carries and delivers the baby for the birth parents, but otherwise has no claim or maternal relationship to the baby. Some of the ethical issues in this situation are the same as with in vitro fertilization, but some are also concerned that some surrogates are paid. Paying women to have babies elicits the idea that babies can be bought and sold, which is illegal. There is also the ethical argument of a weakening of the family system because the significance of shared love through conception is not a part of the birth.[6] Conversely, some consider surrogates as providing a valuable service to families who are unable to have children independently.

- Organ transplantation—refers to the removal of a damaged or improperly functioning organ and replacing it with a healthy donor organ. Typical organ transplants involve kidneys, livers, and hearts, but other organs such as pancreas and lungs are also transplanted. Depending on the type of organ transplanted, the donor may be living or deceased. Sometimes living family members are able to donate to their loved one, but if not, the sick individual typically is placed on a waiting list until a matching donor is found. Considerations of acceptance for the donor list are based on age, comorbidity, medication compliance, and severity of the condition. Comorbidity refers to the patient having more than one health concern, such as being a diabetic and hypertensive; medication compliance occurs when the patient takes all medications as indicated on a regular and routine basis. The ethical concerns here are about fair distribution. Someone receives and someone does not. Who gets to make the decision? Should the decision be made by age of the recipient? Should the decision be based on the length of time the individual has waited? Or perhaps the decision should be based on the severity of the condition. In other words, how long will the individual survive without the organ? Many other ethical issues related to organ transplantation exist, and the debate is not likely to end any time soon.

- Care of prisoners—refers to the care prisoners receive while incarcerated. Prisoners have constitutional rights ensuring that all necessary medical treatments are provided. Treatment is not based on prison length of stay, the crime committed, or the cost involved in the services. Because payment for the services is provided through taxes paid by U.S. citizens, this creates an ethical dilemma for some. Some argue that when a person commits a crime he or she should not be rewarded with free health care, particularly when many law-abiding citizens cannot afford to pay for similar services. Some also argue that the resources used in prisoners' treatment are scarce and would be better used on individuals who contribute to society. All of these reasons, and perhaps others, constitute ethical concerns regarding the prison population and free health-care services.

- Genetic intervention—refers to the use of genetic engineering to alter or modify a defective gene. In many instances the positives of this technology would seem to outweigh any potential negatives. With genetic intervention, the possibility exists to eradicate certain genetic diseases because carriers of those diseases could opt not to pass on the genes through conception. On the flip side, some argue that genetic intervention may increase the selection process, such as having all males or specific hair and eye color.[6,7] Who should make these types of decisions? Scientists or potential parents? Other ethical issues concern the right of parents to know about the genetic testing and the possible results, and the obligations of physicians to inform the parents. If parents were told about specific conditions of an unborn child, would embryo selection become popular for those who can afford the testing? Regarding the resources, who should pay for genetic testing—society or individuals?

- Experimental drugs—refers to drugs that have not been approved by the U.S. Food and Drug Administration (FDA) for human use. The United States relies on the FDA to make the decision regarding safety and effectiveness. However, some other countries use experimental drugs to treat patients who have no other option.[6] When there is not an FDA-approved treatment, U.S. patients can make the decision to travel abroad to seek potential remedies. Who should ultimately get to make the decision on treatment if the patient is terminal and will likely die without treatment?

- Life support—refers to the use of a machine known as a ventilator that assists or replaces spontaneous breathing for a patient. Ventilators can be used for short periods of time, such as in surgery, or for much longer periods. Individuals who are typically placed on long-term ventilators are those who have suffered a serious condition such as a stroke or heart attack or were involved in an accident. Some of these individuals are independently comatose and others are induced in a comatose state for medical reasons, such as swelling on the brain. The short-term use of the ventilator rarely causes any ethical issues, but for those who are dependent on the machine for months or years, ethical issues arise. For individuals who have advance directives indicating their wishes, such as do-not-resuscitate orders, their decisions may be difficult for loved ones to accept but are legally binding. Those without advance directives present quite a different situation. Some of the concerns involve the age of the person, the physical condition before the coma, quality of life, family wishes, resources, chances of recovery, and many other ethical concerns. In many cases, families have been ripped apart when having to make a decision on whether to "pull the plug" on the ventilator and when. Who should be in the decision-making position—family or medical staff?

As you can see from the ethical issues discussed, many situations require individuals to look at the medical implications in addition to human values. Fortunately, in many instances there are clearly defined laws that help individuals face many ethical dilemmas. Other times, the patients themselves have completed instructions regarding their wishes, with which family members must abide. The worst ethical dilemmas are those where there are neither laws nor instructions to provide

Ethical dilemma

Read the case study at the end of the chapter and think about how you would address the problem.

guidance and the decision, if any, becomes a joint effort between the health-care professional and patient's family.

Legal/Ethical Issues

Ethical dilemmas can occur when individuals are faced with making a decision based on the best interest of self or others. In this scenario, we may look to the legal system to help alleviate the burden. It would seem logical that if something is legal it must be ethical, or if something is ethical it must be legal. Unfortunately, this perception is far from reality. There are times when ethics and legality go hand in hand; however, there are other times when they are total opposites. For example, a business owner may hire a less qualified family member for a job when someone else is a better candidate. This situation is not illegal, but many consider it unethical. Conversely, it is illegal to drive over the posted speed limit; however, many might not consider it unethical to speed in the case of emergency situations such as driving to the hospital. Legally, the individual is indeed speeding and deserves a traffic ticket; however, many people would disagree and say the circumstances surrounding the speeding make issuing a ticket unethical. Again, the reason that we may view these situations differently are based on our own perceptions, which create gray areas in decision-making.

Personal Traits

Health-care work is a challenging but rewarding career. One of the challenges is being involved in the decision-making that occurs daily. As a health professional you will be faced with decisions that could potentially affect someone's life. Many of these challenges are based on ethical and legal concerns. Before beginning the task of confronting ethical and legal issues in health care, one needs to examine personal traits that may affect the overall decision-making process. Our personal traits include those core characteristics that make up who we are. These characteristics are the attributes we use when viewing the world. Typically, these characteristics are stable and change very little over time. Of course, there are some exceptions to the rule, but you can pretty much expect your behavior to be based on these core personal characteristics, which, in turn, will affect your behavior in the workplace. Some of the personal characteristics include your reputation, morals, honesty, and respect.[3]

Reflection

Can you think of other scenarios where something may be legal but unethical, or vice versa?

Reputation

A person's **reputation** may affect the ability to not only obtain a job in health care but also to keep that job. Your reputation is the view of how others see you, whether positive or negative. When seeking a career in health care, your reputation may greatly affect your marketability. If you have a tarnished reputation, it might preclude you from obtaining employment in the health-care environment because those looking to hire may fear you having a negative impact on the company, or otherwise not fitting in with the environment. Companies, like individuals, have reputations at stake as well. With the growth of technology and the many public markets available, companies are now beginning to use social media as an avenue for employee selection. Therefore, professionals should work hard daily to uphold the reputation of the company along with their own personal reputation.

Morals

Morals are the ideas or beliefs about how to behave in ways that are considered right and virtuous by most people. A person's morals work much like a compass that leads one in a direction that person considers being right. Although morals differ from person to person, an individual has to make that determination alone. For example, we all would consider stealing as an immoral act; however, the nature of the act might change the minds of some individuals. If the thievery was based on hunger, some would still consider it immoral whereas others would not. Morals help the individual to determine right from wrong and to stay on a chosen track. Individuals without morals are generally not concerned with right and wrong and may lose sight of the best interest of the patient in favor of their own, potentially causing great harm and irreversible damage. Morals also greatly affect honesty and trustworthiness, important professional characteristics employers seek in their potential employees.

Honesty

As in other professions, dishonesty and deceit occur in health-care environments. Dishonesty in health care can be defined in much the same way as in any other business. Dishonesty includes lying, cheating, theft, deception, falsifying records, and taking credit for work not delivered. The cost of dishonesty can be measured through a direct cost approach and an indirect cost approach. Dishonesty results in legal fees, stolen equipment, lost revenue, and missing supplies—all direct costs for the employer. Having dishonest employees may jeopardize referrals for potential clients or patients, which in turn costs the company money. Indirect approaches such as unauthorized employee breaks or manipulating a time card or hours worked can add up to large amounts of money lost by the company.[3,4] Companies look to hire individuals who do not place the company at risk for an infraction. Health-care professionals should recognize the damage that can be done by dishonesty and strive to be proactive in the fight against it even if that means having to report a coworker for dishonest conduct. Although you may only be held accountable for your own actions, allowing someone else to be dishonest and not reporting it will eventually place you in an uncompromising position. Do not risk your reputation for someone else.

Respect

The ability to garner respect from supervisors, coworkers, and patients is one of the most important qualities for health-care professionals.[1] Respect is earned through consistencies. These consistencies include keeping promises, following through on obligations, and being a dependable employee, among others. If you plan to seek out a career in health care, be sure to gauge the level of respect others have for you. If lacking in this area, try to determine why so that you may do things differently in the future.

Professional Traits

Professional traits are the characteristics or qualities that influence your workplace behavior and can greatly affect your career. Individuals with excellent professional traits may enhance their likelihood of acquiring a job, receiving a promotion, or increasing their salaries. From the company viewpoint, employing professionals who exhibit the desired qualities may boost customer satisfaction, a positive reputation, and repeat business, which boosts company profits. Like personal traits, there are numerous professional traits that one can possess. Some of the more common professional traits include flexibility, emotional stability, empathy, communication skills, accountability, and problem-solving skills.[3,4]

Flexibility

Flexibility refers to being able to adapt to changing environments and disruptions in the workplace. Many fields and industries face change regularly; however, careers in the health-care environment seem to change daily. Advancements in technology, population and demographic shifts, government policy and intervention, and reimbursement changes are just a few of the reasons that health care is constantly changing.[3,4] Employees have to adapt to the changes or be left behind. Professionals who are flexible not only adapt but also embrace the changing environment. These individuals make a smoother transition and create positive energy for others.

Emotional Stability

Emotional stability refers to the manner in which a person behaves even in the face of adversity or potential threats of disruptions. Health care often involves emotionally charged situations. Health-care workers regularly work with illness, terminal conditions, and life-threatening situations.[3,4] These conditions not only affect the patients, but involve the family members as well. Often there may be accusations of neglect, discrimination, incompetence, or disparity from patients or family members. Recognizing that people may often use abusive language in the heat of emotion, emotionally stable professionals manage to remain calm and rational. These professionals understand the stress the patient or family members are facing and recognize that an overreaction on their part only serves to stimulate more aggression. Maintaining composure and rationality help to reduce added stress and enhance patient care by shifting the focus to the patient rather than the disruption.

Empathy

Empathy refers to the ability to relate to someone else's emotions or situation. Empathy, unlike sympathy, projects a feeling of understanding rather than pity for the individual.[4] Being able to empathize with others indicates a confirmation or acknowledgment of the condition while still offering inspiration to continue on rather than giving up. Professionals who are able to empathize with others recognize the pain, whether physical or emotional, that a patient may be coping with and can provide support. Empathetic individuals usually have better relationships with their patients and family members, which increases patient satisfaction.

Communication Skills

Communications skills refer to the ability to communicate effectively verbally, nonverbally, and in written form. In addition, effective communication entails the ability to actively listen with the body and mind. This type of listening is demonstrated by nodding the head appropriately and using eye contact while listening to the patient. Patients need to feel like their health-care professional is truly listening to their needs, beyond just hearing what is said. Sometimes, the nonverbal language may provide more information than what is actually spoken. If you plan to work in health care, you will need to develop effective communication skills to enhance patient care and satisfaction.

Accountability

Accountability refers to individuals taking responsibility for their actions. In all types of work environments, accountability is a vital attribute for employees to possess; however, health-care accountability is more than vital—it is required.[3,4] Accountability indicates that you have completed the activities or task as delegated for the best patient care. Being accountable can be as simple as making an appointment reminder phone call to a patient or as complex as using all possible resources to provide the patient with the ultimate care needed. Regardless of the importance or the complexity of the task, all professionals should be held accountable for their work. If one person fails to complete a task, a domino effect could ensue. Accountability is such an important aspect of health care that the government has intervened by requiring health-care providers to be accountable for patient care in designated populations such as a medically underserved population due to a shortage of providers. The primary-care physician is charged with improving patient outcomes such as fewer hospitalizations, compliance, and reduction in chronic illness by using preventive medicine. The enactment, which ties reimbursement to patient care outcomes, is part of the Health Care and Education Reconciliation Act of 2010 and strengthens the resolution that all professionals need to be accountable. The reason for this enactment by the federal government was based on health-care disparities, delivery systems, and lack of accountability for patient outcomes. Tying reimbursement to patient outcomes was one method of improving accountability.

In addition to accountability in patient care, health-care professionals should be accountable for their roles in health care and accept blame when problems arise. Rather than pointing the finger at others, it is more important to own up to the mistakes and work toward a solution for improvement.

Problem-Solving Skills

Problem-solving refers to the systematic approach to addressing or handling problems or issues. A person with good problem-solving skills recognizes the importance of critical-thinking skills as a requirement in solving problems. Employees who are skilled at solving problems typically are often also creative and divergent thinkers. Health-care professionals, who are frequently faced with problems or concerns, often solve them by thinking "outside the box," especially when resources are scarce. Good problem solvers use a step process that includes identifying the problem, defining the problem, gathering relevant information, developing possible solutions, and making a decision. Having employees with the ability to systematically solve problems is a winning combination for the employee and the organization.

Self-Assessment

Complete this self-assessment to determine your personal and professional approach.

1 = Never

2 = Sometimes

3 = Usually

4 = Always

1. I treat my coworkers/fellow students with respect.
2. I am willing to compromise for the benefit of the team/group.
3. I have an optimistic attitude.
4. I am reliable and my coworkers/fellow students can depend on me.
5. I use assertive communication but not aggressive.
6. I refrain from trying to embarrass or mock others.
7. I dress appropriately for work or school.
8. I use appropriate language at work or in a group environment.
9. I always give my best effort to my coworkers/fellow students when working together.
10. I am honest about my strengths and weaknesses and try to improve as needed.

Reflect on your answers to these questions. If you have all or mostly 3s and 4s, you are doing a great job and should continue on this path. If you have some 1s or 2s, look at the particular statement and determine what you can do differently to improve your results.

Values and Value Conflicts

Values

Although the last chapter in this textbook discusses ethics and values in the health-care environment, this section introduces the concepts to generate thought about how your current value system may fit in a health-care career.[3] This section will help you to recognize the importance of values and how well suited you are for a helping profession. Remember that your values may not always be similar to your patients' or clients' values. Actually, in many cases, there will be differences between your values and other health-care professionals. The key to working as a health-care professional is capably handling these differences so that the impact you have on patients is positive.[3] Will you be able to empathize with patients and understand their plight (situation, position, or condition)? Or do you automatically impose your values without personal regard for someone else?

Values refer to your moral principles or standards and the way you view life or work. Values are influenced by community, family, school, and friends. Our behavior is typically affected by our personal values, which can include both the tangible and the intangible. Tangible values refer to concrete items that you can see, such as a car, a house, or your job title. These types of values are materialistic in nature and will differ from person to person.[1] One person may place more value on having a large, expensive home; someone else may value the type of car driven.

Intangible values refer to concepts rather than concrete items. These values include love, happiness, independence, and freedom. Some individuals value independence and prefer to live and work alone, as opposed to individuals who would rather work and live with others.

Values Conflict

Values conflict occurs when there is a reaction based on individual difference in values.[1] An example might involve an individual who condones occasional recreational drug use who works with someone who is totally opposed to the idea. Both individuals have their own values, and because their values are conflicting, problems may ensue. Depending on the nature of the conflict, some people may decide it is better to ignore the situation. However, when working in health care, particularly with patients, ignoring the individuals with whom you clash is not an option because you are obligated to provide the best possible care at all times. When a patient and a health-care professional clash, it may create tension and feelings of distrust within the patient. It is important, then, as a professional that you do not further jeopardize the relationship by forcing your own agenda.[1] Remember that in this situation, the concern should be for the patient, not you. However, you do not have to forsake your own values. You can still be honest with the patient without force or coercion. If you feel the clash in values is too much for you to resolve, it is in the best interest of the patient that you make a referral to another health-care professional. An example of a clash may occur when a patient asks for pain medicine refills too frequently. The provider may be uncomfortable with this situation due to suspicion of misuse. In this scenario, the better option for both the patient and provider would be a referral.

SUMMARY

Working in health care can be the most rewarding experience you could imagine. However, there are many issues that may provoke some soul searching and level-headed thinking. Being a health-care professional means you accept these challenges and opportunities and always address them professionally. If you have solid personal and professional qualities and clear values and ethics, you will have a foundation that ensures first-class health-care service to your patients. This does not mean you will not stumble and fall occasionally; it just means you will be able to stand up and walk again.

CASE STUDY: AN ETHICAL DILEMMA

You are a marriage counselor and have been working with couples for about 10 years. You have a successful business and have earned a good reputation for your client confidentiality and respect. You have prided yourself on never letting your values interfere in the counseling process. Recently, you accepted a referral from another counselor who was unable to take on any new clients. Before accepting the referral, you were provided information about the married couple and learned they were a same-sex couple. Although this was your first same-sex couple, you automatically accepted the referral and made an initial appointment so you and the couple could meet to discuss the counseling process. Your appointment was today at 2:00 p.m. at which time you met the couple and discussed therapies, time commitments, and expected progress. You found the couple to be pleasant, but you felt some reservations about counseling them. Although you have always been respectful of individual differences, your religious beliefs and background begin to color your thinking. You were raised to believe that only a man and a woman should become a married couple, and now you are unsure about what decision to take with this couple as clients. You like to think that you are nonjudgmental and are a libertarian regarding modern acceptance of differences, but already you feel somewhat disloyal to your values. What should you do? Should you openly discuss your values with the clients and hope that you can work through the issues?

Questions

1. Should you not say anything and see if you are able to put your feelings aside?

2. Should you tell them that you have a full load and will be unable to provide them with the needed sessions? (You know this is not true, but you do not want to offend them.)

3. Should you refer them to another therapist?

Review Questions

1. An individual's _____ works like a compass and points them in the right direction.
   - A. Thoughts
   - B. Morals
   - C. Character
   - D. Personal qualities

2. _____ is based on how others see you.
   - A. Professionalism
   - B. Ethics
   - C. Attitude
   - D. Reputation

3. If a person behaves irrationally, he or she is emotionally stable.
   - A. True
   - B. False

4. Empathy and sympathy are basically the same things.
   - A. True
   - B. False

5. What constitute an individual's moral standards or principles?
   - A. Values
   - B. Ethics
   - C. Trust
   - D. Reliability

6. Another term for taking responsibility is:
   - A. Independent
   - B. Honesty
   - C. Stability
   - D. Accountability

7. According to Kohlberg, the _____ moral level of development refers to self-interest and rewards.
   - A. Postconventional
   - B. Preconventional
   - C. Conventional
   - D. All of the above

8. _____ refers to using diplomacy and good judgment.
   - A. Discretion
   - B. Privacy
   - C. Values
   - D. Morals

9. Attitudes can be positive or negative.
   - A. True
   - B. False

10. A reliable person is always _____.
    - A. Trustworthy
    - B. Emotionally stable
    - C. Consistent
    - D. Ethical

Glossary of Key Terms

Ethical—refers to situations or scenarios that address moral principles or standards

Values—refers to concepts or beliefs influenced by family, friends, or experiences that guide our decision-making

Ethics—refers to standards or principles that guide our behavior

Discretion—refers to diplomacy and the use of good judgment, particularly when dealing with private and personal issues

Reputation—the view or perspective that others have about us

Morals—refers to standards that guide us in the right direction

Emotional stability—refers to the manner in which an individual may behave rationally when faced with adversity

Empathy—refers to the ability to place ourselves in someone else's situation

Values conflict—refers to the internal conflict that occurs when our value system is compromised or threatened

Davis*Plus*   Additional Resources are available online at www.davisplus.com

References

1. de Janasz S, Dowd K, Schnedier B. *Interpersonal Skills in Organizations*, 4th ed. New York, NY: McGraw-Hill; 2012.

2. Robbins S, Hunsaker P. *Training in Interpersonal Skills,* 4th ed. Upper Saddle River, NJ: Pearson Prentice Hall; 2006.

3. Longest B, Darr K. *Managing Health Services Organizations and Systems,* 6th ed. Baltimore, MD: Health Professions Press; 2014.

4. Makely S. *Professionalism in Health Care: A Primer for Career Success,* 2nd ed. Upper Saddle River, NJ: Pearson-Prentice Hall; 2005.

5. Corey G, Corey M, Patrick M. *Issues and Ethics in the Helping Professions,* 4th ed. Pacific Cove, CA: Brooks/Cole Publishing; 1993.

6. Munson R. *Intervention and Reflection: Basic Issues in Medical Ethics,* 8th ed. Belmont, CA: Thomson Higher Education; 2008.

7. Bolin R. Genetic intervention: the ethical challenges ahead. Center for Bioethics and Human Dignity, Trinity International University. https://cbhd.org/content/genetic-intervention-ethical-challenges-ahead. Accessed December 15, 2014.

CHAPTER 31

Professionals Working Together

Patricia Royal, EdD

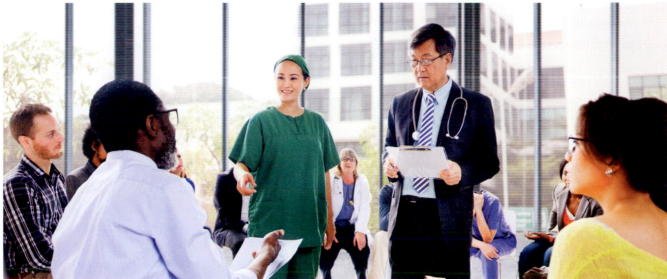

Learning Objectives

After reading this chapter, students should be able to:

- Discuss the importance of health-care teams
- Define the characteristics of good teams
- Explain the importance of interpersonal skills
- Discuss the ramifications of team obstacles
- Define ethics and the importance of it in health-care teams

Key Terms

- Nonverbal communication
- Accommodation
- Avoiding
- Collaborating
- Compromising
- Competing
- Transformational leaders
- Transactional leaders
- Organizational ethics
- Ethical dilemma

Introduction

Throughout this text, the concept of interprofessional approaches to health care has been discussed on various levels. The importance of interprofessional care has been addressed through many disciplines, and the recognition of working in health-care teams has been established within each profession. This last chapter examines the characteristics of high-performing teams, discusses the interpersonal skills needed for working in interprofessional health-care teams, and examines the barriers that may be encountered as a successful team player. The last part of the chapter focuses on ethics and ethical decision-making.

Characteristics of a High-Performing Health-Care Team

High-performing teams meet goals in a timely manner by making the most effective and efficient use of resources.

There are many aspects to examine when determining characteristics of a high-performing health-care team. Some of these characteristics include the following[1-3]:

- Team structure
- Purpose and goal
- Psychological, personal, and professional characteristics of the team members
- Communication
- Accountability
- High-level interpersonal skills

Team Structure

Team structure involves aspects related to the organization of the team. Some things that should be taken into account when considering the health-care team structure include size, team leadership, and experience of the team.

The size of the health-care team can help or hinder overall progress. Although interprofessional teams can consist of many disciplines as determined by the nature of the patient's illness, there may be instances where the number of participants should be minimized to ensure higher performance. On the other hand, a team that is too

---

Case Application: Team 1, Trauma Center

Kennedy Memorial Hospital is a midsize public facility operating as the only hospital in the county of Johnsonville. The hospital has a trauma center, a women's and children's hospital, and a cancer center. Each of the different divisions has its own interprofessional team that works to ensure quality care.

Team: physician, surgeon, surgical technician, nurse, radiographer, social worker, occupational therapist, physical therapist, and dietitian. Not all team members are needed for every patient, but each team member remains a part of the team.

Jonathan is a 39-year-old man who was involved in a motor vehicle accident. He is transported by emergency medical services (EMS) to the hospital with life-threatening injuries. EMS stabilizes him as much as possible, but the injuries are critical and he is rushed to the trauma center. On arrival, the radiographer completes a brain scan, which indicates swelling on the brain. This is an urgent concern and requires immediate surgery. The trauma team (surgeon, surgical technician, and nurse) work together to begin the first surgery. In addition to the brain injury, Jonathan's left arm has severe lacerations with tendon and ligament involvement requiring additional surgeries when appropriate. After the lifesaving brain surgery has successfully been completed, the physician calls the team together for the care plan meeting. He explains that although Jonathan is expected to recover, there are still many hurdles that will challenge him. Together the team begins to discuss the next steps for Jonathan. Each member of the team discusses recommendations based on his or her specific discipline. The interprofessional plan of care for Jonathan includes the following:

- Surgeon—repair torn tendons and ligaments as soon as possible
- Radiographer—complete another series of x-rays to ensure the brain has completed recovered

- Nurse—monitor Jonathan's vital signs, manage pain, administer medications, and update team as needed
- Physical therapy—work with Jonathan to increase his arm range of motion and mobility
- Occupational therapy—assess Jonathan for temporary adaptive appliance for employment purposes and activities of daily living
- Social worker—discuss employment concerns and financial issues and provide supportive counseling
- Dietitian—assess Jonathan for nutritional needs to ensure optimal healing

Discussion questions:

1. What is the benefit of having diverse team members to provide Jonathan's care?

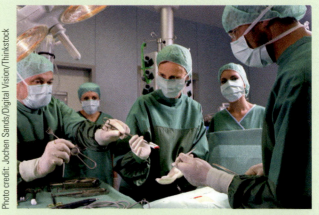

Photo credit: Jochen Sands/Digital Vision/Thinkstock

Performing surgery requires a team of professionals working together to achieve a successful outcome. Because teams are interdependent, they rely on each member and are held accountable as both individuals and a team.

2. Are you able to determine the leader of the interprofessional team? Why is this person the leader?

3. Provide justification for the team meeting. How does it affect quality care?

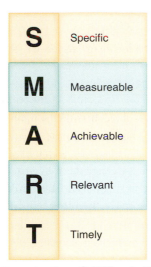

S	Specific
M	Measureable
A	Achievable
R	Relevant
T	Timely

FIGURE 31-1 Effective goal setting—SMART goals. High-performing teams are effective in setting and achieving goals. Goal setting should include specific, measurable, attainable, realistic, and timely (SMART) goals. If all of these components are accounted for, the team is more likely to be successful.

small may not provide enough input to enhance quality care. The team should be large enough to achieve the best results but small enough to be able to reach a consensus on decisions. Team size should generally be between 6 and 10 participants; however, other factors might affect the optimal size, such as patient condition and availability of team members.[1]

One of the advantages to creating interprofessional health-care teams is shared leadership that produces a holistic approach; however, this does not mean that there are no leaders within the team. Leadership on an interprofessional team is an important element of the team and should be addressed early in the team formation. Typically, the primary-care provider serves as the team leader, but there may be times when a professional of a different discipline may serve as leader. The lead role is one of great responsibility to both the patient and the team.

Team members may change depending on the needs of the patient. As a patient's condition changes, some disciplines may be needed more whereas others are needed less or not at all. This is typical in health-care teams because the patient's needs change with time and progression of the disease or condition. Conversely, some health-care teams remain the same, such as those assigned to the overall quality enhancement programs at health-care facilities. These teams do not necessarily handle direct patient care, but rather the overall protocols surrounding specific treatments and procedures. These types of teams generally remain intact, with some variability as employee turnover and retention occurs, or as designated at the beginning of the developmental stage.

Purpose and Goal

The purpose and goal of the health-care team should be clearly defined to ensure that members fully understand their roles and responsibilities.[4,5] When determining purpose and goals, attributes such as specific and measurable objectives need to be considered. For example, in patient care the overall purpose may be to improve patients' health; however, without some type of specific measure, it may be difficult to determine improvement. Therefore, using an objective (e.g., 80% of hypertensive patients will see a reduction of 10 points for systolic blood pressure over the next 6 months) provides both a specific goal and a measure to determine success. The goals and objectives are determined by using a realistic perspective that the patient can achieve by following specific orders prescribed by the medical provider.

Psychological, Personal, and Professional Characteristics of the Members

Health-care teams are made up of individual members of differing characteristics and various disciplines. Even individuals who work in the same discipline may not have characteristics in common other than a shared knowledge of the specific field. Therefore, it is important to recognize the team's diversity and seek ways to appreciate that diversity.

Psychological Characteristics

Psychological characteristics include traits such as personality, motivation, self-awareness, and attitude. These traits are relatively stable and do not change much over time.[1,3] Therefore, it would not be reasonable to expect individual team members to dramatically change these aspects of themselves, so learning to work with all types of personalities is the appropriate action to building successful teams.

Personal Characteristics

Personal characteristics include attributes such as gender, age, race, and disabilities. Most of these characteristics are not situational, meaning they will usually not change. These characteristics shape the individual and contribute to the success of the team by providing diversity, which helps to ensure creativity needed for problem-solving and decision-making.[3]

Case Application: Team 2, Women's Center

Team: physicians (obstetrics and pediatric), nurse, dietitian, social worker, health educator, and pharmacist. Not all team members are needed for every patient, but all remain part of the team.

Rhonda is a 43-year-old pregnant woman in active labor who has been admitted to the women's center. Rhonda is 28 weeks pregnant and the baby is in fetal distress. Because of Rhonda's age and condition of uncontrolled hypertension, her pregnancy was classified as *at-risk*. Additionally, Rhonda has miscarried three other times; however, each of those pregnancies terminated within 2 months of conception. Believing this might be their last opportunity to have a child, Rhonda and her husband have been ecstatic about this pregnancy. Thus, despite her medical history and her doctor's warning, they decided not to terminate the pregnancy. Rhonda has been bedridden for the past month because of extreme edema (swelling) in her feet and legs and rapid weight gain. She was also diagnosed with preeclampsia at her last visit to the doctor. (Eclampsia is a serious, potentially fatal condition that may cause seizures.) On admittance to the women's center, the doctor tells Rhonda that her condition is deteriorating and that the baby must be delivered immediately. The main objective at this point is to deliver the baby safely and then reassess Rhonda's vital signs. The surgeon completes a cesarean section (C-section) immediately. The baby girl is taken to the neonatal intensive care unit (NICU) for assessment while Rhonda is monitored. The next day, the interprofessional team meets to discuss the plan of care for both mother and baby.

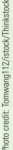

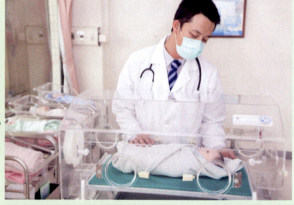

Rhonda's baby will be placed in a neonatal unit such as the one shown. The medical staff will monitor the baby for any sign of distress.

Each member of the team discusses recommendations based on his or her specific discipline. The interprofessional plan of care includes the following:

- Obstetrician—explain the purpose of the emergency C-section and provide updates on the mother's progress.

- Nurse—monitor the patient's vital signs, manage pain, administer medications, possibly remove Foley catheter next day (depending on patient's improvement), remove intravenous line next day, have patient sit up on side of bed as able, and update team as needed.

- Health educator—Rhonda is unable to breastfeed at this time due to her own health condition, but the health educator will meet with her and discuss the importance of breastfeeding (especially for a premature baby), offer support and instructions on breastfeeding, and provide information about formula if Rhonda decides to bottle-feed. The health educator will discuss car-seat safety with both parents and ensure the availability of a seat when baby is discharged.

- Dietitian—meet with mother and discuss diet for breastfeeding moms, provide information on low-salt diet for hypertension, and discuss nutritional needs for new mothers.

- Pharmacist—visit mother and confirm maintenance medications and discuss new medications prescribed since birth of baby.

- Pediatrician—assess and monitor baby's needs, meet with mom to discuss progress and special instructions as needed.

- Neonatal nurse—monitor baby's vital signs, encourage and assist mom with breastfeeding, support mom in holding/handling baby, assist mom with bathing baby when appropriate, demonstrate diaper changing if needed, and update team as needed.

Discussion questions:

1. Does this scenario reflect purpose and goal?

2. What is the primary goal of the team in this scenario? Why?

3. What is the secondary goal? Why?

4. Can you think of a time when the goals in this scenario may be reversed?

Professional Characteristics

Psychological and personal characteristics may remain stable with little deviation; however, professional characteristics change over time. Examples of professional characteristics include education and training, professional experience, job

Reflection

Have you ever been involved in a group or team where someone had a negative attitude? If so, how did it affect the team? How did the team work through the issue?

Case Application: Team 3, Cancer Center

Team: oncologist, radiation therapist, surgeon, surgical technician, dietitian, nurse, health educator, occupational therapist, physical therapist, and pharmacist. Not all team members are needed for every patient, but all remain part of the team.

Karina is a 31-year-old woman who has recently been diagnosed with breast cancer. She is a single mom of two children, ages 3 and 5. Recently separated from her husband, Karina works full time to provide for her children, but even with the child support payments she receives from the children's father, she is barely able to make ends meet. Although she moved to a new area because of her marriage, Karina decided to stay in the area after her separation because she likes her job and coworkers. However, it means that she has no familial support but is now involved in a situation where family is desperately needed. Karina found a lump in her breast about 3 months ago. She immediately made an appointment with her primary-care provider, who sent her for a mammogram. The mammogram indicated a pea-size mass in her left breast and a biopsy was ordered. Unfortunately, the results of the test came back positive for stage 2 breast cancer. A total body scan was completed to determine if lymph nodes are involved and if the cancer has spread to other organs. The scan revealed one lymph node that tested positive but otherwise the results were negative. Karina will need to meet with the oncologist to discuss her options. In addition to her health concerns, Karina is anxious about work, child care, and finances. She realizes that her sick time is limited at work, she has very little emotional support, and her budget is already stretched.

The interprofessional team meets to discuss options for Karina. Each member of the team discusses recommendations based on his or her specific discipline. Following is some of the conversation among the team members who will be involved in Karina's care.

Oncologist (Dr. B): "Since the lymph involvement was negative except for the area closest to the breast involvement, my recommendation is removal of the left breast along with radiation."

Radiation therapist (Dr. M): "I disagree with that recommendation. If Karina has radiation, her breast should not be removed. She is young and other than the cancerous lump, she is healthy. I realize there is the possibility that chemotherapy may be needed depending on her response to radiation; however, that should be used as a last resort."

Oncologist (Dr. B): "I certainly understand your position, Dr. M, and of course I will mention both options to Karina. You are right. She is healthy but I would not want to see her go through this problem again. It is ultimately up to her. I will let her know the advantages and disadvantages of both options. Perhaps she could meet with both of us at the same time."

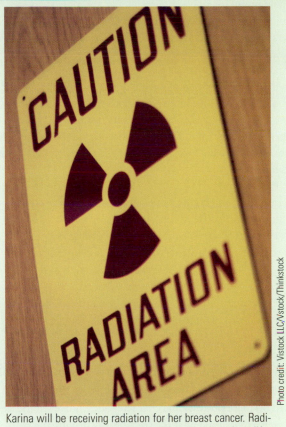

Photo credit: Vstock LLC/Vstock/Thinkstock

Karina will be receiving radiation for her breast cancer. Radiation is used to treat many forms of cancer and can be a lifesaver; however, there are dangers related to unnecessary exposure. The caution sign alerts visitors about the radiation area and possible exposure.

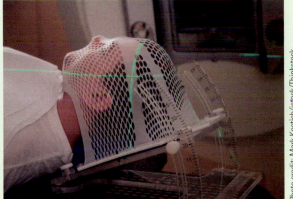

Photo credit: Mark Kostich/istock/Thinkstock

Radiation therapy is used to treat many types of cancer, such as Karina's breast cancer. It is also commonly used for treatment of brain cancer as shown here.

Social worker (Ms. K): "I don't know the best medical treatment for Karina, but I do know she has a lot of concerns about work and finances. I spoke briefly with her last week when she had her body scan. She was asking about time out of work. Maybe I can speak with her after she meets with you, Dr. K. I can provide some supportive counseling regarding her

(continued)

options. I can provide her with additional information regarding mastectomy support groups should she decide to take that route. Also she will need to learn about financial resources to assist her with needed services such as wigs for hair loss and resources for child care."

Dietitian (Ms. P): "Ms. K, I think your discussion with her will definitely provide some answers, and meeting with both Drs. B and M will ensure that she is fully informed about options. Regardless of her decision about surgery, I will still need to provide her nutritional advice about radiation and food choices that work best to reduce nausea and increase energy levels."

Physical therapist (Mr. O): "If Karina does opt for the surgery, I will meet with her and discuss an exercise regimen that will involve the muscles around the left arm. I will also explain the importance of continuing an exercise plan to maintain muscle mass and enhance stamina needed to endure the radiation. My concern is whether her decision will be made based on her financial situation and work issues. What do you all think?"

Pharmacist: "Mr. O, I think that is a valid question considering Karina is a single mom with very little financial resources.

Keep in mind that she does not have family here to assist with the children either. Ms. K, when you meet with her, could you ask about the possibility of having a family member engaged in the conversation, if only by phone? When I meet with Karina to discuss the side effects of radiation and medications to reduce nausea, I will see if she has any specific questions related to costs of the medications and report back at our next meeting."

The interprofessional team finalizes their thoughts and plans for Karina as Dr. B prepares for the initial meeting with Karina. Discussion questions:

1. How does each team member ensure accountability while still working as a team?

2. What do you think would happen if one of the members neglected his or her duties?

3. Interprofessional teams require meetings, which can be time consuming. Do you think the time spent justifies the quality care? Why?

4. How might this scenario be different without an interprofessional team?

satisfaction, professional socialization, and status in the health-care team. Leaders often emerge, whether planned or not, based on these professional characteristics; however, the leader of interprofessional health-care teams is usually the primary-care provider. The primary-care provider is typically educated, skilled, and knowledgeable in the expert area of the patient's condition, and has passed the required licensing examination required by medical associations. Depending on the diagnosis, the primary-care provider may consult with specialists regarding the patient's diagnosis and treatment, but usually still maintains the leadership role in the overall patient care.

Communication

As with any team effort, communication is always an important element; however, in interprofessional health-care teams, communication is vital to ensuring quality care. Communication structures include the methods used in the communication process such as routine meetings, as-needed meetings, or brief verbal communications without specific agendas.[5] The communication processes include how feedback is delivered and the method used for any conflict resolution or problem-solving measures.

Accountability

Accountability refers to the members' acceptance of individual and collective responsibility for the team's success. The team members must not only know their roles and responsibilities, but also understand how they contribute to

the cohesiveness of the group. The team members have skills independent of one another; therefore, they are accountable to their respective disciplinary bodies for ethics and standards of care. However, the team must remain supportive of the decisions and actions of the entire group to enhance quality care and team success.

High-Level Interpersonal Team Skills

Health-care teams are only as effective as what the individual members bring to the team. One of the most important elements to team success is the individual's interpersonal team skills. Interpersonal skills can enhance team cohesion and ensure progress. Some of the more effective interpersonal skills that help make a team successful include the following[1,6]:

- Effective communication skills
- Self-awareness
- Problem-solving skills
- Ability to provide effective feedback
- Time management skills
- Confliction resolution skills
- Negotiation skills
- Leadership skills
- Persuasion skills
- Ability to work in diverse groups

Interpersonal Skills

A question that might be asked is whether interpersonal skills can be taught or, similar to personality characteristics, are relativity stable and change very little over time. One school of thought views interpersonal skills much like personalities, and as such are deeply rooted in humans and not likely to change.[7] Conversely, another school of thought indicates that these skills can be taught and learned, and over time become a natural part of us.[6] There is no evidence that suggests that teaching interpersonal skills will always produce effective leaders and team members; however, there is research that proposes interpersonal skills can be taught and, when practiced routinely, can produce successful results in managerial performance.[6] Interpersonal skills are often taught in college and university programs, and are a required part of the curriculum needed to meet program certification.[6] The key element is not the teaching aspect, but the application technique. Within the course framework of a curriculum that teaches interpersonal skills, there is usually a practical piece that calls for students to complete activities such as case studies, role plays, simulations, and other exercises that engage them in interpersonal skill development. Additionally, many programs use internships to further student development of the skills taught in class. The practice of these skills increases the probability that the skills will become part of the students' tool kit after graduation and carry over into their careers.

Effective Communication Skills

When people think of communication skills, their first thought is often verbal communication. Although verbal or oral communication is certainly a vital part of communication, there are other elements that are just as important. These elements include the ability to listen and the ability to discern between verbal and nonverbal communication.

An individual with effective communication skills understands the importance of listening to others. Listening goes further than just hearing words, and it involves more than just the ears. To be effective in listening, the individual needs to not only hear words but process them while using other cues, such as **nonverbal communication.** There are three dimensions to listening: the hearing of the words (sensing), the processing or evaluation of the words, and the responding to the words.[1] The processing or evaluation requires another element, which is nonverbal communication. We may hear someone say something, but body language may tell us something different. Because over 50% of interpersonal communication is conveyed nonverbally,[1] it is extremely important to learn to recognize when the two are not in alignment. Nonverbal communication can include

facial expressions, eye contact or avoidance, smiles, body movements, tone, pitch and volume of voice, and many other elements. Individuals working in health care must learn to discern both verbal and nonverbal communication. In health care the patient's nonverbal communication cues may help provide some direction for the physician. For example, if asked about pain level, a patient may respond that the pain is not too bad, but at the same time, there may be a grimace on the patient's face. An observant health-care professional will pick up on the discrepancy and probe further. Similarly, health-care team members should look to each other for both verbal and nonverbal cues when forming a consensus on patients' treatments, care plans, and interventions.

Self-Awareness

Self-awareness is the concept of knowing and understanding your strengths and weaknesses. It involves knowing your preferences, motivations, and personality,[1] and recognizing the way these traits influence your judgment, decisions, and relations with others. Essentially, self-awareness is the impact your feelings have on your behavior and your ability to control the behavior when it is not appropriate. Being self-aware enables you to predict your behavior to a certain degree. There will always be times when the unexpected happens, causing the need for altered judgments or decisions; however, self-aware individuals are typically consistent in their behavior regardless of the circumstances.

One way to increase self-awareness is by self-analysis, which requires individuals to view themselves objectively. Although a somewhat difficult task for most, self-analysis will help individuals understand their behavior and possibly implement new behavioral or cognitive changes in the future. Behavior is usually associated with the way we view situations based on our perspectives, and self-analysis allows us to view the situation in a new perspective.

Problem-Solving Skills

Possessing successful problem-solving skills is a definite attribute for individuals working in health-care teams. As can be expected, problems do occur, not only in the work environment, but also within the group itself. Solving problems appropriately can be a rather long process; however, solving the problems in the correct manner may reduce potential troubles. Rather than take the quick and easy way out, one should consider taking the time to analyze the problem to determine the most beneficial solution. One of the most important steps to problem-solving is solving the correct problem by identifying and analyzing it effectively. Often we try to solve a problem that is superficial and does not get to the root of the issue, or we try to solve the wrong problem. Problem identification and analysis helps to examine the problem through other viewpoints so the group can reach consensus on the action plan.

Effective Feedback

Effective feedback is an important and valuable element in team building. Feedback provides individuals with details about how well someone is doing a task or could relay information about changes that need to be made in the job; hence feedback can be positive or negative. The more important element of feedback is the manner of delivery. Tips to keep in mind when delivering feedback include the following[1,6]:

- Keep the focus on the specific behavior and not the individual person.
- Keep the feedback nonjudgmental.
- Provide feedback in a timely manner.
- Keep feedback constructive.
- Keep feedback in balance by providing both positive and negative comments.
- Present feedback in the most appropriate place.

Time Management Skills

Time management skills are always an important acquisition for any individual but are appreciated even more so within health-care teams because of the ever-changing nature of the environment. How time is spent and managed may be critical in health care because medical (or patient) needs often occur quickly and must be addressed immediately. Time management skills allow us to allocate our time

and resources to achieve the desired goal. Effective time management skills allow individuals to create a balance between career and personal life, which reduces stress levels. Productivity levels are increased with time management skills because mental energy or effort is directed toward achieving goals or objectives. Team members with effective time management skills are an asset to all teams because they are able to prioritize, delegate, and complete tasks in the most effective and efficient manner.

Conflict Resolution Skills

Conflict resolution skills are considered by some to be the most important skill for organizational effectiveness.[8] The ability to handle conflict in one situation is interchangeable with handling conflict in other environments. The skills learned and used in conflict management can be applied to all kinds of settings because conflict is not a matter of if, but rather a matter of when. Types of conflicts that may occur include personality clashes, issues with roles and responsibilities, workloads, or scheduling concerns. Because conflict is certain to occur, being equipped with the appropriate skills will reduce the potential for further misunderstandings.

Conflict is not necessarily a negative thing. Today's view of conflict proposes that positive results can occur from conflict, such as creativity, innovation, renewed energy, and change.[1] The manner in which the conflict is handled predicts the negative or positive outcomes. Therefore, learning how to manage conflict is important in all relationships—work or personal.

Many factors can lead to conflict. Some include miscommunication, limited resources, differences in attitudes and values, and differences in goals and objectives. There are several useful strategies for handing conflict, but the type of strategy is dependent on the relationship between the individuals. An individual or group must keep in mind the importance of the relationship and the ramifications that might surface after the conflict resolution occurs. For example, one type of strategy is **accommodation,** which means you *accommodate,* or allow room for the individual's opinion, action, or method.[1] This strategy works well if the relationship is more important than the actual conflict; however, accommodation can only work a certain number of times because it can be perceived by one or both parties as a win-lose outcome.

Tips and Tools

Examine your problem-solving skills by completing this activity at the end of the chapter.

Reflection

Think about how you manage your time for family, school, sports, friends, and self. Do you have a strategy that works best for you?

Avoiding is another conflict management strategy that focuses on the relationship more than the conflict. People may avoid any type of conflict because they are fearful of damaging the relationship. Individuals using this strategy hope the conflict goes away without intervention. This strategy will work occasionally; however, the problem is never really addressed, so issues remain unresolved.

The most successful conflict strategy is **collaborating,** because this process involves all participants and provides equal representation, allowing both sides to win. Typically, a team can meet the goals and objectives and solve the conflict by using the creativity of the team. Collaborating improves the commitment from each person because of the ownership involved in the decision and outcome. The disadvantage to collaborating is the time constraints. Depending on the conflict, time may be of the essence, which prevents a collaborative approach.[1]

Compromising in conflicts provides a method of keeping harmonious relationships intact because both parties have a say in the solution. Each of the parties gives and takes to reach an agreement; however, creativity could be stifled because the solution is not based on new solutions or ideas. Compromising on every conflict may create more conflicts because neither party is ever completely satisfied.[1]

Competing is a conflict management strategy that creates a win-lose scenario. One party wins while another loses. The positives to this strategy are the sense of self-power and winning it all; the negatives involve the possibility of alienating others and losing it all.[1] There are times when this type of strategy is needed, such as a situation involving a child refusing to take medications. No other strategy would work effectively in this scenario, so competing is the best option.

Each of these strategies has both advantages and disadvantages, and no one strategy works best for all situations. Therefore, learning the various strategies will allow one to select the most appropriate choice when needed.

Tips and Tools

To further develop your conflict management skills, complete this activity at the end of the chapter.

Reflection

Think about the way you handle conflicts with your family. The family relationship needs to be preserved, but at the same time, you do not want to always give in; so what type of strategy do you think is most beneficial? Why?

Negotiation Skills

Negotiation, much like conflict, is a part of life and will happen in work and personal lives. Learning how to be a good negotiator may result in "win-win" situations, which can be advantageous for many reasons. Negotiation begins with a shared interest between two or more individuals; the next phase is the back-and-forth negotiation process until an agreement is met.[1,6] Benefits of good negotiation skills include the possibility of obtaining a pay raise, a new job, a promotion, scarce resources, or any other item deemed worthy.

Negotiation skills can be learned and then polished to improve the overall odds of success. However, negotiation is not to be used in every aspect of life or work. One needs to determine the importance of the objective before deciding to negotiate. Once the determination has been made, the next step is to decide the best you can possibly achieve and the least you can accept. Having this information in advance will help you set the stage for the negotiation to begin. For example, if you want to purchase a car, you might not automatically agree to the sticker price. You need to determine the most that you can afford to pay for the car and the least amount of money the dealer may accept. Of course, this is where planning comes into play. This information needs to be determined before you enter the negotiation process. Typically, there is a back-and-forth progression until both parties either agree or one walks away. Although simplistic in the sense of negotiating the purchase of a car, negotiation skills can transfer to more complex issues such as vying to obtain resources within your health-care facility. Once the technique has been developed it can be used in many avenues.

Leadership Skills

To understand the skills associated with leadership, the term itself needs to be defined. There are many ways in which individuals define *leadership,* but the basic definition is the ability an individual (or individuals) has that inspires followers or influences others toward a goal or social change. Although many theories exist, there does not appear to be any proven theories that determine what makes leaders successful in their roles.[8,9] Therefore, determining effective leadership is dependent on certain characteristics or qualities that enhance the ability to lead others. Some of the characteristics, such as effective communication and self-awareness, have been discussed; others include the following[10,11]:

- Honesty
- Confidence
- Commitment
- Intuition
- Resourceful

- Organized
- Consistent
- Open-minded

Two primary types of leaders are typically acknowledged. The first one is **transformational leaders.** These individuals tend to be more visionary and provide more direction toward the overall objective by setting goals, clarifying expectations, and persuading others to look beyond self-interest and think about the group benefit. Transformational leaders use empowerment to encourage individuals to act on the vision. Some famous transformational leaders include George Washington, Abraham Lincoln, Martin Luther King, Jr., Steve Jobs, and Nelson Mandela.

Transactional leaders are more prone to task-oriented behaviors and tend to use reward and punishment as ways to achieve the objective. Transactional leaders use people as resources by hiring the right people for the positions and directing them toward the objective. As opposed to transformational leaders, transactional leaders are not focused on change but rather maintaining the current status quo. Some famous transactional leaders include Charles de Gaulle, John F. Kennedy, Dwight D. Eisenhower, and Ronald Reagan.

Regardless of the leadership style an individual selects, it is important to recognize that not everyone can be a leader. Without someone to follow, progress will not take place. When there is a tendency for everyone to lead, conflicts may occur and create tension within the team. Therefore, when working in teams of any sort, there is a give-and-take philosophy—sometimes you lead, and sometimes you follow.

Ability to Work in Diverse Groups

Within today's marketplace, we are fortunate to have a diverse group of workers. This diversity represents professional characteristics such as specialties along with personal diversity such as ethnicities. Although the importance of diversity in all jobs is significant, it is more important in health care because all individuals will need health care at some point in their lives. Fortunately, the health-care workers come from diverse backgrounds as well, which benefits all patients. Diversity in health care allows for cultural and gender sensitivities to be addressed while also providing equality in the workforce. The health-care team benefits by having diverse members, but it also sometimes creates tension when team

Reflection

Can you think of any famous people who might fit into the transformational leadership style? What characteristics makes this individual(s) stand out as transformational?

members do not have any experience working in diverse teams. Recognition of diversity and learning to respect the differences propels the team in a positive direction. The greater the diversity, the greater the creativity is within the team, which ultimately provides a more holistic approach to health care.

Team Obstacles

Just as there are benefits to teamwork, there are also obstacles that the team must work together to overcome. Learning and practicing the skills needed to be a good team member can be transferred to any type of team environment; likewise, lessons gained while learning to overcome the obstacles can transfer to all types of team settings. There are a myriad of obstacles to working in teams; some of the more common include the following[1,6]:

- Lack of defined purpose or goal
- Lack of trust
- Lack of objectivity
- Competition
- Lack of resources or support

Lack of Defined Purpose or Goal

As mentioned, having a clearly defined purpose or goal will propel a team toward meeting objectives. The lack of defined goals may create tension, frustration, lack of enthusiasm, and stagnation. Without progression or momentum, team members become indecisive and lack direction. When the team is not moving forward, it is probably moving backward. The longer the team remains static, the more likely team members will lose interest or enthusiasm, resulting in absenteeism. When part of the team is missing, stagnation may occur. Therefore, it is important to make sure everyone commits to the purpose or goal to ensure movement toward the objective.

Lack of Trust

Teams, unlike groups, are expected to emerge from separate entities to create a whole. Although this solidarity does not mean that everyone agrees 100% with all thoughts, ideas, and suggestions, it does mean that the team is probably unanimous in their solution or recommendations and has worked as a unit to reach the decision. It is much like a sports team: when working cohesively, the focus is not on who scored the winning point, but rather the win itself. The same holds true for teams; however, for this unit to become one, there must be trust within the entire team. Each member must be able to rely on the other members' participation, responsibility for their roles, and commitment to keeping the team's interest in mind. Like sports teams, trusting and supporting your fellow team members are the key elements to a job well done. Without trust, the team will not survive.

Lack of Objectivity

Effective teamwork requires individuals to put aside personal judgment and bias to become open-minded to others' ideas. It is difficult to truly listen to others when our minds are already closed to new ideas. One of the major advantages to teamwork is the notion that each person has something to bring to the table; however, if the table is already full with your own ideas, there is no room left for others. Being objective does not mean that your ideas are not important; it means that everyone's ideas deserve the same respect as yours.

Competition

Competition should never exist in teams, particularly health-care teams. The ultimate goal for health-care teams is to improve patient care, and the focus should be on this objective. There are times when the focus may shift because egos get in the way of progress. Individual egos should be checked at the door and left there to ensure competition within the group does not occur.

Lack of Resources or Support

Regardless of how well the team works together, if resources or support are not available, the team will fail. It is important that adequate resources be available and support from managers or supervisors be addressed early in the process. The best solutions to problems will not ensure success unless the solutions are within reach.

Ethics in Health-Care Teams
Individual Ethics vs. Organizational Ethics

As previously stated, ethics are based on our own perceptions and value systems. We rarely even think about them unless we are presented with a situation that tests our ethics or causes us to question them. We face these types of challenges in both our personal and professionals lives, but whereas in our personal lives we may allow ourselves to be governed by our own personal standards, the workplace standards may dictate differently. These situations are known as **organizational ethics** and they represent the culture of the organization.[1] It is fair to assume that most organizations are ethical and their employees, in turn, are ethical. Unfortunately, there may be times when individual ethics and organizational

ethics are at odds. When these two systems collide, you may be faced with either conforming to the culture or standing out to make a statement. Either decision could produce anxiety and place you at risk for job dissatisfaction.

Guidelines for Making Ethical Decisions

Whether working in a health-care team or within an organization, there are some guidelines or tools that will enhance your ethical decision-making. Guidelines are designed to augment your own abilities rather than take away from them. Your values and perceptions will still play a major role in the ethical decision process; these guidelines provide some other options or ways of viewing the situation[1,6]:

- Code of ethics—most professional disciplines have a code of ethics, which provides a written code or statement regarding professionalism. Some organizations have their own internal code of ethics that can be used when ethical conflict occurs.

- Consider all costs or consequences—when considering the **ethical dilemma,** be sure to view the solution through many lenses. Rather than settling on one possibility, think through several and play the "What if. . . ?" game. With each solution, consider all possible ramifications and ask, "What if . . . ?"

- Seek consultation from others—it is important to remember that most people have gone through similar situations as you and their expertise may help you through yours.

- Ethics training courses—if possible, attend ethics training courses, especially those that might be available at your place of employment.

- Ethical decision-making framework—several models are available that will take you step by step through the decision process. These models enhance your thinking and processing abilities by providing steps and rules for before proceeding to the decision.

- Use your intuition—regardless of the decision made, if you feel in your gut that something is wrong, it probably is. Use that gut feeling to help you recognize when decisions made are not right for you.

The role of ethics, especially in health care, cannot be overstated. When making decisions that may potentially affect someone's health, or even life, it is not wise to leave anything to chance. Take the time needed to address all issues and possible consequences before embarking on a journey that could change someone's life—for the better or for the worse.

SUMMARY

This chapter has discussed many important aspects of working successfully as a health-care team. As a potential future health-care professional, you should understand the importance of interprofessional teams. No one discipline, in itself, has all the right answers to all the possible questions. The adage "It takes a village to raise a child" lends some truth to health care—"It takes an interprofessional team to treat a patient."

EXERCISES

Exercise 31-1: Role Play

Case

Martha is a 59-year-old woman who recently had a fall that resulted in a fractured hip requiring surgery.

Medical History

Two surgeries—appendix in early teens and hysterectomy at 39, which was due to ovarian cancer. Patient is insulin-dependent diabetic requiring one injection per day. In addition to the insulin, patient is on a statin drug (that she admits she sometime misses due to costs) for cholesterol. Other medicines are over-the-counter vitamins and a low-dose aspirin.

Blood pressure: 170/91 mm Hg (blood pressure is high).

Weight: 168 pounds.

Height: 5 feet 4 inches.

Total cholesterol: 245 (cholesterol should be less than 200).

Family history—widowed with one grown child who lives in another state, has an older sister living in nearby town, no other family members.

Social history—social drinker, currently smokes cigarettes (1 pack per day).

Work history—patient works in retail sales and must continue working due to insurance benefits. She states that she would not be able to afford the insurance on an individual basis due to her previous cancer diagnosis, weight, and diabetes.

The health-care team consists of the primary-care provider, surgeon, nutritionist, physical therapist, social worker, and pharmacist. Remember that the patient is also part of the team and should be included.

The roles should be decided at least a day in advance for the team to have ample time to read the case and reflect on the readings from previous chapters. Each discipline should have some idea of what their roles might entail in a real case similar to this one.

The team will role play the scenario and discuss options for the patient. The team will develop an interprofessional plan of care (IPOC). Afterward, the remaining students will discuss some of the following issues.

Questions for discussion:

1. Who, if anyone, took the leadership role?
2. Was the patient involved in the IPOC?
3. How did the team members respond to each other?
4. Were any important details left out of the plan?
5. Were all team members open to hearing ideas from other members?

Exercise 31-2: Effective Communication

Case

Dr. Jones takes pride in having a diverse patient population. One day Jose comes in for a visit. Dr. Jones has only seen Jose a couple of times and cannot remember much about him. Jose is a non–English-speaking citizen; therefore, he brings in his 10-year-old son to interpret. According to the patient chart, Jose has flu-like symptoms. Dr. Jones asks Jose several questions about his symptoms and Jose nods his head to each question. Jose's son does not say anything, so Dr. Jones assumes everything is fine. Dr. Jones' diagnosis is a severe case of flu and Jose will need to take at least three different medications for 2 weeks. Additionally, Jose was to purchase an over-the-counter drug to use for his cough. Dr. Jones gave the prescription to Jose and asks if he understood. Jose nodded his head. Jose comes back to the office after 2 weeks for a follow-up visit. This time, Jose's wife, who speaks English, accompanies him. Dr. Jones notices that some of Jose's symptoms have not cleared up. He asks Jose if he took all the medicines and Jose nods. Jose's wife speaks up and says, no, this is not correct. He only took two of the prescribed medications and even those he did not finish. Dr. Jones is confused about this situation because he thought Jose understood all of the directions.

Questions for discussion:

1. Identify the problem(s) in this patient scenario.

2. Why did Dr. Jones think Jose understood everything?

3. How could this scenario have been different?

Exercise 31-3: Problem-Solving

Read the following case and develop strategies to solve the problems.

Case

The small island of Trouble has many problems that have affected the population's health, education, economics, and safety. Here are the facts about the island:

Trouble is located about 225 miles from the nearest land and is only accessible by boat. There are only 1,068 residents on the island. Of the 1,068, almost 60% are either not old enough to work, are unemployed, or are too old to work, which means the remaining residents have to support the majority of the population. Jobs are available for those who are able and old enough to work. Because there are only three health-care providers on the island, there is always a waiting line at the health-care facilities and making an appointment is difficult. Therefore, some of the preventive measures such as vaccines and routine testing go undone. Recently, there was an epidemic of bird fever and many residents contracted the disease, requiring antibiotics that are in very short supply. Without the antibiotic, the disease is sometimes fatal. Education is also a major concern because many of the students are dropping out of school at around age 15 for employment to help support their families. With the number of dropouts, the school system is considering shutting one school down due to the expense of maintaining both. If one of the schools is closed down, some residents would not be able to attend the other one because of distance and lack of personal or public transportation. Also with the closing of the school, many school employees would be out of work. Other issues with the island are lack of clean water and poor sanitary conditions.

In developing solutions for the island of Trouble, consider the following questions:

1. What are the most pressing issues at this time?

2. How do you prioritize the needs of the community?

3. What are some possible ways to solve some of these problems?

4. What overall strategic plan would you implement if you were the leader of the island?

Exercise 31-4: Conflict Management

This activity is best suited for a team of five or six students. You are to read the following case and individually prioritize the tasks. Then as a group, you are to rank order the tasks.

Case

You and six others have chartered a small private boat for the day. The group has decided to travel to a remote island to explore for a few hours before heading back home. The island is approximately 180 miles from your home. Right before you reach the island, the boat develops engine trouble and you barely make it to the island. As you drift into the island the captain tells everyone the engine has died and he does not have the necessary tools to even attempt to make repairs. The radio is not working either; therefore, he cannot call for help. He does assure you that if the boat is not returned within 48 hours the authorities will be notified. Thinking about the possibility of being shipwrecked for 2 days, a couple of the passengers begin to panic. As the panic begins to subside somewhat, you all realize that one of your group members is severely sunburned. Another person in the group continues to scream and yell with fear. It is time for you to decide what you are going to do. As a group, you are asked to rank in order of importance the following tasks that will be completed.

1. Explore the island and lagoons.

2. Treat the sunburn victim.

3. Search for food.

4. Create an action plan.

5. Calm the hysterical person.

6. Build a fire.

7. Search for drinking water.

8. Erect a netted shelter to keep the insects out.

9. Send up a flare. (You only have one.)

10. Make straw mats for sleeping.

You *must* reach a group consensus regarding the order of importance of these tasks. You will have 15 minutes to complete the activity.

Questions for discussion:

1. How did you reach your agreement?

2. Was the decision unanimous or did you have to negotiate any tasks?

3. Did you use any conflict strategies? If so, which ones?

4. Did the team work together in a cohesive manner?

5. If there was conflict, do you think it was functional or dysfunctional?

Exercise 31-5: Examining Your Value System

1. Spend a few minutes thinking about your personal values. What words would you use to describe yourself?

2. Based on the words you used to describe yourself in question 1, create your personal mission statement that you feel adequately describes you.

Exercise 31-6: Ethical Issues

Case 1: Religious Differences

A 7-year-old child has been taken to the emergency department for abdominal pains, nausea, vomiting, and fever of 103°F. Blood work indicates that the white blood cell count is extremely high, which indicates infection. On examination, the diagnosis is acute cholecystitis. The surgeon relays the message to the parents that the child needs to have a cholecystectomy (removal of gallbladder) immediately. In the process of preparing for the surgery, the child needs to have a blood type and crossmatch for potential blood transfusion should the need arise. The parents refuse to allow the child to have the blood type and crossmatch because their religious beliefs do not allow blood transfusions. The surgeon explains that this procedure is for precautionary reasons, and more than likely the child will not need blood. The parents still refuse to allow the surgery if there is any possibility that the child will need blood.

Questions for discussion:

1. Identify the ethical issues in the case.

2. How do the parents' religious beliefs affect the child's medical needs?

3. What are your suggestions for solving this ethical dilemma?

4. Do you think this type of case actually occurs? Explain your response.

Case 2: Money vs. Quality Care

Janice is a 39-year-old woman who works full time as a waitress at a local restaurant. In addition to her regular job, Janice is a part-time student at the local community college. Her goal is to obtain her associate degree in nursing. Janice does not have insurance because the restaurant is not required to offer insurance based on the size of the business. Janice did have a private insurance policy but it lapsed about 3 months ago due to nonpayment of premiums. Janice visits her doctor, Dr. James, and is told she has an unusual bacterial infection and will need treatments. One treatment (option 1) has serious side effects and will require missed days of work and school, but costs less money. Another treatment (option 2) has fewer side effects and the treatment time is actually less; however, this option is more costly. Because Janice does not have health insurance, Dr. James only tells her about the one treatment option, thinking that Janice would opt for that one anyway. During recovery, one of Janice's coworkers comes to visit and inquires about Janice's treatment option. Janice relays the information to her coworker, who tells Janice that she heard about someone else having the same condition but was offered another treatment option. Janice decides to research the infection and treatment options and realizes that her coworker was correct about the two options.

Questions for discussion:

1. Does this action violate patient rights?

2. Was this decision by Dr. James ethical?

3. How do you think Janice feels after finding out the truth?

4. Do you think this type of behavior actually occurs?

Review Questions

1. What is the optimal size for an effective team?

    A. Three members

    B. Four to five members

    C. Four to six members

    D. Six to ten members

2. An attribute of professional characteristics is:

    A. Job satisfaction

    B. Age

    C. Motivation

    D. Attitude

3. _____ of interpersonal communication is conveyed nonverbally.

    A. 10%

    B. 25%

    C. 55%

    D. 60%

4. Knowing and understanding your strengths and weaknesses is a product of:

    A. Motivation

    B. Personality

    C. Communication skills

    D. Self-awareness

5. In delivering effective feedback, one should:

    A. Relay only positive comments

    B. Wait several weeks before presenting the feedback

    C. Provide your own opinion and judgments

    D. Focus on the behavior, not the person

6. The accommodation strategy for addressing conflict involves:

    A. One wins and one loses

    B. Everyone wins

    C. No one wins

    D. This strategy does not exist

7. The two primary types of leadership styles are:

   A. Transformational and transitional

   B. Transactional and transitional

   C. Transactional and transformational

   D. Stationary and situational

8. The concept of objectivity refers to:

   A. Knowing yourself

   B. Being open to other ideas

   C. Stating the importance of your opinions

   D. Being effective in negotiation

9. _____ should never exist in teams.

   A. Negotiation

   B. Conflict

   C. Competition

   D. Ethics

10. Individual ethics are based on:

    A. Ethics training courses taken

    B. Legality

    C. Perceptions and value systems

    D. Organizational culture

Glossary of Key Terms

Nonverbal communication—communication that takes places when a person is not speaking but does relay a message, such as a frown or lack of eye contact

Accommodation—a conflict resolution strategy used when preserving the relationship is more important than getting your way; uses the "you win, I lose" philosophy

Avoiding—a conflict strategy used when you do not want to deal with the conflict

Collaborating—a conflict strategy used that takes more time when resolving conflict, but is beneficial to both parties because it is a "win-win" situation for both

Compromising—a conflict strategy used when both parties split the difference

Competing—a conflict strategy used when both parties try to win regardless of the outcome

Transformational leaders—a type of leadership style where the leader focuses on change for the better and motivates others to become change agents

Transactional leaders—a type of leadership style where the leader uses rewards and punishment to justify a change or to establish a purpose for no change

Organizational ethics—the values, behaviors, and beliefs of employees within an organization as influenced by culture and practice

Ethical dilemma—condition that warrants us to make a decision based on judgments, not facts

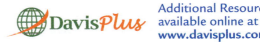
Additional Resources are available online at www.davisplus.com

References

1. de Janasz S, Dowd K, Schneider B. *Interpersonal Skills in Organizations,* 3rd ed. San Francisco, CA: McGraw-Hill Irwin; 2009.

2. Poulton B, West M. The determinants of effectiveness in primary health care teams. *J Interprofessional Care.* 1999;13(1):7–17.

3. Yaffe M, Dulka I, Kosberg J. Interdisciplinary health-care teams: What should doctors be aware of? *Can J CME.* 2001;13(5): 153–160.

   www.stacommunications.com/journals/cme/ images/cmepdf/may01/workingteams.pdf.
   Accessed July 11, 2014.

4. Borrill C, Carletta J, Carter A, et al. *Report. The Effectiveness of Health Care Teams in the National Health Service.* Aston University, University of Glasglow, and University of Leeds; 1999.

5. Grumbach K, Bodenheimer T. Can health care teams improve primary care practice? *J Am Med Assoc.* 2004;291(10):1246–1251.

6. Robbins S, Hunsaker P. *Training in Interpersonal Skills,* 4th ed. Upper Saddle River, NJ: Pearson Prentice Hall; 2006.

7. Fiedler F. *A Theory of Leadership Effectiveness.* New York, NY: McGraw-Hill; 1967.

8. Tjosvold D, Johnson D. *Productive Conflict Management: Perspectives for Organizations.* New York, NY: Irvington Publishers; 1983.

9. Weiss D, Tilin F, Morgan M. *The Interprofessional Health Care Team.* Burlington, MA: Jones & Bartlett Learning; 2014.

10. Prive T. Top 10 qualities that make a great leader. Forbes. 2012.

    www.forbes.com/sites/tanyaprive/2012/12/19/ top-10-qualities-that-make-a-great-leader/.
    Accessed July 16, 2014.

11. Holden Leadership Center, University of Oregon. Leadership characteristics.

    http://leadership.uoregon.edu/resources/ exercises_tips/skills/leadership_characteristics.
    Accessed July 16, 2014.

Other Health-Related Professions

Other health-related disciplines are listed separately because they are not typically educated in the same programs generally recognized as health sciences (medicine, nursing, or allied health), which are educated using the medical model. Most, if not all, of these other health-related programs are classified as either arts and sciences or health and human performance in academic schools. Although some professions may be hands-on, such as massage therapy, most of these professions provide a supportive role for patients and families, rather than the hands-on approach. The supportive approach combined with the direct patient approach ensures holistic care to patients and families.

- Health education
- Forensic science
- Massage therapy
- Psychology
- Medical science
- Surgical technology
- Veterinary medicine

Health Education

Introduction

Health educators provide an important service to patients, clients, and other health professionals. Their contribution to the improvement of overall health stems from the education and training they provide to individuals and communities. Not only do health educators teach positive behaviors, they also develop application strategies for individual use. Some health educators conduct needs assessments for further development of needed programs within the communities.

Health educators, like many other health-care professions, work in a variety of settings and perform a variety of tasks. Their roles/tasks include the following[1,2]:

- Promote health education programs
- Conduct workshops, trainings, and conferences
- Develop materials for individuals or for health facilities
- Conduct evaluations of health education programs
- Create and distribute reports, pamphlets, bulletins, and other materials for public use
- Create and maintain databases for public and private companies and health facilities
- Provide supervision of professional and technical staff

Work settings for health educators include the following[1,3]:

- Doctor's offices
- Public health departments
- Hospitals
- Government
- Schools, colleges, and universities
- Social advocacy organizations
- Outpatient care centers
- Ambulatory care centers
- Nonprofit organizations

Education

Typically, health educators need a bachelor's degree for entry-level positions; however, some positions, such as those in public health promotion and federal government, require a master's degree. Educational institutions may require a doctoral degree in health education if teaching in that discipline. Although not common in every state, there are times when community health workers hold a high school diploma in addition to previous work experience.[1,4]

Licenses and Certifications

Few states require that health educators be licensed or certified; however, some employers do require certifications. Certifications can be obtained at the bachelor's or master's level. These certifications are offered by the National Commission for Health Education Credentialing. Depending on the educational component, health educators can become a certified health education specialist (CHES) or a master certified health education specialist (MCHES). To preserve certification, health educators must complete 75 hours of continuing education every 5 years.[1]

Salary and Employment Outlook

Salaries for health educators vary according to job settings, education levels, and work regions. In 2013, the median salary for health educators was $49,210 and for community health workers it was $34,620.[4] The higher-paying jobs were, in general, medical and surgical hospitals; the lower-paying jobs were in community food and housing services and individual and family services. The exception to the salary averages is in the federal executive branch, which pays the highest salary for all health educators.[4]

The job outlook for 2012–2022 is expected to be a 21% increase, which is faster than average. The large increase is thought to be a result of an overall effort to reduce health-care costs by educating individuals about healthy behaviors.[1,4]

With the projected job outlook and the overall need for more health-care services, the choice of becoming a health educator is certainly a positive move. The variety in jobs and work settings, along with the growth potential, promotes a pleasant outlook for individuals looking to become health educators.

Forensic Science

Introduction

For anyone interested in criminology, forensic science is an excellent field. The term *forensic* refers to law, and individuals working as forensic scientists may analyze evidence in crime scene investigations that will later be used in a court of law.[5,6] Forensic scientists examine the physical evidence provided by police or other legal entities who are involved in solving a crime. The forensic scientist prepares a report that will be used in a court of law for criminal cases.

There are many avenues for anyone interested in forensics. Unlike the crime scenes in many television shows, some forensic scientists may never see the crime scene. Rather than collecting evidence from the scene of the crime, the forensic scientist may spend most of the day in the laboratory examining evidence brought in by authorities. Other forensic scientists may spend time examining fingerprints taken from a crime scene. Other areas of concentration for individuals who are interested in forensic science include the following[5,6]:

- Toxicology—refers to examination of blood and tissues for determination of alcohol or drug use, or other types of toxins.
- Polygraphs—also known as "lie detectors," these instruments are useful when questioning witnesses. Forensic scientists are trained to detect deception by measuring certain internal body functions such as blood pressure rates.
- Document examination—investigates forgeries, document tampering, handwriting analysis, and other areas of fraud.

- Chemistry—individuals working in this area analyzes physical evidence such as blood spatters that help to identify how the crime was committed.
- Firearms identification—refers to the matching characteristics between firearms and bullets, which identifies the firearm used in a crime.
- Toolmark identification—involves identifying the tool such as an axe that may be used in a crime. This area also includes explosives identification.

Work environments for forensic scientists include crime laboratories (city, county, and state) and federal agencies such as Postal Inspection Service, Health and Human Services, Department of Justice, and Drug Enforcement Administration. Some private laboratories also employ forensic scientists, as well as some colleges and universities. [5,6]

Education

The minimum entry level for most forensic scientists is a bachelor's degree in the natural sciences and on-the-job training. Some individuals may hold a master's degree in forensic science or another similar field such as criminology or psychology. For advancement purposes such as a laboratory director, a doctorate degree is usually preferred. [5,6]

Licenses and Certifications

Typically, license and certifications are not common; however, a few universities offer some type of certifications whether at the undergraduate or graduate level. Additionally, some professional associations offer voluntary certification. These types of certifications ensure professional competence in specific fields of forensic science.[6]

Salary and Employment Outlook

Salaries vary according to job settings, specialties, and work regions. In 2012, the median salary for forensic science technicians was $52,840.

The job outlook for 2012–2022 is expected to grow around 6%, which is slower than average. One of the reasons for the projected low increase is due to the considerable interest in forensic science a few years ago that helped lead individuals down that path, which saturated the market. The peak in interest was thought to be influenced by the increase in crime scene investigation made popular by the media.[6,7]

For detail-oriented individuals who are strong in math and science, a career path in forensic science may be a natural fit. Additionally, if you are inquisitive and enjoy putting pieces of the puzzle together, forensic science is definitely a good choice. Although typical work hours are about 40 per week, there may be times when overtime is required and night shifts are expected; however, the work can be exciting, challenging, and rewarding.

Massage Therapy

Introduction

Massage therapists provide treatment to clients who suffer from muscular pain and stress. Some clients see the massage therapist for wellness maintenance. A massage therapist manipulates the muscles and soft tissues to reduce pain, improve circulation, or increase relaxation. They assess clients for range of motion and muscle strength to provide the most comprehensive treatment plan.[8] Massage therapists also provide educational techniques to improve posture, improve stretching abilities, and enhance the client's relaxation skills. Massage therapists also develop treatment plans, refer clients to other health professionals when necessary, and collaborate with others to ensure quality care.[4,8]

Massage therapists work in a variety of settings. They work in both public and private environments such as hospitals, fitness centers, and spas. The traveling massage therapist will travel to the client's home to provide treatment. Of course, in this situation, the therapist has to provide appropriate equipment such as a table and chair, which increases the potential for their own injuries.[8]

Education

States vary on the educational requirements and standards for massage therapists. Generally, to become a massage therapist, postsecondary education and at least 500 study hours are required. In addition to the classroom education, the student is required to complete direct hands-on practice of massage techniques. Some colleges offering massage therapy programs offer specialties or concentrations in specific treatment approaches such as neuromuscular therapy.[8]

Licenses and Certifications

As with education, states vary on the licensing or certification requirements; however, most states do regulate massage therapy even if only at the local level. States that do regulate massage therapy require students to pass an approved program and take a licensing or certification examination, which may be a state or national examination. There are two nationally recognized examining boards: the Massage and Bodywork Licensing Examination and the National Certification Board for Therapeutic Massage and Bodywork.[9]

Salary and Employment Outlook

Like many other professions in health care, salaries for massage therapists vary according to job settings and work regions. In May 2012, the median annual salary for massage therapists was $39,970. The higher-paying industries for massage therapist include general medical and surgical hospitals, ambulatory health-care services, and specialty hospitals.[4,8]

The job outlook for 2012–2022 is a projected growth of 23%, which is much faster than average for all occupations. An aging population has helped to create a greater need for massage therapists. As the demand for services increases, opportunities for massage therapists will likewise increase.[4,8]

For individuals who enjoy direct client care, massage therapy is definitely a career to consider. The projected growth expected in the field provides security, and the potential for being self-employed is higher than many other health-care professions. Conversely, the work is physically demanding and repetitive-motion problems do occur more often in this type of work. Therefore, as in any career, one has to weigh the benefits and challenges carefully before embarking on a career path.

Psychology

Introduction

Psychology is a health-care discipline that involves the scientific study of cognitive, emotional, and social behaviors. A practitioner of psychology, a psychologist, observes people's behavior to understand the way mental functions affect behaviors. Psychologists also study the relationship between individuals and their environments by using observation and interpretation skills. The field of psychology has many specialty branches, such as social psychology, organizational psychology, behavioral psychology, abnormal psychology, developmental psychology, and counseling psychology, among many others.[10,11] Depending on the type of psychology in which one is trained, the tasks and responsibilities may deviate greatly; however, following are some general tasks that psychologists may perform.[10,11,12]

- Provide therapeutic counseling for individuals, groups, or families
- Provide crisis management therapy
- Analyze data to diagnose the client's problem(s)
- Provide psychosocial assessments
- Conduct interviews to gather information
- Supervise others
- Consult with other health professionals

- Develop treatment plans
- Conduct research
- Refer clients to other health professionals

Work settings for psychologists include the following[10]:

- Private and public health-care facilities
- School systems
- Institutional systems
- Mental health agencies
- Research and development
- Federal programs
- Colleges, universities, and professionals schools
- Private practice

Education

Individuals may receive a bachelor's, master's, or doctoral degree in psychology; however, practicing psychologists generally are required to hold an advanced degree. The minimum degree for case management is typically a bachelor's degree. Individuals working directly with clients typically are required to hold a license or certification, which can only be achieved by completing advanced degrees. In addition to the educational requirement there are internship requirements to be completed before being awarded the degree.[12]

Licenses and Certifications

Most of the states in the United States require licensure or certification to practice psychology. States do vary on the licensing requirements; however, for a clinical psychologist title, an individual must hold a doctoral degree in psychology, have completed an internship, and have at least 1 to 2 years of supervised professional experience and have passed the licensing examination. Individuals may also hold certifications in specialty areas such as psychoanalysis. For most states, once licensed, psychologists are required to complete continuing education to maintain their licensure. Information regarding specific state requirements can be obtained from the Association of State and Provincial Psychology Boards at www.asppb.net.[12]

Salary and Employment Outlook

There is great variability in salaries for psychologists due to education, working environments, licensure, and client population; however, the median salary for psychologist in May 2012 was $69,280. The higher-paying industries include offices of health-care practitioners and scientific research and development services.[10,11]

The job outlook for employment in psychology is projected to grow 12% from 2012 to 2022, which is about as fast as average for all occupations. Individuals holding doctoral degrees in school psychology and specialty degrees will have the best prospects.[10,11]

If you are a good listener and enjoy helping others, you might want to consider a career in psychology. Like many health professions, the rewards of helping others can definitely be felt when you are able to see someone's life change for the better.

Medical Science

Introduction

Medical scientists, also referred to as medical researchers, study diseases and prevention, conduct research, and engage in clinical investigations or trials to improve the overall health of humans.[13] There are many areas or specializations in which medical scientists can be employed; therefore, work descriptions vary depending on the environment. Some of the tasks and duties associated with medical scientists include the following[13,14]:

- Evaluating the effects of pesticides, gases, parasites, and drugs
- Conducting studies and investigations of human and animal health for prevention of disease(s)
- Preparing and analyzing cell, organ, and tissues samples to examine toxicity or bacteria levels
- Publishing scholarly work in scientific journals and applying for research grants
- Developing new equipment and instruments for medical applications
- Examining methods of immunizations and standardizing the dosages
- Investigating the performance of specific drugs against diseases

Work environments where medical scientists may work include the following:

- Hospitals
- Colleges or universities
- Private and public laboratories
- Research centers
- Pharmaceutical companies

Areas in which medical scientists may specialize include the following[13,14]:

- Oncology—cancer research focusing on prevention and cure

- Gerontology—research on aging and health improvements for older adults
- Immunology—research on effects of chemicals and drugs on the immune system
- Pharmacology—research and development of new medications
- Toxicology—research on the effects and safety of drugs, dangers of household chemicals, and effects of other poisonous substances

Education

Although some medical scientists may have a master's graduate degree only, the degree requirement for working in this environment is typically a PhD. Some individuals have both a PhD and MD degree, especially if they work in clinical research with patients. These joint degrees provide both the clinical skills and the research skills needed to engage fully in this work environment. Students who wish to pursue this line of work would need to focus on biology, physical sciences, chemistry, and mathematics in undergraduate school to improve their chances of being accepted into one of the required programs for this career.[13]

Licenses and Certifications

Individuals working with patients and administering drugs need a license to practice as a physician. Other medical scientists do not need licenses or certifications if conducting research only.

Salary and Employment Outlook

In 2013, the average salary for all medical scientists was $79,840. The higher-paying positions were those working in pharmaceuticals and medicine manufacturing; the lower-paying positions were in colleges and universities and state jobs.[14]

The job outlook for employment as a medical scientist is projected to grow 13% from 2012 to 2022. This rate of growth is about as fast as the average for all occupations. As the aging population grows, the reliance on medicines will increase, which will affect the projected growth rate in the future.[13,14]

If your skill set includes critical thinking, complex problem-solving, judgment and decision-making, and scientific knowledge, a career as a medical scientist might be right for you. Keep in mind that you also should enjoy educational learning because this career will require an advanced degree.

Surgical Technology

Introduction

Surgical technicians or technologists are members of the operating team who assist the surgeon in delivering patient care. They are supervised by the surgeon, surgeon assistant, anesthesiologist, or registered nurse. They help set up the operating room, adjust lights and equipment, and pass supplies and instruments to surgeons.

Tasks that the surgical technician (surg tech) may perform include the following[15,16]:

- Prepare patients for surgery
- Provide assistance as needed to surgery team
- Count sponges, needles, and instruments before and after operations
- Sterilize equipment in the operating room
- Pass the instruments and supplies to the surgeon
- Hold retractors and cut sutures
- Position patients on the operating table
- Move patients to and from the operating room
- Suction surgical sites
- Restock operating room after surgery

Surgical technicians usually work in hospitals or surgery centers. Typically they work in 8- or 12-hour shifts. Although rewarding, the job can be somewhat demanding due to the shift work, long hours, and strength needed for positioning a patient or equipment. Surgical technicians need physical stamina due to the long hours of standing for extended periods.[15]

Education

The typical surgical technician is expected to either complete an associate degree or certification. The length of time needed for becoming a surgical technician ranges from several months to 2 years. Programs may be offered at community colleges, vocational schools, colleges, or universities, and even some hospitals provide the required education. Program accreditation is offered by the Commission on Accreditation of Allied Health Education Programs (CAAHEP) and the Accrediting Bureau of Health Education Schools (ABHES). For those interested in pursuing a career in surgical technology, taking courses in anatomy, biology, and medical terminology will be beneficial before beginning the program.[15,16]

Licenses and Certifications

There is no license required for individuals working as surgical technicians; however, certifications are available and may be required depending on the state. Two credentialing organizations offer certifications: the National Board of Surgical Technology and Surgical Assisting and the National Center for Competency Testing. Both of these organizations require individuals to complete continuing education to preserve certification.[15,16]

Salary and Employment Outlook

In 2013, the average salary for all surgical technicians was $42,720. The higher-paying positions were based on education rather than employment location. Individuals with an associate degree were paid the highest, and those with no degree were paid the lowest.[16]

Job security is an added bonus for individuals looking for careers as a surgical technician. The projected job outlook is expected to grow 30% from 2012 to 2022, which is significantly higher than the average for all occupations. One reason for the projected growth is based on the improved safety outcomes for surgeries, which results in more operations as treatment options for diseases and injuries.[15]

For individuals who enjoy direct patient care, but do not want the added responsibility and educational requirement associated with advanced training, surgical technicians are a great option. If you are a detail-oriented person who has a high stress tolerance and are flexible in your work scheduling, you might want to explore the career path for surgical technology. It is a fast-paced and rewarding career that is expected to provide many job opportunities for years to come.

Veterinary Medicine

Introduction

Veterinary medicine is a profession that blends health care and love of animals into a rewarding career. Individuals who love animals and the helping profession might enjoy this career because they are able to spend their time diagnosing and treating diseases in animals. Veterinarians work in laboratory environments, conduct urinalysis and blood counts, prepare and administer vaccines, and perform surgeries. Veterinarians work with all types of animals and perform a variety of tasks. Some of the job duties and tasks include the following.[17,18]

- Diagnose animals to detect disease or injuries
- Prescribe medications
- Perform surgery
- Suture and administer first aid
- Prepare vaccines and serums

- Consult, educate, and advise the community and animal owners about diseases and the risk to humans and other animals
- Assist in the birthing process for large animals such as horses or cows
- Euthanize animals when necessary

Veterinarians typically work in clinics but often travel to farms when problems arise with livestock. Some veterinarians work in research laboratories; others teach in colleges or universities. Many veterinarians have their own practice and work long hours due to emergencies. Although rewarding, the job of a veterinarian can also be physically demanding due to animal bites, scratches, risk of infection, and the lifting requirements associated with providing animal care.[17]

There are several avenues for veterinarians to consider when deciding on a career. Possibilities include small animal veterinarian, large animal veterinarian, emergency veterinarian, equine veterinarian, and veterinarian medicine doctor.[17]

Education

The required education for veterinary medicine depends on the career path chosen. For those seeking the veterinarian medicine doctor (VMD) or the doctor of veterinary medicine (DVM), the educational requirements are a doctoral degree from an accredited college of veterinary medicine. For specialty areas such as surgery, some additional education may be required beyond the doctoral degree. Students wishing to enter this area need strong skills in math, science, and animal science.[17,18]

For those interested in animal care, but not the advanced education or full responsibility of care, veterinary technician provides another option. These individuals work with veterinarians by assisting them with various tasks such as surgery. To become a veterinary technician, an associate degree, training in vocational schools, or on-the-job training is typically required. Some clinics may offer apprenticeship programs.[17]

Licenses and Certifications

Although the licensing requirements differ from state to state, all states in the United States require prospective veterinarians to pass the North American Veterinary Licensing Examination after the completion of an accredited degree program. In addition to the national examination, most states require a state examination as well.[17]

Certifications for specialties, such as surgery, are offered by the American Veterinary Medical Association. Although not required to practice veterinary medicine, the certification does indicate exceptional skills in particular areas. A residency program must be completed to sit for the certification examination.[17]

Salary and Employment Outlook

In 2013, the average salary for veterinarians was $86,640 and the average salary for veterinary technicians was $30,500. These numbers may vary depending on the type of work environment and specialties involved.[18]

The projected employment outlook for veterinarians is expected to grow at a rate of 12% from 2012 to 2022, which is about average for all jobs. One area in particular that may grow more than others is employment of veterinarians working as inspectors in the food supply to ensure health for both animals and humans.[17]

The projected employment outlook for veterinary technicians is expected to grow at a rate of 22% from 2012 to 2022, which is much higher than the average of all occupations. One explanation for the higher rate for technicians is because there are typically three or four technicians working for each veterinarian.[17]

To be an effective veterinarian or veterinary technician, one must enjoy working with animals. Although there is contact with humans, the primary work is with the animals. Individuals must also be able to tolerate the physical attributes such as lifting and handling of animals of all sizes. Like many careers in health care, the rewards will be plentiful.

References

1. Bureau of Labor Statistics, U.S. Department of Labor. Occupational outlook handbook, 2014–2015 edition. Health educator.
   http://www.bls.gov/ooh/community-and-social-service/health-educator.htm.
   Accessed July 30, 2014.

2. Health educator career information. About Careers.
   http://careerplanning.about.com/od/exploringoccupations/p/health-educator.htm.
   Accessed July 30, 2014.

3. What is a health educator? Society for Public Health Education.
   www.sophe.org/sophe/pdf/what_is_a_health_educator.pdf.
   Accessed July 30, 2014.

4. Summary report for:_21-1091.00-health educators. O*net Resource Center.
   www.onetonline.org/link/summary/21-1091.00.
   Accessed July 30, 2014.

5. Torpey E. Careers in forensics: analysis, evidence, and law. *Occupational Outlook Quarterly*. Bureau of Labor Statistics. 2009;53(1):14–19.
   www.bls.gov/careeroutlook/2009/spring/art02.pdf.
   Accessed August 18, 2014.

6. Bureau of Labor Statistics, U.S. Department of Labor. Occupational outlook handbook, 2014–2015 edition. Forensic science technicians.
   www.bls.gov/ooh/life-physical-and-social-science/forensic-science-technicians.htm.
   Accessed August 8, 2014.

7. Who are we? American Board of Forensic Document Examiners.
   https://www.abfde.org/index.html.
   Accessed August 18, 2014.

8. Bureau of Labor Statistics, U.S. Department of Labor. Occupational outlook handbook, 2014–2015 edition. Massage therapists.
   www.bls.gov/ooh/healthcare/massage-therapists.htm.
   Accessed August 19, 2014.

9. National Certification Board for Therapeutic Massage and Bodywork.
   www.ncbtmb.org.
   Accessed August 19, 2014.

10. Bureau of Labor Statistics, U.S. Department of Labor. Occupational outlook handbook, 2014–2015 edition. Psychologists.
    www.bls.gov/ooh/life-physical-and-social-science/psychologists.htm.
    Accessed August 20, 2014.

11. O*net Resource Center. Counseling Psychologists.
    http://onetonline.org/summary/19-3031.03.
    Accessed August 20, 2014.

12. American Psychological Association.
    www.apa.org.
    Accessed August 20, 2014.

13. Bureau of Labor Statistics, U.S. Department of Labor. Occupational outlook handbook, 2014–2015 edition. Medical scientist.
    www.bls.gov.ooh/life-physical-and-social-science/medical-scientist.htm.
    Accessed September 10, 2014.

14. Medical Scientist. O*net Resource Center.
www.onetonline.org/link/summary/19-1042.00.
Accessed September 10, 2014.

15. Bureau of Labor Statistics, U.S. Department of
Labor. Occupational outlook handbook, 2014–2015
edition. Surgical technologists.
www.bls.gov/ooh/healthcare/surgical-technologists.
htm.
Accessed September 10, 2014.

16. Surgical technologists. O*net Resource Center.
www.onetonline.org/lin/summary/29-2055.00.
Accessed September 10, 2014.

17. Bureau of Labor Statistics, U.S. Department of
Labor. Occupational outlook handbook, 2014–2015
edition. Veterinarians.
www.bls.gov/ooh/healthcare/veterinarians.htm.
Accessed September 11, 2014.

18. Veterinarians. O*net Resource Center.
www.onetonline.org/link/summary/29-1131.00.
Accessed September 11, 2014.

INDEX

Note: Page numbers followed by **b**, **f** or **t** refer to boxes, figures, or tables, respectively.

A

AAA. *See* American Academy of Audiology (AAA)

AABB. *See* American Association of Blood Banks (AABB)

AAC. *See* Augmentative and alternative communication (AAC)

AACP. *See* American Association of Colleges of Pharmacy (AACP)

AAMA. *See* American Association of Medical Assistants (AAMA)

AAMC. *See* Association of American Medical Colleges (AAMC)

AARC. *See* American Association for Respiratory Care (AARC)

AART. *See* American Association of Radiologic Technicians (AART)

ABG. *See* Arterial blood gas (ABG)

ABHES. *See* Accrediting Bureau of Health Education Schools (ABHES)

Abortion, as ethical issue in health care, 341

Academic settings, athletics trainers and, 118

Academy of Dispensing Audiologists (ADA), 129

Academy of Nutrition and Dietetics, Dietetics Practice Groups (DPG), 169

Accidental Death and Disability: The Neglected Disease of Modern Society (Report), 175

Accountability
   health-care teams and, 353
   as professional trait, 344–345

Accreditation
   allied health professionals and, 57
   audiology and, 136
   definition of, 267
   forensic science and, 366
   health information management and, 191
   health related disciplines and, 365
   health services management and, 202–203
   massage therapy and, 367
   physical therapy and, 241–242
   process of, 196, 207
   radiography and, 262
   veterinary medicine and, 370–371

Accreditation Council for Education in Nutrition and Dietetics, 169

Accreditation Review Commission on Education for the Physician Assistant, Inc. (ARC-PA), 250

Accrediting body representative, 188

Accrediting Bureau of Health Education Schools (ABHES), 212, 217

ACPE. *See* American Council on Pharmaceutical Education (ACPE)

Acquired communication disorder, 324, 332

Activities of daily-life, 221, 230

Acute care, 15

Acute-care hospital, physical therapy in, 236–237

ADA. *See* Academy of Dispensing Audiologists (ADA); American Dental Association (ADA); American Disabilities Act of 1990 (ADA)

Addams, Jane, 314

Addiction, 278, 288

ADIME. *See* Assessment, diagnosis, intervention, monitoring, and evaluation (ADIME)

Administrative health-related career, characteristics of, 7, 7f

ADN. *See* Associate degree registered nurse (ADN)

Adult family homes, 30

Advanced EMTs (AEMTs), 173, 182

Advanced practice nurse, role of, 96

Advocacy, 291, 297, 321

AEMTs. *See* Advanced EMTs (AEMTs)

Affiliated health careers, characteristics of, 7, 7f

Affordable Care Act, 22, 46, 81, 83, 221, 225, 230

AHIMA. *See* American Health Information Management Association (AHIMA)

AIDS awareness symbol, 18

AIDS patients facilities, 30

AIHC. *See* American Interprofessional Health Collaborative (AIHC)

AIHS. *See* Association of Interprofessional Healthcare Students (AIHS)

Alcott, Louisa May, 91

Allied health professions
   definition of, 55–56, 60
   education and, 57
   employment trends of, 57–58
   not identified in textbook, 56b
   opportunities and challenges in, 58–59
   origin of, 56–57, 56f
   professional associations and relationships, 57
   salaries and job settings for, 58
   sampling of fields and statistics, 59t

Allied Health Professions Personnel Training Act of 1967, 56

Allopathic medicine, 79

Alzheimer patients' facilities, 30

Ambulance technicians, 175

Ambulance volantes, 174, 183

Ambulatory care facilities
   description and definition of, 28–29, 32

history of, 29

types of, 29

Ambulatory surgical center (ASC), 29

Ameigh, Rex, 264

American Academy of Audiology (AAA), 129, 136

American Association for Respiratory Care (AARC), 304, 309

American Association of Blood Banks (AABB), 146

American Association of Colleges of Pharmacy (AACP), 110

American Association of Medical Assistants (AAMA), 211, 217

American Association of Radiologic Technicians (AART), 259

American Auditory Society, 136

American College of Health Care Administrators (ACHCA), 207

American Council on Pharmaceutical Education (ACPE), 110

American Counseling Association, 292

American Dental Association (ADA), 151, 157

American Dental Education Association, 158

American Disabilities Act of 1990 (ADA), 230

American Health Information Management Association (AHIMA), 188, 196

American Hospital Association (AHA), 17, 23, 32

American Interprofessional Health Collaborative (AIHC), 72

American League for Nursing, 99

American Medical Association (AMA), 52, 61, 78

American Medical Technologists (AMT), 146, 211, 217

American Nurses Association, 52, 99

American Occupational Therapy Association (AOTA), 221, 223, 226

American Physical Therapy Association (APTA), 235–236

American Recovery and Reinvestment Act (ARRA), 190

American Registry of Medical Assistants (ARMA), 210, 217

American Registry of Radiologic Technologists (ARRT), 261, 272, 276

American Rehabilitation Counseling Association (ARCA), 298

American Society for Clinical Laboratory Science (ASCLS), 146

American Society of Clinical Pathologists (ASCP), 138

American Society of Radiologic Technologists (ASRT), 259, 261, 267, 276

American Society of Superintendents of Training Schools for Nurses, 92

American Society of X-Ray Technician (ASXT), 259

American Speech-Language-Hearing Association (ASHA), 136, 332

Americans with Disabilities Act, 225

American Therapeutic Recreation Association (ATRA), 279, 281, 288

AMT. *See* American Medical Technologists (AMT)

Anatomy, 238, 244

Ancillary and paramedical workers, 56

Angioplasty, 264

Antibiotics, development of, 47–48

AOTA. *See* American Occupational Therapy Association (AOTA)

APIE process. *See* Assessment, planning, implementation, and evaluation (APIE) process

Apothecary, 50, 50f, 52

APTA's Guide to Physical Therapist Practice, 236

ARCA. *See* American Rehabilitation Counseling Association (ARCA)

ARC-PA. *See* Accreditation Review Commission on Education for the Physician Assistant, Inc. (ARC-PA)

ARMA. *See* American Registry of Medical Assistants (ARMA)

Armstrong, Missy, 280

ARRA. *See* American Recovery and Reinvestment Act (ARRA)

ARRT. *See* American Registry of Radiologic Technologists (ARRT)

Arterial blood gas (ABG), 302, 310

Artificial femoral head, invention of, 16

Arts and Crafts Movement, 221, 222

ASAHP. *See* Association of Schools of Allied Health Professions (ASAHP)

ASC. *See* Ambulatory surgical center (ASC)

ASCLS. *See* American Society for Clinical Laboratory Science (ASCLS)

ASCP. *See* American Society of Clinical Pathologists (ASCP)

ASHA. *See* American Speech-Language-Hearing Association (ASHA)

Ashbee, Charles Robert, 221

ASRT. *See* American Society of Radiologic Technologists (ASRT)

Assessment, diagnosis, intervention, monitoring, and evaluation (ADIME), 164, 165f, 169

Assessment, planning, implementation, and evaluation (APIE) process, 278, 288

Assessment(s)
  definition of, 88, 99
  of hospice services, 87
  psychosocial, 313, 315, 321
  self-, 8, 345

Assisted-living facilities, 30

Assistive technology (AT), 290, 292, 297

Associate degree registered nurse (ADN), 96

Association of American Medical Colleges (AAMC), 79

Association of Collegiate Schools of Nursing, 92

Association of Interprofessional Healthcare Students (AIHS), 72

Association of Schools of Allied Health Professions (ASAHP), 60–61

ASXT. *See* American Society of X-Ray Technician (ASXT)

Athletic trainers (ATs)
  attributes of, 121
  certification and licensure, 120–121
  continuing education and, 122
  "A Day in the Life" of, 115–116
  education and, 119–120
  employment by industry of, 120t
  salary of, 120
  scope of practice for, 117–118, 118t
  vs. personal trainer (trainer), 117b
  work settings for, 118–119b

Athletic training. *See also* Athletic trainers (ATs)
  challenges in, 121–122
  introduction to, 117
  state regulation of, 120–121
  trends in, 121
  working with medical personnel, 122

Athletic Training Education Competencies, 120

ATRA. *See* American Therapeutic Recreation Association (ATRA)

ATs. *See* Athletic trainers (ATs)

Attendance, professional ethics and, 339

Attire, professional ethics and, 340

Attitude, professional ethics and, 339

AuD. *See* Doctor of audiology (AuD)

Audiologists
  characteristics of, 133
  "A Day in the Life" of, 127–128
  education and, 130–131
  licensure, 132
  role of, 133–134t, 135
  salary of, 132
  scope of practice for, 129–130
  specialties, work settings, and roles, 133–134t

Audiology. *See also* Audiologists; Hearing
  case study, 134–135
  challenges in, 132
  description of, 128–129
  introduction to, 128–129
  trends in, 132

Augmentative and alternative communication (AAC), 327

Aural rehabilitation, 328

Autonomous practice, 236, 244

Autonomy, 291, 297, 338

Avoiding, as conflict management strategy, 357

B

Baccalaureate-prepared social workers, 319

Bachelor of Science degree in nursing (BSN), 96

Banting, Frederick, 15

Barter system, 33, 34f

Barton, Clara, 91

Beneficence, as principle of ethics in health care, 338

Best, Charles, 15

Bickerdyke, Mary Ann, 91

Bilik, S. E., 117

Biopsychosocial model, 82, 83

Blogs, on dietetics, 170

Blood banks/blood banking, 29. *See also* Immunohematology (blood bank)

Blue Cross Blue Shield, 15, 35

Board-certified specialist in dietetics, 167

Board examinations, respiratory care and, 304, 310

Board of Certification (BOC), 119, 120, 125, 169

Body systems
  cardiovascular and pulmonary, 241
  lymphatic and integumentary, 241
  musculoskeletal, 240
  neuromuscular, 240–241
  physical therapy and, 239–240, 244

Bone densitometry, 260, 267

BSN. *See* Bachelor of science degree in nursing (BSN)

Burkett, Tony, 142

C

CAAHEP. *See* Commission on Accreditation of Allied Health Education Programs (CAAHEP)

CAATE. *See* Commission on Accreditation of Athletic Training Education (CAATE)

CAHR. *See* Council for the Advancement of Hospital Recreation (CAHR)

Cancer treatment, radiation therapy in, 271

Canfield, Norton, 129

Cantor, Eddie, 15

Capitation, 81, 83

Capnography, 175, 183

Cardiopulmonary, 303, 310

Cardiopulmonary resuscitation (CPR), 175, 183

Cardiopulmonary system, 303

Cardioscope/defibrillator, 175, 176f, 183

Cardiovascular interventional technologist (CVIT), 264, 267

Cardiovascular intervention technology, 260, 267

CARE. *See* Medical Imaging and Radiation Therapy (CARE)

Care, definition of, 99

Career in health professions
  aptitude and, 5–6

characteristics of specific health-care
professions, 8
expectations of, 3–4
health-care and, 6–7, 6f, 7f
introduction to, 3
personality and, 4–5
skills and, 4
work interests and, 5
work values and, 5
Care of prisoners, as ethical issue in health care, 342
Care plan, 87
Care team, 70, 71
CARF. *See* Commission on Accreditation
of Rehabilitation Facilities (CARF)
Carhart, Raymond, 129
Case management, 291, 297, 316, 321
Case study
athletic training preparing for lacrosse team,
123–124
audiologists working with other team
members, 134–135
dentists and interprofessional collaboration, 156
emergency services integration with other
services, 181
ethical issues and level of nursing care, 97–98
ethics in health-care, 346
health-care team of clinical laboratory
scientists and physician, 144
health information managers and plan of care,
194–195
health professionals as part
of interprofessional team, 71
information services managers handling
patient care, 205–206
interprofessional care, 66
medical assistants and interpersonal
collaboration, 215–216
occupational therapists and interprofessional
collaboration, 228–229
physical therapists and interprofessional
collaboration, 243
physician assistants involvement with health
professionals, 253
radiation therapists implementation
of therapy plan, 273–274
radiographs of lumbar spine, 266
recreational therapists therapy treatment,
286–287
refilling medications for multiple chronic
problems patients, 109
respiratory therapists interaction with other
disciplines, 309
role of doctors and health professions
in health care, 82
social workers and interprofessional
collaboration, 320
speech-language pathologists and success
in therapy, 331
treating type 2 diabetes mellitus, 168

CCC. *See* Certificate of Clinical Competence
(CCC)
Centers for Medicare and Medicaid Services, 23,
32, 40
Certificate of Clinical Competence (CCC),
329, 332
Certification. *See also* Accreditation
athletic trainers and, 120–121
Board of Certification (BOC), 119, 120,
125, 169
clinical laboratory scientist and, 139, 140, 145
definition of, 145
forensic science and, 366
health educators and, 366
health information management and, 191
health services management and, 202–203
massage therapy and, 367
medical scientists and, 369
national, 124
process of, 196, 207
psychology and, 368
recreational therapist and, 283
surgical technicians and, 369–370
veterinary medicine and, 370–371
Certified medical assistant (CMA), 212, 217
Certified pulmonary function technologist
(CPFT), 307
Certified respiratory therapist (CRT), 305, 306
Certified therapeutic recreation specialist
(CTRS), 278, 287
CHAIIM. *See* Commission on Accreditation
for Health Information and Informatics
Management Education (CHAIIM)
Chain, Ernst Boris, 15
CHAMPUS. *See* Civilian Health and Medical
Program of the Uninformed Services
(CHAMPUS)
Charnley, John, 16
Chemistry, forensic science and, 366
Cherkasky, Martin, 64
Child, family, and school social workers,
316, 319
Child and family social worker, 321
Children's Health Insurance Program (CHIP),
36, 38f, 40
CHIP. *See* Children's Health Insurance
Program (CHIP)
Chronic disease management, 278, 288
Cigarette smoking, report on health and, 16f
Civilian Health and Medical Program of the
Uninformed Services (CHAMPUS), 38
Clark, Barney, 18
Client, definition of, 315
Clinical audiologist, 127–128
Clinical chemistry
in clinical laboratory science, 139
definition of, 145
role of clinical laboratory scientist in,
141–142

Clinical laboratory science. *See also* Clinical
laboratory scientist (CLS)
areas of specialization, 139
case study, 144
challenges in, 141
introduction to, 138–139
required characteristics in, 141
trends in, 140–141
Clinical laboratory scientist (CLS)
baccalaureate degree and, 140
certification/license, 139, 140, 145
continuing education and, 140
"A Day in the Life" of, 137–138
description of, 145
education and, 139–140
interaction with health professionals, 144
role in clinical chemistry, 141–142
role in clinical hematology, 142
role in immunohematology, 142
role in immunology, 143
role in microbiology, 143–144
role in molecular biology, 144
salary for, 140
scope of practice for, 139
Clinical laboratory technician, 140, 145
Clinical nurse specialist (CNS), 93
Clinical pharmacy practitioner, 105–106, 110
Clinical Simulation Examination (CSE), 305
Clinical Social Work Association (CSWA), 322
Clinical social workers, 318–319
Clinicians. *See* Providers
Cloning, 18
CLS. *See* Clinical laboratory scientist (CLS)
CMA. *See* Certified medical assistant
(CMA)
CME. *See* Continuing medical education
(CME)
CNS. *See* Clinical nurse specialist (CNS)
COA. *See* Cost of attendance (COA)
Cochlear implants, 128, 136
CODA. *See* Committee on Dental Accreditation
(CODA)
Code of ethics, 359
CoEMSP. *See* Committee on Accreditation of
Educational Programs for EMS Professions
(CoEMSP)
Cohen, Dotty, 121
Collaboration, 252, 357
Collaborative environment
clear roles and, 69
effective communication and, 68–69
mutual trust and, 69
support and, 69
values and, 69–70
Commission on Accreditation for Health
Information and Informatics Management
Education (CHAIIM), 191, 196
Commission on Accreditation of Allied Health
Education Professions, 175

Commission on Accreditation of Allied Health Education Programs (CAAHEP), 57, 61, 183, 212, 217

Commission on Accreditation of Athletic Training Education (CAATE), 119–120, 125

Commission on Accreditation of Rehabilitation Facilities (CARF), 279, 288

Commission on Rehabilitation Counselor Certification (CRCC), 298

Commission on the Health Needs of the Nation, 56

Committee on Accreditation of Educational Programs for EMS Professions (CoEMSP), 175, 183

Committee on Dental Accreditation (CODA), 150

Communication. *See also* Communication aspects
  health-care teams and, 353
  nonverbal, 363
  skills, as professional trait, 344, 355

Communication aspects
  language and, 325–326
  speech and, 324–325

Communication disorder, 324, 332

Community-based experience, interprofessional education models and, 68

Community hospitals, 27, 32

Community integration, 288

Community nutrition, 162, 169

Community paramedicine, 174, 179, 182, 183

Community pharmacy, 103, 110

Community skills, 279, 288

Competence, professional ethics and, 339–340

Competing, as conflict management strategy, 357

Competition, teams and, 359

Compromising, as conflict management strategy, 357

Computed tomography (CT), 258, 260, 262, 267, 270

Computed tomography (CT) technologist, 263

Conflict resolution skills, 356

Consultant/technical authority, 66

Consumers, 291, 292, 295, 297

Continuing education, definition of, 145

Continuing medical education (CME), 183, 254

Conventional level, in moral development, 338–339

Coordinated dietetics program (CP), 161, 169

Coordinator of effort/point of contact, 66

CORE. *See* Council on Rehabilitation Education (CORE)

Cost of attendance (COA), 79

Council for the Advancement of Hospital Recreation (CAHR), 281

Council on Academic Accreditation in Audiology and Speech-Language Pathology, 328

Council on Rehabilitation Education (CORE), 298

Council on Social Work Education, 322

CP. *See* Coordinated dietetics program (CP)

CPFT. *See* Certified pulmonary function technologist (CPFT)

CPR. *See* Cardiopulmonary resuscitation (CPR)

CRCC. *See* Commission on Rehabilitation Counselor Certification (CRCC)

Creativity, collaborative environment and, 69

Credentials/credentialing
  Athletic training/athletic trainers and, 120–121
  audiologists and, 132
  Board of Certification (BOC), 119, 120, 125, 169
  clinical laboratory science and, 139, 140, 145
  definition of, 95, 99
  as document or certification, 99
  forensic science and, 366
  health information management and, 191
  health services management and, 202–203, 207
  medical science and, 369
  physician assistants and, 251
  process, 194, 196, 267
  psychology and, 368
  radiography and, 259
  speech language pathologists and, 329

Critical-care therapists, role of, 306–307

CRT. *See* Certified respiratory therapist (CRT)

CSE. *See* Clinical Simulation Examination (CSE)

CSWA. *See* Clinical Social Work Association (CSWA)

CT. *See* Computed tomography (CT)

CTRS. *See* Certified therapeutic recreation specialist (CTRS)

CT technologist. *See* Computed tomography (CT) technologist

Cultural awareness, didactic model and, 68

Cumming, Kate, 91

Cummings, Doyle, 106

Curie, Marie, 14

Curiosity, collaborative environment and, 70

CVIT. *See* Cardiovascular interventional technologist (CVIT)

Cytotechnologist, 57, 60

D

Daily-life activities, 221, 230

Dally, Clarence Madison, 259

DAT. *See* Differential Aptitude Test (DAT)

Davis, Michael, 200

DDS. *See* Doctor of dental surgery (DDS)

Deductible, 35

Delegation of Services Agreement, 249

Dental caries, 151, 151f, 157

Dental hospital consultation, 150, 157

Dental hygienist, 151, 155, 157

Dental professions. *See also* Dentist, general
  case study, 156
  challenges in, 153–154
  dental diseases and conditions, 151
  introduction to, 150–151
  trends in, 153

Dental specialist, 155–156, 157

Dentist, general
  "A Day in the Life" of, 149–150
  description of, 157
  education and, 152–153
  evaluation and treatment of oral health, 156
  qualities of, 154
  role of, 154–155, 156
  salary of, 154
  scopes of practice for, 151–152

Department of Health and Human Services (DHHS), 38, 179, 183–184, 196, 208

Developmental communication disorder, 324, 332

DHHS. *See* Department of Health and Human Services (DHHS)

DI. *See* Dietetic internship program (DI)

Diagnosis, 238, 244

Dialysis machine, 16f

Dialysis units, 29

Didactic program in dietetics (DPD), 161, 162, 169

Didactic programs, 67–68

Dietetic internship program (DI), 161, 169

Dietetics. *See also* Registered dietitians (RDs)/ registered dietitian nutritionists (RDNs)
  case study, 168
  challenges in, 164
  introduction to, 160–161
  role of board-certified specialist in, 167
  trends in, 163

Differential Aptitude Test (DAT), 6

Disability accommodations, 295, 297

Disability management, 292, 297

Discipline(s)
  collaborative environment and, 69
  in interprofessional teams, 65–67

Discretion, professional ethics and, 340, 347

District hospitals. *See* Rural hospitals

Diverse groups, health-care teams and, 358

Dix, Dorothea, 91

DMD. *See* Doctor of dental medicine (DMD)

DNP. *See* Doctor of nursing practice (DNP)

DNSc. *See* Doctor of nursing science (DNSc)

DO. *See* Doctor of osteopathic medicine (DO)

Dock, Lavinia, 88

Doctorally prepared nurse, role of, 97

Doctor of audiology (AuD), 130, 136

Doctor of dental medicine (DMD), 152

Doctor of dental surgery (DDS), 152

Doctor of nursing practice (DNP), 97

Doctor of nursing science (DNSc), 97

Doctor of osteopathic medicine (DO), 259, 267
Doctor of science in nursing (DScN), 97
DPD. *See* Didactic program in dietetics (DPD)
Drug rehabilitation centers, 30
Drugs, generic *vs.* brand-name, 17
DScN. *See* Doctor of science in nursing (DScN)
Dye, Deanna, 239
Dysphagia, speech-language pathologist and, 328, 332

E

Early evidence-based period, medicine in, 47
ECG. *See* Electrocardiogram (ECG)
Economic Opportunity Act of 1964, 21
Economy
    in early 1970s, 18
    during the Great Depression, 20
    health-care environment and, 11
ED. *See* Emergency department (ED)
Edison, Thomas Alva, 259
Educational standards and accreditation, of allied health professions, 57
EEG technician, 57, 60
EENEP. *See* Expanded Food and Nutrition Education Program (EENEP)
Effective communication, as element of collaborative environment, 68–69
EHRs. *See* Electronic health records (EHRs)
Electrocardiogram (ECG), 173, 182
Electronic health records (EHRs), 67, 81, 83, 188, 190, 196
Electronic medical record (EMR), 211
Electrophysiological evaluation, 131, 136
Emergency care unit, 29
Emergency department (ED), 258
Emergency medical services (EMS). *See also* Paramedics
    abilities and skills in, 181
    case study, 181
    continuing education and, 180
    current trends in, 179
    education and, 177–178
    interaction with emergency department, 181
    introduction and description of, 173–174
    profession of, 182
    role of emergency medical technicians, 179–180
    salaries and career opportunities, 178–179
    scope of practice for, 176–177
Emergency medical technicians (EMTs), 173, 182
Emotional intelligence, 95
Emotional stability, as professional trait, 344, 347
Empathy, as professional trait, 344, 347
Employer-sponsored insurance, 34–35, 35f, 40
Employment trends, allied health professions and, 57–58, 58f
Empowerment, 291, 297

EMR. *See* Electronic medical record (EMR)
EMS. *See* Emergency medical services (EMS)
EMTs. *See* Emergency medical technicians (EMTs)
End-of-life decisions, as ethical issue in health care, 341
Endotracheal intubation, 173, 182
Endotracheal tube, 302, 310
End-state renal disease (ESRD), 29
Engel, George, 82, 83
Entertainment/performing arts settings, athletics trainers and, 119
Entry point/referral channel, 66
ESRD. *See* End-state renal disease (ESRD)
Ethical decision, guidelines for making, 359–360
Ethical dilemma, 359
Ethics in health-care
    case study, 346
    definition of, 338, 347
    individual, 338–339
    individual ethics *vs.* organizational ethics, 359
    introduction to, 337–338
    issues of, 337, 340–344
    professionals and, 337–338, 339–340
    professional traits and, 344–345
    role of, 338
    values and value conflicts, 345–346
Euthanasia, as ethical issue in health care, 341
Evaluate, 234, 244
Examination, 239, 244
Exertion tolerance, 234, 244
Expanded Food and Nutrition Education Program (EENEP), 167
Experimental drug, as ethical issue in health care, 342
Externship, 212

F

Family and Medical Leave Act, 19
Family medicine, 46, 52
Fauchard, Pierre, 150
Fedde, Elizabeth, 90
Federal government, health care and, 20–21
Feedback, effective, 356
Fellowship, 80, 83
Fidelity, in delivering health care, 338
Firearms identification, forensic science and, 366
First Aider, 117
Flanagan, Katie Walsh, 123
Fleming, Sir Alexander, 15
Flexibility, as professional trait, 344
Flexner, Abraham, 78
Flexner Report, 56, 78, 92
Fliedner, Theodore, 89
Florey, Sir Howard Walter, 15
Fluency, 325
Flu epidemic, 15
Fluoroscope, 259

Food nutrition labels, 18f
Food-service systems management, 166, 169
Ford, John, 29
Forensic rehabilitation, 298
Forensic science
    education and, 366
    introduction to, 366
    licenses and certifications, 366
    salary and employment outlook, 366–367
Formularies, 108
For profit *vs.* not for profit hospitals, 26–27
Freshley-Lebkuecher, Amy, 264
Fry, Elizabeth, 89
Function, 278, 288
Functional activities, 235, 244

G

Gardasil vaccine, 19
General acute-care therapist, role of, 306
General dentist, 151, 157
General hospitals. *See* Community hospitals
General pediatrics, 46
Generic drug, 17, 23
Genetic intervention, as ethical issue in health care, 342
Genetics, health care and, 11, 13f, 23
Gingival tissue, 151, 157
Glacken, Joan, 142
Goals
    of health-care environment, 14
    health-care teams and lack of, 358
Goldmark Report, 92
Government settings, athletics trainers and, 119
GPA. *See* Grade point average (GPA)
Grade point average (GPA), 106
Great Depression, 17, 20, 21, 35, 91–92
Greer, Annette, 97
Greiger-Brown and colleagues report, 95
Group health insurance plans, 15
Group homes, 30
Group insurance. *See* Employer-sponsored insurance

H

Hall, Herbert, 222
Harper, Jennifer, 273
Health care. *See* Career in health professions; Ethics in health care; Health-care environment; Health-care facilities; Health-care providers; Health-care services; Health-care teams; Professional traits in health care
Health-care administrators, 200, 207
Health Care Education Reconciliation Act of 2010, 19, 21, 23
Health-care environment
    definition and elements of, 11
    determinants of, 13f

education and, 11
federal initiatives, 20–21
goals associated with, 14
health-care reform and, 21–22
heredity and, 12, 13f
historical events and, 14–19
lifestyles, behaviors, and, 12, 13f
medical services and, 13–14
morbidity, mortality, and, 19–20, 20f
natural and human-made environmental
    issues, 12, 13f
socioeconomics and, 12, 13f
war on poverty, 21–22, 64
Health career testing, resources on, 9
Health-care facilities
    ambulatory care facilities, 28–29
    home health and hospice, 30–31
    hospitals, 25–28
    medical and diagnostic laboratories, 31
    nursing and residential care facilities, 29–30
    physician and dental offices, 30
Health-care providers
    billing of, 39
    World War II and, 15
Health-care reform, health-care environment
    and, 21–22
Health-care services. See also Health-care
    services funding
    Children's Health Insurance Program, 36,
        38f, 40
    contact with clinical aspects of patient
        care, 205
    funding sources, 34–35
    managed care, 35–36, 36f, 40
    Medicaid, 36, 37f
    Medicare, 36, 37f
    Medigap, 36
    Nation's Health Dollar, 38
    paying for, 33–34, 34f
    provider billing, 38–39
    retired military and, 38
    Ryan White Program, 37
    Snyder Act and, 37
    uninsured and, 38
    Workers' compensation and, 38
    Health-care settings, athletics trainers and, 118
Health-care social workers, 316, 321
Health-care teams
    accountability and, 353
    cancer center, case application, 353–354
    communication and, 353
    ethics in, 359–360
    exercises, 360–362
    high-performing, characteristics of, 349–350
    interpersonal skills of, 355–358
    obstacles and, 358–359
    psychological, personal and professional
        characteristics of, 351–353
    purpose and goal of, 351

structure, 350–351
    trauma center, case application, 350
    women's center, case application, 352
Health-care workforce, 81
Health Center Program, 21
Health educators
    education of, 366
    licenses and certifications, 365
    roles and tasks, 365
    salary and employment outlook, 365–366,
        366–367
Health informatics, 191
Health information management (HIM). See also
    Health information managers
    accreditation and certification, 191
    case study, 194–195
    challenges in, 192
    contact with other disciplines, 194
    description, 188–190, 196
    job environment for, 190
    knowledge/skills for, 192
    role of associate degree-prepared health
        information technician, 192–193
    trends in, 191–192
Health information managers
    "A Day in the Life" of, 188
    definition of, 188
    education and, 191
    role of baccalaureate-prepared, 193
    role of doctoral-prepared, 194
    role of master's-prepared, 193–194
    salary for, 191
    scope of practice of, 190–191
Health information technician (HIT), 192–193,
    196
Health Information Technology for Economic
    and Clinical Health (HITECH) Act, 190
Health Insurance Portability and Accountability
    Act (HIPAA), 18, 19, 196, 200, 207
Health maintenance organizations (HMOs), 35
The Health Manager's Website, 208
Health Manpower Education Initiative Awards
    (HMEIA), 64
Health-related professions
    forensic science, 366–367
    health education, 365–366
    massage therapy, 367
    medical science, 368–369
    psychology, 367–368
    surgical technology, 369–370
    veterinary medicine, 370–371
Health Resources and Services Administration
    (HRSA), 38, 99
    Bureau of Health Professions/Nursing, 99
    HIV/AIDS Bureau, 41
Health Service Act, 21
Health services management. See also Health
    services managers
    accreditation and certification, 202–203

case study, 205–206
    challenges in, 203
    introduction to, 200–201
    trends in, 203
Health services managers
    baccalaureate-prepared, role of, 203–204
    "A Day in the Life" of, 199–200
    doctoral-prepared, role of, 205
    education and, 202
    job environment for, 201, 201f
    master's-prepared, role of, 204
    medical, role of, 204–205
    as professionals, 200, 207
    salary for, 203
    scope of practice of, 201–202
    skills for, 203
Hearing. See also Hearing loss
    basic and applied research, 130
    conservation, 130
    evaluation of, 127, 136
    expertise, 130
    intraoperative neurophysiological
        monitoring, 130
    National and Nutrition Examination Survey
        and, 132
    speech-language pathologists and, 327–328
Hearing aids, 127, 136
Hearing loss
    definition of, 136
    identification of, 129
    nonmedical treatment of, 129–130
Heart implantation, 18
Hematology, 139, 145
Heredity, 11, 13f
Hesse, Michelle, 163
HHS. See Department of Health and Human
    Services (DHHS)
Higher education institutions
    barriers to effective interprofessional teams, 71
    interprofessional health-care practice and, 70
Hill-Burton Act, 21
HIM. See Health information management
    (HIM)
HIPAA. See Health Insurance Portability
    and Accountability Act (HIPAA)
Hippocrates, 46f, 47, 52
Hippocratic oath, 45, 46f
Hip replacement surgery, 16
Histologic technician, 57, 60
HITECH Act. See Health Information
    Technology for Economic and Clinical
    Health (HITECH) Act
HIV infection, identification of, 17, 18
HMEIA. See Health Manpower Education
    Initiative Awards (HMEIA)
HMOs. See Health maintenance organizations
    (HMOs)
Holistic approach, 65, 291, 297
Holloway, Linda, 294

Home care therapists, role of, 308
Home health, physical therapy in, 237
Home health agencies, 30–31
Honesty
    collaborative environment and, 69
    health care and, 343–344
Hospices/ hospice care, 30–31, 87–88
Hospital Administration: A Career; The Need
    of Trained Executives for a Billion Dollar
    Business, and How They May Be Trained
    (Davis), 200
Hospital pharmacy, 103–104, 110
Hospitals. *See also* Hospital structures; Hospital
    types
    categorization of, 27
    development of, 25
    U.S. hospitals in 2014, 27f
Hospital structures, 25–26
    administrative division of the support
        department, 26
    administrator, 26
    ancillary department, 26
    environment division of the support
        department, 26
    financial department, 26
    governing body, 26
    medical staff department, 26
    nursing department, 26
    support department, 26
Hospital types
    community hospitals, 27
    for profit *vs.* not for profit, 26–27
    public hospitals, 27
    rural hospitals, 27–28
    specialized hospitals, 28
    teaching hospitals, 27
HRSA. *See* Health Resources and Services
    Administration (HRSA)
Human immunodeficiency virus/acquired
    immunodeficiency syndrome, as ethical
    issue in health care, 341
Human-made environmental issues, health-care
    environment and, 11–12, 13f
Humility, collaborative environment and, 70

I

IARP. *See* International Association of
    Rehabilitation Professionals (IARP)
IASWG. *See* International Association for Social
    Work with Groups, Inc. (IASWG)
ICD-10 codes, 193f, 200, 207
IDEA. *See* Individuals with Disabilities
    Education Improvement Act (IDEA)
IEP. *See* Individual educational plan (IEP);
    Individual educational program (IEP)
IHTD. *See* Institute for Health Team
    Development (IHTD)
Image-guided radiation therapy, 270

Imaging centers, 29
Immunohematology (blood bank), 139, 145
Immunology, 139, 145
Inclusion, 291, 297
Individual educational plan (IEP), 230
Individual educational program (IEP), 220
Individual ethics, 338–339
Individuals with Disabilities Education
    Improvement Act (IDEA), 225
Industry settings, athletics trainers and, 119
Informatics, 191
Information communicator, 67
Inhalation therapy. *See* Respiratory therapists
Institute for Health Team Development
    (IHTD), 64
Institute of Medicine (IOM), 23
Institute of Medicine Committee on Quality
    of Heath Care in America, 67
Instrumental activities of daily living, 230
Insurance
    employer-sponsored, 34–35, 35f, 40
    private-pay, 35, 40
Integrated care, 82, 83
Integration, 291, 297
Interdisciplinary education, 64
Internal medicine, 46
International Association for Social Work
    with Groups, Inc. (IASWG), 322
International Association of Rehabilitation
    Professionals (IARP), 298
International Society of Radiographers and
    Radiologic Technologists (ISRRT), 267
Internship, 200, 207
Interpersonal skills, 353, 355–358
Interprofessional care. *See also* Interprofessional
    education
    definition of, 63–64
    disciplines in, 65–67
    holistic approach, 65
    origin of, 63–64
    practice, benefits of, 70
    teams, 64–65, 70–71
Interprofessional collaboration. *See*
    Interprofessional care
Interprofessional education
    community-based experience model, 68
    definition of, 63–64
    didactic program model, 67–68
    interprofessional simulation experience
        model, 68
Interprofessional health-care practice, benefits
    of, 70
Interprofessional practice. *See* Interprofessional
    care
Interprofessional simulation experience, 68
Interprofessional teams, barriers to effective, 70–71
Interventions, 235, 244
Intraoperative neurophysiological monitoring,
    129, 130, 136

Intuition, 360
In vitro fertilization, as ethical issue in health
    care, 341
Iron Lung, 15
Irons, Thomas G., 81
ISRRT. *See* International Society of
    Radiographers and Radiologic
    Technologists (ISRRT)

J

JADA. *See* Journal of the American Dental
    Association (JADA)
Jerman, Eddy C., 259
Johnson, Lyndon, 21
The Joint Commission, 32, 288
Joint Review Committee on Education in
    Radiologic Technology (JRCERT), 267,
    272, 276
Journal of the American Dental Association
    (JADA), 157
JRCERT. *See* Joint Review Committee on
    Education in Radiologic Technology
    (JRCERT)
Justice, as principle of ethics in health care, 338

K

Kaiserwerth
    influence on nurse education in US, 89–90
    Nightingale and, 89
    "Kaiserwerth Motherhouse" (nursing school), 89
Keely, Jennifer, 307
Kennel, Julie, 163
Keogh Hoss, Mary Ann, 280
Kidney dialysis machine, 16
Kinesiology, 238, 244
Kohlberg, Lawrence, 338

L

Laboratory centers, 29
Landsteiner, Karl, 14f
Language, 325–326, 332, 340
Larrey, Baron Dominique Jean, 174, 174f
Laryngoscopy, 179, 183
Leadership skills, 357–358
Legal/ethical issues, health care and, 343
Leisure and play needs, 278, 288
Licensed practical nurse (LPN), role of, 95–96
Licensed vocational nurse (LVN), 96
License(s)/licensures
    audiologists and, 132
    definition of, 145
    forensic science and, 366
    health educators and, 366
    massage therapy and, 367
    medical scientists and, 369
    medicine and, 78–80
    physical therapists and, 241–242

physician assistants and, 251
psychology and, 368
radiography and, 262
recreational therapists and, 283
respiratory therapists and 305
speech language pathologists and, 329
surgical technicians and, 369–370
veterinary medicine and, 370–371
Life span, 235, 244
Lifestyles and behaviors, health-care
    environment and, 11, 13f
Life support, as ethical issue in health care,
    342–343
Linear accelerator, 269, 275
Long-term care pharmacy, 104, 110
LPN. See Licensed practical nurse (LPN)
Lung cancer, cigarette smoking and, 16, 16f
LVN. See Licensed vocational nurse (LVN)
Lybrand, Kelley, 155
Lymphedema, 241, 244

M

Magnetic resonance imaging, 260, 267
Magnetic resonance (MR) technologist, 264–265,
    265f
Mahoney, Mary, 90
Making Health Team Work (Wise), 64
Mammographers, 265, 265f
Mammography, 260, 267
Managed care, 35, 36f, 40
Manual therapy, 235, 244
March of Dimes, 15
Massage therapy
    education and, 367
    introduction to, 367
    licenses and certifications, 367
    salary and employment outlook, 367
Master's-prepared social worker, 318
MCAT. See Medical College Admission Test
    (MCAT)
Mechanical ventilator, 302, 310
Medicaid, 17, 21, 23, 27, 36, 37f
Medical and diagnostic laboratories, 31
Medical assistants
    characteristics for, 214
    "A Day in the Life" of, 210
    education and, 212–213
    evolving role of, 215
    interprofessional collaboration, 215
    role as clinical assistant, 214
    role as office managers, 214
    role as support staff, 214–215
    role in other settings, 215
    salary for, 213
    scope of practice for, 211–212, 211f, 212f
Medical assisting. See also Medical assistants
    case study, 215–216
    challenges in, 213

introduction to, 210–211
    trends in, 213
Medical board specialties, in medicine, 80b
Medical College Admission Test (MCAT), 79, 83
Medical doctor (MD), 259, 267
Medical dosimetrist, 271, 276
Medical first responders, 175
Medical health services manager, role of,
    204–205
Medical Imaging and Radiation Therapy
    (CARE), 262
Medical laboratory scientist, 138
Medical list responders, 175
Medical physicist, 271, 276
Medical records. See Health information
    management (HIM)
Medical researchers. See Medical scientists
Medical scientists
    areas of specialization, 368–369
    education and, 369
    licenses and certifications, 369
    salary and employment outlook, 369
Medical services
    providers and, 13–14
    technology and, 13
Medical social workers, 318
Medical technologists (MTs), 138
Medically underserved areas (MUA), 21
Medically undeserved population (MUP), 21
Medicare, 17, 21, 23, 27, 36, 37f
Medication therapy management, 105
Medicine
    attributes to the practice of, 81
    challenges in, 81
    continuing education and, 80
    education and licensure, 78–79
    health-care team and patient care, 82
    history of, 46–48, 78
    medical board specialties, 80b
    role of physicians, 81
    salary of physicians, 80
    scope of practice, 80
    trends in, 81
Medicine and dentistry-related careers
    (associated health), 6, 6f
Medigap, 36, 40
Melendez, Laura, 214
Mental health and substance abuse social
    workers, 316, 319
Mental health social worker, 321
Microbiology, 139, 145
Middle Ages, medicine in, 47
Midlevel workers, allied health professions as,
    55–56, 60
MIH. See Mobile integrated health care (MIH)
Military settings, athletics trainers and, 119
Minute clinics, 29
Mobile integrated health care (MIH), 174, 175,
    179, 183

Molecular biology, 139, 145
Moloney-Johns, Amanda, 252
Monosky, Keith, 177
Moral development, 338–339
Moral distress, 94–95
Morals, health care and, 343, 347
Moral treatment, 221, 230
Morbidity, 19–20, 23
Morris, William, 221
Mortality, 19–20, 23
Movement, 235, 244
MTs. See Medical technologists (MTs)
MUA. See Medically underserved areas (MUA)
Multidisciplinary care, 51, 52
MUP. See Medically undeserved population
    (MUP)

N

NAACIS. See National Accrediting Agency for
    Clinical Laboratory Science (NAACIS)
NAEMT. See National Association of EMTs
    (NAEMT)
NASW. See National Association of Social
    Workers (NASW)
NATA. See National Athletic Trainers'
    Association (NATA)
National Accrediting Agency for Clinical
    Laboratory Science (NAACIS), 146
National and Nutrition Examination Survey
    (NHANES), 132
National Association of EMTs (NAEMT), 184
National Association of Social Workers
    (NASW), 322
National Athletic Trainers' Association
    (NATA), 117
National Board for Certification in Occupational
    Therapy (NBCOT), 225
National Board for Respiratory Care (NBRC),
    304, 306, 310
National Center for Interprofessional Practice
    and Education, 73
National certification, for athletic trainers,
    119, 123
National Collegiate Athletic Association
    (NCAA), 115
National Commission on Certification
    of Physician Assistants (NCCPA), 249
National Council for Therapeutic Recreation
    Certification (NCTRC), 281, 288
National Council Licensure Examination
    for Registered Nurses (NCLEX-RN), 93
National Council on Rehabilitation Education
    (NCRE), 298
National EMS Education Standards, 177, 183
National Foundation for Infantile Paralysis, 15
National Highway Transportation Safety
    Administration (NHTSA), 175, 183, 184
National Institute of Health (NIH), 21

National League for Nursing, 92
National Library of Medicine, 32
National Mental Health Act, 16
National Registry of EMTs (NREMT), 175, 184
National Rehabilitation Counseling Association (NRCA), 298
Nation's Health Dollar
 expenditures, 38, 39f
 revenues, 38, 38f
Natural environmental issues, health-care environment and, 11–12, 13f
NBCOT. *See* National Board for Certification in Occupational Therapy (NBCOT)
NBRC. *See* National Board for Respiratory Care (NBRC)
NCCPA. *See* National Commission on Certification of Physician Assistants (NCCPA)
NCLEX-RN. *See* National Council Licensure Examination for Registered Nurses (NCLEX-RN)
NCRE. *See* National Council on Rehabilitation Education (NCRE)
NCTRC. *See* National Council for Therapeutic Recreation Certification (NCTRC)
Nebulizer treatments, 302, 310
Negotiation skills, 357
Neighborhood Health Center Guidelines, 64
NHANES, National and Nutrition Examination Survey (NHANES)
NHTSA. *See* National Highway Transportation Safety Administration (NHTSA)
Nightingale, Florence, 48, 52, 89, 90f, 91
Nightingale Training School for Nurses at St. Thomas' Hospital, 89
Nineteenth and twentieth centuries, medicine in, 47–48
Nonclinical respiratory therapists, role of, 308
Nonmaleficence, as principle of ethics in health care, 338
Nonpharmacological intervention, 284, 288
Nonprofit hospitals, 26–27, 32
Nonverbal communication, 355
Notes on Matters Affecting the Health, Efficiency and Hospital Administration of the British Army, 89
NP. *See* Nurse practitioner (NP)
NRCA. *See* National Rehabilitation Counseling Association (NRCA)
NREMT. *See* National Registry of EMTs (NREMT)
NSP. *See* Nursing Society of Philadelphia (NSP)
Nurse aide, role of, 95–96
Nurse practitioner (NP), 259, 267
Nurses. *See also* Nursing; Registered nurses (RN)
 advanced practice, role of, 96
 doctorally prepared, role of, 97
 education and, 91, 99

Florence Nightingale, 89, 90, 90f, 91
licensed practical nurse and nurse aide, role of, 95–96
Mary Seacole, 90
from nurse apprentice training to nurse education
salary of, 94
working with health professionals, 97
Nurse specialist, 93, 99
Nursing
 career, 95
 challenges in, 94–95
 education and, 93–94
 emotional intelligence nursing characteristics, 95
 Great Depression and immigration influence on, 91–92
 history of, 48–49, 49f, 88–89
 influence of Kaiserwerth on nursing education in US, 89–90
 influence of war on, 91
 introduction to, 88
 Kaiserwerth and Nightingale as basis of, 89
 from nurse apprentice training to nurse education, 89
 phases of nursing process, 92f
 scope of practice, 92, 93f
 trends in, 94
Nursing and residential care facilities, 29–30, 32
Nursing Society of Philadelphia (NSP), 48

O

OASID. *See* Old-Age, Survivors, Insurance Disability (OASID)
Obama, Barack, 19f, 21
Obesity, 11
Objectivity, lack of, 359
Obstetrics and gynecology, 46, 52
Occupational Outlook Handbook, Medical and Health Services Managers, 196, 208
Occupational performance, 230
Occupational therapists
 assistant, role of, 227–228, 228f, 230
 collaboration with other disciplines, 228
 "A Day in the Life" of, 220
 definition of, 221–222, 230
 education and, 224–225
 role of, 226–227
 salary for, 225
 scope of practice for, 223–224
Occupational therapy. *See also* Occupational therapists
 case study, 228–229
 challenges in, 226
 introduction to, 221–223
 opportunities, 226, 227
 skills for, 226
 trends in, 225–226

Occupational therapy assistant, role of, 227–228, 228f, 230
Occupations, 230
Office of Interdisciplinary Programs, 64
Old-Age, Survivors, Insurance Disability (OASID), 21
Oncology, 276
Online resources, on health profession careers, 9
Oral and maxillofacial surgery, 152
Oral maxillofacial pathology, 152
Oral maxillofacial radiology, 152
Orchard, Tonya, 163
Organizational ethics, 359
Organ kidney transplant, 16
Organ procurement coordinators, 310
Organ transplantation, as ethical issue in health care, 341–342
Orthodontics, 152
Osteopathic medicine, 79
Osteopathy, 55, 60
Outcomes, 278, 288
Outpatient. *See* Ambulatory care
Outpatient clinic, physical therapy in, 237–238

P

PA. *See* Physician assistant (PA)
PANCE. *See* Physician Assistant National Certifying Exam (PANCE)
Panel, 81
PANRE. *See* Physician Assistant National Recertifying Examination (PANRE)
Paradigm, 92, 99
Paramedical education, 56
Paramedics
 bachelor's degree-prepared, role of, 180
 continuing education and, 180
 "A Day in the Life" of, 172–173
 definition of, 173, 182
 education and, 177–178
 opportunities for, 178–179
 role of, 179–180
 work with emergency department, 181
Passavant, William, 89
Pathologist, 138
Patient, 70, 71, 315
Patient management process, physical therapy and, 239, 240f, 241t
Patient Protection and Affordable Care Act (Obamacare), 21, 22
PCAT. *See* Pharmacy College Admissions Test (PCAT)
PCP. *See* Primary-care provider (PCP)
Pediatric dentistry, 152
Pediatrician, "A Day in the life" of, 77–78
Pediatric orthopedics, 152
Penicillin, discovery of, 5, 15, 20
Periodontal disease, 151, 157
Periodontics, 152

Personal characteristics, of health-care teams, 351

Personality, in health profession careers, 4–5

Personality tests, resources on, 9

Personal Protection and Affordable Care Act of 2010, 179, 183

Personal traits, health care and, 343

Pharmaceutical(s)
 industry, 105, 110
 regulation of, 103–106

Pharmacists. *See also* Clinical pharmacy practitioner
 characteristics required for, 107
 education and, 106–107
 hospital, "A Day in the Life" of, 101–102
 locations and content of practice of, 103–106
 as member of interprofessional care team, 109
 role of, 103
 salary of, 107

Pharmacy. *See also* Pharmacists; Pharmacy technicians
 challenges in, 108
 clinical pharmacy practitioner, 105–106
 community, 103
 definition of, 52
 education and, 106–107
 history of, 49–51, 49f, 50f
 hospital, 103–104
 introduction to, 102–103
 long-term care, 104
 practice, specialized areas of, 105–106
 trends in, 107–108

Pharmacy College Admissions Test (PCAT), 107

Pharmacy technicians
 definition of, 107
 locations and content of practice for, 103–106

Physical therapist (PT)
 characteristics needed for, 242
 collaboration with health professionals, 242
 continuing education and, 238–239
 "A Day in the Life" of, 234
 definition of, 235, 237
 licensure, 241–242
 scope of practice of, 239–240
 specialization areas of, 239
 work settings, 236–238

Physical therapy
 case study, 243
 education and, 238
 introduction to, 235–236
 pathologies and injuries treated in, 242t
 trends, challenges, and aptitude, 242

Physician, role of, 81

Physician and dental offices, 30

Physician Assistant National Certifying Exam (PANCE), 251

Physician Assistant National Recertifying Examination (PANRE), 251

Physician assistant (PA)
 collaboration with other professions, 252
 "A Day in the life" of, 247–248
 definition of, 248, 252
 education and, 250–251
 license for, 251
 salary for, 251
 scope of practice for, 249–250
 skills needed for, 252

Physician assisting
 case study, 250–251
 challenges in, 251–252
 description of, 248
 history of, 248–249
 trends in, 251

Physician extender, 306, 310

Physiology, 238, 244

Plan of care, 66–67, 239, 244

Play. *See* Leisure and play needs

Podiatry, 55, 60

The Poison Prevention Packaging Act of 1970, 17

Polio vaccine, 16, 17f, 20

Polygraphs, forensic science and, 366

Polysomnography therapists, role of, 308

Poorhouses. *See* Nursing and residential care facilities

Postconventional level, in moral development, 339

Poverty, war on, 21–22, 64

PPOs. *See* Preferred provider organizations (PPOs)

Practice setting, physical therapy in, 237, 238

Pragmatics, 326

Preceptors, 119, 124

Preceptors of medical interns, teaching hospitals as, 27, 32

Preconventional level, in moral development, 338

Preferred provider organizations (PPOs), 35

Premedical curriculum, 78–79, 83

Premium, 35

Prepared health information manager
 baccalaureate, role of, 193
 Doctoral, role of, 194
 master's, role of, 193

Prepared health information technician, role of associate degree, 192–193

Prepared health services manager
 baccalaureate, role of, 203–204
 Doctoral, role of, 205
 master's, role of, 204

Primary care professions. *See* Medicine; Nursing; Pharmacy

Primary-care provider (PCP), 46, 259, 267

Primary health-care professions. *See also* Medicine; Nursing; Pharmacy
 definition of, 45–46, 46f, 52
 definition of primary care, 83
 origin of, 45–46, 46f
 vs. primary care provider, 46

Privacy, in delivering health care, 338

Private-pay insurance, 35, 40

Problem-solving skills, 345, 356

Professional associations and relationships, allied health professions and, 57

Professional characteristics, of health-care teams, 352–353

Professional ethics
 attendance and, 339
 attire and, 340
 attitude and, 339
 competence and, 339–340
 definition of, 339
 discretion and, 340
 language and, 340
 social media and, 340

Professionalism. *See* Ethics in health-care

Professional sports settings, athletics trainers and, 119

Professional traits in health-care
 accountability and, 344–345
 communication skills and, 344
 definition of, 344
 emotional stability and, 344
 flexibility and, 344
 problem-solving skills and, 345

Protocols, 173, 183

Provider billing, health-care services and, 38–39

Providers, 13–14, 210, 211, 217

Provider-sponsored organizations (PSOs), 35

PSOs. *See* Provider-sponsored organizations (PSOs)

Psychoacoustics, 131, 136

Psychological characteristics, of health-care teams, 351

Psychology
 education and, 368
 as health-related discipline, 368–369
 introduction to, 367–368
 licenses and certifications, 368
 salary and employment outlook, 368

Psychosocial assessments, 313, 315, 321

PT. *See* Physical therapist (PT)

Public funding
 retired military, 38
 Ryan White Program, 38
 Snyder Act, 38
 workers' compensation, 38

Public Health Security and Bioterrorism Preparedness and response Act of 2002, 18

Public hospitals, 27

Pulmonary function therapists, role of, 307

Pulse oximeter, 175, 183

Q

QM. *See* Quality management technologist (QM)
Quality management technologist (QM), 265
Quality of life, 278, 287

R

Radiation oncologist, 271, 276
Radiation therapists. *See also* Radiation therapy
   collaboration with medical staff, 273
   "A Day in the Life" of, 269–270
   employment conditions for, 272
   expertise of, 271–272
   skill sets and characteristics of, 272
   types and conditions of employment, 272
Radiation therapy
   in cancer treatment, 271
   case study, 273–274
   challenges in, 273 in
   education and, 272
   history of, 271
   modern, 271–272, 276
   trends in, 272–273
Radiographers
   accreditation process, 56
   cardiovascular interventional technologist (CVIT), 264
   characteristics for, 262
   computed tomography (CT) technologist, 263, 263f
   "A Day in the Life" of, 258
   definition of, 259, 267
   education and, 261–262
   interaction with clinical and support staff, 265
   magnetic resonance (MR) technologist, 264–265, 265f
   mammographers, 265
   quality management technologist, 265
   radiologic technologist, role of, 263, 263f
   salary for, 262
   scope of practice for, 261
   x-ray technician and radiologic technologist, 260
Radiography, 56, 60. *See also* Radiographers
   case study, 266
   introduction to, 259–261
   licensure, 262
   trends/outlook, 262
Radiologic technologists. *See* Radiographers
Radiologists, 259, 267
Radiology centers, 29
Radiopharmacy, 105
Range of motion, 234, 244
RCEA. *See* Rehabilitation Counselors
   and Educators Association (RCEA)
RCPs. *See* Respiratory care practitioners (RCPs)
RDNs. *See* Registered dietitians (RDs)/registered
   dietitian nutritionists (RDNs)

RDs. *See* Registered dietitians (RDs)/registered
   dietitian nutritionists (RDNs)
Reading specialists, speech-language pathologists
   and, 326–327
Recreational therapists
   attributes of, 285
   certification and license, 283
   certified therapeutic recreation specialist, 278, 287
   "A Day in the Life" of, 278
   definition of, 278, 279, 287
   education and, 283
   employment of, 279
   role of, 284–285
   salary for, 283
   scope of practice for, 281–283
   working with teams, 285
Recreational therapy. *See also* Recreational
   therapists
   case study, 286–287
   challenges in, 284
   introduction to, 279–281
   overcoming obstacles and, 281
   trends in, 283–284
RECs. *See* Regional extension centers (RECs)
Reed, Wallace, 29
Regional extension centers (RECs), 190
Registered dietitians (RDs)/registered dietitian
   nutritionists (RDNs)
   collaboration with professionals, 167–168
   "A Day in the Life" of, 160
   definitions of, 169
   emerging areas of practice for dietitians, 167
   personality traits and characteristics of, 167
   required education for, 161–162
   role of dietitian in food-service systems
     management, 165–166
   role of RDs in clinical settings, 164
   role of RDs in community settings, 166–167
   salary for, 162–163
   scope of practice for, 162, 162t
   working in long-term care, 164–165, 165f
Registered health information administrator
   (RHIA), 193
Registered medical assistant (RMA), 210,
   212, 217
Registered nurses (RN)
   "A Day in the life" of, 87–88
   description of, 99
   role of, 96
Registered pulmonary function technologist
   (RPFT), 307
Rehabilitation, 7, 7f, 244
Rehabilitation centers, 238
Rehabilitation counseling. *See also* Rehabilitation
   counselors
   case study, 296
   challenges in, 292–293
   characteristics needed for, 293

   introduction to, 290–291
   trends in, 292
Rehabilitation counselors
   "A Day in the Life" of, 290
   education and, 292
   interaction with allied health professionals,
     295
   role in business and industry, 294–295
   role in higher education, 295
   role in mental health and addiction, 294
   role in rehabilitation facilities, 295
   role of baccalaureate-prepared rehabilitation
     specialists, 295
   role of forensic rehabilitation counselor, 295
   role of transition counselors, 294
   role of vocational rehabilitation counselor, 293
   salary for, 292
   scope of practice for, 291–292
   transition vocational rehabilitation
     counselor, 290
Rehabilitation Counselors and Educators
   Association (RCEA), 298
Rehabilitation Movement, 222
Renaissance period, medicine in, 47
Reputation, health care and, 343, 347
Residency, 79–80, 83
Resource manager, 67
Resources, lack of, 359
Respect, health care and, 344
Respiration, 304, 310
Respiratory care/cardiopulmonary. *See also*
   Respiratory therapists
   case study, 309
   definition of cardiopulmonary, 310
   introduction to respiratory therapy, 303–3044
   role of critical-care therapists, 306–307
   role of general acute-care therapist, 306
   role of home care therapists in, 308
   role of nonclinical respiratory therapists
     in, 308
   role of polysomnography therapists, 308
   role of pulmonary function therapists, 307
   role of transport therapists, 307
   trends and challenges in, 305–306
Respiratory care practitioners (RCPs), 303
Respiratory therapists
   characteristics of, 306
   collaboration with nurses and physicians, 308
   continuing education and, 305
   "A Day in the Life" of, 302
   education and, 304–305
   licensure and salary, 305
   scope of practice for, 304
Resuscitation team, 303, 310
Retail clinics, 29
Retired military, health-care services and, 38
RMA. *See* Registered medical assistant (RMA)
RN. *See* Registered nurses (RN)
Robert Wood Johnson Foundation, 64

Robotic surgical device, 18

Roentgen, Wilhelm Conrad, 259

Roles, clear, as element of collaborative
environment, 69

Rollins, Kathryn, 307

Rout, Ayasakanta, 134

Royal, Patricia, 192, 201, 319

Royal Commission for the Health of the Army, 89

RPFT. *See* Registered pulmonary function
technologist (RPFT)

Rural hospitals, 27–28

Ryan White Program, 37

S

Salk, Jonas, 16

"Satellite pharmacies," 101

Scope of practice, in medicine, 80

Seacole, Mary, 90

Seaman, Valentine, 48

Self-assessments, 8, 345

Self-awareness, 355

Semantics, 326

Settings, 88, 99

Shatuuck Report of 1850, 56

A Short History of Nursing (Dock), 89

Shuey, Elaine, 329

Sieveking, Amalie, 89

Sigma Theta Tau, 92

Simulation, 270, 275

Sisters of Charity, 89

Sisters of Hotel-Dieu in Paris, 89

Skilled nursing facility/long-term care, physical
therapy in, 237

Skills, in health profession careers, 4

SLP. *See* Speech-language pathologist (SLP)

Snyder Act, 37

Social media, professional ethics and, 340

Social Security Act of1935, 20

Social work, 316. *See also* Social workers
case study, 320
challenges in, 317–318
characteristics needed for, 317
introduction to, 314–315
trends in, 316

Social workers
baccalaureate-prepared, role of, 319
child, family, and schools, role of, 319, 321
clinical, role of, 318–319
continuing education and, 319–320
"A Day in the Life" of, 313–314
education and, 316
involvement with other disciplines, 320
master's-prepared, role of, 318
medical, role of, 318
mental health and substance abuse, role
of, 319, 321
salary for, 316
scope of practice for, 315

Society for Social Work and Research (SSWR),
322

Society for the Promotion of Occupational
Therapy, 222

Socioeconomics, health-care environment
and, 11, 13f

Specialization, physical therapy and, 238

Specialized hospitals, 28

Speech, 332, 334–325

Speech-language pathologist (SLP)
basic skills for, 330
"A Day in the Life" of, 323–324
education and, 328–329
health-care facility-based, role of, 330
interaction with other professionals, 330
salary for, 329
school-based, role of, 330
scope of practice for, 324

Speech-language pathology. *See also*
Speech-language pathologist (SLP)
additional areas of practice, 326–328
aspects of communication, 324–325, 325f,
326f
case study, 331
challenges in, 330
hearing and, 327–328
introduction to, 324
license/credentials, 329
trends in, 329

Spelman Seminary in Atlanta, 90

SSWR. *See* Society for Social Work and Research
(SSWR)

St. Vincent de Paul, 89

Standing orders, 173, 183

Starr, Ellen Gates, 314

State certification, 121

State Education Agency, 332

State Licensing Agency, 332

State registration, 121

State regulation, 120–121, 124

State Speech-Language Hearing Associations,
332

Strength, 234, 244

Students
barriers to interprofessional teams, 71
interprofessional health-care practice and, 70

Substance abuse centers, 29

Substance abuse social worker, 321

Superintendents, 200, 207

Supervising physician, 249

Supplemental Nutrition Assistance Program
(SNAP), 160

Support, as element of collaborative
environment, 69

Support, lack of, 359

Support services provider, 66

The Surgeon Dentist (Fauchard), 150

Surgical technicians/technologists, 368
education and, 369

introduction to, 369
licenses and certifications, 369–370
salary and employment outlook, 370
tasks of, 369

Surrogate pregnancy, as ethical issue in health
care, 341

Syntax, 325

T

Teaching, physical therapy and, 238

Teaching hospitals, 27, 32

Teams, 64–65, 82

Technical standards, 121, 124

Technicians, assistants, and technologists
(health related) career characteristics,
7, 7f

Technology, as factor in health-care
environment, 13

Tests, on health careers, 9

Therapeutic exercise, 235

Therapeutic recreation, 287

Therapy, 244

Therapy setting, speech-language pathology
and, 328, 328f

Time management skills, 356

Toolmark identification, forensic science
and, 366

Toxicology, forensic science and, 366

The Trainer's Bible (Bilik), 117

Transactional leaders, 358

Trans-fat, battle against, 18

Transformational leaders, 358

Transition, 290

Transition vocational rehabilitation counselor
(TVRC), 290, 297

Transplantation
baboon heart, 18
organ, as ethical issue in health care, 341–342
organ kidney, 16

Transport therapists, role of, 307

Trauma center, high-performing health-care
team case application in, 350–351

Treatment and diagnostics career (direct practice
care), 6, 6f

Truman, Harry, 16

Trust, lack of, 358–359

Trust, mutual, collaborative environment
and, 69

Tubman, Harriet, 91

TVRC. *See* Transition vocational rehabilitation
counselor (TVRC)

U

Uninsured individuals, health-care services
and, 38

Urgent care unit, 29

U.S. Food and Drug Administration (FDA), 18,
19, 23, 103

V

Vaccine, Gardasil, 19
Values
  in assessing health professionals, 345–346
  collaborative environment and, 69–70
  definition of, 347
  in health-care professions, 337, 347
Values conflict, 346, 347
Ventilator-dependent patients' facilities, 30
Veracity, in delivering health care, 338
Veterinary medicine
  education and, 370
  introduction to, 370
  licenses and certifications, 370–371
  profession of, 370
  salary and employment outlook, 371

Vital signs, 234, 244
Vocational Rehabilitation and Employment
  Services (VR&E), 293, 297
Vocational rehabilitation (VR), 290
VR. *See* Vocational rehabilitation (VR)
VR&E. *See* Vocational Rehabilitation
  and Employment Services
  (VR&E)

W

War on poverty, 21–22, 64
Wellness, 278, 288
Wheeze, 309, 310
Whitman, Walt, 91
Wintz, Gregory, 223
Wise, Harold, 64

Women, Infants, and Children (WIC)
  program, 167
The Wonderful Adventures of Mrs. Seacole
  (Seacole), 90
Workers' Compensation, 38
Workforce, 251
Work interests, in health profession careers, 5
Work values, in health profession careers, 5

X

X-ray technician, 260

Z

Zemplinski, Julie, 142
Zostavax vaccine (shingles), 19